Obstetrics Algorithms in Clinical Practice

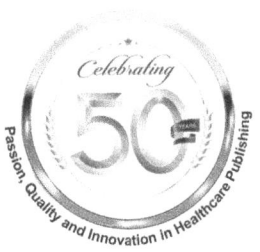

Obstetrics Algorithms in Clinical Practice

Editor
Alok Sharma
MD DHA MICOG
Consultant
Department of Obstetrics and Gynecology
Civil Hospital, Sundernagar
Mandi, Himachal Pradesh, India

Foreword
Professor (Dr) CN Purandare

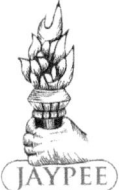

JAYPEE BROTHERS MEDICAL PUBLISHERS
The Health Sciences Publisher
New Delhi | London

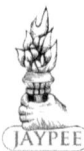 **Jaypee Brothers Medical Publishers (P) Ltd.**

Headquarters
Jaypee Brothers Medical Publishers (P) Ltd
4838/24, Ansari Road, Daryaganj
New Delhi 110 002, India
Phone: +91-11-43574357
Fax: +91-11-43574314
Email: jaypee@jaypeebrothers.com

Overseas Office
J.P. Medical Ltd
83 Victoria Street, London
SW1H 0HW (UK)
Phone: +44 20 3170 8910
Fax: +44 (0)20 3008 6180
Email: info@jpmedpub.com

Website: www.jaypeebrothers.com
Website: www.jaypeedigital.com

© 2020, Jaypee Brothers Medical Publishers

The views and opinions expressed in this book are solely those of the original contributor(s)/author(s) and do not necessarily represent those of editor(s) of the book.

All rights reserved. No part of this publication may be reproduced, stored or transmitted in any form or by any means, electronic, mechanical, photocopying, recording or otherwise, without the prior permission in writing of the publishers.

All brand names and product names used in this book are trade names, service marks, trademarks or registered trademarks of their respective owners. The publisher is not associated with any product or vendor mentioned in this book.

Medical knowledge and practice change constantly. This book is designed to provide accurate, authoritative information about the subject matter in question. However, readers are advised to check the most current information available on procedures included and check information from the manufacturer of each product to be administered, to verify the recommended dose, formula, method and duration of administration, adverse effects and contraindications. It is the responsibility of the practitioner to take all appropriate safety precautions. Neither the publisher nor the author(s)/editor(s) assume any liability for any injury and/or damage to persons or property arising from or related to use of material in this book.

This book is sold on the understanding that the publisher is not engaged in providing professional medical services. If such advice or services are required, the services of a competent medical professional should be sought.

Every effort has been made where necessary to contact holders of copyright to obtain permission to reproduce copyright material. If any have been inadvertently overlooked, the publisher will be pleased to make the necessary arrangements at the first opportunity. The **CD/DVD-ROM** (if any) provided in the sealed envelope with this book is complimentary and free of cost. **Not meant for sale**.

Inquiries for bulk sales may be solicited at: jaypee@jaypeebrothers.com

Obstetrics Algorithms in Clinical Practice

First Edition: **2020**

ISBN: 978-93-89587-53-1

Dedication

To all the Obstetricians who are working day and night around the world and providing care to the Antenatal mothers to make them deliver safely.

Contributors

Aakanksha Kumar MS
Junior Resident
Department of Obstetrics and Gynecology
Bharati Vidyapeeth University Medical College
Pune, Maharashtra, India

Aanya Sharma MBBS
3rd Year Junior Resident
Department of Obstetrics and Gynecology
Indira Gandhi Medical College
Shimla, Himachal Pradesh, India

Abha Rani Sinha MS
Professor
Department of Obstetrics and Gynecology
Shri Krishna Medical College and Hospital
Muzaffarpur, Bihar, India

Ajay Chhabra MD
Associate Professor
Department of Medicine
Government Medical College
Amritsar, Punjab, India

Ajith S MD DGO Dip NB FRCOG
Professor and Head
Department of Obstetrics and Gynecology
Government Medical College
Kannur, Kerala, India

Alok Sharma MD DHA MICOG
Consultant
Department of Obstetrics and Gynecology
Civil Hospital, Sundernagar
Mandi, Himachal Pradesh, India

Alpana V Chhetri MD
Assistant Professor
Department of Obstetrics and Gynecology
College of Obstetrics, Gynecology and Child Health
Kolkata, West Bengal, India

Anjali Gupta MD
Professor
Department of Obstetrics and Gynecology
Pandit Bhagwat Dayal Sharma, Post Graduate Institute of Medical Science
Rohtak, Haryana, India

Anshuja Singla DGO DNB
Associate Professor
Department of Obstetrics and Gynecology
University College of Medical Sciences and Guru Teg Bahadur Hospital
New Delhi, India

Anupama Bahadur DNB MNAMS FICOG
Additional Professor
Department of Obstetrics and Gynecology
All India Institute of Medical Sciences
Rishikesh, Uttarakhand, India

Anuradha Sood MD
Associate Professor
Department of Microbiology
Dr Rajendra Prasad Government Medical College
Kangra, Himachal Pradesh, India

Arshi Syal MBBS
Junior Resident
Department of Obstetrics and Gynecology
Government Medical College and Hospital
Chandigarh, India

Bhaskar Pal MD DNBE FICOG FRCOG
Senior Consultant
Department of Obstetrics and Gynecology
Apollo Gleneagles Hospital
Kolkata, West Bengal, India

Bindiya Gupta MD MAMS FICOG
Associate Professor
Department of Obstetrics and Gynecology
University College of Medical Sciences and Guru Teg Bahadur Hospital
New Delhi, India

Chaitra Thunga A MS DNB
Fellow in Reproductive Medicine
Department of Obstetrics and Gynecology
CRAFT Hospital and Research Centre
Kodungallur, Kerala, India

Charu Yadav MD
Senior Resident
Department of Obstetrics and Gynecology
University College of Medical Sciences and Guru Teg Bahadur Hospital
New Delhi, India

Dilpreet Kaur Pandher MD
Associate Professor
Department of Obstetrics and Gynecology
Government Medical College and Hospital
Chandigarh, India

Esha Gupta MS
Senior Resident
Department of Obstetrics and Gynecology
University College of Medical Sciences and Guru Teg Bahadur Hospital
New Delhi, India

Geetha Balsarkar MD DGO DNB FCPS
Professor and Unit Head
Department of Obstetrics and Gynecology
Seth GS Medical College
Nowrosjee Wadia Maternity Hospital
Mumbai, Maharashtra, India

Geetika Syal MD
Assistant Professor
Department of Obstetrics and Gynecology
Indira Gandhi Medical College
Shimla, Himachal Pradesh, India

Girija Wagh MD FICOG FICS Dip (Endoscopy)
Professor
Department of Obstetrics and Gynecology
Bharati Vidyapeeth University Medical College
Pune, Maharashtra, India

Haresh U Doshi MD PhD (Medicine) FICOG Diploma (USG) PGDCR PDMLS PGDHHM PGCML
Professor and Head
Department of Obstetrics and Gynecology
GCS Medical College, Hospital and Research Centre
Ahmedabad, Gujarat, India

Japleen Kaur MD DNB
Fellowship (Reproductive Endocrinology and Infertility)
Medical Officer
Department of Obstetrics and Gynecology
Postgraduate Institute of Medical Education and Research
Chandigarh, India

JB Sharma MD FRCOG (London) FAMS PhD FICOG MFFP DNB FIMSA
Professor
Department of Obstetrics and Gynecology
All India Institute of Medical Sciences
New Delhi, India

Jyothi Goulay MS (2nd Year)
Junior Resident
Department of Obstetrics and Gynecology
Al-Ameen Medical College
Bijapur, Karnataka, India

Jyotsna Suri MD FICOG
Professor
Department of Obstetrics and Gynecology
Vardhman Mahavir Medical College and Safdarjung Hospital
New Delhi, India

K Aparna Sharma MD
Additional Professor
Department of Obstetrics and Gynecology
All India Institute of Medical Sciences
New Delhi, India

Kalpana Negi MS
Assistant Professor
Department of Obstetrics and Gynecology
Indira Gandhi Medical College
Shimla, Himachal Pradesh, India

Kanica Kaushal MD
Senior Resident
Department of Community Medicine and School of Public Health
Postgraduate Institute of Medical Education and Research
Chandigarh, India

Kartik Syal MD
Associate Professor
Department of Anesthesiology
Indira Gandhi Medical College
Shimla, Himachal Pradesh, India

Kavita Khoiwal MD
Assistant Professor
Department of Obstetrics and Gynecology
All India Institute of Medical Sciences
Rishikesh, Uttarakhand, India

Kiran Guleria MD DNB
Director-Professor
Department of Obstetrics and Gynecology
University College of Medical Sciences and Guru Teg Bahadur Hospital
New Delhi, India

Kunal Kumar Sharma MD DM
Resident
Department of Neuroanesthesia
National Institute of Mental Health and Neurosciences
Bengaluru, Karnataka, India

Latika Chawla MD
Fellow Maternal and Fetal Medicine
Assistant Professor
Department of Obstetrics and Gynecology
All India Institute of Medical Sciences
Rishikesh, Uttarakhand, India

Leena Wadhwa MD DNB FICOG
Professor and IVF Incharge
Department of Obstetrics and Gynecology
ESI Postgraduate Institute of Medical Sciences and
Research and Model Hospital
New Delhi, India

Madhu Gupta MD Phd
Professor
Department of Community Medicine and School of Public Health
Postgraduate Institute of Medical Education and Research
Chandigarh, India

Madhu Nagpal MD FICOG
Professor and Head
Department of Obstetrics and Gynecology
Sri Ram Das Institute of Medical Sciences and Research
Amritsar, Punjab, India

Madhuri Chandra MD DNB FICOG CMCL FAIMER Fellow
Former Professor and Unit Head
Department of Obstetrics and Gynecology
Gandhi Medical College
Bhopal, Madhya Pradesh, India

Manishi Mittal MD FRM
Consultant
Department of Obstetrics and Gynecology
Mittal Maternity and Superspeciality Hospital
Yamunanagar, Haryana, India

Manju Puri MD
Director Professor
Department of Obstetrics and Gynecology
Lady Hardinge Medical College and Smt Sucheta Kriplani Hospital
New Delhi, India

Mansi Dhingra MS RCOG
Consultant
Department of Obstetrics and Gynecology
ESI Postgraduate Institute of Medical Sciences and
Research
Lucknow, Uttar Pradesh, India

Meenakshi Barsaul Chauhan MS
Professor
Department of Obstetrics and Gynecology
Pandit Bhagwat Dayal Sharma, Post Graduate Institute of Medical Sciences
Rohtak, Haryana, India

Minakshi Rohilla MD
Professor
Department of Obstetrics and Gynecology
Postgraduate Institute of Medical Education and Research
Chandigarh, India

Monika Gupta MS DNB FICOG FICMCH MNAMS
Associate Professor
Department of Obstetrics and Gynecology
Vardhman Mahavir Medical College and Safdarjung Hospital
New Delhi, India

Munjal Pandya MS
Assistant Professor
Department of Obstetrics and Gynecology
AMC MET Medical College and Sheth LG Hospital
Ahmedabad, Gujarat, India

Namrata Verma MS
Senior Resident
Department of Obstetrics and Gynecology
Vardhman Mahavir Medical College and Safdarjung Hospital
New Delhi, India

Neha Gupta MS DNB
Fellow in Fetal Medicine
Consultant
Department of Fetal Medicine
Kailash Hospital
Noida, Uttar Pradesh, India

Nivedita Sharma MD
Assistant Professor
Department of Pediatrics
Dr Radhakrishnan Government Medical College
Himachal Pradesh, India

Pancham Chauhan MD Dch
Assistant Professor
Department of Pediatrics
Indira Gandhi Medical College
Shimla, Himachal Pradesh, India

Parag Biniwale MD
Consultant
Department of Obstetrics and Gynecology
Biniwale Clinic
Pune, Maharashtra, India

Parneet Kaur DGO MD
Professor
Department of Obstetrics and Gynecology
Government Medical College
Patiala, Punjab, India

Parul Kotdawala MD FICOG FICMCH MAMS
Endoscopy Surgeon
Department of Obstetrics and Gynecology
VS Hospital and Smt NHL Municipal Medical College
Ahmedabad, Gujarat, India

Parveen Bhardwaj MD DNB
Fellowship in Pediatric Intensive Care
Professor
Department of Pediatrics
Indira Gandhi Medical College
Shimla, Himachal Pradesh, India

Piyush Gautam MD
Associate Professor
Department of Obstetrics and Gynecology
Dr Rajendra Prasad Government Medical College
Kangra, Himachal Pradesh, India

Pradnya Supe MS
Assistant Professor
Department of Obstetrics and Gynecology
Lokmanya Tilak Municipal General Hospital and Lokmanya Tilak Municipal Medical College
Mumbai, Maharashtra, India

Pratima Mittal MD FICOG FRCOG
Professor
Department of Obstetrics and Gynecology
Vardhman Mahavir Medical College and Safdarjung Hospital
New Delhi, India

Priti Samir Vyas MD DGO FCPS MSC (Psychological Counseling and Therapy)
Partner-Director
Sangita Maternity Surgical and Diagnostic Centre, Mumbai
Consultant
Surya Mother and Child Care, KLS Memorial Hospital
Mumbai, Maharashtra, India

Rajesh Kumar Verma MD
Associate Professor
Department of Anesthesiology
Indira Gandhi Medical College
Shimla, Himachal Pradesh, India

Ram Krishan Kaushal MD
Consultant
Department of Pediatrics
Siddhi Vinayak Multispeciality Hospital
Shimla, Himachal Pradesh, India

Rashmi Bagga MD DNB FICOG
Professor
Department of Obstetrics and Gynecology
Postgraduate Institute of Medical Education and Research
Chandigarh, India

Rashmi G Jalvee MS DGO DNB
Assistant Professor
Department of Obstetrics and Gynecology
HBT Medical College and Dr RN Cooper Municipal Hospital
Mumbai, Maharashtra, India

Reena Wani MD FRCOG DNBE FCPS DGO DFP FICOG
Additional Professor and Unit Head
Department of Obstetrics and Gynecology
HBT Medical College and Dr RN Cooper Municipal Hospital
Mumbai, Maharashtra, India

Reeti Mehra MD FIMSA
Associate Professor
Department of Obstetrics and Gynecology
Government Medical College and Hospital
Chandigarh, India

Richa Sharma MD
Associate Professor
Department of Obstetrics and Gynecology
University College of Medical Sciences and Guru Teg Bahadur Hospital
New Delhi, India

Rohini Rao MD
Assistant Professor
Department of Obstetrics and Gynecology
Indira Gandhi Medical College
Shimla, Himachal Pradesh, India

S Sampathkumari MD DGO FICOG FC Diab FIME
Professor
Department of Obstetrics and Gynecology
Government Hospital for Women, Madras Medical College
Chennai, Tamil Nadu, India

Sandeep Sharma MD
Medical Officer (Specialist)
Department of Obstetrics and Gynecology
Dr Radhakrishnan Government Medical College
Hamirpur, Himachal Pradesh, India

Sanjita MS
Senior Resident
Department of Obstetrics and Gynecology
ESI Postgraduate Institute of Medical Sciences and
Research and Model Hospital
New Delhi, India

Saswati Sanyal Choudhury MD FICOG FICMCH FIAOG
Associate Professor
Department of Obstetrics and Gynecology
Gauhati Medical College
Guwahati, Assam, India

Savita Singhal MD DGO
Senior Professor
Department of Obstetrics and Gynecology
Post Graduate Institute of Medical Sciences
Rohtak, Haryana, India

Sayeba Akhter MBBS FCPS (BD) DRH (UK) CMCH (IN) FCPS (PAK) FIAOG (IN) FRCOG (UK)
Professor and CEO
Department of Women's Health
MAMM'S Institute of Fistula and Women's Health (MIFWOH)
Dhaka, Bangladesh

Seema Chopra MD
Additional Professor
Department of Obstetrics and Gynecology
Postgraduate Institute of Medical Education and Research
Chandigarh, India

Shail Kaur MD
Associate Professor
Department of Obstetrics and Gynecology
Punjab Institute of Medical Sciences
Jalandhar, Punjab, India

Shailesh Kore MD DGO
Professor and Head
Department of Obstetrics and Gynecology
Topiwala National Medical College and
BYL Nair Hospital
Mumbai, Maharashtra, India

Shikha Rani MS
Assistant Professor cum maternity and childwelfare officer
Department of Obstetrics and Gynecology
Government Medical College
and Hospital
Chandigarh, Punjab, India

Shalini Gainder MD
Additional Professor
Department of Obstetrics and Gynecology
Postgraduate Institute of Medical
Education and Research
Chandigarh, India

Sharda Patra MD DNB
Professor
Department of Obstetrics and Gynecology
Lady Hardinge Medical College and Smt
Sucheta Kriplani Hospital
New Delhi, India

Shaveta Jain MS
Associate Professor
Department of Obstetrics and Gynecology
Post Graduate Institute of Medical
Sciences
Rohtak, Haryana, India

Shilpi Nain DGO DNB FICOG
Associate Professor
Department of Obstetrics and Gynecology
Lady Hardinge Medical College and
Smt Sucheta Kriplani Hospital
New Delhi, India

Shivani Sharma MD
Registrar
Department of Obstetrics and Gynecology
Postgraduate Institute of Medical
Education and Research
Chandigarh, India

Sruthi Bhaskaran MS
Associate Professor
Department of Obstetrics and Gynecology
University College of Medical Sciences and
Guru Teg Bahadur Hospital
New Delhi, India

Shyjus Puliyathinkal MS FMAS DMAS
FICOG Certificate in da Vinci Robotic Surgical System
Fertility Specialist
Department of Reproductive Medicine
ARMC-IVF Fertility Centre
Kannur, Kerala, India

Smiti Nanda MD
Senior Professor
Department of Obstetrics and Gynecology
Pandit Bhagwat Dayal Sharma, Post
Graduate Institute of Medical Sciences
Rohtak, Haryana, India

Smriti Chauhan MD
Assistant Professor
Department of Microbiology
Dr Radhakrishnan Government Medical
College
Hamirpur, Himachal Pradesh, India

Sneh Kiran MS
Senior Resident
Department of Obstetrics and Gynecology
Indira Gandhi Institute of Medical Sciences
Patna, Bihar, India

Snigdha Kumari MS DNB
Assistant Professor
Department of Obstetrics and Gynecology
ESI Postgraduate Institute of Medical
Sciences and
Research, New Delhi, India

Subhash Chand Jaryal MD
Professor and Head
Department of Microbiology
Dr Rajendra Prasad Government Medical
College
Kangra, Himachal Pradesh, India

Suman Thakur MD
Assistant Professor
Department of Obstetrics and Gynecology
Indira Gandhi Medical College
Shimla, Himachal Pradesh, India

Suman Thakur MD
C&DST LAB
Department of Microbiology
Indira Gandhi Medical College
Shimla, Himachal Pradesh, India

Suparna Grover MD
Associate Professor
Department of Obstetrics and Gynecology
Government Medical College
Amritsar, Punjab, India

Taru Gupta MS DNB
Professor and Head
Department of Obstetrics and Gynecology
ESI Postgraduate Institute of Medical
Sciences and
Research
New Delhi, India

Taruna Sharma MS DNB
Senior Resident
Department of Obstetrics and Gynecology
University College of Medical Sciences and
Guru Teg Bahadur Hospital
New Delhi, India

Vaishali Korde Nayak DGO DNB MNAMS
Professor and HOU
Department of Obstetrics and Gynecology
MIMER Medical College
Pune, Maharashtra, India

Vandana Bhuriya MD
Associate Professor
Department of Obstetrics and Gynecology
Pandit Bhagwat Dayal Sharma, Post
Graduate Institute of Medical Sciences
Rohtak, Haryana, India

Vani Malhotra MD
Professor
Department of Obstetrics and Gynecology
Pandit Bhagwat Dayal Sharma, Post
Graduate Institute of Medical Sciences
Rohtak, Haryana, India

Venus Dalal MD MRCOG (London) DNB
Senior Resident
Department of Obstetrics and Gynecology
All India Institute of Medical Sciences
New Delhi, India

Vidya Thobbi MD FICOG
Professor and Head
Department of Obstetrics and Gynecology
Al-Ameen Medical College
Bijapur, Karnataka, India

Vivek Chauhan MD
Assistant Professor
Department of Medicine
Indira Gandhi Medical College
Shimla, Himachal Pradesh, India

Foreword

It is an age-old saying that the study of mankind is in the books. Frankly speaking, books are the most convenient form for extracorporeal memory, allowing the reader to benefit from knowledge and the work of the experts in the respective field. Today the scientific field is having a veritable explosion in its information which leaves students overwhelmed and confused.

To overcome this confusion in the scientific information, this particular book on *Obstetrics Algorithms in Clinical Practice* is published to address the need of not only undergraduate and postgraduate medical students but also to the private practicing obstetricians. In my opinion, the information presented in this book is in utmost clarity and lucidity that could be used by any practicing obstetrician.

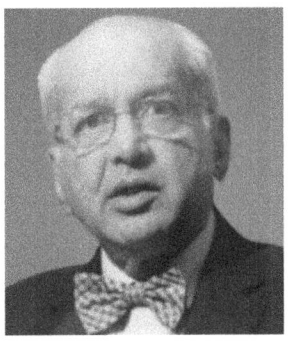

This classic book on *Obstetrics Algorithms* continues to provide the basic knowledge relevant to the practice of obstetrics. Comprehensive in scope, *Obstetrics Algorithms in Clinical Practice* offers contributions from a noted panel of experts and contains an integrated approach that is designed to help deliver the highest possible care to patients.

I have known the editor Alok Sharma from a long time, seeing him evolving as an inspiring editor and a teacher is a great contribution to the obstetrics fraternity. His dedication to critical care obstetrics has led all of us to take better care of our patients, leading to better outcomes for mothers and babies.

Professor (Dr) CN Purandare
MD MA Obst (Ireland) DGO DFP DOBST RCPI (Dublin)
FFIGO FRCOG (UK) FRCPI (Ireland) FACOG (USA) FSLCOG (SL) FTAOG (Tw)
FEBCOG (EU) FDGGG (GER) FEMAO & G (UAE) FAMS FICOG FICMCH PGD MLS (Law)
Hon. Membership Romanian, Colombian and French (CNGOF) ObGyn Societies
Consultant, Obstetrician and Gynecologist
Purandare Hospital, Mumbai, Maharashtra, India
President, FIGO (2015-2018)
Emeritus Dean, Indian College of Obstetricians and Gynaecologists
President, FOGSI (2009)
President, Indian College of Obstetricians and Gynaecologists (2009)
Professor Emeritus, Research Institute for Obstetrics and Gynaecology
Ministry of Health Russian Federation
Editor Emeritus, Journal FOGSI-(JOGI)
Ex Hon. Professor, Department of Obstetrics and Gynecology
Grant Medical College and JJ Hospital, Mumbai
Hon. Consultant, Mumbai Police
Hon. Consultant. Saifee Hospital and BSES Hospital, Mumbai.
Visiting Consultant St. Elizabeth Hospital, Mumbai

Preface

I have welcomed, with enthusiasm, the opportunity to edit this very first edition of the textbook *Obstetrics Algorithms in Clinical Practice*. I have tried to provide a text to help undergraduates, postgraduates, and practitioners to clarify their doubts and to organize some of the intricacies regarding the subject.

I have assembled a group of contributors, nationally with an exceptionally broad range of backgrounds and similar interests. All the contributors have emphasized the latest clinical management approaches with deep understanding. They have all contributed to the same goal, that is, to create a source of information that will help in the care of women in the last phase of pregnancy, during labor, and even after delivery. This book deals with the management of normal and abnormal labor in just algorithm form, to have a quick look in your outpatient department (OPD) or labor room.

No two births are the same and no two mothers have the same changes during pregnancy and labor; therefore, it is important to have a text that deals with planning and anticipating any possible complications during these phases of a woman's life. I have tried my level best to cover all the relevant aspects pertaining to these phases where obstetricians may need guidance in decision making. I hope that the aggregate of my efforts has resulted in a text that will be a worthy resource for those who want to care for pregnant women.

Alok Sharma

Acknowledgments

Giving thanks is a pleasant job, but it is, nonetheless, difficult when one sincerely tries to put such ideas into words. The following humble words of expression and gratitude cannot really convey the deep feelings of my heart. In any attempt to create and produce a textbook of obstetrics and gynecology, one must be fortunate enough to have the assistance and support of many talented professionals, both within and outside the obstetrics and gynecology department. To begin with, I am indebted to all my authors for their generous contributions to this book; all of them, despite their busy schedules, provided recent, up-to-date, and evidence-based chapters on various aspects of Pregnancy, Labor, and Delivery.

I have selected contributors from different parts of India.

It has been a pleasure to work with the dedicated professionals from M/s Jaypee Brothers Medical Publishers (P) Ltd, New Delhi, India. This publisher has been gracious in offering support without any interference whatsoever, and the team has also ensured that the quality of work is superb.

I am deeply indebted to Ms Chetna Malhotra Vohra (Associate Director—Content Strategy) for her unconditional support; she has brought her considerable intelligence, energetic work ethic, and creativity to this edition. Her dedication for creating the best textbook possible equaled my efforts to produce an appropriate style for the textbook.

This textbook would have not seen the light of the day without the untiring efforts of Dr Rajul Jain (Development Editor), who skillfully kept my project on track through an array of potential hurdles.

I acknowledge my respected parents, Smt Dhanwanti Devi Sharma and Hans Raj Sharma, who have laid the foundation stone of literacy in me and given me the courage to face the challenges of the world by inculcating good attributes in me. I thank my wife, Dr Pratibha Sharma, for her tolerance and understanding of the time I spent away from her during my own career and in editing this book. Her constant encouragement, moral support, and love have been a source of inspiration to me for completing this work. I thank my brother, Dr Amit Sharma, for guiding me at every step of the way in shaping the book. Finally, but certainly not last, I thank my lovely daughter, Hiranya, for her immense patience.

—*With love and warm regards*—

Jai Hind

Contents

SECTION 1: MATERNAL DISORDERS

1. **Antiphospholipid Antibody Syndrome** 3
   Kavita Khoiwal, K Aparna Sharma

2. **Hypertensive Disorders of Pregnancy** 7
   Sruthi Bhaskaran, Esha Gupta

3. **Cardiac Disease in Pregnancy** 18
   Ajith S

4. **Anemia in Pregnancy** 23
   Haresh U Doshi

5. **Diabetes in Pregnancy** 33
   Smiti Nanda, Anjali Gupta

6. **Jaundice in Pregnancy: Dilemma in Management** 38
   Sharda Patra

7. **Convulsions in Pregnancy** 47
   Seema Chopra, Arshi Syal

8. **Venous Thromboembolism in Pregnancy** 52
   Vivek Chauhan, Suman Thakur

9. **Shock** 56
   Rohini Rao, Rajesh Kumar Verma, Kunal Kumar Sharma

10. **Advanced Maternal Age** 62
    Vidya Thobbi, Jyothi Goulay

11. **Rh Isoimmunization** 69
    Meenakshi Barsaul Chauhan, Vani Malhotra

12. **H1N1 Infection in Pregnancy** 76
    Suparna Grover, Ajay Chhabra

13. **Zika Virus** 83
    Manishi Mittal

14. **Renal Disorders and Pregnancy** 92
    JB Sharma, Venus Dalal

15. **Thyroid Disorders** 98
    Reena Wani, Rashmi G Jalvee

SECTION 2: ANTENATAL EMERGENCIES

16. **Vomiting in Pregnancy** 103
    Sandeep Sharma

17. **Abdominal Pain in Pregnancy** 107
    Abha Rani Sinha, Sneh Kiran

18. **Bleeding in Early Pregnancy** 111
    Bhaskar Pal, Alpana V Chhetri

19. **Bleeding in Late Pregnancy** 117
    Rashmi Bagga, Japleen Kaur

20. **Preterm Labor** 122
    Madhu Nagpal

21. **Prelabor Rupture of Membranes** 129
    Shyjus Puliyathinkal

22. **Intrauterine Growth Restriction: An Evidence-based Approach** 133
    Minakshi Rohilla, Shivani Sharma

23. **Multiple Gestations in Labor** 139
    Shailesh Kore, Pradnya Supe, Chaitra Thunga

24. **Cervical Insufficiency** 144
    Neha Gupta

25. **Reduced Fetal Movements** 149
    Geetha Balsarkar

26. **Intrauterine Fetal Death** 152
    Savita Singhal, Shaveta Jain

27. **Prolonged Pregnancy** 157
    Suman Thakur

28. **Pregnancy after Lower Segment Cesarean Section** 159
    S Sampathkumari

29. **Pregnancy after Infertility and Assisted Reproductive Technology** 163
    Shalini Gainder, Japleen Kaur

SECTION 3: LABOR

30. **Decision and Induction of Labor** — 171
    Dilpreet Kaur Pandher, Shikha Rani

31. **Augmentation and Management of Labor** — 177
    Leena Wadhwa, Sanjita

32. **Fetal Surveillance during Labor** — 182
    Monika Gupta, Namrata Verma

33. **Pain Relief in Labor** — 188
    Kartik Syal, Geetika Syal

34. **Meconium** — 192
    Anshuja Singla, Charu Yadav

35. **Placental Adhesive Disorders** — 195
    Taruna Sharma, Bindiya Gupta

SECTION 4: DELIVERY

36. **Episiotomy** — 203
    Kalpana Negi, Aanya Sharma

37. **Instrumental Vaginal Delivery** — 208
    Reeti Mehra

38. **Cesarean Section** — 215
    Parul Kotdawala, Munjal Pandya

39. **Breech** — 220
    Kiran Guleria, Richa Sharma

40. **Transverse Lie** — 224
    Vaishali Korde Nayak, Parag Biniwale

41. **Cord Prolapse** — 229
    Taru Gupta, Mansi Dhingra, Snigdha Kumari

42. **Shoulder Dystocia** — 233
    Anupama Bahadur

43. **Injuries of Birth Canal** — 236
    Manju Puri, Shilpi Nain

44. **Postpartum Hemorrhage** — 244
    Sayeba Akhter

45. **Retained Placenta** — 252
    Vandana Bhuriya

46. **Maternal Collapse** — 256
    Pratima Mittal, Jyotsna Suri

47. **Uterine Inversion** — 260
    Parneet Kaur

48. **Sepsis and Septic Shock** — 270
    Latika Chawla

SECTION 5: POSTPARTUM PERIOD

49. **Puerperal Pyrexia** — 277
    Shail Kaur

50. **Secondary Postpartum Hemorrhage** — 282
    Saswati Sanyal Choudhury

SECTION 6: NEONATE

51. **Care of Healthy Newborn** — 287
    Piyush Gautam, Nivedita Sharma

52. **Care of Preterm Newborns** — 293
    Pancham Chauhan

53. **Neonatal Resuscitation** — 298
    Parveen Bhardwaj

54. **Neonatal Jaundice** — 304
    Ram Krishan Kaushal

SECTION 7: MISCELLANEOUS

55. **Teenage Pregnancy** — 313
    Priti Samir Vyas

56. **Blood and Blood Component Therapy** — 318
    Dilpreet Kaur Pandher, Alok Sharma

57. **Patient Communication** — 322
    Girija Wagh, Aakanksha Kumar

58. **Biomedical Waste Management Rules** — 326
    Anuradha Sood, Smriti Chauhan, Subhash Chand Jaryal

59. **How to Curb Maternal Mortality in India** — 329
    Madhu Gupta, Kanica Kaushal

60. **Needle-prick Injury** — 334
    Madhuri Chandra

Index — *339*

Section 1

Maternal Disorders

- **Antiphospholipid Antibody Syndrome**
  Kavita Khoiwal, K Aparna Sharma

- **Hypertensive Disorders of Pregnancy**
  Sruthi Bhaskaran, Esha Gupta

- **Cardiac Diseases in Pregnancy**
  Ajith S

- **Anemia in Pregnancy**
  Haresh U Doshi

- **Diabetes in Pregnancy**
  Smiti Nanda, Anjali Gupta

- **Jaundice in Pregnancy: Dilemma in Management**
  Sharda Patra

- **Convulsions in Pregnancy**
  Seema Chopra, Arshi Syal

- **Venous Thromboembolism in Pregnancy**
  Vivek Chauhan, Suman Thakur

- **Shock**
  Rohini Rao, Rajesh Kumar Verma, Kunal Kumar Sharma

- **Advanced Maternal Age**
  Vidya Thobbi, Jyothi Goulay

- **Rh Isoimmunization**
  Meenakshi Barsaul Chauhan, Vani Malhotra

- **H1N1 Infection in Pregnancy**
  Suparna Grover, Ajay Chhabra

- **Zika Virus**
  Manishi Mittal

- **Renal Disorders and Pregnancy**
  JB Sharma, Venus Dalal

- **Thyroid Disorders**
  Reena Wani, Rashmi G Jalvee

Antiphospholipid Antibody Syndrome

Kavita Khoiwal, K Aparna Sharma

INTRODUCTION

Antiphospholipid antibody (APLA) syndrome is an acquired autoimmune disorder defined by the presence of antiphospholipid antibodies with vascular thrombosis and/or recurrent pregnancy loss (RPL) or placental insufficiency. The incidence of APLA syndrome in women with RPL is 15%.[1]

CLASSIFICATION

- Antiphospholipid antibody syndrome is classified as primary and secondary APLA syndrome.
- Secondary APLA syndrome occurs when it is associated with any of the diseases shown in **Algorithm 1**.

PATHOPHYSIOLOGY

An adverse pregnancy outcome related to APLA syndrome such as RPL and/or intrauterine fetal growth restriction is due to abnormal placentation, local inflammatory destruction, and thrombosis of placental bed vessels.
- Abnormal placentation **(Algorithm 2)**
- Thrombosis **(Algorithm 3)**

DIAGNOSTIC CRITERIA

The diagnostic criteria for antiphospholipid antibody syndrome is shown in **Algorithm 4**.
- At least one of the clinical criteria and one of the laboratory criteria should meet to consider the diagnosis of APLA syndrome.

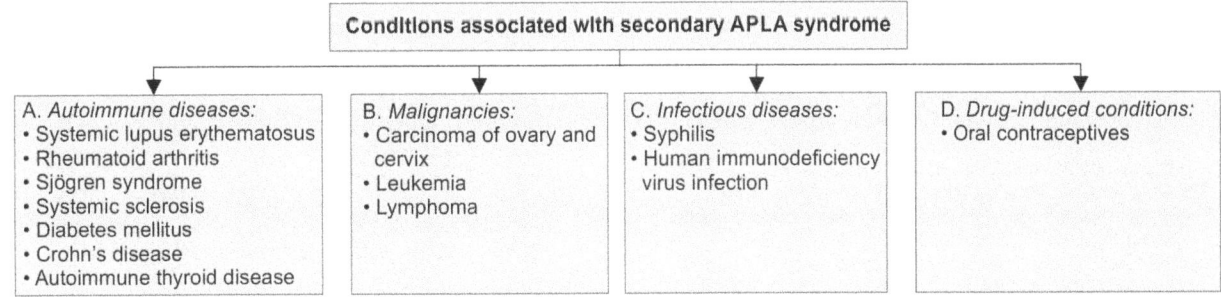

Algorithm 1: Conditions associated with secondary antiphospholipid antibody (APLA) syndrome.

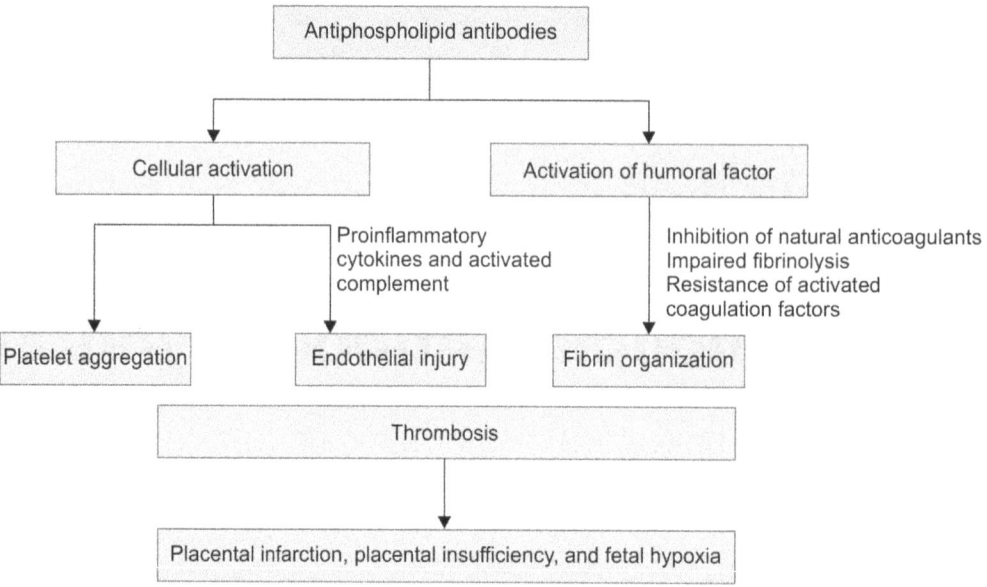

Algorithm 2: Pathogenesis of abnormal placentation.

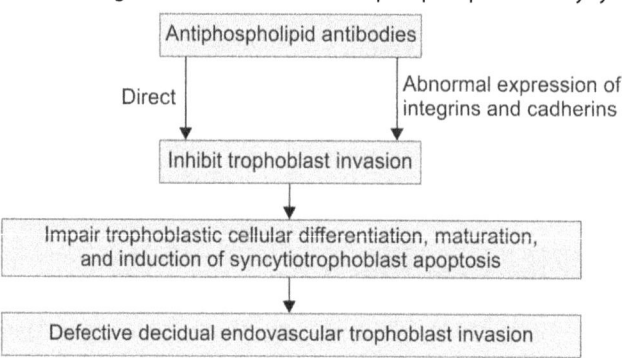

Algorithm 3: Pathogenesis of thrombosis in antiphospholipid antibody syndrome.

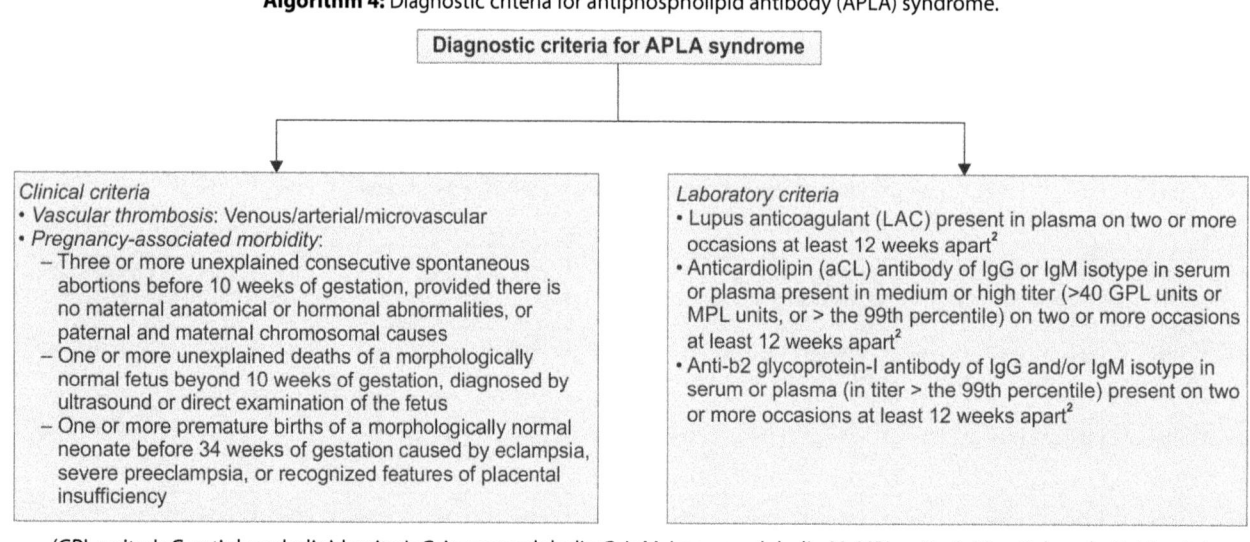

Algorithm 4: Diagnostic criteria for antiphospholipid antibody (APLA) syndrome.

(GPL units: IgG antiphospholipid units; IgG: immunoglobulin G; IgM: immunoglobulin M; MPL units: IgM antiphospholipid units)

- Lupus anticoagulant is more specific while anticardiolipin (aCL) and anti-b2GP-I are more sensitive.[3]

MANAGEMENT

The goal of management is to improve maternal and fetal outcome. It depends upon the individual clinical scenario as shown in **Algorithm 5**.

- Unfractionated heparin (UFH) with low-dose aspirin (75–150 mg) provides the highest success rate.[4]
- Aspirin should be started preconceptionally and UFH from the day the pregnancy test is positive at the dose of 5,000 U (7,500 U if weight >80 kg) subcutaneously twice a day.
- Low molecular weight heparin (LMWH; 40 mg subcutaneously once a day) is the treatment of choice for RPL associated with APLA syndrome.
- LMWH is as safe as UFH. Its advantages over UFH include once-daily dose, less intensive monitoring, and lower risk of heparin-induced thrombocytopenia and osteoporosis.[5]

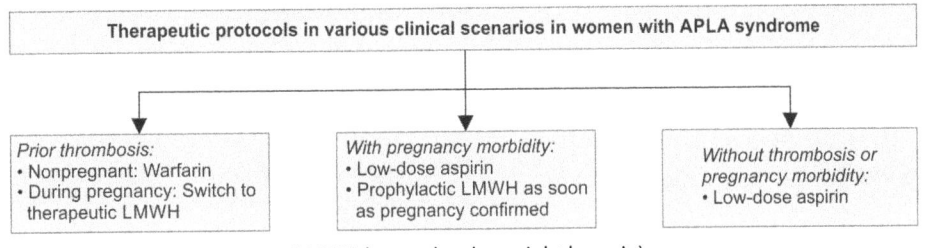

Algorithm 5: Therapeutic protocols in various clinical scenarios in women with antiphospholipid antibody (APLA) syndrome.

(LMWH: low molecular weight heparin)

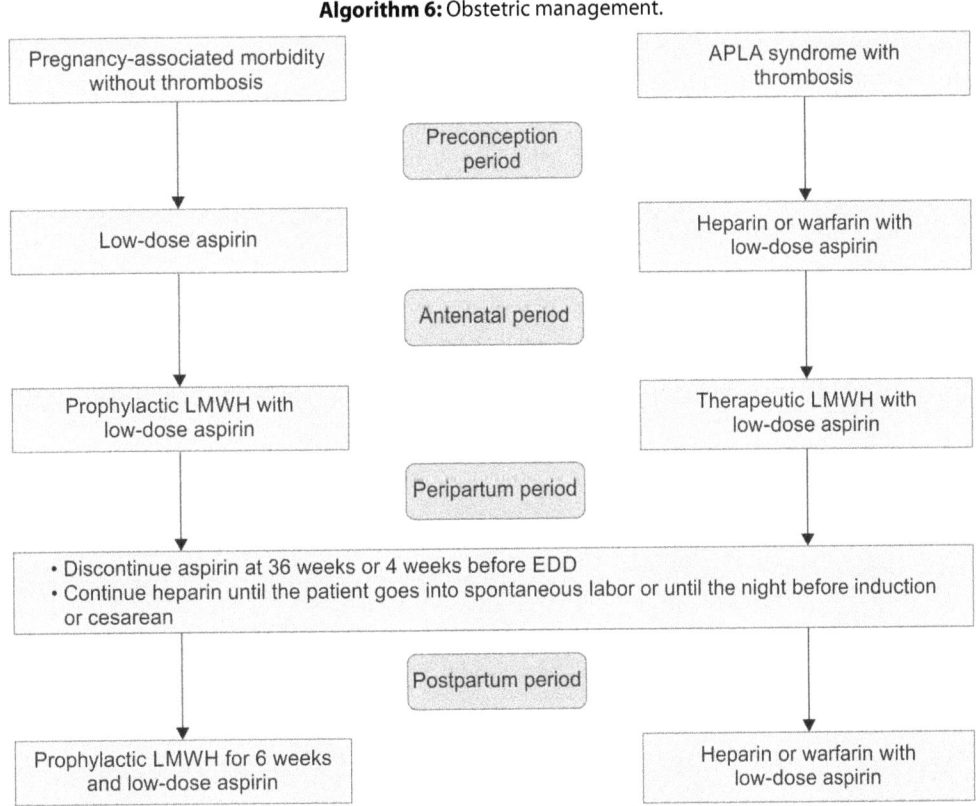

Algorithm 6: Obstetric management.

(APLA: antiphospholipid antibody; EDD: expected date of delivery; LMWH: low molecular weight heparin)

Obstetric Management

Algorithm 6 summarizes the obstetric management in women with APLA syndrome.

Antepartum Surveillance

- Routine antepartum testing
- Daily fetal kick counts, twice-weekly nonstress test, and weekly biophysical profile
- Serial ultrasonography (USG) for fetal growth monitoring.

Peripartum Management

- Neuroaxial anesthesia is safe only after 12 hours of the last prophylactic dose and 24 hours of the last therapeutic dose of LMWH.[6]
- Subcutaneous UFH is not a contraindication to neuroaxial anesthesia.

Postpartum Management

- Initiate early ambulation in women who had a vaginal delivery and use pneumatic compression stocking for women who had a cesarean section.
- Restart low-dose aspirin and heparin, to be given for 4–6 weeks postpartum.[2]
- Calcium supplements should be given along with heparin.
- Estrogen-containing contraceptive pills should be avoided.
- These women have a lifelong risk of thrombosis and stroke and should be kept on follow-up with the collaboration of the hematologist.

REFERENCES

1. Rai RS, Regan L, Clifford K, et al. Antiphospholipid antibodies and beta-2-glycoprotein-I in 500 women with recurrent miscarriage: results of a comprehensive screening approach. Hum Reprod. 1995;10:2001-5.
2. Branch DW, Holmgren C, Goldberg JD. Antiphospholipid syndrome. American College of Obstetricians and Gynecologists Practice Bulletin Number 132. Obstet Gynecol. 2012;120:1514-21.
3. Galli M, Luciani D, Bertolini G, et al. Lupus anticoagulants are stronger risk factors for thrombosis than anticardiolipin antibodies in the antiphospholipid syndrome: a systematic review of the literature. Blood. 2003;101:1827-32.
4. Ziakas PD, Pavlou M, Voulgarelis M. Heparin treatment in antiphospholipid syndrome with recurrent pregnancy loss: a systematic review and meta-analysis. Obstet Gynecol. 2010;115:1256-62.
5. Greer IA, Nelson-Piercy C. Low-molecular-weight heparins for thromboprophylaxis and treatment of venous thromboembolism in pregnancy: a systematic review of safety and efficacy. Blood. 2005;106:401-7.
6. Horlocker TT, Wedel DJ, Benzon H, et al. Regional anesthesia in the anticoagulated patient: defining the risks (the second ASRA Consensus Conference on Neuraxial Anesthesia and Anticoagulation). Reg Anesth Pain Med. 2003;28:172-97.

Chapter 2

Hypertensive Disorders of Pregnancy

Sruthi Bhaskaran, Esha Gupta

INTRODUCTION

Hypertensive disorders of pregnancy complicate 10–15% of pregnancies worldwide and are an important cause of severe morbidity, long-term disability, and death among both mothers and their babies.[1] Among the hypertensive disorders that complicate pregnancy, preeclampsia and eclampsia stand out as major causes of maternal and perinatal mortality and morbidity.

In this chapter, we have discussed the management protocols of this condition **(Table 1)**.

Table 1: Diagnostic criterion for preeclampsia.[2]	
Blood pressure (BP)	• Systolic blood pressure (SBP) ≥ 140 mm Hg or diastolic blood pressure (DBP) ≥ 90 mm Hg on two occasions at least 4 hrs apart after 20 weeks pog with a previously normal BP • Systolic blood pressure of 160 mm Hg or higher, or diastolic blood pressure of 110 mm Hg or higher on two occasions at least 4 hours apart while patient is on bed rest (unless antihypertensive therapy is initiated before this time)
And	
Proteinuria	≥300 mg/24 hr urine collection (or this amount extrapolated from a timed collection Or Pr/cr ratio ≥ 0.3 Dipstick reading of 1+ (used only if other quantitative methods not available)
Or in absence of proteinuria, new-onset hypertension with new-onset severe features of preeclampsia	
Severe features of preeclampsia (any of these findings)	
Thrombocytopenia (platelet count <100,000/µL)	
Impaired liver function tests (≥ twice), severe persistent right upper quadrant or epigastric pain unresponsive to medication and not accounted by alternative diagnoses, or both	
Progressive renal insufficiency (S. Cr > 1.1 mg/dL or doubling of serum creatinine)	
Concentration in absence of renal disease	
Pulmonary edema	
New-onset cerebral or visual disturbances	

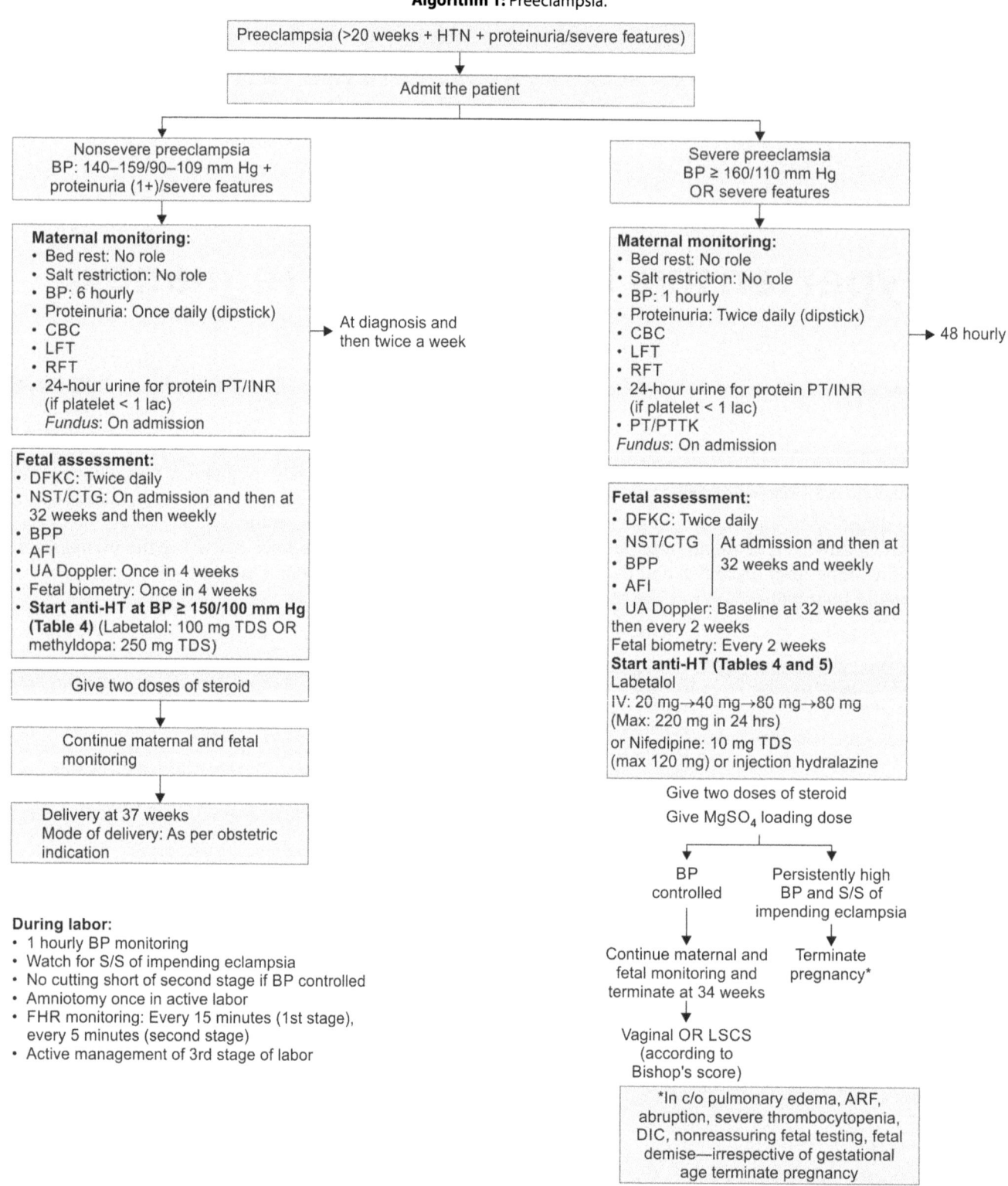

Algorithm 1: Preeclampsia.

Contd...

Contd...

After delivery
- *BP monitoring*: 6 hourly
- *Anti-HT*: Restart if BP ≥ 150/100 mm Hg
- Methyldopa, if already in use should be substituted
- No restriction of angiotensin-converting enzyme (ACE) inhibitors, B-blockers, and dose should be readjusted
- Avoid diuretics during lactation
- *Discharge*: After 72 hours if BP controlled with/without anti-HT
- Follow-up after 1 week and 6 weeks
- *Contraception*: Avoid oral contraceptive pills (OCPs)
- Recurrence risk of preeclampsia: 16% (preeclampsia), 25% [severe preeclampsia, eclampsia, or Hemolysis, elevated liver enzymes and low platelet count syndrome (HELLP)]

(AFI: amniotic fluid index; ARF: acute renal failure; BP: blood pressure; BPP: biophysical profile; CBC: complete blood count; CTG: cardiotocography; DFKC: daily fetal kick count; DIC: disseminated intravascular coagulation; FHR: fetal heart rate; HTN: hypertension; IV: intravenous; LFTs: liver function tests; LSCS: lower segment cesarean section; NST: nonstress test; PT: prothrombin time; RFT: renal function test; TDS: three times daily)

Table 2: Nonsevere preeclampsia (BP: 140–159/90–109 mm Hg + proteinuria (1+)/severe features).

	ACOG (2019)[2]	NICE (2019)[3]	Proposed
Definition: BP	140–159/90–109 mm Hg	Mild: 140–149/90–99 mm Hg Mod: 150–159/100–109 mm Hg	140–159/90–109 mm Hg
Proteinuria	1+	1+	1+
Antenatal monitoring	Home/hospital if: • AFI <5 cm • BPP <6/10 • EBW <5th percentile • PROM	Hospital	Hospital
Salt restriction	No	No	No
Strict bed rest	No	No	No
BP monitoring	Twice weekly	6 hourly	6 hourly
Test for proteinuria	At time of diagnosis	At time of diagnosis	At time of diagnosis and then daily
CBC, LFT, RFT	At time of diagnosis and then once a week	At time of diagnosis and then twice a week	At time of diagnosis and then twice a week
Fundus	At time of diagnosis	–	At time of diagnosis
Fetal monitoring: DFKC by mother	Daily	Daily	Twice daily
NST/CTG BPP	At time of diagnosis and then twice a week Only if NST is nonreactive	At time of diagnosis and then once a week	At time of diagnosis and then fortnightly up to 34 weeks and then weekly
UA doppler	Only if FGR suspected	At time of diagnosis and then every 2 weeks	At time of diagnosis and then fortnightly up to 34 weeks and then weekly (if FGR suspected)
AFI	Once weekly	At time of diagnosis and then every 2 weeks	At time of diagnosis and then fortnightly up to 34 weeks and then weekly
Fetal biometry	Every 3 weeks	At time of diagnosis and then every 2 weeks	At time of diagnosis and then fortnightly up to 34 weeks and then weekly
Anti-HT agents	Not recommended	Start at BP ≥ 150/100 mm Hg	Start at BP ≥ 150/100 mm Hg
Timing of delivery	37 weeks	37 weeks	37 weeks
Mode of delivery	Fetal presentation and cervical status	–	As per obstet indication

Contd...

Contd...

	ACOG (2019)[2]	*NICE (2019)[3]*	*Proposed*
During labor: BP monitoring	Continuous	1 hourly	1 hourly
FHS monitoring	Continuous	Continuous	½ hourly in 1st stage and every 15 min in 2nd stage
Cut short 2nd stage	–	Not recommended	Not recommended
Early amniotomy	–	–	Not recommended
Active management of 3rd stage			Recommended
Postnatal care: • BP monitoring • Anti-HT • Discharge • Follow-up		• 6 hourly while in hospital and then on alternate day for 2 weeks • Continue • When BP is controlled • After 2 weeks	• 6 hourly while in hospital and then daily • Continue • After 72 hrs if BP controlled with or without anti-HT • After 1 week and then at 6 weeks

(ACOG: American College of Obstetricians and Gynecologists; AFI: amniotic fluid index; BP: blood pressure; BPP: biophysical profile; CBC: complete blood count; CTG: cardiotocography; DFKC: daily fetal kick count; EBW: expected body weight; FHS: fetal heart sound; IUGR: intrauterine growth restriction; LFTs: liver function tests; NICE: National Institute of Health and Care Excellence; NST: nonstress test; PROM: premature rupture of membranes; RFT: renal function test; UA: umbilical artery)

Table 3: Severe preeclampsia (BP ≥ 160/110 OR severe features).

	ACOG[2]	*NICE[3]*	*Proposed*
Maternal monitoring	Admit	Admit	Admit
BP monitoring	Every 10 mins × 1 hr, then every 15 mins × 1 hr, then every 30 mins × 1 hr then four times daily	Every 15–30 minutes until BP is less than 160/110 mm Hg, then at least four times daily	Every 15–30 minutes until BP is less than 160/110 mm Hg, then at least four times daily
I/O charting	8 hourly	–	1 hourly
Lab tests (CBC, LFT, RFT, 24 hr urine)	Daily	Three times a week	Alternate day/twice a week
Fundus examination	At the time of diagnosis	–	At the time of diagnosis
Aim: To prolong pregnancy up to	34 weeks	34 weeks	34 weeks
Fetal monitoring: DFKC	Daily	–	Daily
NST/CTG	Daily	Weekly	At admission and then at 32 weeks, then every week
BPP	Twice weekly	–	At admission and then at 32 weeks, then every week
UA Doppler	Every 2 weeks if IUGR is suspected	Every 2 weeks	Baseline at 32 weeks and then every 2 weeks
AFI	Twice weekly	Every 2 weeks	Every week
Fetal biometry	Every 2 weeks	Every 2 weeks	Every 2 weeks
Acute Mx with anti-HT	Labetalol/nifedipine/hydralazine	Labetalol/nifedipine/hydralazine	Labetalol/nifedipine/hydralazine/prazosin
MgSO$_4$ prophylaxis	Yes	Yes	Yes (give loading dose + maintenance if patient delivers)
Timing of delivery Mode of delivery	34 weeks <32 weeks: LSCS >32 weeks: vaginal/LSCS Depending on Bishop score	34 weeks	34 weeks if no complications and BP controlled with anti-HT Vaginal/LSCS depending on Bishop score

Contd...

Contd...

	ACOG[2]	NICE[3]	Proposed
During labor: BP monitoring	Continuous	Continuous	Hourly
FHR monitoring	Continuous	Continuous	15 minutes in the first stage, every 5 minutes in second stage
Cut short 2nd stage	–	Not recommended	Not recommended If BP controlled
Early amniotomy	No role	No role	Amniotomy once in early active labor
Active management of 3rd stage			Recommended
Postnatal care: BP monitoring		6 hourly while in hospital and then on alternate day for 2 weeks	6 hourly while in hospital and then daily
Anti-HT		Continue	Continue
Discharge		When BP is controlled	After 72 hrs if BP controlled
Follow-up		After 2 weeks	After 1 week

(ACOG: American College of Obstetricians and Gynecologists; AFI: amniotic fluid index; BP: blood pressure; BPP: biophysical profile; CBC: complete blood count; CTG: cardiotocography; DFKC: daily fetal kick count; FHR: fetal heart rate; IUGR: intrauterine growth restriction; LFTs: liver function tests; LSCS: lower segment cesarean section; NICE: National Institute of Health and Care Excellence; NST: non-stress test; RFT: renal function test; UA: umbilical artery)

Table 4: Common oral antihypertensive agents in pregnancy.[4]

Drug	Dosage	Comments
Labetalol	200–2,400 mg/day orally in two to three divided doses. Commonly initiated at 100–200 mg twice daily	• Potential bronchoconstrictive effects • Avoid in women with asthma, pre-existing myocardial disease, decompensated cardiac function, and heart block and bradycardia
Methyldopa	500–3,000 mg/day orally in two to four divided doses. Commonly initiated at 250 mg twice or three times daily	May not be as effective as other medications, especially in control of severe hypertension. Use limited by side effect profile (sedation, depression, dizziness)
Nifedipine	30–120 mg/day orally of an extended-release preparation. Commonly initiated at 30–60 mg once daily (extended-release)	• Do not use sublingual form • Immediate-release formulation should generally be reserved for control of severe, acutely elevated blood pressures in hospitalized patients. Should be avoided in tachycardia

Table 5: Antihypertensive agents used for urgent blood pressure control in pregnancy.[4]

Drug	Dosage	Comments	Onset of action
Labetalol	10–20 mg IV, then 20–80 mg every 10–30 minutes to a maximum cumulative dosage of 300 mg; or constant infusion 1–2 mg/min IV	• Tachycardia is less common and fewer adverse effects than other agents • Avoid in women with asthma, pre-existing myocardial disease, decompensated cardiac function, and heart block and bradycardia	1–2 minutes
Hydralazine	5 mg IV or IM, then 5–10 mg IV every 20–40 minutes to a maximum cumulative dosage of 20 mg; or constant infusion of 0.5–10 mg/hr	Maternal hypotension, headaches, and abnormal fetal heart rate tracings; may be more common than other agents	10–20 minutes
Nifedipine	10–20 mg orally, repeat in 20 minutes if needed; then 10–20 mg every 2–6 hours; maximum daily dose is 180 mg	May observe reflex tachycardia and headaches.	5–10 minutes

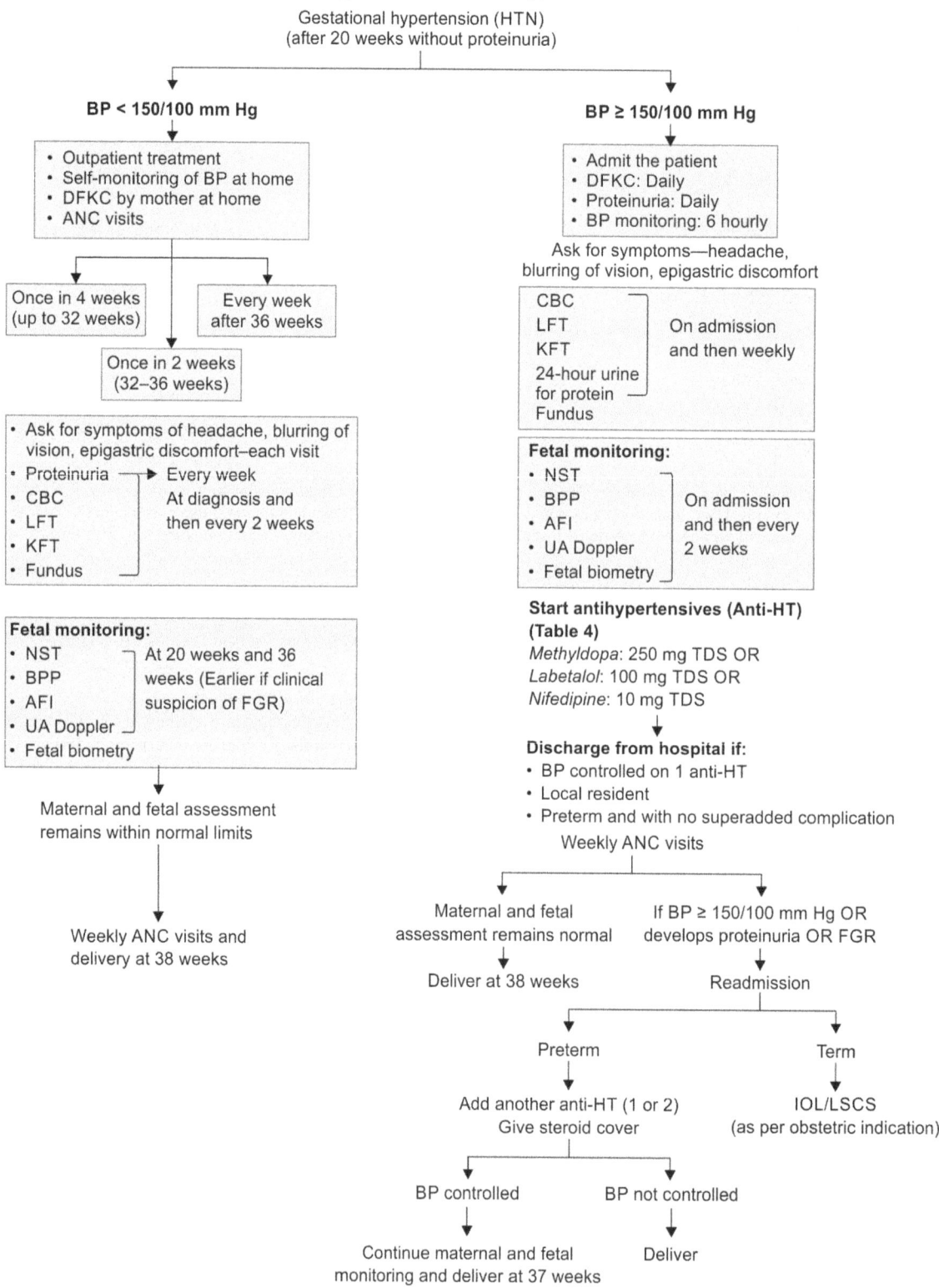

Algorithm 2: Gestational hypertension.

Contd...

Contd...

During labor
- 1 hourly BP monitoring
- No cutting short of second stage if BP controlled
- No early amniotomy
- *FHR monitoring*:
  - ½ hourly (1st stage)
  - 15 minutes (2nd stage)
- Active management of 3rd stage of labor

After delivery
- *BP monitoring*: Once daily
- *Anti-HT*: May not be required
  - Restart if BP ≥ 150/100 mm Hg after 24 hrs
  - Methyldopa should not be used
- No restriction of ACE inhibitors, B-blockers, and dose should be readjusted
- Avoid diuretics during lactation
- *Discharged*: After 72 hours if BP controlled or patient is on anti-HT treatment
- FU after 1 week and 6 weeks
- *Recurrence risk*:
  - Gestational HTN: 16–47%
  - Preeclampsia: 2–7%

(AFI: amniotic fluid index; ANC: antenatal care; BP: blood pressure; BPP: biophysical profile; CBC: complete blood count; DFKC: daily fetal kick count; FGR: fetal growth restriction; IOL: induction of labor; KFT: kidney function test; LFTs: liver function tests; LSCS: lower segment cesarean section; NST: nonstress test; RFT: renal function test; UA: umbilical artery)

ECLAMPSIA

Admit the patient.
History from attendant: Duration of pregnancy, number of fits, history of epilepsy, history of fits or HTN in previous pregnancy, drug therapy.
Call for help.

↓

- **Avoid maternal injury**: Railed cot
- **Maintain**: Airway—Left lateral position, suction of secretions, padded tongue blade
  Breathing: Oxygen by mask (6–8 L/min)
  Circulation: Evaluate PR and BP
- **Examination: GPE**—Conscious/unconscious
  PR/BP/RR/PE
  B/L chest: Clear/crepts
- **Make IV lines patent** (No. 18 Cannula)
- Sample should be sent for CBC, LFT, RFT, and cross-match
  Fluids: Not > 80 mL/hr OR 2 l/24 hrs
  Crystalloids (RL, NS) preferred over colloids (Haemaccel, albumin, dextran)

↓

- **Do P/A**: Abdominal wall edema
  Fundal height, liquor, contractions
  FHR auscultation
- **Do Foley's catheterization**
- **Do P/V**: Dilatation, cervical status, memb, Bishop

Give $MgSO_4$ loading f/b maintenance

Pritchard regime (IM)	**Zuspan regime (IV)**
4 g (20%) of $MgSO_4$ IV bolus over 10–15 min f/b 10 g (50%) deep IM (5 g in each buttock) f/b maintenance; 5 g IM in alternate buttock 4 hourly till 24 hrs of delivery or last seizure whichever occurred later	4–6 g of $MgSO_4$ diluted in 100 mL of NS over 15–20 min f/b maintenance dose of 1 g/hr IV infusion till 24 hrs of delivery or last seizure whichever occurred later (5 g $MgSO_4$ in 500 mL of NS at the rate of 22 d/min, i.e. 1 g/hr)

If seizure reoccurs: Give 2 g of $MgSO_4$ bolus over 5 min OR Increase the rate of infusion to 1.5–2 g/hr

Seizure reoccurs: Give phenobarbitone 300 mg IV over 5 min
Monitor for Mg toxicity: Look for

- Respiratory rate (>12 breaths/min)
- Deep tendon reflexes (+)
- Urine output (>30 mL/hr)

↓

If toxicity occurs: Stop $MgSO_4$
Give Ca gluconate 1 g (10 mL) of 10% over 10 min IV (if there is respiratory depression)
NO DIURETICS if urine output decreased.

↓

Start phenytoin (prior ECG should be done), loading dose: 10–15 mg/kg at the rate of 50 mg/min (600 mg in 300 mL NS over ½ hr f/b 300 mg in 200 mL NS over ½ hr f/b), maintenance dose of 100 mg IV 8 hourly

- **Start anti-HT**: Labetalol 20 mg IV stat → 40 mg IV → 80 mg IV → 80 mg IV every 20 min if BP not controlled. Max dose being 220 mg/24 hrs. Once BP is controlled and patient is conscious start oral labetalol 200 mg TDS.

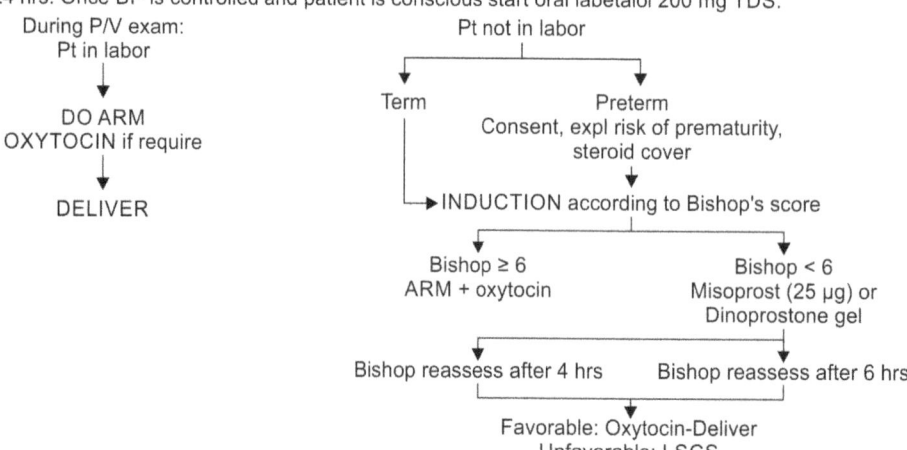

Contd...

Contd...

During delivery
- Bed delivery
- *Cut short 2nd stage of labor:* Forceps/ventouse
- Active management of 3rd stage
- Be vigilant for PPH

After delivery
- Continue $MgSO_4$ maintenance
- *BP monitoring*: Hourly for 24 hrs and then 6 hourly if controlled
- I/O charting 6 hourly
- Restart anti-HT after 24 hrs if BP ≥ 150/100 mm Hg (labetalol/atenolol/nifedipine) with readjusted dose
- Patient to be discharged after 1 week if no complication
- FU after 1 week

(ARM: artificial rupture of membranes; BP: blood pressure; FHR: fetal heart rate; GPE: general physical examination; HTN: hypertension; IM: intramuscular; IV: intravenous; LSCS: lower segment cesarean section; NS: normal saline; PE: preeclampsia; PR: pulse rate; RFT: renal function test; RL: Ringer's lactate)

CHRONIC HYPERTENSION (BEFORE CONCEPTION OR BEFORE 20 WEEKS WITHOUT PROTEINURIA)[4]

Preconceptional Counseling

- Explain risks associated with chronic HTN and superimposed preeclampsia
- Stop ACE inhibitors, ARB, mineralocorticoid antagonists
- Tests: CBC, platelet count, LFT, KFT, serum electrolytes, and TSH; Urine for protein (dipstick, 24 hr protein), urine c/s; fundus examination; USG: B/L kidneys and adrenals

Section 1
Maternal Disorders

Aim

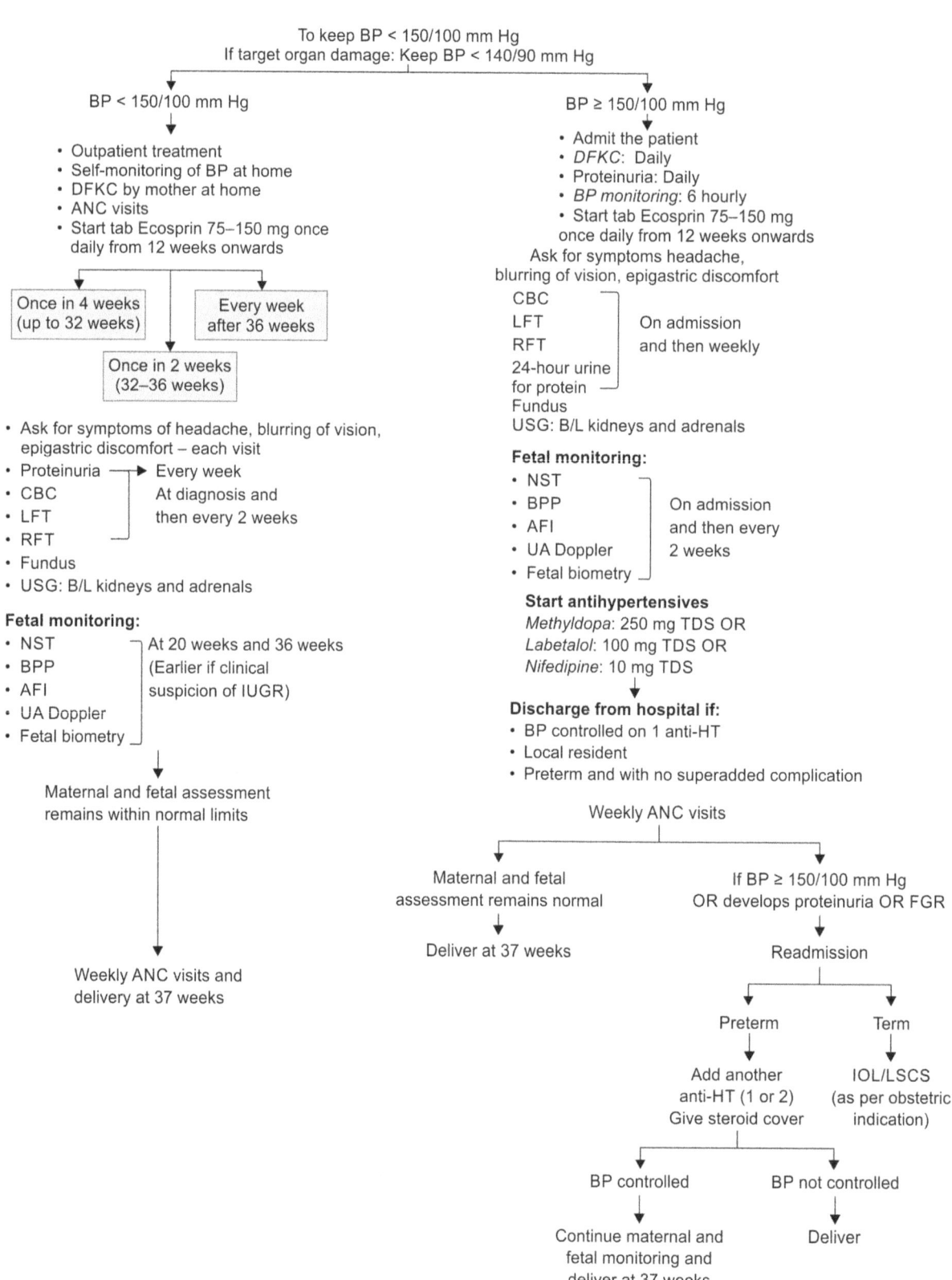

Contd...

Contd...

During labor
- 1 hourly BP monitoring
- No cutting short of second stage if BP controlled
- No early amniotomy
- *FHR monitoring*:
  - ½ hourly (1st stage)
  - 15 minutes (2nd stage)
- Active management of 3rd stage of labor.

After delivery
- *BP monitoring*: Once daily
- *Continue anti-HT*: Methyldopa should not be used
- No restriction of ACE inhibitors, B-blockers, and dose should be readjusted
- Avoid diuretics during lactation
- *Discharged*: After 72 hours if BP is controlled or patient is on anti-HT treatment.
- FU after 1 week and 6 weeks.

(AFI: amniotic fluid index; ANC: antenatal care; BP: blood pressure; BPP: biophysical profile; CBC: complete blood count; DFKC: daily fetal kick count; FHR: fetal heart restriction; IOL: induction of labor; IUGR: intrauterine growth restriction; LFT: liver function test; LSCS: lower segment cesarean section; NST: nonstress test; RFT: renal function test; USG: ultrasonography; UA: umbilical artery)

REFERENCES

1. World Health Organization. WHO Recommendations for Prevention and Treatment of Pre-eclampsia and Eclampsia. Geneva: World Health Organization; 2011.
2. ACOG Practice bulletin no. 202: gestational hypertension and preeclampsia. Obstet Gynecol. 2019;133(1):e1-25.
3. National Institute for Health and Care Excellence. Hypertension in pregnancy: diagnosis and management: NICE guideline. London, UK: National Institute for Health and Care Excellence; 2019.
4. ACOG practice bulletin no. 203. Chronic hypertension in pregnancy. Obstet Gynecol. 2019;133(1):e26-50.

Chapter 3

Cardiac Disease in Pregnancy

Ajith S

INTRODUCTION

Cardiac diseases complicate about 1% of pregnancies. There are some symptoms and signs in normal pregnancies that mimic cardiac diseases **(Boxes 1 and 2)**.

Functional classification based on four symptoms (fatigue, dyspnea, palpitation, and chest pain) is described in **Table 1**.

Box 1	Pregnancy changes that mimic cardiac diseases.

Symptoms
- Dyspnea
- Fatigue
- Palpitation

Signs
- Pedal edema
- Shifting of apex to left and cephalad
- Bounding peripheral pulse
- Prominent neck veins
- Increase in intensity of first sound (S1)
- Physiologic third heart sound (S3)
- Functional systolic murmurs
- Internal mammary venous hum

Electrocardiogram (ECG)
- Left axis deviation
- ST depression

Chest X-ray
- Apparent cardiomegaly
- Straightening of left border

Box 2	Symptoms and signs in cardiac diseases.

Symptoms
- Orthopnea
- Paroxysmal nocturnal dyspnea
- Hemoptysis
- Cyanosis

Signs
- Diastolic murmur
- Systolic murmur > Grade 3, thrill
- Fibrillation
- *ECHO:* Valvular lesions, congenital defects, cardiomyopathy

Table 1: New York Heart Association (NYHA) classification.	
Class 1	No limitation of physical activity
Class 2	Slight limitation of activity, feels discomfort on moderate activity
Class 3	Marked limitation of physical activity, comfortable at rest, but feels symptoms with ordinary activities
Class 4	Symptoms even at rest. All cases of previous cardiac failure and atrial fibrillation, past and present, are included in this class

COMMON CARDIAC DISEASES

- In developing countries:
  - Rheumatic valvular disease
  - Congenital heart disease (CHD, surgically corrected and uncorrected)

- In the United Kingdom, cardiac disease is the leading indirect cause of maternal mortality.[1] The causes are:
  - Myocardial infarction (MI)
  - Dissection of thoracic aorta
  - Cardiomyopathy.

Complications
- Cardiac failure
- Infective endocarditis
- Worsening of New York Heart Association (NYHA) class
- Thromboembolism
- Arrhythmias

Box 3 Common risk period for cardiac failure.
- Pregnancy at 28–30 weeks, when blood volume peaks
- During labor due to uterine contraction and pain
- Postpartum due to shunting of blood from placental bed

Box 4 Precipitating factors for cardiac failure.
- Respiratory infection
- Anemia
- Hypertension
- Multiple pregnancies
- Thyrotoxicosis
- Atrial fibrillation
- Acute febrile illness

Box 5 Predictors of cardiac complications (CARPREG scale).
- NYHA class 3 and 4
- Cyanosis
- Left atrial/ventricular obstruction as indicated by:
  - Mitral valve area < 2 cm²
  - Aortic valve area < 1.5 cm²
  - Peak left ventricular outflow gradient > 30 mm Hg
- LV dysfunction (EF < 40%)
- History of cardiac failure, arrhythmia, stroke, and transient ischemic attack

Table 2: World Health Organization (WHO) risk assessment classification of cardiac disease in pregnancy.

WHO I low risk	• Pulmonary stenosis, PDA, MVP • Surgically corrected ASD, VSD
WHO II medium risk	• Unoperated ASD, VSD • Repaired TOF • Most arrhythmias
WHO II–III (depending on individual)	• Hypertrophic cardiomyopathy • Marfan's syndrome without aortic dilatation • Aorta <45 mm in aortic disease with a bicuspid aortic valve • Repaired coarctation
WHO III high risk	• Mechanical valve • Unrepaired congenital heart disease (CHD) • Other complex CHDs • Fontan circulation • Marfan's syndrome with aortic dilatation 40–45 mm • Aortic dilatation 45–50 mm in bicuspid aortic valve
WHO IV (pregnancy-contraindicated)	• PAH of any cause (primary pulmonary hypertension, Eisenmenger syndrome) • Severe systemic ventricular dysfunction (LVEF <30%, NYHA III, IV) • Previous peripartum cardiomyopathy with any residual impairment of left ventricular function • Severe mitral stenosis, severe symptomatic atrial stenosis • Marfan's syndrome with aortic root dilatation >45 mm • Aortic dilatation > 50 mm in bicuspid aortic valve • Native severe coarctation

(ASD: atrial septal defect; LVEF: left ventricular ejection fraction; MVP: mitral valve prolapse; NYHA: New York Heart Association; PAH: pulmonary arterial hypertension; PDA: patent ductus arteriosus; TOF: tetralogy of Fallot; VSD: ventricular septal defect)

Box 6 Preconceptional management.
- Women with a high mortality rate above 25% should be advised against pregnancy
- Congenital heart disease (CHD) and severe mitral stenosis should be surgically corrected before planning pregnancy
- Correct anemia
- Counseling regarding chance of inheritance of CHD to offspring (5%), genetic transmission of Marfan's syndrome, dilated cardiomyopathy, and familial hypertrophic cardiomyopathy

Box 7 Conditions in which surgical correction prior to pregnancy recommended.
- Severe MS/MR
- Severe AS/AR
- Large ASD/VSD
- PDA with pulmonary hypertension
- TOF
- Severe coarctation of aorta

(AR: aortic regurgitation; ASD: atrial septal defect; MR: mitral regurgitation; MS: mitral stenosis; NYHA: New York Heart Association; PDA: patent ductus arteriosus; TOF: tetralogy of Fallot; VSD: ventricular septal defect)

- Termination of pregnancy should be considered in conditions where pregnancy is contraindicated.
- Second-trimester termination is dangerous and should be discouraged.

Antepartum management is shown in **Algorithm 1**.

Algorithm 1: Antepartum management.

Evaluation in a tertiary center by cardiologist and obstetrician
↓
Accurate diagnosis, NYHA class assessment, risk stratification, maternal and fetal risk assessment, review of medications
↓
- *Counseling*: Limitation of physical activity, salt-restricted diet, avoid stress, avoiding and early treatment of respiratory infection, early recognition and treatment of anemia, asymptotic bacteriuria, and hypertension
- Regular monitoring of Hb, BP, fetal growth
- Monitor for evidence of cardiac failure, arrhythmia

(BP: blood pressure; Hb: hemoglobin; NYHA: New York Heart Association)

Consider doing Fetal Echocardiography in Pregnant Women with Congenital Heart Disease

- *NYHA class I and II:* Can be managed on OP basis, but as pregnancy advances, the functional class may worsen; hence reassess at every visit.
- *Class III and IV:* Need hospital admission.

INTRAPARTUM MANAGEMENT (ALGORITHM 2)

- Most women will have spontaneous onset of labor at or near term.
- *Induction may be required for obstetric indication:* Mechanical methods (such as Foley catheter) and prostaglandins are used for cervical priming. Oxytocin infusion should be given in a higher concentration to avoid fluid overload.
- Spontaneous vaginal delivery is desirable.
- Cesarean section is done on obstetric indications. But if the woman cannot tolerate the hemodynamic changes associated with labor (e.g. Eisenmenger syndrome, severe cardiac dysfunction, cardiac failure, aortic dissection, coarctation of aorta), elective cesarean section should be considered before term when the mother is stable.

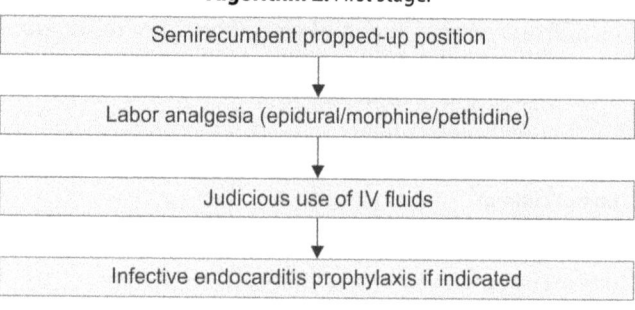

Algorithm 2: First stage.

Semirecumbent propped-up position
↓
Labor analgesia (epidural/morphine/pethidine)
↓
Judicious use of IV fluids
↓
Infective endocarditis prophylaxis if indicated

(IV: intravenous)

Box 8 | Infective endocarditis prophylaxis.

Antibiotic regimen
- Inj. ampicillin 2 g IV + Inj. gentamicin 1.5 mg/kg IV in active labor
- Followed 6 hrs later Inj. ampicillin 1 g IV or amoxicillin 2 g oral

If allergic to penicillin
- Inj. vancomycin 1 g IV over 1–2 hrs + Inj. gentamicin 1.5 mg/kg IV
- Or cefazoline/ceftriaxone 1 g IV
- Or clarithromycin/azithromycin 500 mg oral
- Or clindamycin 600 mg oral

American Heart Association (AHA) and American College of Obstetricians and Gynecologists (ACOG) recommend IE prophylaxis only for high-risk women:
- Women with prosthetic valves
- Prior endocarditis
- CHD unrepaired/repaired within 6 months
- Patients with cardiac transplantation
- *Contraindications for epidural analgesia (CATPIE):*
  - Coarctation of aorta
  - Aortic stenosis (AS)
  - Tetralogy of Fallot (uncorrected)
  - Pulmonary hypertension
  - Idiopathic hypertrophic subaortic stenosis
  - Eisenmenger syndrome

Second Stage of Labor

Cut short the second stage with outlet forceps or ventouse.

Third Stage of Labor

- Oxytocin should be used for AMTSL (active management of the third stage of labor) and ergometrine avoided.
- Inj. Frusemide 40 mg given IV after placental expulsion.
- Continue close monitoring for 24 hours after delivery.

CONTRACEPTION

- Barrier methods are safe.
- Estrogen-containing pills increase the risk of thromboembolism and should be avoided.
- Progesterone-only pills and depot medroxyprogesterone acetate (DMPA) may be considered.
- Intrauterine contraceptive devices (IUCDs) may give rise to bleeding or infection and should be used with caution.
- For sterilization, vasectomy may be preferred to tubectomy.

SPECIAL SITUATIONS

Mitral Stenosis
- Most common acquired valvular lesion.
- Moderate or severe mitral stenosis (MS) is poorly tolerated in pregnancy **(Box 9)**.
- Maternal complications in MS are pulmonary edema, congestive cardiac failure, atrial fibrillation (AF), and embolization.

Box 9	Severity of mitral stenosis.

- *Mild:* 2.5–4 cm^2
- *Moderate:* 1.5–2 cm^2
- *Severe:* <1.5 cm^2

Box 10	Management of mitral stenosis.

- *Moderate/severe mitral stenosis:* Valvotomy or valve replacement
- Reduce heart rate with digoxin and beta-blockers
- Reduce fluid overload and pulmonary congestion with diuretics
- Penicillin prophylaxis against rheumatic fever
- Surgical interventions such as balloon mitral valvotomy may be required in intractable or recurrent pulmonary edema, usually done in second trimester

Mitral Regurgitation

- Regurgitant lesions have better prognosis.
- Management is to avoid fluid overload, use of diuretics, and treatment of AF.
- Valve replacement prior to pregnancy is recommended in symptomatic women with AF, ejection fraction < 50%, and pulmonary systolic hypertension.

Aortic Stenosis

- Mild-to-moderate AS is generally well tolerated in pregnancy.
- *Valve area is <1 cm^2 (severe):* High chance of maternal mortality.
- Severe AS should be corrected prior to pregnancy.
- If uncorrected, may require balloon valvotomy during pregnancy. Hypotension, hypovolemia, and fluid overload should be avoided.

Prosthetic Valves

- Women with prosthetic mechanical valve need anticoagulation (not required in women with bioprosthetic valve)
  - *Warfarin:* Drug of choice in a nonpregnant state.
- The risk is highest between 6 and 12 weeks' gestation.
- Warfarin has less risk of maternal thromboembolism compared to unfractionated heparin and low molecular weight heparin (LMWH).

Warfarin Complications (If Dose > 5 mg/day) **(Algorithm 3)**
- *First trimester:* Warfarin embryopathy (epiphyseal stippling, hypoplasia of nasal bones and limbs, and chondromalacia)
- *Second trimester:* Late fetal loss
- *If given prior to or during labor:* Fetal and maternal hemorrhage

Cardiomyopathy

- *Hypertrophic cardiomyopathy:*
  - Autosomal dominant
  - Pregnancy generally well tolerated
  - In those symptomatic before pregnancy: Arrhythmia, syncope, and maternal death can occur.
  - May require beta-blockers
  - Hypotension (as in epidural block) and hypotension [(as in postpartum hemorrhage (PPH)] should be avoided.
- *Dilated cardiomyopathy*
  - Right and/or left ventricle is dilated and systolic function is reduced.
  - Pregnancy is poorly tolerated.
  - There is 7% mortality with NYHA class III or IV.
- *Peripartum cardiomyopathy*
  - LV systolic dysfunction and heart failure present in the last month of pregnancy and the first 5 months postdelivery.
  - Rare
  - Signs and symptoms of LVF
  - It is a diagnosis of exclusion.
  - *ECHO:* Ejection fraction < 45% and LV end-diastolic dimension > 2.7 cm/m^2.
  - *Treatment:* Beta-blockers, diuretics, hydralazine (hydralazine in postpartum period), and digoxin. Prophylactic anticoagulation may be required.
  - Mortality 5–10%.
  - Complete recovery in about 50%. Subsequent pregnancy after recovery is associated with relapse if the LV systolic function is not fully recovered.
  - There is no consensus regarding recommendation for future pregnancies.[2]
  - Combined pills are generally contraindicated.

Algorithm 3: Complications of warfarin.

```
                          Warfarin
                   ┌─────────┴─────────┐
                 <5 mg              >5 mg
                   │                   │
    Continue warfarin (with close     Switch to dose adjusted s/c LMWH throughout the first
    monitoring of INR) till            trimester ideally before 5 weeks. It has to be given
    36 weeks along with low-dose       twice daily with monitoring of anti-Xa activity
    aspirin. Dose adjusted
    s/c LMWH from 5 to 12 weeks is
    an alternative for those
    who want to avoid fetal risk of warfarin
                                         │
                    Timing of transition of warfarin to LMWH at 36 weeks
                    may need to be individualized for women at high risk
                    of preterm delivery, e.g. multiple pregnancies, previous
                                    preterm delivery

         Last dose of LMWH is given 24 hours before planned induction or cesarean

    12 hours after cessation of LMWH, IV UFH is started at    Intermittent prophylactic dose of LMWH
    1,000–1,250 units per hour (18 units/kg/hr) and           (e.g. enoxaparine 40 mg s/c once daily)
    infusion rate adjusted to keep target APTT at least
                   twice control

    IV UFH is stopped prior to delivery; timing of stopping   Stop prophylactic LMWH 12 hours prior to
    UFH is difficult to decide. If planning cesarean, stop    cesarean or epidural analgesia
                   4–6 hours prior

                                                              Stop prophylactic LMWH 12 hours prior to
                                                              cesarean or epidural analgesia

         IV UFH or s/c LMWH should be resumed within 4–6 hours of delivery if there are no bleeding complications.
                              Warfarin may be started from day 5 to 7
```

(INR: international normalized ratio; LMWH: low molecular weight heparin; UFH: unfractionated heparin)

Acute Pulmonary Edema: Management
- Oxygen by mask
- Semirecumbent position
- Digitalization, especially if there is AF
- Intravenous diuretic (frusemide)
- Parenteral morphine
- Emergency valvotomy/valvuloplasty in tight MS with intractable/recurrent pulmonary edema

Genetic and Prepregnancy Counseling

- Risk of CHD in mothers with CHDs 3–50% depending on the type of CHD, compared to 1% in normal.
- Children of parents with Marfan's syndrome, hypertrophic cardiomyopathy or long QT syndrome have an inheritance risk of 50%.
- Women with cardiac disease should be managed in a tertiary center by a team consisting of cardiologist, obstetrician, anesthesiologist, and neonatologist.

REFERENCES

1. Nanda S, Nelson-Piercy C, Mackillop L. Cardiac disease in pregnancy. Clin Med. 2012;12(6):553-60.
2. Gelson E, Johnson M, Gatzoulis M, et al. Cardiac disease in pregnancy. Part 2: acquired heart disease. Obstet Gynaecol. 2007;9:83-7.

Chapter 4

Anemia in Pregnancy

Haresh U Doshi

BACKGROUND

- As per NFHS-4 (2015–2016), anemia in pregnancy is average 50.3%. It is more common in the rural population (52.1%) as compared to urban population (45.7%).[1]
- Iron is an important micronutrient which is essential for various functions in the human body. It is essential for cellular growth and differentiation, oxygen binding, transport and storage, enzymatic reactions, immune function, cognitive function, mental and physical growth, etc.
- As iron cannot be synthesized in the body, it has to be replaced by consuming it in the diet.
- Globally, 614 million women aged 15–49 years were affected by anemia. India had the largest number of women impacted. In India more than half of all women of reproductive age have anemia.[2]
- Widespread awareness of taking folic acid pre-pregnancy and in early pregnancy has made vitamin B12 deficiency more prominent in present times.
- An estimated 38% of pregnant women are affected by anemia worldwide, translating into 32 million women globally.[3]
- World Health Organization (WHO) attributes about 591,000 perinatal deaths and 11,500 maternal deaths globally to iron-deficiency anemia.[4]
- Anemia is directly responsible for 15–20% of all maternal deaths and in another same percentage of deaths, it is indirectly involved. Apart from this, maternal morbidity is considerable.
- World bank analysis of the global burden of disease in 1993 ranked iron-deficiency anemia as the leading cause of loss of disability-adjusted life years (DALYs) for females aged 15–44 years across the globe.

ANEMIA IN PREGNANCY

A. Deficiency anemia (e.g. iron, vitamin B12, folate)
B. Hemoglobinopathies
C. Hemorrhagic anemia
D. *Hemolytic anemia:* Congenital or acquired
E. Anemia of chronic disease
F. Aplastic anemia

Deficiency anemias and hemoglobinopathies are discussed.

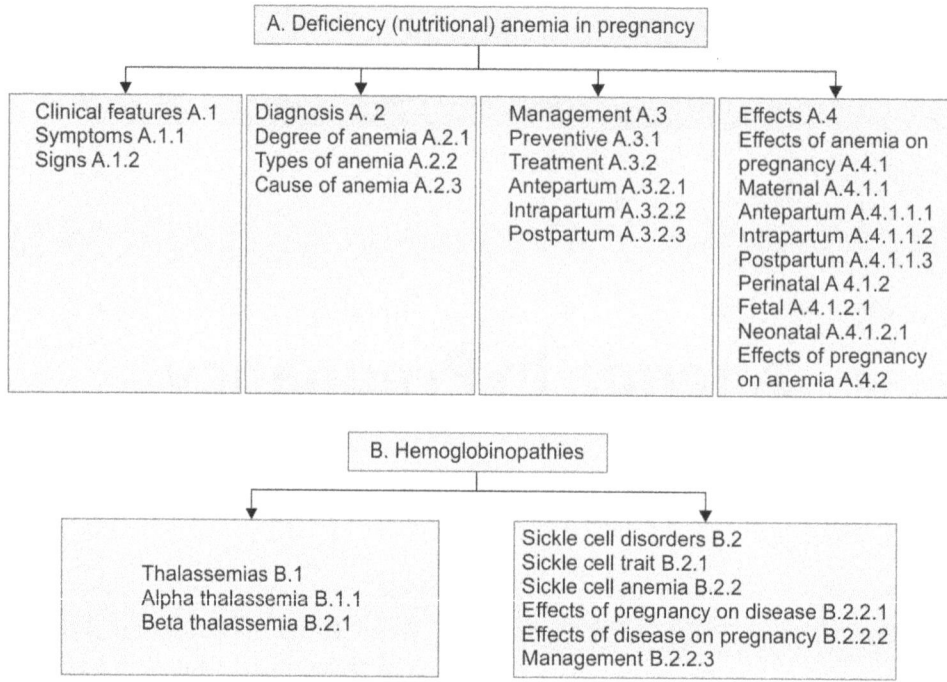

A. DEFICIENCY (NUTRITIONAL) ANEMIA IN PREGNANCY

Clinical Features A.1

Symptoms A.1.1

- May be asymptomatic
- Fatigue, weakness, lassitude, impaired work capacity
- Dizziness, giddiness, headache, insomnia
- Dyspnea on exertion, palpitation, anorexia, dyspepsia
- Edema of ankles.

Signs A.1.2

- Pallor of skin and mucous membrane. In severe anemia, there is even loss of color of palmar creases.
- There may be glossitis, stomatitis, and dysphagia.
- Koilonychia (changes in nails: initially brittleness and dryness, later there is flattening, and finally concavity, i.e. spoon-shaped nails).
- Tachycardia.

Diagnosis A.2

Degree of Anemia A.2.1

- Clinical estimation can be erroneous. Hemoglobin (Hb) estimation is used for diagnosis.

Acid hematin (Sahli's) and cyanmethemoglobin are commonly used methods.
- Hemoglobin below 11.0 g% suggests pathological anemia in pregnancy. Modified WHO definition considers Hb% <11.0 g% in the first and third trimester and <10.5 g% in the second trimester as anemia.
  Values of mild, moderate, and severe degrees as per Indian Council of Medical Research (ICMR) are:[5]
  - *Mild anemia:* 10–10.9 g%
  - *Moderate anemia:* 7–9.9 g%
  - *Severe anemia:* 4–6.9 g%
  - *Very serve:* <4.0 g%.
- Red blood cell (RBC) count <3.2 million and packed cell volume (PCV) <30% suggest anemia.

Types of Anemia A.2.2

- *Peripheral smear (PS):* To study the morphology of RBCs. It shows microcytic hypochromic picture in iron-deficiency anemia. RBCs are smaller in size with central pallor. Also, there is anisocytosis (variation in size) and poikilocytosis (variation in shape). PS may also help in diagnosing malarial parasites. Reticulocyte count may be slightly raised. Occasionally, target cells are present.
  Other causes of microcytic anemias include thalassemia, anemia of chronic disease, sideroblastic anemia, and lead poisoning.

- *Hematological indices:* These are mean corpuscular volume (MCV), mean corpuscular hemoglobin (MCH), and mean corpuscular hemoglobin concentration (MCHC). Their values in iron-deficiency anemia as compared to normal are as follows:

	Normal values	Iron-deficiency anemia in pregnancy
Hb	12.0–16.0 g%	<11.0 g%
RBC count	4–5 million/mm^3	<3.2 million/mm^3
PCV	32–36%	<30%
MCV	75–100 µm^3	<75 µm^3
MCH	25–33 pg	<25 pg
MCHC	30–36%	<30%

- Usually, the above investigations are sufficient. Specific investigations for iron deficiency include serum iron, total iron-binding capacity (TIBC), percentage saturation (Se. iron/TIBC), and serum ferritin level.

In fact, decreased ferritin level is the first feature of iron deficiency.

	Normal values	Iron-deficiency anemia in pregnancy
Serum iron	60–120 µg/dL	<60 µg/dL
TIBC	300–350 µg/dL	>400 µg/dL
Percentage saturation	20–45% (1/3rd average)	<16%
Serum ferritin	15–200 µg/L (ng/mL)	<12 µg/L
Transferrin receptors	2–4 mg/L	Increased
FEP	0–35 µg/dL	Increased
Stainable bone marrow	Present	Absent

- Free erythrocyte protoporphyrin (FEP) is not routinely carried out.
- Transferrin receptors level is a newer investigation now available. It increases early in case of iron deficiency and is more sensitive than even ferritin.
- *Bone marrow examination:* This is not routinely done. It is only indicated in: (1) refractory anemia; and (2) aplastic/hypoplastic anemia. In iron-deficiency anemia, iron stores are absent.

Cause of Anemia A.2.3

For diagnosing the cause, a detailed history is also important, e.g. food habits, obstetric history (multipara, short intervals), gynecological history (menorrhagia), history of malaria/worms.

- *Urine examination:* Routine and microscopy (culture studies if required) are done for diagnosing urinary tract infection (UTI), asymptomatic bacteriuria, hematuria, etc.
- *Stool examination:* Ova (eggs) and cysts and for occult blood. Eggs of hookworm are segmented (four blastomeres) and float in saturated solutions of common salt.
- *Serum proteins:* Hypoproteinemia.

Special tests may be carried out in megaloblastic and other rare anemias.

Serum folate and serum vitamin B12 in megaloblastic anemia.

Recommended dietary allowance and values in deficiency anemias are as follows:

Recommended dietary allowance (RDA)			
	Nonpregnant	Pregnancy	Lactation
FA	180 µg	400 µg	280 µg
Vitamin B12	2.0 µg	2.2 µg	2.6 µg
	FA	Vitamin B12	
Normal level	5–20 ng/mL	150–900 pg/mL	
Deficiency	<3 ng/mL	<100 pg/mL	

Management A.3

Preventive A.3.1

General preventive measures are:
- Screening of adolescent girls in school and giving iron supplements.
- Education and motivation for taking a diet rich in iron.
    - Dietary sources rich in iron are green leafy vegetables (spinach, mustard, fenugreek, etc.), cereals (whole wheat, bajra, jowar, ragi), pulses (green peas, beans, groundnuts), fruits like apples and bananas, jaggery, dates, and in nonvegetarian diet liver and meat.
- Change in food habits, i.e. avoiding tea or coffee for at least 2 hours after meals.
- Prevention of hookworm and malaria. For hookworm, albendazole 400 mg stat or mebendazole 100 mg bid for 3 days is recommended. For malaria prophylaxis, weekly two tablets of chloroquine (300 mg base) are given from the second trimester onward in endemic areas.

- Keeping an adequate interval between pregnancy (>2 years minimum) and avoiding prolonged lactation without iron supplement.
- Fortification of food by iron, i.e. 30–36 mg iron should be added per kilogram of wheat flour.[6]
- Fortification of common salt by iron.
- Cooking in iron utensils is helpful.[7]

Iron prophylaxis: Government of India (Ministry of Health & Family Welfare) has recommended at least 100 mg of elemental iron + 0.5 mg FA/day for 100 days to every pregnant woman and the same amount for 6 months postpartum.

World Health Organization recommends 60 mg elemental iron with 0.4 mg FA/day throughout pregnancy and 3 months postpartum.

Treatment A.3.2

Antepartum A.3.2.1
- *Mild anemia:* Two iron-folic acid (IFA) (100 mg of iron with 0.5 mg of folic acid) tablets/day for 100 days and 6 months postpartum
- *Moderate anemia:* Parenteral iron therapy + oral FA
- *Severe anemia:* Parenteral iron therapy or blood transfusion (PCV) depending upon gestational age
- *Very severe anemia:* PCVs with diuretics
- Dietary advice, adequate rest, regular follow-up, and repeat investigations are recommended.

Intrapartum A.3.2.2
- Blood is kept cross-matched and ready.
- Prolonged labor is avoided. The second stage is cut short by instrumental delivery if required.
- Parenteral fluids are restricted. Oxytocin, if required, should be given in a concentrated manner.
- Proper antiseptic precautions are a must.
- Active management of the third stage of labor is done.

Postpartum A.3.2.3
- Iron and FA are given for 6 months.
- In moderate-to-severe anemia, parenteral iron should be given.
- Blood is given when there is severe hemorrhage during delivery or cesarean section and postpartum anemia with decompensation.

Iron therapy:
- Oral
- Parenteral

- *Oral iron therapy:*
  - It is cheap, safe, and effective in most of the cases.
  - Different common iron salts with their elemental iron content are mentioned in **Table 1**.

Table 1: Oral iron preparations.

Salt	Tablet	Elemental iron
Ferrous sulfate	200 mg	60 mg (30%)
Ferrous fumarate	200 mg	66 mg (33%)
Ferrous gluconate	320 mg	36 mg (12%)
Ferrous succinate	100 mg	35 mg (35%)
Ferric ammonium citrate	125 mg	25 mg (17–22%)
Ferrous ascorbate	100 mg	
Iron polymaltose complex	100 mg	
Carbonyl iron	90 mg	
Sodium feredetate	231 mg	
Hb preparation	2.1 g	(0.33%)

  - Ferrous salts are three times readily absorbed than ferric salts.
  - Ferrous sulfate is the cheapest and well-absorbed form of iron.
  - Ferrous gluconate is well tolerated but it has low iron content (36 mg in 320 mg tablet).
  - Ferrous fumarate is the most commonly used salt in commercial preparations.

Ferrous ascorbate is a synthetic molecule of ascorbic acid and iron and as ascorbate makes stable chelate with iron, there is no dissociation in the gastrointestinal (GI) tract, so there is no action of food inhibitors. Tablets containing 100 mg elemental iron are available for use.

Sustained-release (SR) or time-release (TR) preparations have less GI side effects but lesser iron is released in the main absorptive area, i.e. duodenum and upper jejunum and so less is absorbed.

Gastric delivery system (GDS) contains ferrous sulfate in a gel-forming polymer matrix, so the tablet floats in the stomach for 5–12 hours releasing a small amount of iron to the main absorptive area (i.e. duodenum). It is claimed that three times more iron is absorbed with less side effects.

Carbonyl iron: Here, iron is obtained by thermal decomposition of iron pentacarbonyl which when heated above its boiling point decomposes to give iron and carbon monoxide. Iron thus obtained has high purity (>98%), very fine spherical size (<5 u), and uniform particle size. It is easily absorbed and less toxic than ionized forms of iron such as iron sulfate.

Sodium feredetate: It contains ferric sodium ethylenediaminetetraacetic acid (EDTA). It contains iron in an unionized form. It is not astringent and does not discolor teeth. Its absorption is less affected by food inhibitors like phytates. It is also available as a chewable tablet.

Ferrous bisglycinate chelate: It is a chelated form of iron, where two molecules of amino acid glycine are bound to a molecule of iron. It does not cause gastric irritation and constipation.

IPC complex: It is ferric hydroxide polymaltose complex. It is nonionic and it does not stain the teeth. There is no metallic taste and no interaction with food or other drugs. It is safe as it does not generate free radical. Along with iron, most of the commercial preparations contain other hematopoietic factors like FA, vitamin B12, vitamin C, zinc, etc.

Iron prescription:
- If there is a swallowing problem or intolerance, use liquid preparation (less side effects but staining of teeth may be a problem).
- Tablet is to be taken on an empty stomach or 1 hour after the meal.
- Tea, coffee to be avoided for 2 hours after taking iron.
- Taking vitamin C helps in absorption.
- Calcium salts (except calcium carbonate and calcium citrate) and antacids should be avoided.

Recent Cochrane review confirmed that intermittent iron supplementation is as effective as daily iron for prophylaxis and it increases compliance as side effects are less.[8]

Response:
- Reticulocyte count increases by 7–10 days.
- Hb% rises at 10–14 days. About 1 g%/week rise in Hb occurs from the second week onward.

Side effects of oral iron:
- *Upper GI tract:* Nausea, gastric discomfort, loss of appetite, and eructation. Staining of teeth particularly in the liquid preparation.
- *Lower GI tract:* Constipation, diarrhea, and flatulence.

Parenteral iron therapy: It is indicated when:
- Intolerance to oral iron
- Noncompliance to oral iron
- Poor absorption of oral iron (malabsorption syndrome, dysentery, etc.)
- No response to oral iron after 4 weeks in a confirmed case of iron-deficiency anemia
- Some cases of moderate or severe anemia (6–8 g Hb) very late in pregnancy.

Preparations:
- Iron sucrose: (100 mg/5 mL) or (50 mg/2.5 mL)
- Ferric carboxymaltose.
  Iron sorbitol citric acid complex (I/M) and iron dextran: 2 mL (I/M), 10 mL (I/V), ampoules preparations are not used now due to side effects and severe anaphylactic reactions, respectively.
- *Iron sucrose:*
  - It is a category B drug. It is given diluted 200 mg in 200 mL of normal saline and given I/V over 30 minutes.
  - Dose calculation is total iron = 2.4 × weight in kg (prepregnancy) × deficit of Hb in grams.
  - 500 mg should be added for pregnancy.
  - It is safe, effective, and well-tolerated.
  - Test dose not recommended. However, some authorities prefer to give a test dose.
  - Maximum 200 mg per dose is given repeated up to three times a week.
  - Iron sucrose is dissociated by the reticuloendothelial system into iron and sucrose. The released iron increases Hb. 75% sucrose is excreted by the kidney in 24 hours.
  - It is claimed that there is a rapid rise of Hb than oral iron, i.e. after 1 week and also rapid build-up of iron stores.[9]
  - It cannot be given I/M due to alkaline pH (>10) as it causes muscle damage.
  - It is not stable in dextrose, so it cannot be diluted in dextrose.
- *Ferric carboxymaltose:*
  - It is a newer formulation of parenteral iron. Contains 50 mg/mL in 10 mL vial.
  - 1,000 mg in 250 mL normal saline can be given over 15 minutes.
  - It was initially recommended for postpartum use only safety during pregnancy, it is now established and approved by the FDA (2013).
  - Side effects are nausea, dizziness, headache, and hypertension.

Erythropoietin: Recombinant human erythropoietin is mainly useful for anemia in patients with renal disease and on cancer chemotherapy. In pregnancy as such erythropoietin levels are increased. It is useful in resistant anemia when iron supplementation fails to raise Hb as an alternative to blood transfusion. It is given 150 IU/kg subcutaneously thrice a week with iron supplements.

Blood transfusion: It is indicated in iron-deficiency anemias in the following cases:
- Severe anemia (Hb <7.0 g) at any gestational age.
- Moderate anemia beyond 36 weeks and when there is failure of response to iron therapy.
- *Severe hemorrhage:* Antepartum hemorrhage (APH), postpartum hemorrhage (PPH), rupture uterus, and cesarean section.
- Thalassemias and sickling disorders in pregnancy.

Whole blood transfusion should not be used. Packed cells transfusion is better than whole blood as patient will have less: (1) volume overload, (2) less transfusion reactions; and (3) components separated from whole blood can be used for other patients. Properly grouped, typed, and "X"-matched PCV should be used. It is administered slowly taking 4 hours for one unit, along with diuretics.

Exchange transfusion: This is particularly indicated in severe anemia with congestive cardiac failure (CCF).

Packed cell volumes (PCVs) are transfused (minimum three units) through one antecubital vein and simultaneously whole blood is withdrawn from the opposite femoral vein. Blood withdrawn should be 200 mL more than the amount transfused, i.e. keeping negative balance.

Adverse reactions to blood transfusion:
- *Transfusion reactions:* The most dangerous is an acute hemolytic reaction due to mismatched transfusion which can be fatal. These are mentioned in **Table 2**.

Table 2: Transfusion reaction.	
Reaction	Risk per unit
Acute fatal hemolytic	1:1,00,000
Delayed hemolytic	1:1,000
Febrile (nonhemolytic)	1–4:100
Allergic (urticarial)	1–4:100
TRALI	1:5,000
Anaphylactic	1:1,50,000
(TRALI: transfusion-related acute lung injury)	

- *Infections:*
  - *Viral:* Hepatitis B, Hepatitis C, human immunodeficiency virus (HIV), human T-cell lymphotropic virus (HTLV), cytomegalovirus
  - *Bacterial:* Syphilis, gram-negative bacteria
  - *Parasitic:* Malaria
- *Volume overload:* If whole blood is transfused in chronic severe anemia and if a diuretic is not used.
- *Others:* These include hypothermia, citrate toxicity, hyperkalemia secondary to increased potassium in stored cells, hypocalcemia (secondary to binding of calcium by citrate-based anticoagulant), iron overload (in thalassemia), and disseminated intravascular coagulation (DIC; dilution coagulopathy in massive blood transfusions), and rarely air embolism.

Effects A.4

Effects of Anemia on Pregnancy A.4.1

Maternal A.4.1.1
- *Antepartum A.4.1.1.1*
  - Increased susceptibility to infection
  - Preeclampsia may be related to malnutrition
  - Cardiac failure at 30–34 weeks of pregnancy
  - Preterm labor (three times greater risk).
- *Intrapartum A.4.1.1.2*
  - Uterine inertia
  - PPH: Even moderate blood loss can lead to collapse
  - Cardiac failure
  - Shock.
- *Postpartum A.4.1.1.3*
  - Cardiac failure
  - Puerperal sepsis
  - Subinvolution
  - Failing lactation
  - Chronic ill-health and backache.

Perinatal: A.4.1.2
- Prematurity[10]
- Intrauterine growth restriction (IUGR) (three times increased risk)
- Increased perinatal deaths
- Decreased iron stores in the neonate (Hb level in the fetus or neonate is not affected in anemic mother).

Effects of Pregnancy on Anemia A.4.2

Deficiency anemias worsen during pregnancy due to increased demand of nutrients.

B. HEMOGLOBINOPATHIES

It is a collective term used for genetic (autosomal recessive) disorders affecting the globin portion of the hemoglobin molecule. Hemoglobin consists of heme (haem) + globin. Globin is made up of two pairs of peptide chains each attached to heme complex.

They are diagnosed by Hb electrophoresis.

- *Naked Eye Single Tube Red cell Osmotic Fragility (NESTROF) test:* Beta-thalassemia (β-thalassemia) trait.
- *Sickle test:* Sickle cell syndromes.

Thalassemias B.1

There is reduced or absent synthesis of structurally normal globin chains (quantitative defect). Depending upon which synthesis is affected, it is called alpha-thalassemia (α-thalassemia) or beta-thalassemia (β-thalassemia).

The incidence of thalassemia in pregnancy for all races is 1 in 300–500.

Alpha Thalassemia B.1.1

Normal individual genotype is α α/α α. The defect in α (alpha) thalassemia is of deletion type. The disease severity increases as the deletion of gene increases. The different types are:

- α α/α: Silent carrier
- α-/α-α Thalassemia minor, - -/α–mild hemolytic anemia
- - - / α - HbH disease, tetramer of β chains (β4) moderate-to-severe hemolytic anemia.
- - -/- - Homozygous α thalassemia Hb Barts [tetramer of gamma chains (γ4)] hydrops fetalis
- *Silent carrier state:* No clinical or hematological abnormality is evident.
- *α thalassemia minor (α -/α -, α α/- -):*
  - Mild microcytic, hypochromic anemia, but usually patients tolerate pregnancy well.
  - Oral iron and folic acid are given. Parenteral iron should never be given.
  - Blood transfusion may be required.
  - Diagnosis is made by low MCV and MCH but serum iron and serum ferritin levels are normal or raised (cf. iron-deficiency anemia) and HbA2 <3.5% on electrophoresis (cf. β thalassemia).
  - If both the parents are minor, the fetus may be major (25%). Here, prenatal diagnosis has a role.

- *HbH disease (α -/- -):*
  - HbH results due to deletion of three genes leading to tetramer of beta chains (β4).
  - These individuals have normal expectancy but chronic hemolytic anemia of moderate-to-severe degree exists.
  - Anemia worsens during pregnancy and blood transfusions are often required.
  - The disease severity varies from β-thalassemia intermedia to β-thalassemia major.
- *Homozygous α thalassemia (α thalassemia major) (- -/- -):*
  - Due to the deletion of all four genes, α chain is not synthesized at all.
  - Tetramer of gamma chains (4γ), i.e. Hb Barts occurs.
  - Hb Barts has very increased affinity for oxygen so it does not deliver it to fetus adequately. Fetus suffers from hypoxia and develops hydrops (nonimmune) and dies in utero. Thus, pregnant patient with α thalassemia major is not seen.
  - Patient can develop severe preeclampsia if the fetus is having thalassemia major.

Beta Thalassemia B.2.1

It results from decreased (β+) or absent (β0) synthesis of beta chain.

Unlike α chain, it is a single gene from each parent and not pairs, so genotype of a normal individual is β/β.

- *Heterozygous β-thalassemia:* β-thalassemia minor
- *Homozygous β-thalassemia:* β-thalassemia major

In India, it is more found in Kutchhi people (Gujarat) and in Sindhi and Lohana community.

- *β-thalassemia major:*
  - In intrauterine life, main Hb is HbF (α 2 gamma 2) so the fetus is not much affected (unlike homozygous × thalassemia). But after birth, the normal replacement of HbF by HbA does not occur due to absence of β-chain. This leads to increased production of α chains. Tetramer of α chains (α4) occurs which is insoluble and precipitates inside the cell (Heinz bodies) and interferes with erythropoiesis, alters cell membrane function, and leads to hemolysis and severe anemia.
  - The child requires repeated blood transfusions. Iron load increases secondary to multiple transfusions and increased absorption from the GI tract due to hypoxia. Iron deposition (hemosiderosis) leads to

liver, cardiac, and endocrinal dysfunction. Growth is stunted. Hyperplastic bone marrows particularly frontal bossing and maxillary prominence gives typical "thalassemia facies." They die early due to intercurrent infections and cardiac failure. Survival beyond teens is uncommon. Also, they are infertile due to gonadal dysfunction. So pregnancy with β-thalassemia major is rare.
  - However, with better transfusion facilities and iron-chelating therapy (desferrioxamine), few pregnancy cases have been reported.
  - Due to high maternal mortality in such cases, medical termination of pregnancy (MTP) is strongly indicated.
- **β-thalassemia intermedia:**
  - This applies to clinical conditions where the disease is much less intense than β-thalassemia major but severe than minor.
  - The several possibilities to explain this intermediate condition are coinheritance of OC thalassemia (OC × β-thalassemia), HbE β-thalassemia.
  - Hemolytic anemia requiring intermittent but not regular, blood transfusion occurs.
- **β-thalassemia minor:**
  - May be asymptomatic and may go unrecognized during pregnancy.
  - Mild microcytic hypochromic anemia which does not respond to iron therapy.
  - Hb remains around 7–8 g% and occasionally blood transfusion may be required.
  - Parenteral iron should never be given.
  - Low MCV (<65), low MCH, with normal or high serum iron and serum ferritin will be found.
  - HbA2 >3.5% by Hb electrophoresis confirms β-thalassemia (however, concomitant iron deficiency common in our country may decrease HbA2 and lead to difficulty in diagnosis).
  - Different Hbs carry different electrical charges so they can be separated and measured by electrophoresis.
  - It is important to check the husband's status and if he is also minor, the fetus has 1 in 4 (25%) chances of developing β-thalassemia major. So prenatal diagnosis of such fetus and termination of pregnancy is advisable for primary prevention of β-thalassemia major.
  - Prenatal diagnosis is done by fetal DNA analysis from trophoblast obtained by chorionic villi sampling (>10 weeks gestation) or from amniocytes obtained by amniocentesis (>15 weeks gestation). Fetal blood sampling is done by ultrasonography (USG)-guided cordocentesis (18–20 weeks).
  - In utero stem cell transplantation and gene therapy are under research.

Sickle Cell Disorders B.2

Sickle Cell Trait B.2.1

Unlike thalassemia, here there is a structural defect in the globin chain, but its rate of synthesis is normal. Hundreds of Hb variants have been described those affecting beta chain are more common and sickle cell hemoglobin (HbS) is the most common.

Sickle cell hemoglobin is transmitted by autosomal recessive gene. The heterozygous state is called sickle cell trait (HbAS), while homozygous state is called sickle cell anemia or sickle cell disease (HbSS).

Pathophysiology: The name sickle is given because RBCs containing HbS on deoxygenation assume the shape of a sickle. HbS is soluble in oxygenated state but in a reduced (deoxygenated) state, it gets polymerized (aggregates). This leads to sickle shape of RBC. On oxygenation again, depolymerization occurs. But repeated sickling and de-sickling lead to cell membrane damage and RBC become permanently sickled (even in oxygenated state).

The sickle cells are rigid and cannot pass through microcirculation like normal RBCs. The blockage of small vessels leads to microinfarcts, painful vaso-occlusive crisis, and end-organ damage. These abnormal RBCs are filtered in the spleen (trapped and destroyed). The life span of such RBCs is hardly 15–20 days (normal 120 days).

In sickle cell anemia, there is no normal HbA, but in sickle cell trait >50% is HbA. So in patients of HbAS, clinical manifestations are rare except under conditions of extreme hypoxia. HbF has some protective effect to sickling. HbF present in the same RBC prevents polymerization of HbS on deoxygenation and prevents sickling. It is about 2–20% in patients with HbSS.

Sickle Cell Trait in Pregnancy B.2.1

- No effect on pregnancy. Half of the patients may not be aware of the disease due to its asymptomatic nature.
- Patients may have mild anemia (normocytic). Hb usually remains between 7 g% and 10 g%.
- Iron and folic acid supplements should be given.

- Urinary tract infection (pyelonephritis) risk is doubled.
- People with sickle cell Hb are immune to malaria as malaria parasites are trapped and killed along with sickled RBCs. This is the reason why sickle cell is common in malaria endemic regions, e.g. Africa. Nature offers protection by causing mutagenic change in the gene for the globin chain to produce HbS.
- If sickle cell trait is diagnosed in mother, counseling is done and husband's Hb is checked for HbS. If he is also having HbS trait prenatal diagnosis is offered to couple to detect 25% chances of fetus having sickle cell anemia. Prenatal diagnosis is done if found homozygous state in the fetus (HbSS), MTP is advised.

Sickle Cell Anemia (HbSS) B.2.2

- The disease starts right from childhood, at 3-6 months of age when HbF is normally replaced by normal HbA (here HbSS).
- Chronic hemolytic anemia is present with Hb ranging between 6 g% and 9 g%.
- Crisis is precipitated by infection, cold, exercise dehydration, acidosis, stress, and high altitude.

Different crisis are:
- *Painful crisis:* Due to vascular occlusion of various organs by capillary thrombosis resulting in infarction. Severe pain can occur in the abdomen, chest, back, bones, and joints.
- *Aplastic crisis:* It is not infrequent during pregnancy. It may be due to viral or bacterial infection.
- *Hemolytic crisis:* Acute hemolysis
- *Splenic sequestration crisis:* It is common in children. Auto splenectomy occurs by adulthood. Rapidly enlarging spleen with abdominal pain occurs.
- *Megaloblastic crisis:* Due to folate deficiency particularly during twin pregnancy.

Treatment of crisis includes oxygenation, narcotic analgesics, hydration by I/V fluids, antibiotics, and blood transfusion (PCV or exchange transfusion to reduce HbS <30%).

Due to repeated microinfarcts, patients may have renal damage, chronic lung disease, cardiac dysfunction, retinopathy, bony deformity, central nervous system (CNS) damage, and leg ulcers.

Effects of disease on pregnancy B.2.2.1
- *Maternal:*
  - *Severe anemia:* Due to extra burden of pregnancy on a chronic hemolytic state.
  - *Sickling crisis:* Increased, but severity and frequency are unpredictable
  - *Preeclampsia:* Increased incidence (15%).
  - *Infections:* Pyelonephritis, pulmonary infections, and puerperal sepsis are more common.
- *Perinatal:*
  - Abortion
  - Prematurity
  - *IUGR:* Due to severe anemia or poor perfusion of placenta
  - Stillbirth

Overall, perinatal mortality increases by seven times.

Effects of pregnancy on disease B.2.2.2
- As such, there is no direct effect, but patients are more likely to have a crisis during late pregnancy, delivery, and puerperium.

Maternal mortality can be as high as 25%.

Management B 2.2.3
- *Antenatal management:*
  - Counseling of the patient regarding disease and risk of complications.
  - Hematologist should be consulted.
  - *Frequent antenatal visits:* Every 2 weeks in second trimester and every weekly in third trimester.
  - Folic acid 5 mg is given to all. Iron is only indicated if deficiency is confirmed.
  - Fetal surveillance should begin at 32-34 weeks by serial USG and weekly nonstress tests (NSTs).
  - *Investigations:* Routine pregnancy investigations +Hb electrophoresis + renal function tests (RFTs) and liver function tests (LFTs).
  - Prophylactic blood transfusion is controversial. It is given every 6 weeks. Some authorities prefer blood transfusion only when the need arises, i.e. crisis or severe anemia. The purpose of prophylactic transfusion is to keep Hb around 10-11 g% and HbS around 30-40%.
- *Intrapartum:*
  - The patient is managed on the same lines as a cardiac patient.
  - Continuous oxygen is given.
  - Good hydration is ensured if required by I/V fluids.
  - Continuous electronic fetal monitoring is advisable.
  - Lower segment cesarean section (LSCS) is done only for obstetric indications. Some patients may have bony deformities.

- Regional (epidural) anesthesia is preferred to general anesthesia (GA).
- Proper antibiotic cover is a must.
- *Postpartum:*
  - Breastfeeding is not contraindicated.
  - Antibiotics are continued.
- *Contraception:*
  - Sterilization is advised even with one child due to short life span of the mother.
  - Oral pills are contraindicated due to thrombo-embolic risks. Progesterone-only contraceptives can be given.
  - Intrauterine contraceptive device (IUCD) is contraindicated for risk of infection and bleeding.
  - Barrier contraceptives are preferred.
- *Important:*
  - 1 pint of blood raises Hb by 0.8–1.2 g%.
  - 1 g of Hb can combine with 1.34 mL of O_2.
  - One transferrin molecule binds two atoms of iron.
  - Total iron bound to transferrin in the blood is 3–4 mg.
  - 1 mL of red cells contain 1.1 mg iron.
  - Antidote to iron are desferrioxamine and deferiprone (L1). Desferrioxamine is given S/C or I/V infusion, while deferiprone (L1) has the advantage of the oral route and low cost.
  - *Advantages of physiological anemia (hemodilution) include:* (1) postpartum loss of RBCs is reduced, (2) blood viscosity is reduced, and (3) increases gaseous exchange at placental level. (4) Overall increase in blood volume copes up with decreased peripheral resistance and increased cardiac output of pregnancy.

REFERENCES

1. National Family Health Survey IV, 2015-16. Ministry of Health & Family Welfare. Government of India.
2. Development Initiatives, 2017. Global Nutrition Report 2017: Nourishing the SDGs. Page 36. Bristol, UK: Development Initiatives.
3. Steven GA, Finucane MM, De-Regil LM, et al. Global, regional, and national trends in haemoglobin concentration and prevalence of total and severe anemia in children and pregnant and non-pregnant women for 1995-2011: a systematic analysis of population-representative data. Lancet Glob Health. 2013;1:e16–25.
4. Ezzati M, Lopez AD, Rodgers A, et al. Comparative Quantification of Health Risks. Global & Regional Burden Attributed to Selected Major Risk Factors. Geneva: World Health Organization; 2004.
5. Indian Council of Medical Research. Evaluation of the National Nutritional Anaemia Prophylaxis Programme. Task Force Study. New Delhi: ICMR; 1989.
6. Baltussen R, Knai C, Sharan M. Iron fortification & iron supplementation are cost effective interventions to reduce iron deficiency in four subregions of the world. J. Nutr. 2004;134:2678-84.
7. Adish AA, Esrey SA, Gyorkos TW, et al. Effects of consumption of food cooked in iron pots on iron status & growth of young children: a randomized trial. Lancet. 1999;353:712-6.
8. Pena Rosas JP, DeRegil LM, Garcia Casal MN, et al. Intermittent oral iron supplementation during pregnancy. Cochrane Database Syst Rev. 2015;10:CD009997.
9. Bhandal N, Russel R. Intravenous versus oral iron therapy for postpartum anemia. BJOG. 2006;113(11):1248-52.
10. Liberman E, Ryan KJ, Monson RR, et al. Association of maternal hematocrit with preterm labour. Am J Obstet Gynecol. 1988;159(1):107-14.

Chapter 5

Diabetes in Pregnancy

Smiti Nanda, Anjali Gupta

INTRODUCTION

Diabetes can be pre-existing or carbohydrate intolerance with onset or first recognition during pregnancy which is then called gestational diabetes mellitus (GDM).

INCIDENCE

The incidence of GDM is 3.8–17.9% depending on geographical location and diagnostic criteria.[1]

RISK FACTORS

- Advanced maternal age (>30 years)
- Multiparity
- Obesity [body mass index (BMI) >30 kg/m^2]
- Ethnicity
- Physical inactivity
- Previous GDM or macrosomia
- History of stillbirth
- History of congenital anomaly
- Polycystic ovarian syndrome
- Family history of diabetes

PATHOPHYSIOLOGY

The pathophysiology of GDM is shown in **Figure 1**.

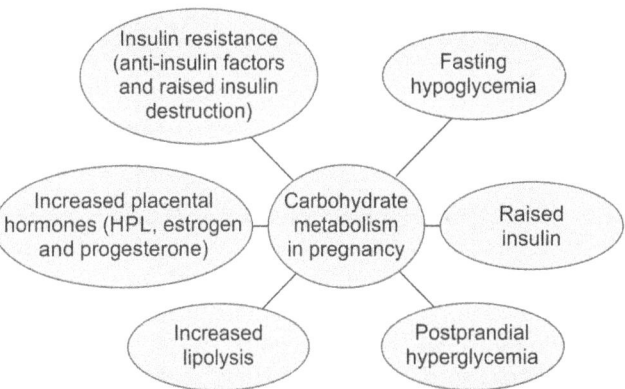

Fig. 1: Pathophysiology of gestational diabetes mellitus. (HPL: human placental lactogen)

SCREENING AND DIAGNOSIS

Why to Screen?

- *Two generations are at risk:* Mother and offspring.
- Women are at increased risk of future diabetes (type 2 DM).
- Treatment of GDM may improve a woman's quality of life and perinatal morbidity.

How to Screen?

The optimal screening approach is controversial. The screening ranges from selective screening of average and high-risk individuals to universal diagnostic testing of the

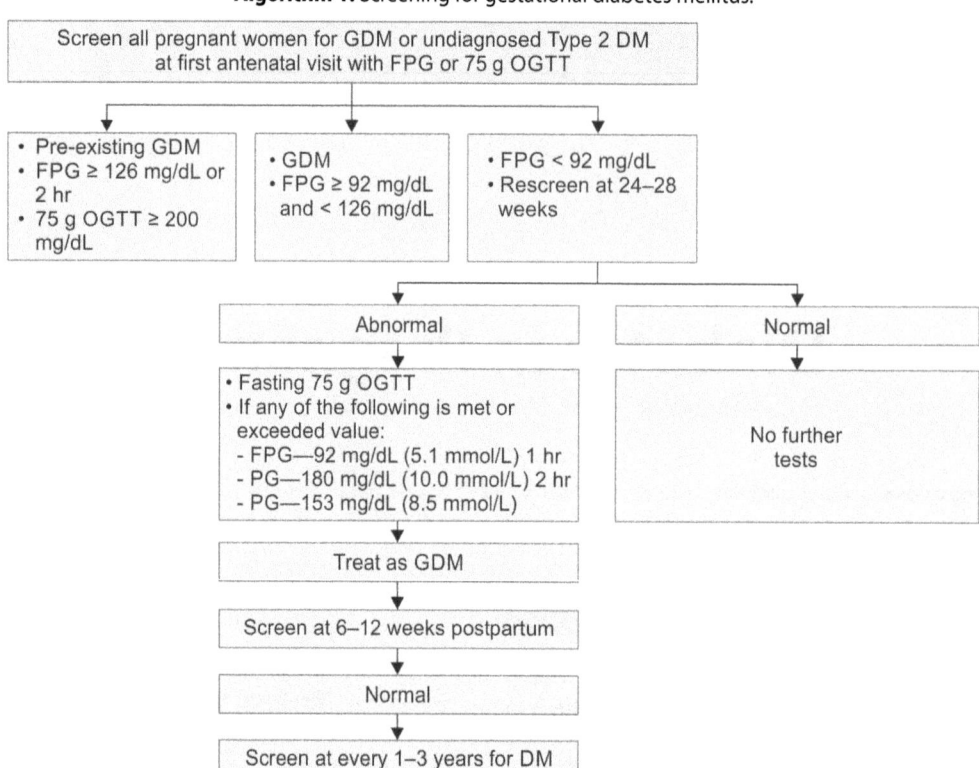

Algorithm 1: Screening for gestational diabetes mellitus.

(FPG: fasting plasma glucose; GDM: gestational diabetes mellitus; OGTT: oral glucose tolerance test)

entire population depending on the risk of diabetes in the population. Various associations have described the screening for diabetes (DIPSI 2009,[2] WHO 2013,[3] IADSP 2010,[4] ACOG 2013,[5] ADA 2016,[6] NICE 2015[7]). The authors recommend universal screening using fasting 2 hours 75 g oral glucose tolerance test (OGTT) or fasting plasma glucose (FPG) at the first antenatal visit and fasting 75 g OGTT at 24-28 weeks **(Algorithm 1)**. Complications of diabetes in pregnancy are shown in **Table 1**.

Table 1: Complications of diabetes in pregnancy.

Maternal	Fetal
Preeclampsia	Abortions
Premature labor	Congenital anomalies (CVS, CNS, skeletal, renal, GIT, and others)
Polyhydramnios	Macrosomia
UTI and moniliasis	IUGR
Operative delivery	Stillbirth
Recurrence: 33-50%	Shoulder dystocia
	Birth trauma
Long-term complications of GDM	
Type 2 diabetes (50% risk within 22-28 years)	
Cardiovascular disease	

(CNS: central nervous system; CVS: cardiovascular system; GDM: gestational diabetes mellitus; GIT: gastrointestinal tract; IUGR: intrauterine growth restriction; UTI: urinary tract infection).

MANAGEMENT

Preconceptional Care

Joint consultation of endocrinologist, obstetrician, and dietician is required. Evaluate and treat diabetic complications (retinopathy, nephropathy, neuropathy, and hypertension).

Counseling

- Counsel regarding congenital anomalies, obstetrical, fetal, and neonatal complications.
- Advise contraception until glycemic control is achieved (FPG < 95 mg/dL, 1 hour ≤140 mg/dL, 2 hours ≤120 mg/dL). Avoid pregnancy if HbA1c >10%.
- Folic acid supplementation 5 mg/day.
- Weight reduction to achieve BMI < 27 kg/m^2.
- Assess blood sugar control.
- Do baseline investigations (blood glucose, HbA1c, renal function tests, ophthalmoscopy).

Management

- Lifestyle modification
- Medication/insulin

- Blood sugar monitoring
- Antepartum surveillance.

Lifestyle Modification

- Physical activity
- Regular exercise (walking for 30 minutes after a meal)
- Medical nutrition therapy
- Advise to take three major meals and three minor meals. Diet should contain carbohydrate 50%, protein 20%, and fat 25–30%. The calorie intake, based on BMI, is given in **Table 2**. The target values for glucose are given in **Table 3**.

Table 2: Calorie intake based on body mass index (BMI).

BMI (based on weight before pregnancy) (kg/m²)	Calorie intake (kcal/kg)
<19	35
19–27	30
>27	25

Table 3: Target values for glucose.

Fasting	≤95 mg/dL (5.3 mmol/L)
1-hour postprandial	≤140 mg/dL (7.8 mmol/L)
2-hours postprandial	≤120 mg/dL (6.7 mmol/L)
Either 1- or 2-hours glucose levels are acceptable.	

Pharmacological Therapy

Pharmacological therapy is shown in **Algorithm 2**.

Algorithm 2: Pharmacological therapy.

> Medical therapy if blood glucose targets not met with diet or exercise within 1–2 weeks
> ↓
> Insulin/oral (metformin—start at dose 500 mg/day, max 2500 mg/day; glyburide—start at 2.5 mg/day, max 10 mg twice a day (First line/equally effective)

Total daily dose of insulin required is 0.7–1.0 units/kg. Half of this is given as single, long-acting insulin (e.g. glargine and detemir) and the other half in three divided doses at mealtime as rapid-acting insulin (e.g. lispro and aspart).

Monitoring Blood Glucose

- Pregnant women on multiple insulin injections are advised to test their fasting, premeal, 2 hours postmeal, and 2:00 AM–3:00 AM (seven samples) blood glucose levels daily during pregnancy.
- Pregnant women are advised to test their fasting and 2-hour postmeal blood glucose levels (four samples) daily during pregnancy if they are on diet and exercise therapy or taking oral therapy or single-dose intermediate- or long-acting insulin.

Antenatal Surveillance

Antenatal surveillance is shown in **Algorithm 3**.

Algorithm 3: Antenatal surveillance.

> Joint management by endocrinologist, obstetrician, and dietician
> Measure HbA1c levels at the time of diagnosis
> Retinal and renal assessment at the first antenatal visit if pre-existing DM
> ↓
> If diabetes retinopathy diagnosed at booking, additional retinal assessment at 16–20 weeks
> ↓
> USG scan at 18–20 weeks and again retinal assessment at 28 weeks
> ↓
> Antenatal visit every 1–2 weeks throughout pregnancy
> ↓
> USG monitoring of fetal growth and AFI every 4 weeks from 28 to 36 weeks
> ↓
> Fetal kick count from 28 weeks onward
> ↓
> NST twice weekly or weekly modified BPS starting at 32–34 weeks
> ↓
> Antenatal steroids for fetal lung maturity (if gestation <34 weeks). Blood glucose level monitoring intensified in next 72 hours if the woman on insulin

(BPS: biophysical profile score; NST: nonstress test; USG: ultrasonography; HbA1c: hemoglobin A1c; AFI: amniotic fluid index)

Intrapartum Management

- *Induction of labor:* No morning dose of insulin is given.
- Monitor blood glucose every 1–2 hours (maintain between 4 mmol/L and 7 mmol/L).
- If not maintained, start I/V 5% dextrose at a rate of 125 mL/min and insulin infusion from a syringe pump as shown in **Table 4**.

Table 4: Insulin requirement during labor.

Blood glucose (mg/dL)	Insulin (U/hr)	Infusion rate (mL/hr)
Up to 100		
101–140	1.0	1.0
141–180	1.5	1.5
181–220	2.0	2.0

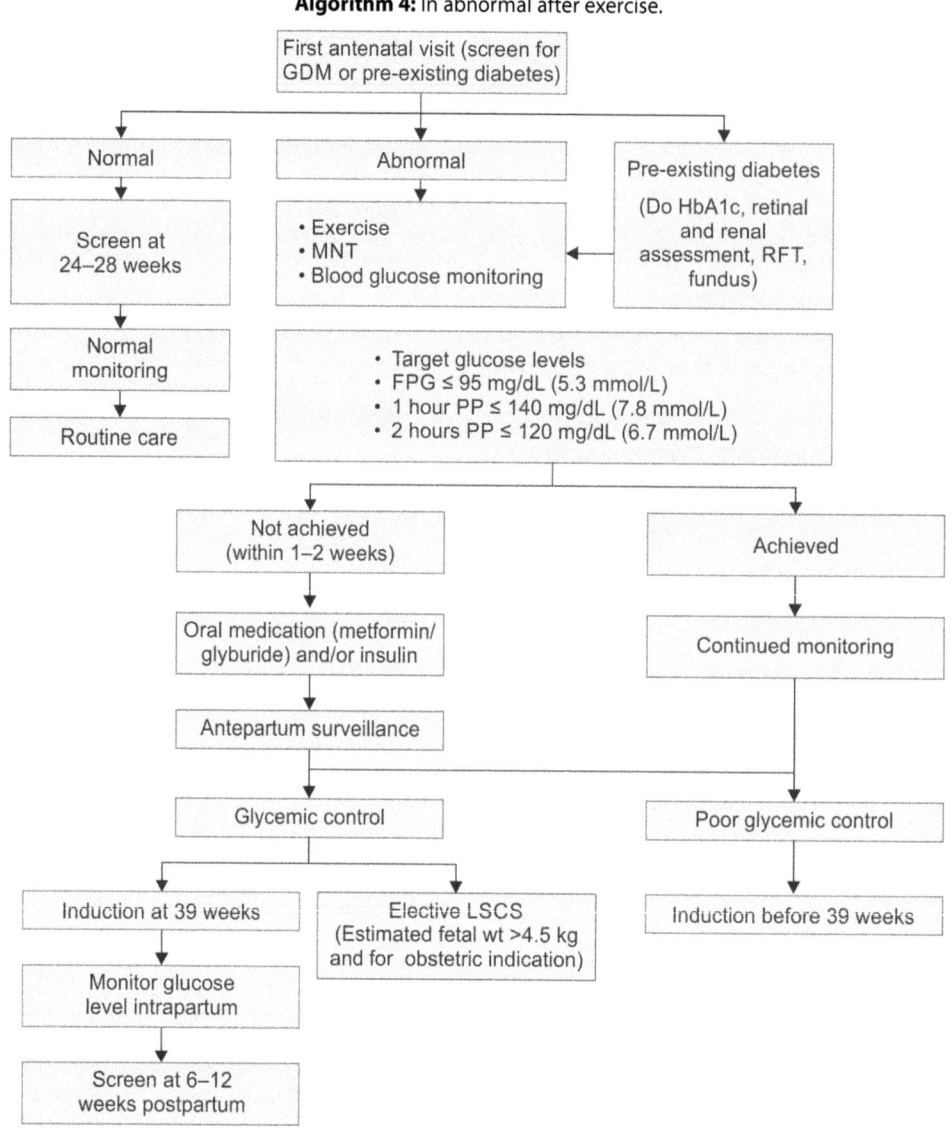

Algorithm 4: In abnormal after exercise.

(GDM: gestational diabetes mellitus; LSCS: lower segment cesarean section; MNT: medical nutrition therapy; RFT: renal function tests)

Neonatal Care

- *Neonates*: Blood glucose testing at 2–4 hours after birth.
- Breast-feeding within 30 minutes of birth and at intervals of every 2–3 hours.

Postnatal Care

In GDM, insulin may not be required immediately after expulsion of placenta. Women with insulin-treated pre-existing diabetes should reduce their insulin immediately after birth and monitor their blood glucose level **(Algorithm 4)**.

REFERENCES

1. Raja MW, Baba TA, Hanga AJ, et al. A study to estimate the prevalence of gestational diabetes mellitus in an urban block of Kashmir valley (North India). Int J Med Sci Public Health. 2014;3:191-5.

2. Seshiah V, Sahay BK, Das AK, et al. Gestational diabetes mellitus—Indian guidelines. J Indian Med Assoc. 2009; 107(799-802):804-6.
3. World Health Organization. Diagnostic Criteria and Classification of Hyperglycemia First Detected in Pregnancy. Geneva: World Health Organization; 2013.
4. International Association of Diabetes and Pregnancy Study Groups Consensus Panel, Metzger BE, Gabbe SG, et al. International association of diabetes and pregnancy study groups recommendations on the diagnosis and classification of hyperglycemia in pregnancy. Diabetes Care. 2010;33:676-82.
5. Committee on Practice Bulletin-Obstetrics. Practice Bulletin No 137: gestational diabetes mellitus. Obstet Gynecol. 2013; 122:406-16.
6. American Diabetes Association. Diabetes management guidelines. Diabetes Care. 2015;38:S1-13.
7. NICE Guidelines. (2015). Diabetes in pregnancy. Management of diabetes and its complications from preconception to postnatal period. [online] Available from nice.org.uk/guideline/ng3 [Last accessed on August, 2019].

Chapter 6

Jaundice in Pregnancy: Dilemma in Management

Sharda Patra

CAUSES OF JAUNDICE IN PREGNANCY

Jaundice in pregnancy may occur due to varied causes **(Algorithm 1)** which may be induced due to pregnancy like intrahepatic cholestasis, acute fatty liver, hemolysis, elevated liver enzyme levels, low platelet count (HELLP) syndrome, and hyperemesis gravidarum, or pre-existing liver disease which worsens during pregnancy or liver disease coincidental with pregnancy causes like viral hepatitis.[1] Viral hepatitis is the most common cause of jaundice during pregnancy followed by intrahepatic cholestasis of pregnancy (IHCP) but the incidence may be a little variable depending on geographical location.[2] Among the hepatitis viruses, hepatitis E virus is most commonly detected during pregnancy. It causes severe liver dysfunction during pregnancy and is associated with very high fetomaternal morbidity.[3]

Jaundice affects pregnant women in all trimesters of pregnancy, but some liver diseases which occur during the third trimester and are associated with increased maternal–perinatal morbidity and mortality are acute fatty liver of pregnancy (AFLP), HELLP syndrome, acute viral hepatitis, and hepatic rupture due to severe preeclampsia.[3]

Workup of a Pregnant Woman with Jaundice

A proper diagnostic approach to the jaundiced patient begins with a careful history and physical examination, and screening laboratory studies **(Algorithm 1)**. An exhaustive and comprehensive history is mandatory. Provisional differential diagnosis of jaundice in pregnancy based on history is illustrated in **Algorithm 2**. An extremely detailed general physical and systemic examination needs to be done looking for the level of consciousness and response to verbal commands, distribution, and severity of icterus in skin, sclera, and conjunctiva. Presence of anemia, rash, bleeding diathesis, swelling of feet, and vital signs like temperature, pulse, and blood pressure need to be noted. Abdominal examination should be carefully done to look for enlarged, tender liver, ascites, enlarged spleen, venous distension, bruit or rub, and reduced liver dullness. The uterine size including fetal weight, presentation, and fetal heart sound should be assessed. Biochemical tests include complete blood count and peripheral smear, liver function tests (LFTs) (serum bilirubin, serum transaminases, serum albumin), coagulation profile-specific tests [serum lactic dehydrogenase (S-LDH) if hemolysis is suspected, serum bile acids for IHCP], and viral serology. A differential diagnosis is formulated and appropriate further testing is performed to narrow the diagnostic possibilities.[4] A provisional diagnosis on the basis of the clinical presentation **(Algorithm 2)** should be made till the time the viral serology reports are available so as not to delay the management of the patient.[5] A pregnant woman with jaundice may present to a clinician in various ways and at various periods of gestation. She may present with excessive nausea/vomiting in first trimester that suggests hyperemesis gravidarum or acute viral hepatitis. If such a lady presents in second or third trimester, the differentials would

Chapter 6
Jaundice in Pregnancy: Dilemma in Management

Algorithm 1: Causes of jaundice in pregnancy.

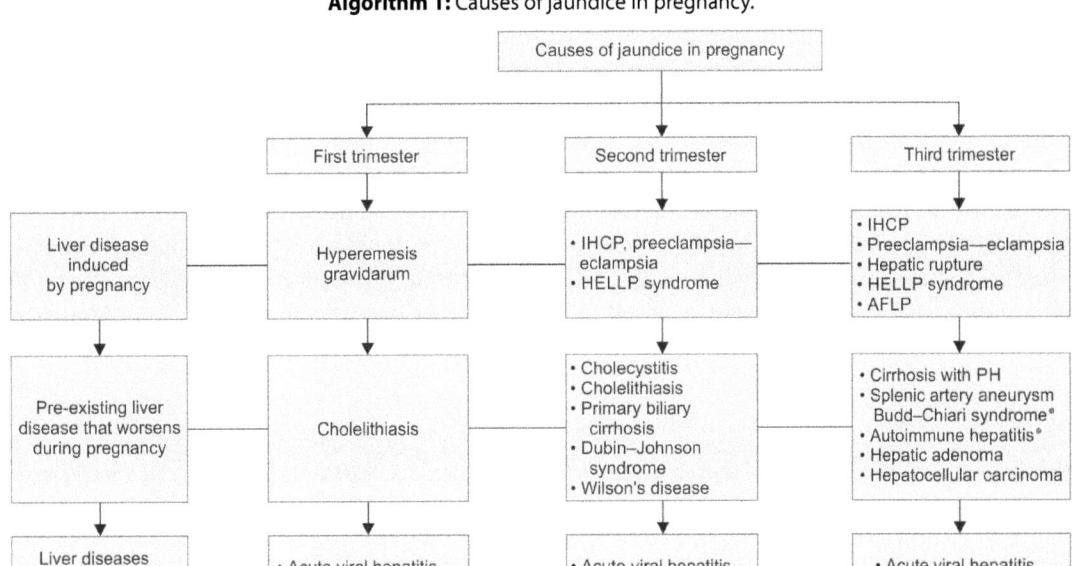

*Most commonly manifests in postpartum period.
(AFLP: acute fatty liver of pregnancy; HELLP: hemolysis, elevated liver enzymes and low platelet count syndrome; IHCP: intrahepatic cholestasis of pregnancy; PH: portal hypertension)

Algorithm 2: Algorithmic initial workup of a pregnant woman presenting with jaundice in pregnancy.

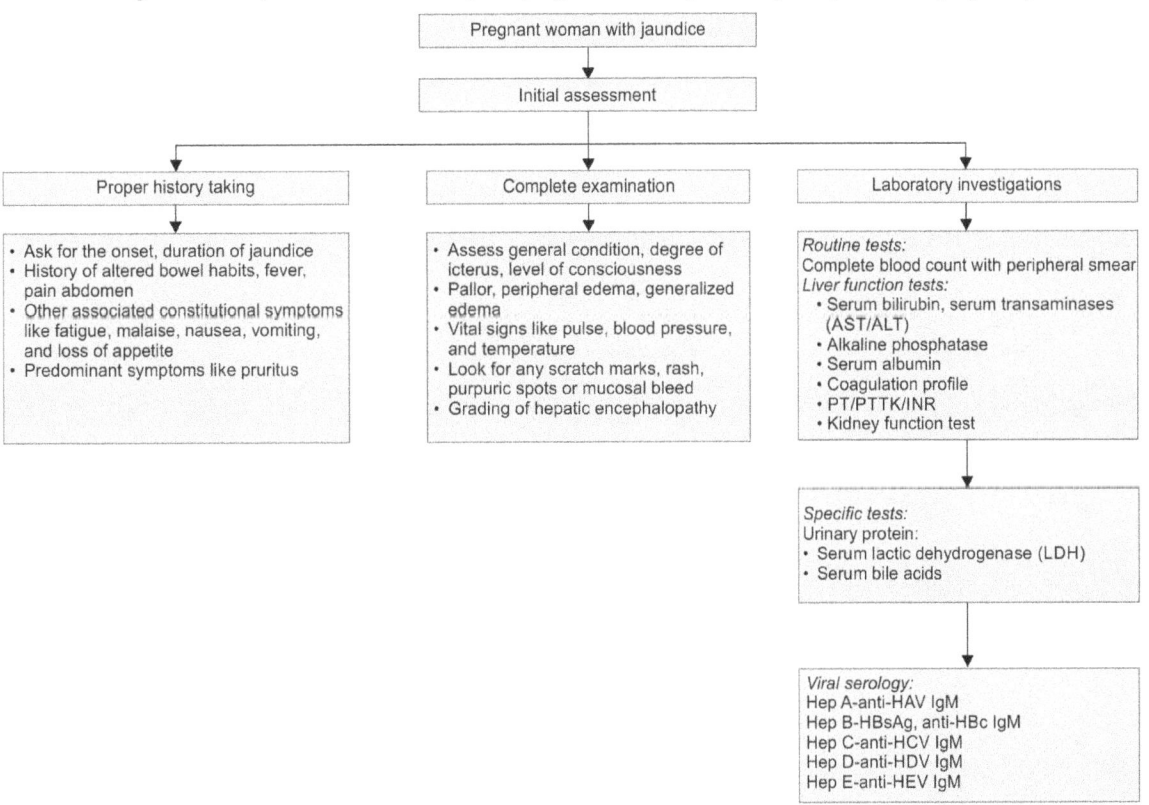

(AST: aspartate aminotransferase; ALT: alanine aminotransferase; INR: international normalized ratio; PT: prothrombin time; PTTK: partial thromboplastin time)

be acute viral hepatitis, AFLP or severe preeclampsia. If a pregnant lady presents with jaundice and pruritus it is likely that she is suffering from intrahepatic cholestasis of pregnancy or acute viral hepatitis. If the woman has associated right upper quadrant mild pain then she is suffering from acute viral hepatitis or AFLP. If the pain is severe and also associated with fever, it is likely that the woman may be suffering from cholelithiasis. But if there is no fever and just the right upper quadrant pain in a pregnant woman with jaundice, she may be suffering from HELLP syndrome, severe preeclampsia, hepatic hematoma, or hepatic rupture. The last and most severe type of presentation is when a pregnant woman with jaundice comes with disordered sensorium or unconscious state. In this case, it is most likely to be fulminant hepatic failure secondary to acute viral hepatitis. In some cases, it may be due to AFLP and hepatic failure or post-eclamptic unconsciousness. A history of convulsion prior to unconsciousness clinches its diagnosis. The diagnosis becomes clearer based on the laboratory investigation as is given in **Algorithm 3**.

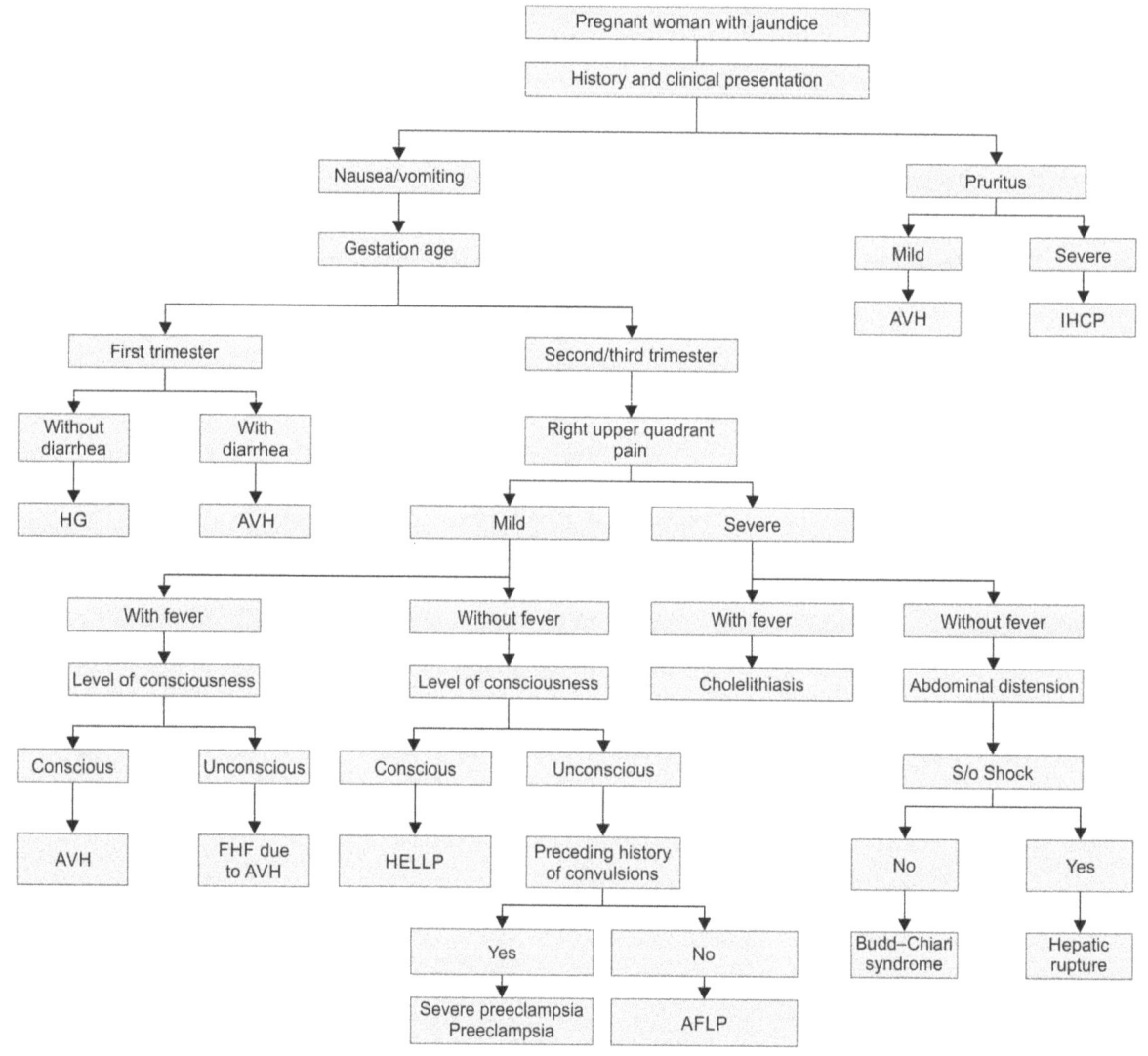

Algorithm 3: Algorithm of the workup of a pregnant woman presenting with jaundice basing on history and clinical presentation.

(AFLP: acute fatty liver of pregnancy; AVH: acute viral hepatitis; FHF: fulminant hepatic failure; HELLP: hemolysis, elevated liver enzymes and low platelet count syndrome; HG: hyperemesis gravidarum; IHCP: intrahepatic cholestasis of pregnancy)

MANAGEMENT

Mostly women with acute viral hepatitis when progress to fulminant hepatic failure (FHF) presents with severe jaundice with moderately elevated LFTs, hepatic encephalopathy, and disseminated intravascular coagulation (DIC) with a positive viral serology. There is no role of termination of pregnancy and most often the majority of the affected patients go in spontaneous labor. The management comprises of supportive therapy with anticoma regime correction of coagulation defect and caution during delivery to prevent postpartum hemorrhage (PPH) either due to atony or trauma to vagina or cervix. In severe preeclampsia, there is severe hypertension with significant proteinuria with mild jaundice and mildly elevated LFTs whereas in HELLP syndrome, presence of significant thrombocytopenia with/without preeclampsia, mild jaundice with hemolytic anemia, mild elevation of LFTs, absent DIC, and absent neurological symptoms (hepatic encephalopathy) clinches the diagnosis. This should be differentiated from certain hematological conditions like hemolytic uremic syndrome (HUS) and thrombotic thrombocytopenic purpura (TTP). In HUS and TTP, the predominant features are sepsis, DIC, with microangiopathic hemolytic anemia, thrombocytopenia, renal failure, and neurological disturbances. Liver dysfunction is usually mild and this is due to hemolysis. The management options in these conditions require an immediate termination of pregnancy to prevent the maternal–fetal complications.[6-8]

In AFLP, the presence of coagulation failure in absence of hepatic encephalopathy, renal failure in a pregnant woman at third trimester of pregnancy, with mild jaundice, mild elevation of LFTs with or without thrombocytopenia, no hemolysis with leukocytosis (up to 30,000), hypoglycemia, hypocholesterolemia, hypolipidemia, and a negative viral serology points toward the diagnosis. However, to differentiate it from FHF due to viral hepatitis, a positive viral serology confirms the latter. Hepatic rupture should be suspected in a pregnant woman with known

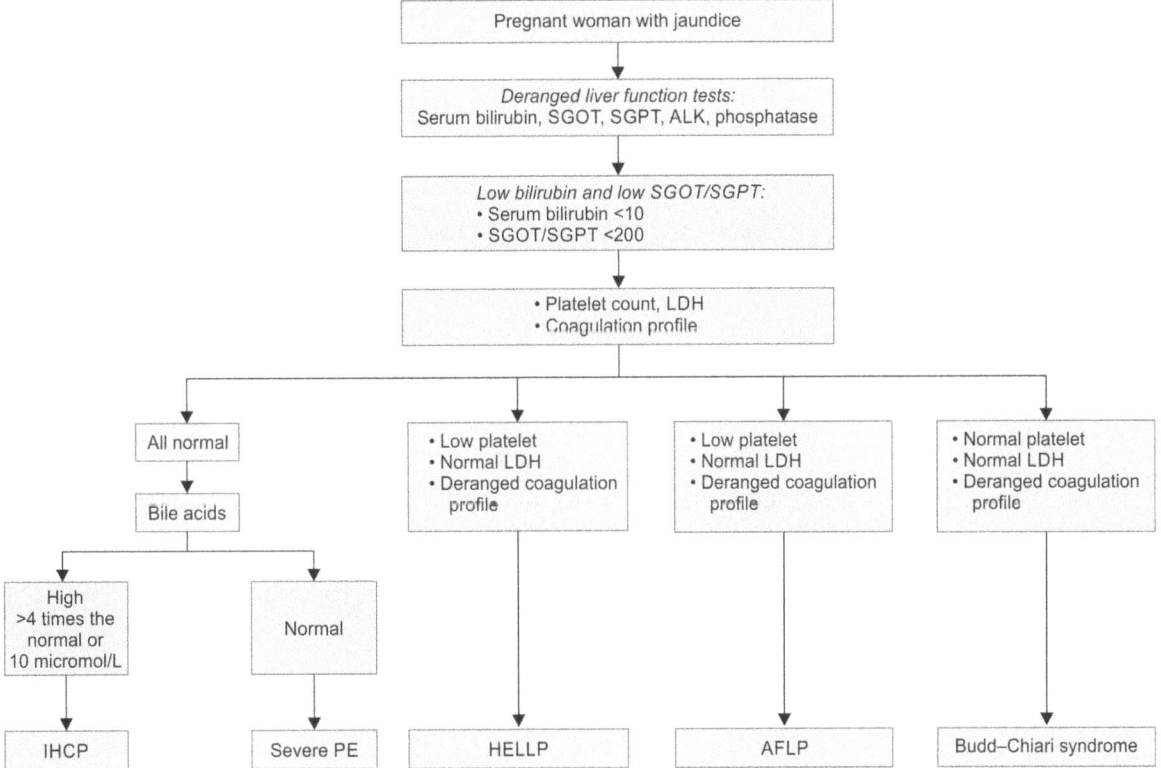

Algorithm 4: Algorithm of the workup of a pregnant woman presenting with mild jaundice based on laboratory investigations.

(AFLP: acute fatty liver of pregnancy; ALK: alkaline; HELLP: hemolysis, elevated liver enzymes and low platelet count syndrome; IHCP: intrahepatic cholestasis of pregnancy; LDH: lactic dehydrogenase; PE: preeclampsia; SGOT/SGPT: serum glutamic oxaloacetic transaminase/serum glutamic pyruvic transaminase)

preeclampsia, who develops sudden onset upper abdominal pain typically shoulder pain with features of shock with bleeding diathesis with hepatic encephalopathy. Delivery is the preferred method of management in these disorders because it can be lifesaving to mother except in acute viral hepatitis. A less mild form of jaundice in pregnancy may present with hyperemesis gravidarum and intrahepatic cholestasis of pregnancy, the diagnosis of these two conditions is easy. Hyperemesis gravidarum suspected in a pregnant woman who in first trimester of pregnancy presents with intractable nausea and vomiting, dehydration with mild jaundice with mildly elevated liver enzymes and the biochemical abnormality reverses with correction of dehydration, improvement in nutrition, and cessation of vomiting. It is to be differentiated from acute viral hepatitis and thyrotoxicosis. In IHCP, the presentation is usually in third trimester of pregnancy in which the woman presents with itching characteristically on palms and soles which becomes more severe and distressing at night, with mild jaundice with mild elevation of LFTs and increased levels of serum total bile acids.[9,10] The symptoms resolve within 48 hours of delivery **(Algorithms 4 to 6)**.

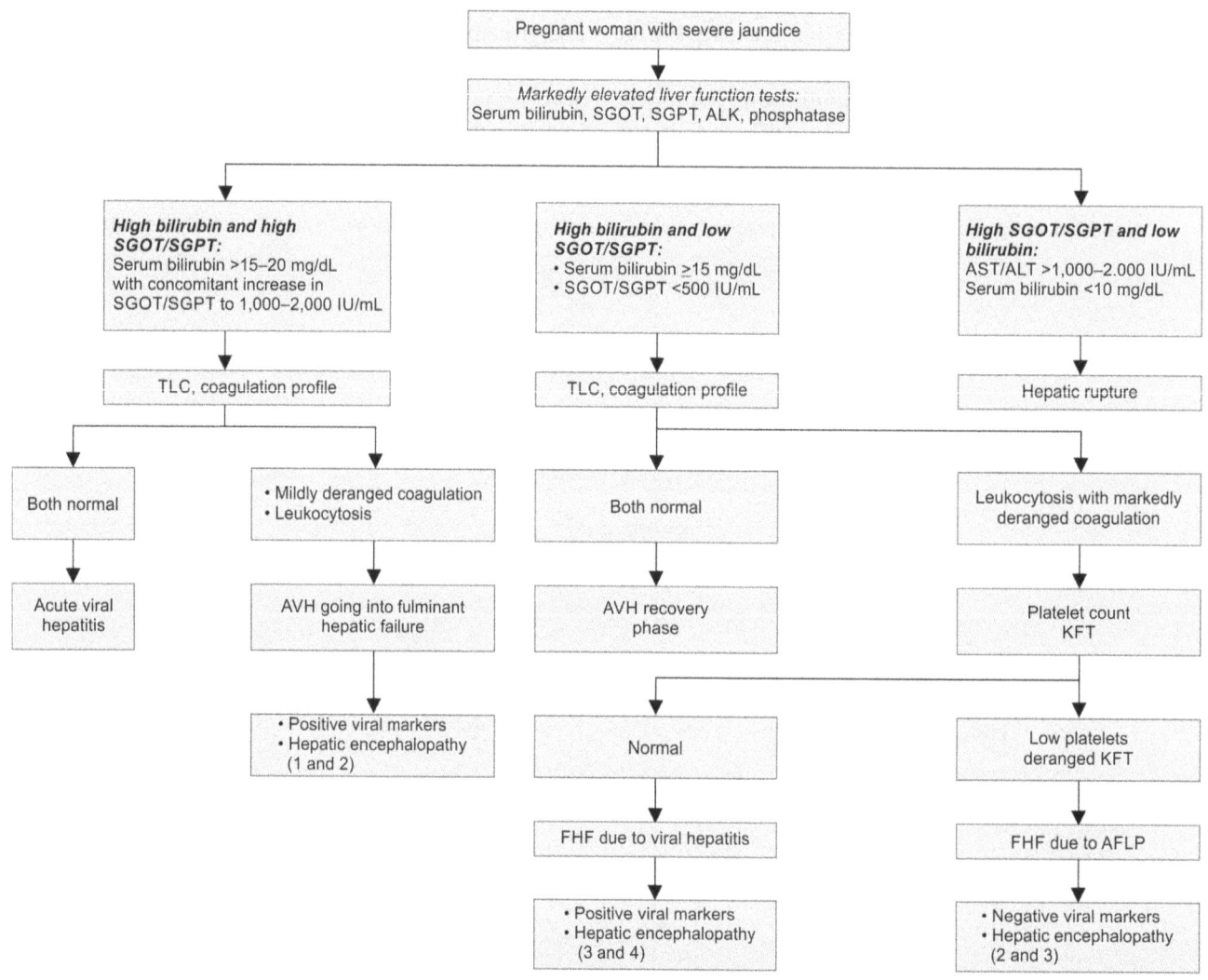

Algorithm 5: Algorithm of the workup of a pregnant woman presenting with severe jaundice based on laboratory investigations.

(AFLP: acute fatty liver of pregnancy; ALK: alkaline; AST/ALT: aspartate aminotransferase/alanine aminotransferase; AVH: acute viral hepatitis; FHF: fulminant hepatic failure; KFT: kidney function test; SGOT/SGPT: serum glutamic oxaloacetic transaminase/serum glutamic pyruvic transaminase; TLC: total leukocyte count)

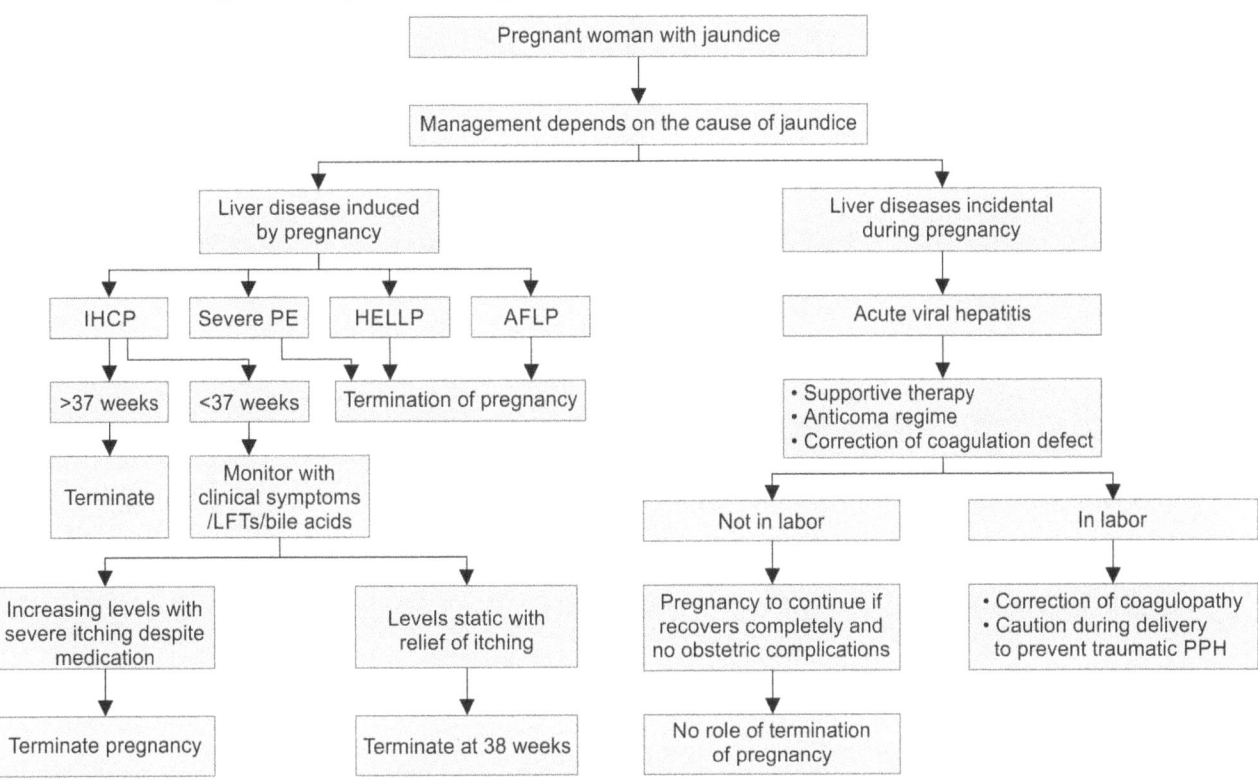

Algorithm 6: Algorithm of management of a pregnant woman presenting with mild jaundice.

(AFLP: acute fatty liver of pregnancy; HELLP: hemolysis, elevated liver enzymes and low platelet count syndrome; IHCP: intrahepatic cholestasis of pregnancy; LFTs: liver function tests; PE: preeclampsia; PPH: postpartum hemorrhage)

Management of a Pregnant Woman with Fulminant Liver Failure

If a pregnant lady with jaundice comes in labor to an obstetrician, there can be following scenarios—mild jaundice with borderline deranged LFTs and normal coagulation, severe jaundice with mildly or grossly deranged liver enzyme levels with normal coagulation, severe jaundice with mildly or grossly deranged liver enzyme levels but with coagulopathy, severe jaundice with altered sensorium, i.e. in hepatic encephalopathy **(Algorithms 7A and B)**.

The management in such cases mainly depends on the etiology of jaundice and the gestation at which the patient is presenting with the liver dysfunctions. In the first case, where patient is stable and there is mild jaundice with mildly deranged liver functions, the lady needs to be fully evaluated for etiology and usually are cases with cholestasis of pregnancy or viral hepatitis. They can be most conservatively managed with anticoma regimen, close monitoring of the LFTs till she attains term with termination of pregnancy for routine causes. The second case, where there is severe jaundice with severely deranged liver functions, maybe due to severe viral hepatitis or AFLP or even HELLP syndrome. It is very critical to establish the etiology in this case as the management depends on the etiology. In case it turns out to be viral hepatitis, the treatment is supportive and termination of pregnancy is only for routine causes. But in the case of AFLP and HELLP, liver dysfunction will be resolved only with pregnancy termination. In that case, irrespective of period of gestation, labor needs to be induced and pregnancy terminated. The blood and blood components need to be kept arranged and precautions to be followed to prevent and tackle postpartum hemorrhage.[8-10]

In the third case in which the jaundiced pregnant lady at presentation is in altered sensorium or already in liver failure, management will require a combined and coordinated effort by the intensivist, obstetrician, hepatologist, neonatologist, and if necessary, the transplant team.

Section 1
Maternal Disorders

Algorithm 7A: Algorithm of management of a pregnant woman presenting with severe jaundice with suspected liver failure: medical management.

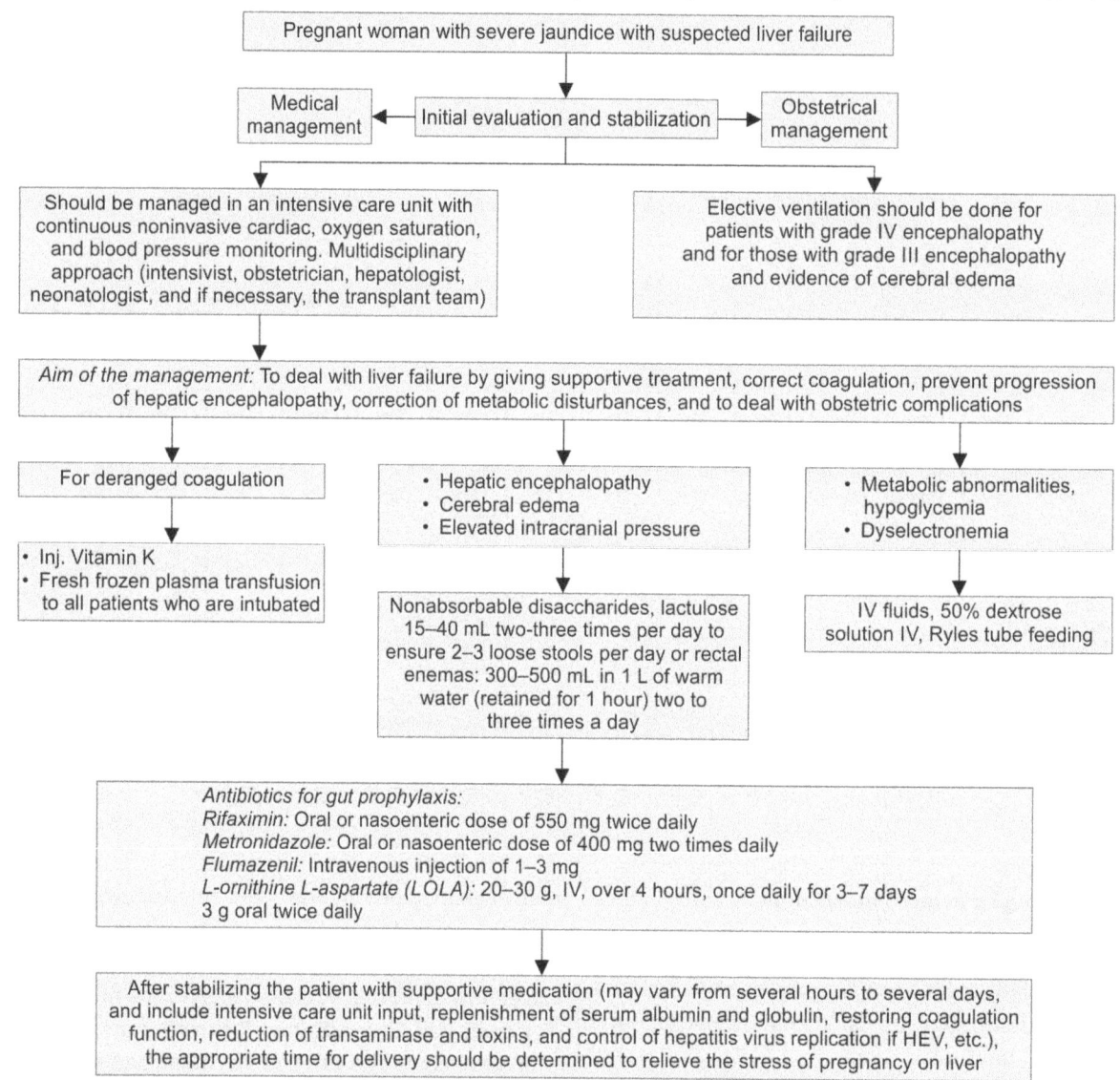

(HEV: hepatitis E virus; IV: intravenous)

It is primary to stabilize the patient, maintain optimum hemodynamics, treat cerebral edema/intracranial hypertension if present, evaluate for any infections and do prompt antimicrobial treatment, correct coagulopathy, do volume replacement, give vasopressor support and ensure adequate renal perfusion, correct hypoglycemia, dyselectrolytemia, and give adequate nutrition supplementation. Intensive care management of such a patient should be focused on the diagnosis and etiology specific treatment. A high index of suspicion should be kept for pregnant patients presenting with altered mental status, deranged LFTs, and coagulopathy. Such patients need multidisciplinary approach in tertiary center and may even require liver transplantation in severe cases.[11-13]

CONCLUSION

Thus the management of jaundice in pregnancy do present with many dilemmas from diagnosis to its management. However, an in-depth understanding of the physiological changes during pregnancy, ability to identify and treat liver disorders, and a proper vigilance in recognizing clinical

Algorithm 7B: Algorithm of management of a pregnant woman presenting with severe jaundice with suspected liver failure: obstetrical management.

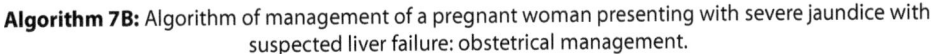

```
                Pregnant woman with severe jaundice with suspected liver failure
                                  │
                ┌─────────────────┴──────────────────┐
            In labor                              Not in labor
                │                                     │
       Obstetrical management          Usually 80–90% go into spontaneous labor
                                       within 24–48 hours. In almost all with FHP,
                                       it is associated with intrauterine fetal death
                                                      │
                                       No role of termination of pregnancy
                                       to stop the progression of disease

                                       Indications for termination of pregnancy
```

- The preferable mode of delivery is vaginal
- As most of the patients with FHF have deranged coagulation hence peripartum fresh frozen plasma should be transfused to keep INR at <2
- Dose is 15 mL/kg body weight (3–4 units) stat followed by 2 units every 8 hours till at least 24 hours after delivery
- Avoid massive FFPs transfusion

During delivery

- Caution should be taken to prevent traumatic PPH
- Certain practices like sweeping/stretching of perineum during second stage, and fundal pressure should be avoided
- Timely episiotomy should be given in primigravidas to prevent perineal tears
- Avoid instrumental delivery for prevention of vaginal laceration and if used should be used with caution preferably ventouse
- The genital tract carefully should be explored for any tears after delivery of the placenta and those with bleeding if due to cervical and/or vaginal lacerations should be recognized and should be managed with primary suturing and or vaginal packing for 24 hours. Balloon tamponade should be used to control atonic PPH
- Prophylactic use of uterotonics to prevent atonic PPH
- Proper hemostasis should be maintained during episiotomy repairs
- Vaginal packing should not be done as routine as this lead to more lacerations
- Delivery should always be conducted by an experienced obstetrician

Indications for termination of pregnancy:
- Patient stabilized with a steady state of laboratory indices, such as coagulation function, serum albumin, transaminase, total bilirubin, etc.) for 24–48 hours and associated with PPROM, IUD, or postdated pregnancy
- No improvement in clinical conditions with deterioration of hepatic encephalopathy requiring liver transplant in centers with availability of transplant facility

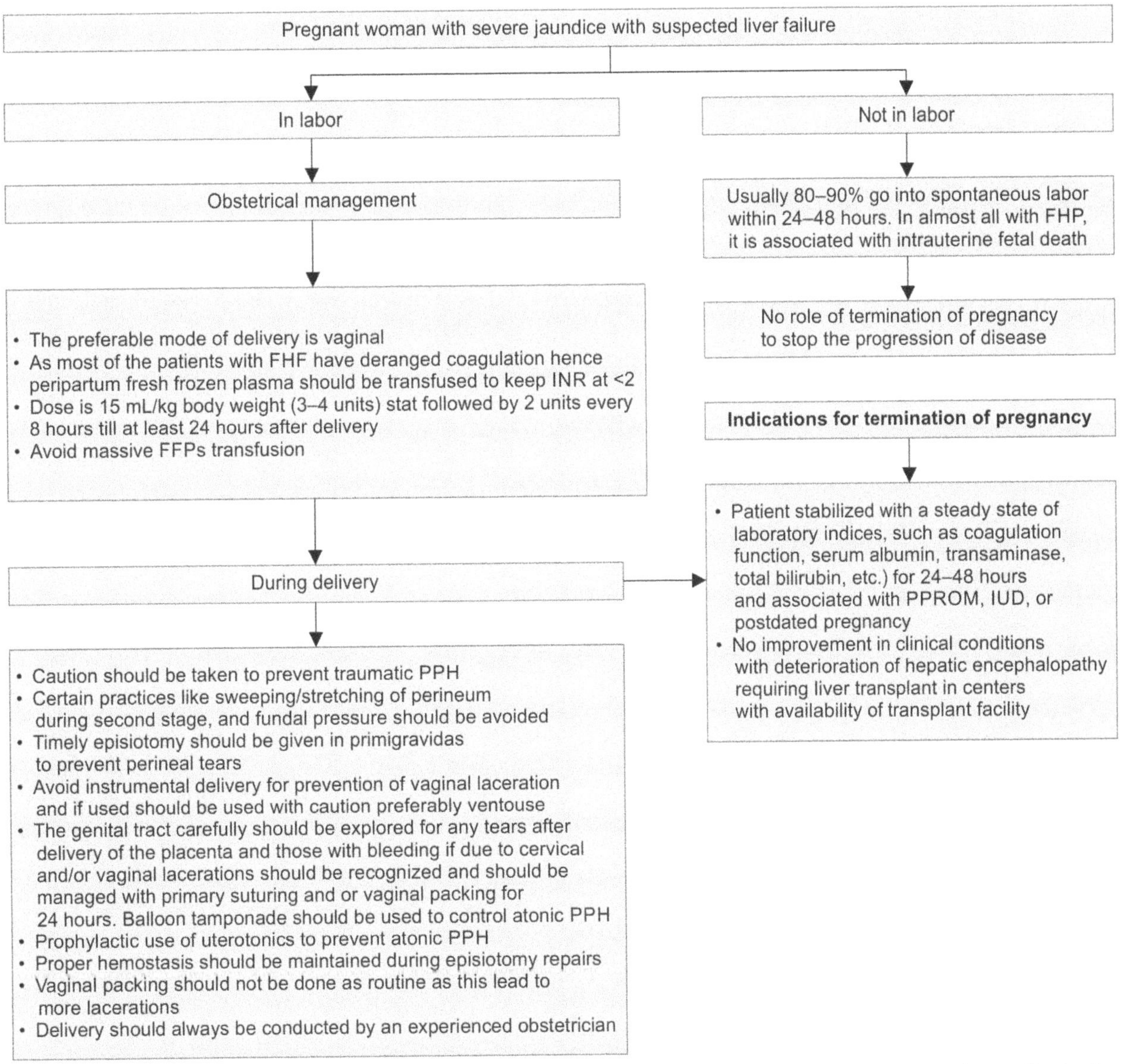

(FFP: fresh frozen plasma; FHF: fulminant hepatic failure; FHP: fulminant hepatitis in pregnancy; INR: international normalized ratio; IUD: intrauterine device; PPH: postpartum hemorrhage; PPROM: preterm premature rupture of the membrane)

and laboratory abnormalities in a timely manner along with a coordinated team approach management involving the primary care physician, obstetrician, hepatologist, and a transplant surgeon can to some extent promote a favorable maternal and fetal outcome.

REFERENCES

1. Fagan EA. Disorders of the liver, biliary system and pancreas. In: de Swiet M (Ed). Medical Disorders in Obstetric Practice, 4th edition. Oxford: Blackwell Science; 2002. pp. 282-345.
2. Thapa BR, Walia A. Liver function tests and their interpretation. Indian J Pediatr. 2007;74:663-71.
3. Patra S, Kumar A, Trivedi SS, et al. Maternal and fetal outcomes in pregnant women with acute hepatitis E virus infection. Ann Intern Med. 2007;147:28-33.
4. Jamjute P, Ahmed A, Ghosh T. Liver function test and pregnancy. J Matern Fetal Neonatal Med. 2009;22(3):274-83.
5. Chitra R. Jaundice in pregnancy. In: Trivedi SS, Puri M (Eds). Management of High Risk Pregnancy: A Practical Approach. New Delhi. Jaypee Brothers Medical Publishers (P) Ltd; 2009. pp. 348-68.

6. Nelson-Piercy C. Liver disease. In: Nelson-Piercy C (Ed). Hand Book of Obstetric Medicine, 4th edition. London, UK: Informa Healthcare; 2010. pp. 193-212.
7. Gimson AES. Liver and gastrointestinal diseases during pregnancy. In: Warrell DA, Cox TM, Firth JD (Eds). Oxford's Text Book of Medicine, 5th edition. Oxford, UK: Oxford University Press; 2011. pp. 421-6.
8. Puri M, Patra S, Singh P, et al. Factors influencing occurrence of postpartum haemorrhage in pregnant women with hepatitis E infection and deranged coagulation profile. Obstet Med. 2011;4:108-12.
9. Shi Z, Li X, Yang Y, et al. Obstetrical management of fulminant viral hepatitis in late pregnancy. Reproductive Sys Sexual Disord. 2012;1:102.
10. Castello H, Schoch L, Grogan TA. Acute liver failure in an obstetric patient: challenge of critical care for 1 patient. Crit Care Nurse. 2013;33:48-56.
11. Bittencourt PL, Terra C, Parise ER, et al. Intensive care management of patients with liver disease. Arq Gastroenterol. 2015;1:55-72.
12. Patra S. Approach to a pregnant woman presenting with jaundice. In: Puri M (Ed). Clinical Methods in Obstetrics & Gynaecology. New Delhi: Jaypee Brothers Medical Publishers; 2015. pp. 118-27.
13. Tran TT, Ahn J, Reau NS. AGA ACG clinical guideline: liver disease and pregnancy. Am J Gastroenterol. 2016;111(2): 176-94.

Chapter 7

Convulsions in Pregnancy

Seema Chopra, Arshi Syal

INTRODUCTION

Epilepsy is one of the most common neurological disorders in pregnancy characterized by recurrent, unprovoked seizures, with a prevalence of 0.5–1%.[1] About one-third of women with epilepsy (WWE) are in the reproductive age group.[2] Therefore, as per an estimate, 3–5 births/1000 will be to WWE.[1] On antiepileptic drugs (AED), seizures are well controlled in the otherwise healthy people who have epilepsy, and therefore expect to participate fully in life experiences, including procreation. The risk of death is increased tenfold in pregnant WWE compared with those without the condition.[3] WWE constitute a vulnerable group who need special obstetric care **(Algorithm 1)**.

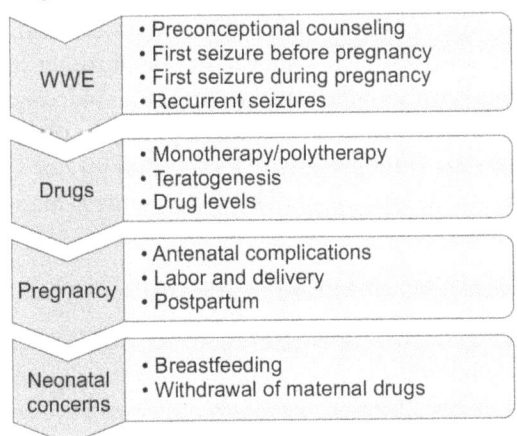

Algorithm 1: Obstetric care of women with epilepsy.

PRECONCEPTIONAL COUNSELING

Women with epilepsy, who are seizure-free for at least 10 years (last 5 years off AEDs) and those who had childhood epilepsy syndrome and now are treatment-free as adults, are considered as not having epilepsy any longer.[4] The aim of preconceptional counseling in WWE is to have an optimal obstetrical outcome **(Algorithm 2)**.

FIRST SEIZURE IN PREGNANCY

Classification of the epilepsy syndrome is important in order to start the appropriate AED, to determine prognosis in pregnancy, and to identify and prevent the factors of seizure deterioration **(Algorithm 3)**.

Especially after 20 weeks of gestation, when there is uncertainty whether seizure is secondary to epilepsy or eclampsia, magnesium sulfate is the drug of choice for eclamptic seizures, until a definitive diagnosis is reached.[5]

The differential diagnoses include cerebral venous sinus thrombosis, posterior reversible leukoencephalopathy syndrome (PRES), space-occupying lesions, and reversible cerebral vasoconstriction syndrome. Other medical disorders like syncope due to cardiac arrhythmia, aortic stenosis, carotid sinus sensitivity, vasovagal syncope, and metabolic causes such as hypoglycemia, hyponatremia, and Addisonian crisis need exclusion for first presentation of seizures in pregnancy.[6]

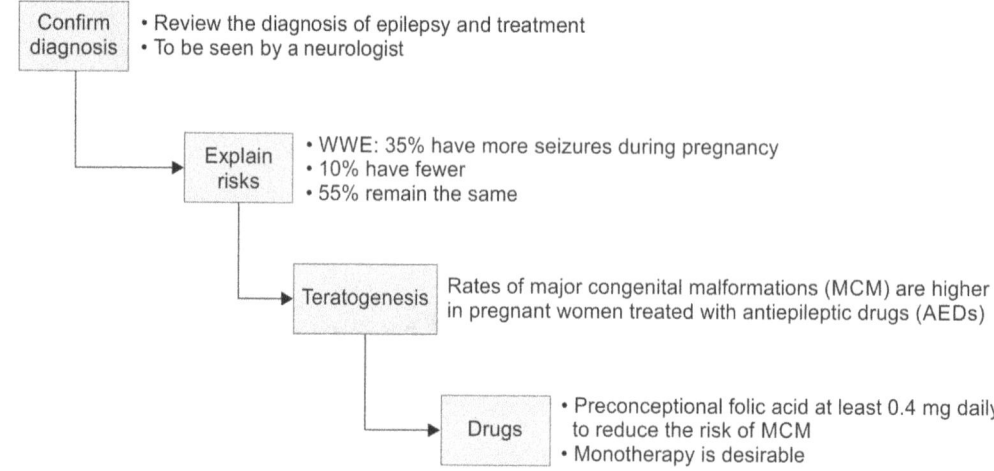

Algorithm 2: Preconceptional counseling for women with epilepsy (WWE).

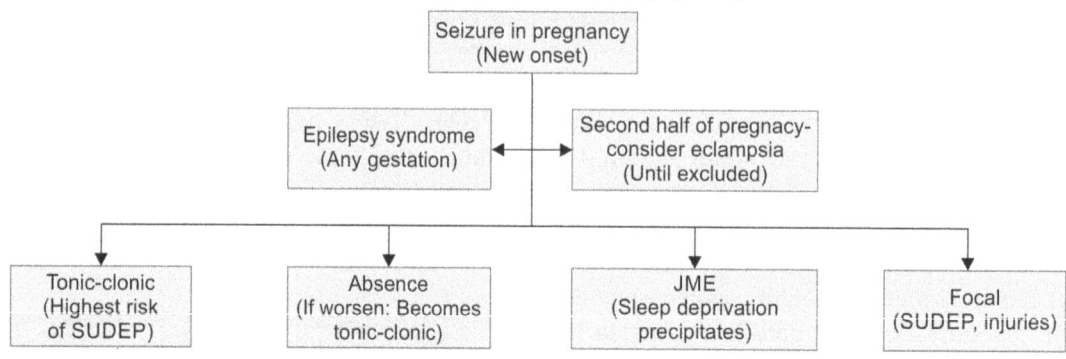

Algorithm 3: Classifying seizure in pregnancy.

(JME: juvenile myoclonic epilepsy; SUDEP: sudden unexpected death in epilepsy)

SUDEP, more common with tonic-clonic seizures, is tenfold more common in pregnant WWE, and is defined as "sudden, unexpected, witnessed or unwitnessed, nontraumatic, and nondrowning death in patients with epilepsy, with or without evidence for a seizure and excluding documented status epilepticus, in which postmortem examination does not reveal a toxicologic or anatomic cause for death."[7]

Co-recurrent seizures: Approximately 35% of WWE have more seizures during pregnancy, 10% have fewer, and 55% remain the same.[8]

The data from the EURAP (International Registry of Antiepileptic Drugs and Pregnancy) study showed that pregnant women with idiopathic generalized epilepsies were more likely to remain seizure-free (74%) than those with focal epilepsies (60%).[9]

ANTIEPILEPTIC DRUGS[10]

In WWE with an unplanned pregnancy, change in the dose or type of AED may be needed in order to minimize the fetal risks. But AEDs should not be abruptly stopped or changed without discussion with the woman regarding the risk of seizures. Even sodium valproate is still the drug of choice for certain epilepsies even though not safe for fetus, and a discussion of risks and benefits is mandatory **(Algorithm 4)**.[11]

Teratogenicity of Antiepileptic Drugs

Higher teratogenic risk is associated with higher AED levels and polytherapy. The lowest effective dose of monotherapy should be used for optimal control of convulsive seizures with minimal risk of physical injury to the fetus or the infant.[12]

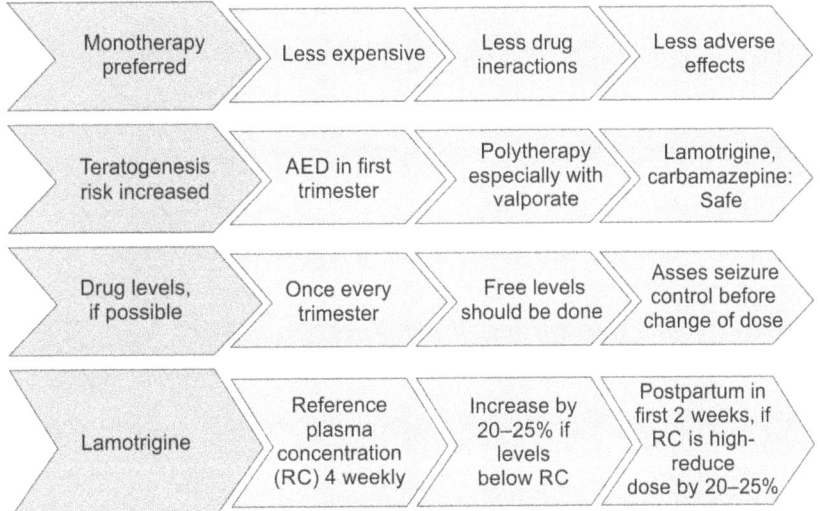

Algorithm 4: Drugs in pregnancy in women with epilepsy (WWE).

Major congenital malformations (MCM) reported with AEDs are that sodium valproate leads to neural tube defects, facial cleft, and hypospadias; phenobarbital and phenytoin cause cardiac malformations; and phenytoin and carbamazepine are associated with cleft palate in the fetus.[11]

Risk of MCM is fourfold higher with valproate in polytherapy, and the prevalence is two to threefold higher after risk adjustments in women prescribed valproate.[13]

COMPLICATIONS IN PREGNANCY (ALGORITHM 5)

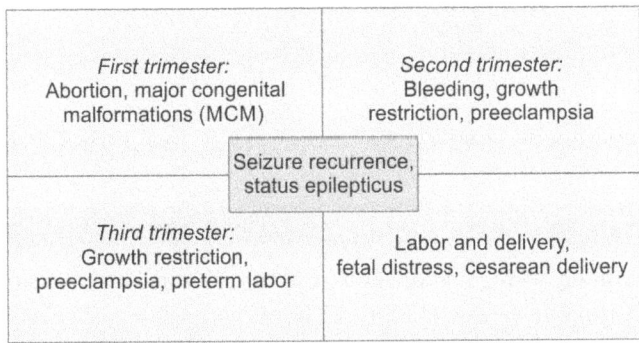

Algorithm 5: Antenatal complications in WWE.

The risks of antenatal complications during pregnancy in WWE are higher in those on AED than those without.

The diagnosis of epilepsy in pregnancy is not an indication for elective cesarean section or induction of labor. An uncomplicated labor and delivery is the usual expected outcome in WWE.[11]

INTRAPARTUM MANAGEMENT (ALGORITHM 6)

Antiepileptic drugs should not be withheld during labor. A parenteral alternative should be given if oral is not tolerated. In WWE, at high risk of seizures in the peripartum period, long-acting benzodiazepines such as clobazam can be considered.[11] About 1–2% of WWE in labor experience tonic-clonic seizures and within 24 hours postpartum in another 1–2%. The EURAP registry reported seizures in 3.5% of WWE in labor.[14]

In WWE, any seizure lasting more than 5 minutes represents a high risk of progressing to status epilepticus, which is a life-threatening medical emergency, and it affects around 1% of pregnancies in WWE.[15]

LABOR ANALGESIA/ANESTHESIA

Transcutaneous electrical nerve stimulation (TENS), Entonox®, and regional analgesia (epidural, spinal, combined spinal-epidural) are safe for labor analgesia in WWE.[16] Diamorphine should be preferred to pethidine as pethidine is metabolized to norpethidine, which is known to be epileptogenic in high doses to patients with normal renal function.[17]

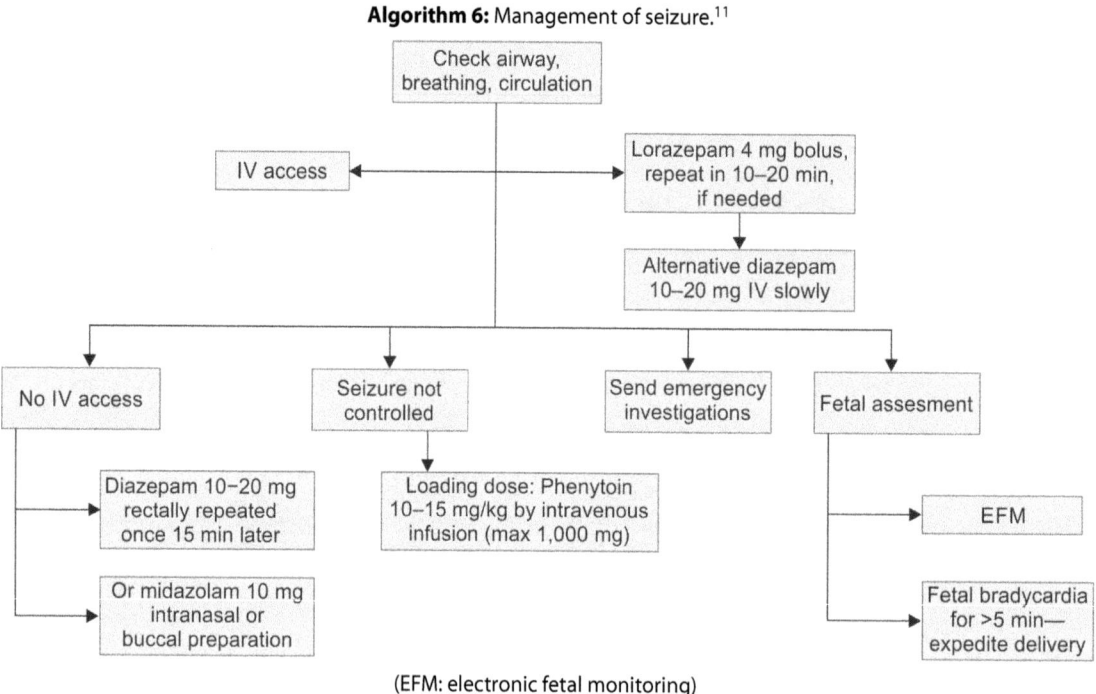

Algorithm 6: Management of seizure.[11]

(EFM: electronic fetal monitoring)

Algorithm 7: Medical management of eclamptic seizure.

Nonepileptic seizures	• Treat as eclampsia • Magsulf 4 g IV loading dose over 5 min • IV infusion 1 g/hr till 24 hrs postseizure or delivery whichever is later
Recurrent seizure	• Repeat magsulf 2–4 g over 5 min (RCOG) • Repeat 2 g bolus, twice if needed (Clinical practice guidelines) • Full IV or IM magsulf (WHO guidelines)
Uncontrolled/Refractory seizure: Lasting 5–30 min	• Phenytoin • Phenobarbital: 20 mg/kg IV at 50–100 mg/kg • Valporate sodium: 20–40 mg/kg IV at 10 mg/kg/min • Levetiracetam: 1,500–3,000 mg IV over 15–20 min
Status epilepticus: Seizure for >30 min	• Intubate • Midazolam: 0.2 mg/kg IV q5 min till seizures stop, then 2 mg/min • Propofol: 1–2 mg/kg q 5 min loading dose (max 10 mg/kg) then 1–10 mg/kg/hr at <50 mg/min • Thiopental: 2–7 mg/kg at <50 mg/min

In case general anesthesia is required, avoid pethidine, ketamine as they lower seizure threshold and sevoflurane which may have epileptogenic potential.[18]

NONEPILEPTIC SEIZURE

Treat all nonepileptic seizures, such as those without a past history of epilepsy, especially >20 weeks of gestation as eclampsia until proven otherwise **(Algorithm 7)**.

POSTPARTUM PERIOD

Women with generalized and partial seizures are at high risk of seizure exacerbation 72 hours peripartum especially in those who had seizures in the month before pregnancy.[19]

Avoid sleep deprivation, which can precipitate seizures. The intake AEDs should be continued as prescribed and adjust dose if increased in pregnancy, within 10 days of delivery to avoid postpartum toxicity.

NEONATAL CONCERNS

Vitamin K (1 mg IM) at birth to prevent hemolytic disease of newborn.[11]

Breastfeeding not contraindicated. AEDs such as phenobarbital, carbamazepine, phenytoin, lamotrigine, oxcarbazepine, and topiramate, have an umbilical cord to maternal serum AED concentration (US) that is close to one, suggesting free transfer of AED across the placenta, thus no withdrawal symptoms in infant. The fetal accumulation is mildly increased for levetiracetam, sodium valproate, and gabapentin.[20] On follow-up, no effect on cognitive outcomes is seen in children of mothers on AED.

CONTRACEPTION

- Cu IUCD, LNG-IUS—recommended.
- *Oral pills:* AEDs being enzyme inducers, failure rates are threefold higher, or use a higher dose of estrogen, or use along with barrier method.

REFERENCES

1. Edey S, Moran N, Nashef L. SUDEP and epilepsy-related mortality in pregnancy. Epilepsia. 2014;55:e72-4.
2. Adab N, Chadwick DW. Management of women with Epilepsy during pregnancy. Obstet Gynaecol. 2006;8:20-5.
3. Yerby MS. Quality of life, epilepsy advances, and the evolving role of anticonvulsants in women with epilepsy. Neurology. 2000;55:S21-31.
4. Fisher RS, Acevedo C, Arzimanoglou A, et al. ILAE official report: a practical clinical definition of epilepsy. Epilepsia. 2014;55:475-82.
5. Altman D, Carroli G, Duley L, et al. Do women with pre-eclampsia, and their babies, benefit from magnesium sulphate? The Magpie Trial: a randomised placebo-controlled trial. Lancet. 2002;359:1877-90.
6. Beach RL, Kaplan PW. Seizures in pregnancy: diagnosis and management. Int Rev Neurobiol. 2008;83:259-71.
7. Nashef L. Sudden unexpected death in epilepsy: terminology and definitions. Epilepsia. 1997;38(Suppl s1)1:S6-8.
8. Schmidt D, Beck-Mannagetta G, Janz D, et al. The effect of pregnancy on the course of epilepsy: a prospective study. In: Janz D, Dam M, Richens A (Eds). Epilepsy, Pregnancy and the Child. New York: Raven Press; 1982.
9. Battino D, Tomson T, Bonizzoni E, et al. Seizure control and treatment changes in pregnancy: observations from the EURAP epilepsy pregnancy registry. Epilepsia. 2013;54:1621-7.
10. Sabers A. Algorithm for lamotrigine dose adjustment before, during, and after pregnancy. Acta Neurol Scand. 2012;126(1):e1-4.
11. Royal College of Obstetricians and Gynaecologists. Epilepsy in Pregnancy: RCOG Green-top Guideline No. 68. London, UK: Royal College of Obstetricians and Gynaecologists; 2016.
12. Tomson T, Xue H, Battino D. Major congenital malformations in children of women with epilepsy. Seizure. 2015;28:46-50.
13. Petersen I, Collings SL, McCrea RL, et al. Antiepileptic drugs prescribed in pregnancy and prevalence of major congenital malformations: comparative prevalence studies. Clin Epidemiol. 2017;9:95-103.
14. Pennell PB. EURAP outcomes for seizure control during pregnancy: useful and encouraging data. Epilepsy Curr. 2006;6:186-8.
15. EURAP Study Group. Seizure control and treatment in pregnancy: observations from the EURAP epilepsy pregnancy registry. Neurology. 2006;66:354-60.
16. Uczkowski KM. Labor analgesia for the parturient with neurological disease: what does an obstetrician need to know? Arch Gynecol Obstet. 2006;274:41-6.
17. Arinella MA. Meperidine-induced generalized seizures with normal renal function. South Med J. 1997;90:556-8.
18. Billington M, Kandalaft OR, Aisiku IP. Adult status epilepticus: a review of the prehospital and emergency department management. J Clin Med. 2016;5(9):74.
19. Thomas SV, Syam U, Devi JS. Predictors of seizures during pregnancy in women with epilepsy. Epilepsia. 2012;53:e85-8.
20. Chen L, Liu F, Yoshida S, et al. Is breast-feeding of infants advisable for epileptic mothers taking antiepileptic drugs? Psychiatry Clin Neurosci. 2010;64:460-8.

Chapter 8

Venous Thromboembolism in Pregnancy

Vivek Chauhan, Suman Thakur

INTRODUCTION: FACTS ABOUT VENOUS THROMBOEMBOLISM IN PREGNANCY

- Venous thromboembolism (VTE) that includes deep venous thrombosis (DVT) and pulmonary embolism (PE) increases morbidity and mortality in pregnant females.
- Risk of DVT is higher in pregnancy than in a nonpregnant state.
- Risk of DVT is even higher till 12 weeks' postpartum than that in pregnancy.
- Females at risk for DVT or prior VTE need prophylaxis during pregnancy and postpartum.
- Treatment and prophylaxis of VTE during pregnancy is challenging for both the fetus and the mother.

The chapter describes important considerations for treatment and prevention of VTE before, during, and after pregnancy based upon the guidelines published by various societies.

EPIDEMIOLOGY

Venous thromboembolism does not list among the top five causes of maternal mortality in the developing world though it is the fifth leading cause responsible for 9.2% of all maternal deaths in the United States.[1,2] Prevalence of VTE ranges from 0.5 to 2.2 per 1,000 deliveries.[3] PE can lead to sudden death, and thus its diagnosis is often missed in the developing countries.

PATHOGENESIS

Pregnancy and postpartum state fulfill the criteria of Virchow's triad for venous thrombosis **(Algorithm 1)**.

CLINICAL PRESENTATION

Eighty percent pregnant females with DVT have lower extremity discomfort and edema.[5] Tachycardia, tachypnea, dyspnea, and lower extremity pain or swelling are common complaints in many pregnant females; thus, they have poor specificity for predicting VTE.

Mnemonic for Symptoms of DVT: LEFT

- *L*: Left lower extremity symptoms
- *E*: Edema (mid-circumference difference between right and left more than 2 cm)
- *FT*: First trimester of presentation

When LEFT was studied, for presence of one symptom, 16% had DVT; for two or three symptoms, 58% had DVT.[6]

DIAGNOSIS

The diagnostic algorithm for suspected VTE during pregnancy is shown in **Algorithm 2**.

TREATMENT AND PROPHYLAXIS

The recommendations that follow for treatment and prophylaxis of VTE have been selected by the author from

Algorithm 1: Virchow's triad for venous thrombosis.[4]

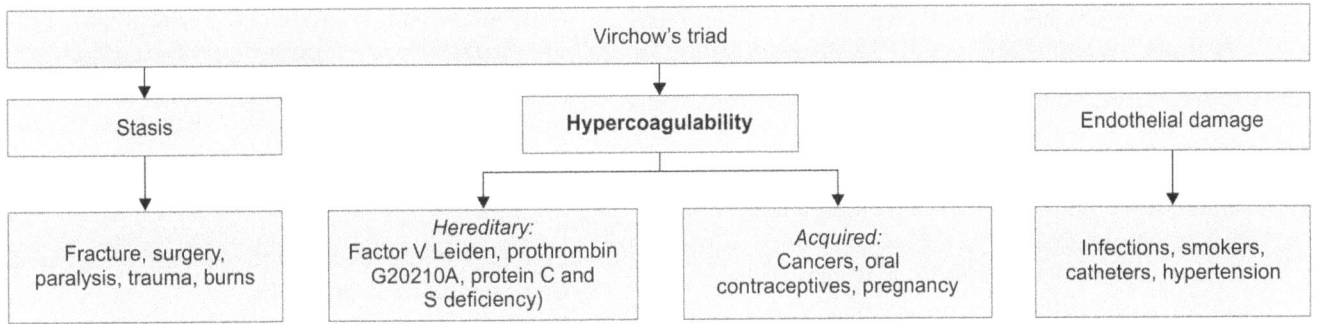

Algorithm 2: Diagnostic algorithm for suspected venous thromboembolism (VTE) during pregnancy.

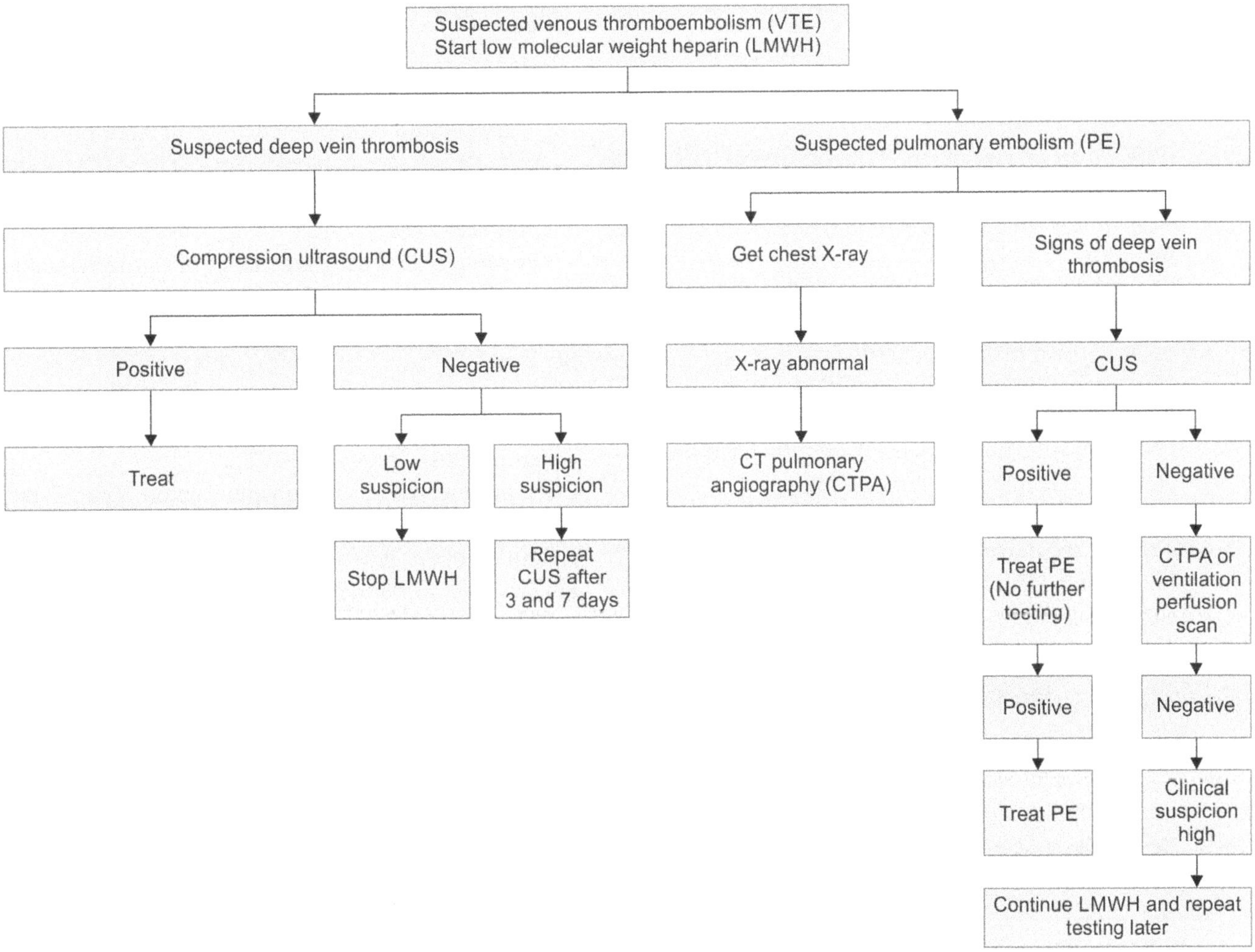

the published practice guidelines by the American College of Gynecologists and Obstetricians (ACOG),[5,7] Society of Obstetricians and Gynecologists of Canada (SOGC),[8] and Royal College of Obstetricians and Gynecologists (RCOG).[9-11] For more details and variations, please refer to the original guidelines.

Choice of Anticoagulant

- Stop warfarin as soon as pregnancy is confirmed (preferably within 2 weeks of conception).
- Heparin is the preferred anticoagulant for use during pregnancy. Low molecular weight heparin (LMWH) is preferred over unfractionated heparin (UFH) for use during pregnancy.

- Oral Xa inhibitors and direct thrombin inhibitors should be avoided during pregnancy.
- Postpartum warfarin, LMWH, and UFH are compatible with breast-feeding.

Treatment of Acute Venous Thromboembolism

- Hospitalization for the first few days after diagnosis of VTE is recommended.
- Low molecular weight heparin is recommended at once- or twice-daily dosages to treat VTE during pregnancy.
- *Thrombolysis indications during pregnancy:*
  - Life-threatening PE
  - Limb-threatening DVT
- *UFH is preferred over LMWH in VTE in the following circumstances:*
  - Near term (anticipated delivery)
  - Anticipated surgery or thrombolysis (massive PE)
- *Role of graded compression stockings:*
  - Recommended for symptom relief in acute proximal DVT
  - Below-knee graduated elastic stocking is recommended for 2 years in confirmed DVT
- *Duration of treatment with heparin:*
  - Low molecular weight heparin is to be given for the rest of the pregnancy and minimum 6 weeks postpartum or until at least 3 months have been completed in total (whichever is longer).
- *Possible indications to be considered for inferior vena cava (IVC) filter during acute VTE:*
  - Recurrent VTE despite anticoagulation.
  - Contraindications to anticoagulation.

PROPHYLAXIS

- *General recommendations:*
  - Every female must receive individualized risk assessment for VTE
  - Repeat risk assessment must be performed at every hospitalization during pregnancy or postpartum
- *Testing for thrombophilias:*
  - Routine screen for inherited thrombophilias is not recommended on first VTE during pregnancy
  - Test for proteins C, S and antithrombin following first VTE during pregnancy if family history of thrombophilias is positive or VTE occurs at unusual sites
  - Testing is recommended for antiphospholipid antibodies in unprovoked VTE during pregnancy
- *Clinical surveillance during pregnancy and postpartum:*
  - Heterogeneous factor V Leiden or prothrombin gene mutation with previously diagnosed thrombophilias without VTE
- *Clinical surveillance during pregnancy with 6 weeks postpartum prophylaxis:*
  - Protein C or S deficiency with previously diagnosed thrombophilias without VTE
  - Previous provoked VTE, not due to estrogen
- *Antepartum prophylaxis with LMWH with 6 weeks postpartum prophylaxis:*
  - Compound heterozygosity with or without previous VTE
  - Homozygosity for factor V Leiden or prothrombin gene mutation with or without previous VTE
  - Antithrombin deficiency with or without previous VTE
  - Antiphospholipid antibodies with or without previous VTE
  - Previous VTE during pregnancy or estrogen intake
  - Previous unprovoked VTE
- *Higher dose low molecular weight heparin for prophylaxis*
  - Two or more previous VTE episodes.
  - Antithrombin deficiency or antiphospholipid antibodies with previous VTE.
- Offer prophylaxis during hospitalization if unrelated to labor or active bleeding and discontinue after the resolution of the cause.
- For assisted reproduction and multiple clinical risk factors, consider antepartum prophylaxis.
- Cesarean delivery
  - *Emergency cesarean:* 10 days LMWH prophylaxis postdelivery.
  - *Elective cesarean:* Consider 10 days LMWH prophylaxis if additional risk factors positive.
  - Place pneumatic compression devices before cesarean if not on thromboprophylaxis already.
- Other general considerations
  - Advise all women to stop injecting LMWH once they think they are in labor.
  - Discontinue LMWH 24 hours prior to planned delivery.
  - In high-risk women for recurrent VTE, switch to UFH before delivery which is withheld 4–6 hours prior to delivery or epidural injection.

- Get platelet counts for women on prophylaxis with heparins before labor or cesarean.
- Withheld neuraxial blockade for 10–12 hours after the last dose of LMWH and 4–6 hours of UFH.
- Resume anticoagulation after 4–6 hours of vaginal delivery or 6–12 hours after cesarean delivery.
- Prophylactic LMWH can be started 4 hours after neuraxial catheter removal provided there is full neurological recovery and no evidence of active bleeding or coagulopathy.

REFERENCES

1. WHO. Maternal mortality. [online] Available from: http://www.who.int/mediacentre/factsheets/fs348/en/. [Last accessed on September, 2019].
2. CDC. (2017). Pregnancy Mortality Surveillance System. Pregnancy. Reproductive health. [online] Available from: https://www.cdc.gov/reproductivehealth/maternalinfanthealth/pmss.html [Last accessed on September, 2019].
3. Bates SM, Middeldorp S, Rodger M, et al. Guidance for the treatment and prevention of obstetric-associated venous thromboembolism. J Thromb Thrombolysis. 2016;41:92-128.
4. McMaster Pathophysiology Review. Etiology of venous thromboembolism – Virchow's triad | [online] Available from: http://www.pathophys.org/vte/pe-virchow-2/ [Last accessed on September, 2019].
5. James AH, Tapson VF, Goldhaber SZ. Thrombosis during pregnancy and the postpartum period. Am J Obstet Gynecol. 2005;193(1):216-9.
6. Chan W-S, Lee A, Spencer FA, et al. Predicting deep venous thrombosis in pregnancy: out in "LEFt" field? Ann Intern Med. 2009;151(2):85-92.
7. James A, Committee on Practice Bulletins—Obstetrics. Practice Bulletin no. 123: thromboembolism in pregnancy. Obstet Gynecol. 2011;118(3):718-29.
8. Branch DW, Holmgren C, Goldberg JD, et al. Practice Bulletin no 132: antiphospholipid antibody syndrome. Obstet Gynecol. 2012;120(6):1514-21.
9. Chan W-S, Rey E, Kent NE, et al. Venous thromboembolism and antithrombotic therapy in pregnancy. J Obstet Gynaecol Can. 2014;36(6):527-53.
10. Royal College of Obstetricians and Gynaecologists. Thrombosis and embolism during pregnancy and the puerperium, reducing the risk (Green-top Guideline No. 37a). [online] Available from: https://www.rcog.org.uk/en/guidelines-research-services/guidelines/gtg37a/ [Last accessed on September, 2019].
11. Royal College of Obstetricians and Gynaecologists. Thrombosis and embolism during pregnancy and the puerperium, the acute management of (Green-Top Guideline No. 37b). [online] Available from: https://www.rcog.org.uk/en/guidelines-research-services/guidelines/gtg37b/ [Last accessed on September, 2019].

Chapter 9

Shock

Rohini Rao, Rajesh Kumar Verma, Kunal Kumar Sharma

INTRODUCTION

Shock is defined as the failure of circulation, which is life-threatening. It is characterized by low perfusion of vital organs due to low cardiac output.

TYPES OF SHOCK (ALGORITHM 1)

- *Hemorrhagic:* It occurs when uncontrolled bleeding leads to blood loss amounting to more than 20% of the total blood volume. This uncorrected loss makes the heart incapable of providing sufficient cardiac output to the vital organs of the body.
- *Endotoxic/septic:* It occurs due to gram-negative bacteria that enter the bloodstream and triggers the inflammatory pathway resulting in hyperdynamic cardiovascular response with high cardiac output and low systemic vascular resistance (SVR).[1]
- *Anaphylactic:* It occurs due to release of inflammatory chemical mediators within the patient's body in response to a triggering allergen. The generalized vasodilatation and airway edema lead to circulatory and respiratory failure.
- *Neurogenic:* It occurs due to disruption of autonomic pathways within the spinal canal. Therefore, the patient loses his ability to trigger compensatory mechanisms for shock. The patient develops hypotension due to decreased SVR, which leads to pooling of blood in lower limbs. Bradycardia occurs due to uninhibited vagal activity. The level of spinal cord injury determines the respiratory pattern in such a patient.[2]
- *Cardiogenic:* It occurs due to failure of myocardial cells and musculature to effectively pump the cardiac output. This is commonly seen after myocardial infarction or cardiac failure.

Algorithm 1: Types of shock.

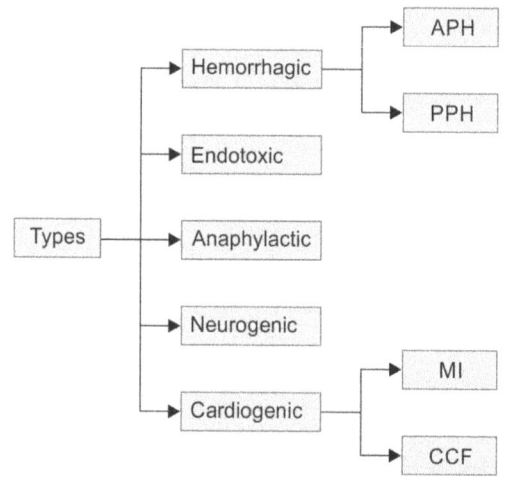

(APH: antepartum hemorrhage; CCF: congestive cardiac failure; MI: myocardial infarction; PPH: postpartum hemorrhage)

The type of shock most commonly encountered in obstetric practice is hemorrhagic shock. Its classification as per Advanced Trauma Life Support (ATLS) guidelines is depicted in **Algorithm 2**.

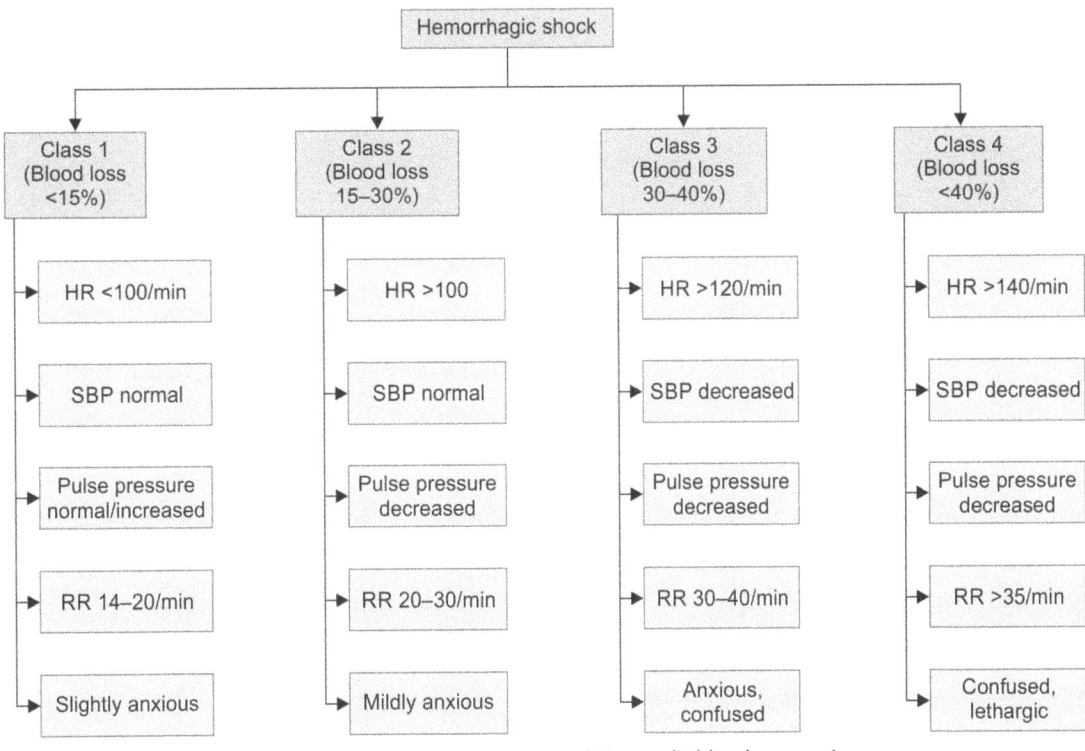

Algorithm 2: Classification of hemorrhagic shock as per advanced trauma life support (ATLS) guidelines.

(HR: heart rate; RR: respiratory rate; SBP: systolic blood pressure)

ASSESSMENT OF BLOOD LOSS IN HEMORRHAGIC SHOCK

Absolute accuracy in blood loss estimation is difficult in an obstetric patient due to mixing up of irrigational saline and amniotic fluid in the suction drain. However, many newer methods have come up for predicting the blood loss to the nearest possible accuracy. These are as depicted in **Algorithm 3**.

RECOMMENDATIONS FOR BLOOD TRANSFUSION IN HEMORRHAGIC SHOCK

Blood oxygen content and oxygen delivery to the tissues are a function of hemoglobin concentration. The compensatory physiologic responses offset the negative effect of anemia on oxygen transport. Tachycardia and increased stroke volume combine to increase cardiac output. The blood viscosity and SVR decrease, thereby augmenting blood flow to tissues. An increase in tissue oxygen extraction is also seen.

However, when hemoglobin concentration falls to 5 g/dL, SVR decreases whereas heart rate, stroke volume, and cardiac index increase. Oxygen transport rate and mixed venous oxyhemoglobin saturation decrease at this hemoglobin level of 5.0 g/dL.

Various guidelines pertaining to the transfusion trigger are given in **Table 1**.

RISKS OF BLOOD TRANSFUSION (ALGORITHM 4)

- *Hemolytic reactions:* ABO incompatibility results in intravascular hemolysis, which manifests clinically as fever, chills, nausea, chest pain, and flank pain along with signs such as hypotension, tachycardia, disseminated intravascular coagulation, and hemoglobinuria.
- *Transfusion-related lung injury:* The criteria for labeling the patient with this outcome involves the presence of acute-onset hypoxemia, $PaO_2/FiO_2 < 300$, $SpO_2 < 90\%$, bilateral infiltrates on chest X-ray, occurrence of

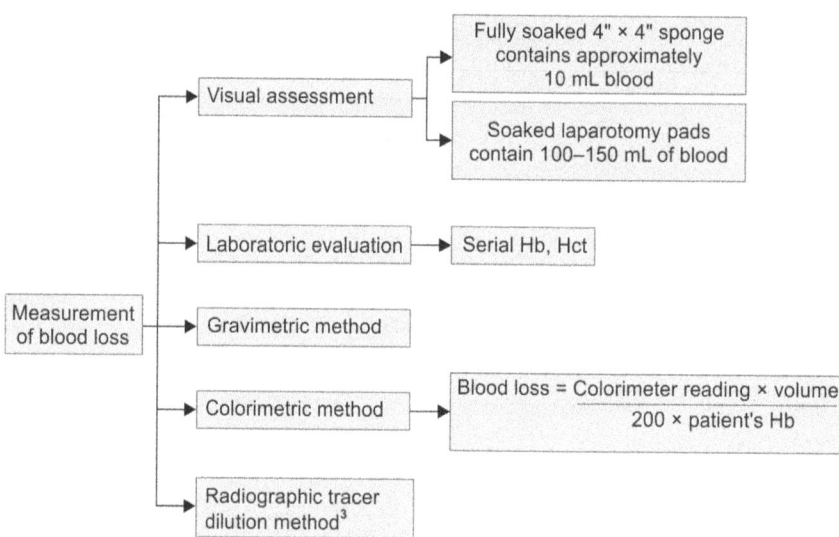

Algorithm 3: Measurement of blood loss.

Table 1: Guidelines pertaining to transfusion trigger.		
Habibi recommendations[4]	*Hébert recommendations*[5]	*ASA guidelines*[6]
Transfuse blood if: • Hb ≤ 8 g/dL in all types of patients • Hb ≤ 10 g/dL in patient of IHD, emphysema • Hb ≤ 10 g/dL with autologus blood • Hb ≤ 12 g/dL in ventilator-dependent patient • If blood loss > 20% blood volume in adults • Blood loss ≥ 100 mL in pediatric patients	Transfuse blood if: • Hb ≤ 10 g/dL in unstable angina and anterior wall MI • Hb between 10 g/dL and 12 g/dL in critically ill patients	• Transfusion of blood solely based on Hb levels is not indicated • See the coexisting pathology of the patient • Transfusion is always required if Hb ≤ 6 g/dL • If Hb is between 6 and 10 g/dL, the blood transfusion depends on complications of inadequate oxygenation and patient's cardiovascular status • Transfusion is rarely required if Hb > 10 g/dL

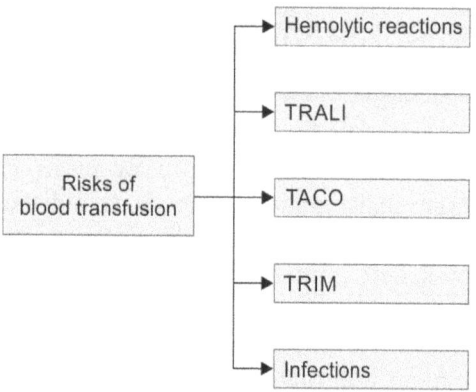

Algorithm 4: Risks of blood transfusion.

(TACO: transfusion-associated circulatory overload; TRALI; transfusion-related acute lung injury; TRIM: transfusion immunomodulation)

symptoms within 6 hours of blood transfusion, and no evidence of left atrial hypertension.

- *Transfusion-associated circulatory overload:* It occurs in 1-6% of blood transfusion patients. Its incidence increases with the amount of plasma transfused. It is seen in young patients, especially during correction of coagulopathy associated with severe hemorrhage.
- *Transfusion-related immunomodulation:* It is seen with allogeneic blood transfusion. The recipient develops immune tolerance, generalized immune suppression, and exhibits microchimerism, which predispose him to autoimmune diseases.
- *Infections:* Screening of donor blood by nucleic acid amplification technology has helped in decreasing the

risk of viral transmission of human immunodeficiency virus (HIV) and hepatitis C virus (HCV). However, cytomegalovirus (CMV) and Creutzfeldt-Jakob disease (CJD) may still be transmitted. Bacterial contamination can occur with platelet transfusion as the platelets are stored at warmer temperatures; hence, culture-negative platelets should be used to decrease the incidence of sepsis.

MANAGEMENT OF HEMORRHAGIC SHOCK IN AN OBSTETRIC PATIENT (ALGORITHMS 5 TO 8)

The patient has to be assessed globally. We assess the hemodynamic, respiratory, and uterotonic options for managing these patients.

Airway management: It primarily involves classifying the severity of shock followed by initiation of appropriate airway interventions. The core key points of management are administration of high-flow oxygen, laboratory evaluation of arterial blood gases, and endotracheal intubation in case of oxygenation failure.

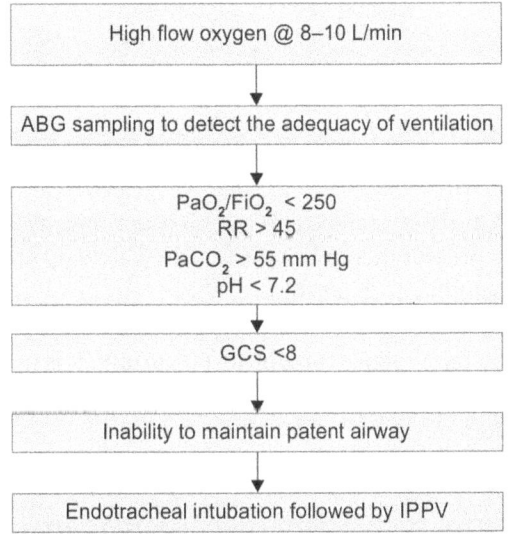

Algorithm 5: Airway management.

(ABG: arterial blood gas; GCS: Glasgow coma scale; IPPV: intermittent positive pressure ventilation)

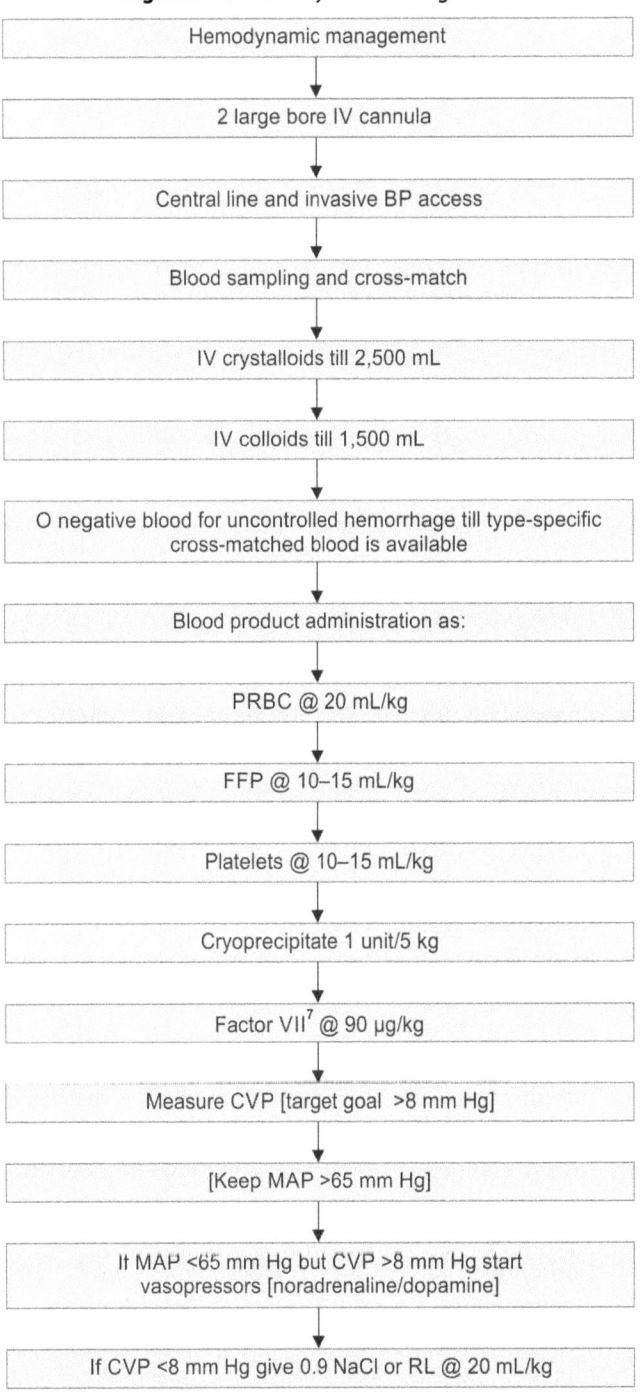

Algorithm 6: Hemodynamic management.

(CVP: central venous pressure; FFP: fresh frozen plasma; MAP: mean arterial pressure; PRBC: packed red blood cells)

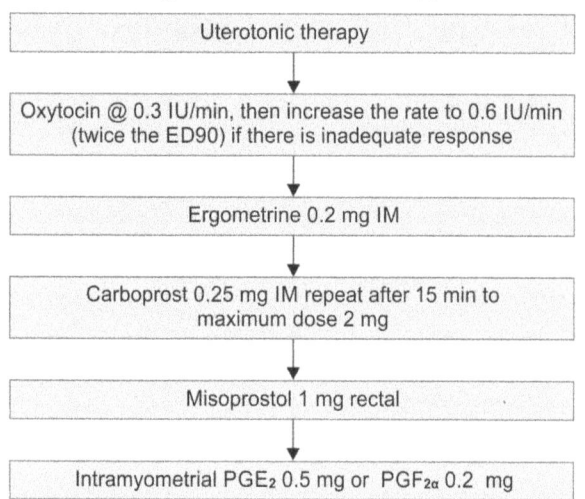

Algorithm 7: Uterotonic therapy.

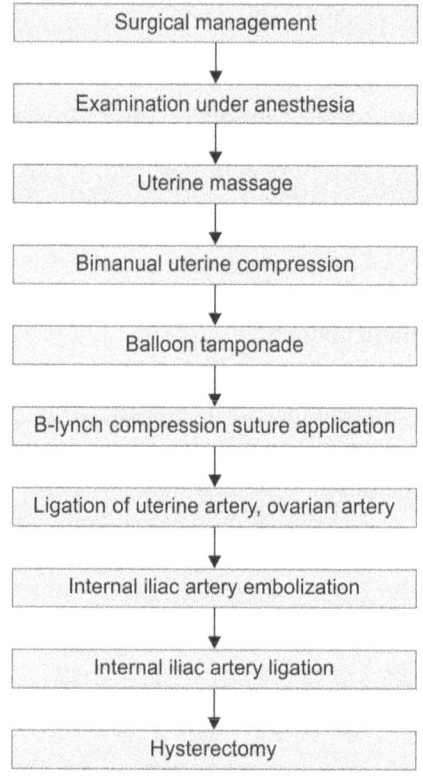

Algorithm 8: Surgical management of PPH.

Uterotonic therapy, as shown in **Algorithm 7**, *is given by the following drugs:*

- *Oxytocin:* Injecting 10–40 IU of oxytocin into a 1 L crystalloid solution and infusing the solution at an unspecified rate can lead to detrimental scenarios in hypovolemic hemorrhagic patients. Administration of phenylephrine can mitigate the adverse hemodynamic consequences of oxytocin. It is advocated to administer prophylactic oxytocin at a rate of 0.3 IU/min (the ED90) and increase the rate to 0.6 IU/min (twice the ED90) if there is inadequate response.
- *Methylergonovine:* Dose is 0.2 mg IM. Bolus intravenous administration is *not* recommended due to high incidence of nausea and vomiting. The uterotonic effect usually lasts for 2–4 hours. It produces tetanic uterine contractions and for this reason, it is restricted to postpartum use. Side effects are vasoconstriction, hypertension, myocardial ischemia, and infarction due to coronary vasospasm, cerebrovascular accidents, seizures, and death.
- *Carboprost (15-methyl prostaglandin $F_2\alpha$):* The recommended dose is 0.25 mg (250 µg), administered intramuscularly, which can be repeated every 15–30 minutes; the total dose should not exceed 2 mg. Side effects such as bronchospasm, abnormal ventilation-perfusion ratio, increased intrapulmonary shunt fraction, and hypoxemia are seen in susceptible patients.
- *Misoprostol (prostaglandin E1 analog):* A dose of 600–1,000 µg per rectum is commonly administered; administration via oral, buccal, and sublingual routes has been described. Adverse effects such as fever, chills, nausea, vomiting, and diarrhea can occur.
- Intramyometrial PGE_2 0.5 mg or $PGF_{2\alpha}$ 0.2 mg.

MANAGEMENT OF NEUROGENIC SHOCK

Besides the IV crystalloids or colloids used for resuscitation, the vasopressor therapy comprises the following drugs:
- *Dopamine:* 5–25 µg/min.
- *Phenylepinephrine:* 100–180 µg/min initially, followed by a maintenance dose of 40–60 µg/min. It is used as a second-line therapy in a patient who is not responding to dopamine.
- *Atropine:* 20 µg/kg IV for severe bradycardia.

MANAGEMENT OF ENDOTOXIC SHOCK (ALGORITHM 9)

- *IV crystalloids:* 30 mL/kg initially to target a mean arterial pressure (MAP) of 65 mm Hg.
- Do not use hydroxyethyl starch for intravascular volume replacement in these patients.

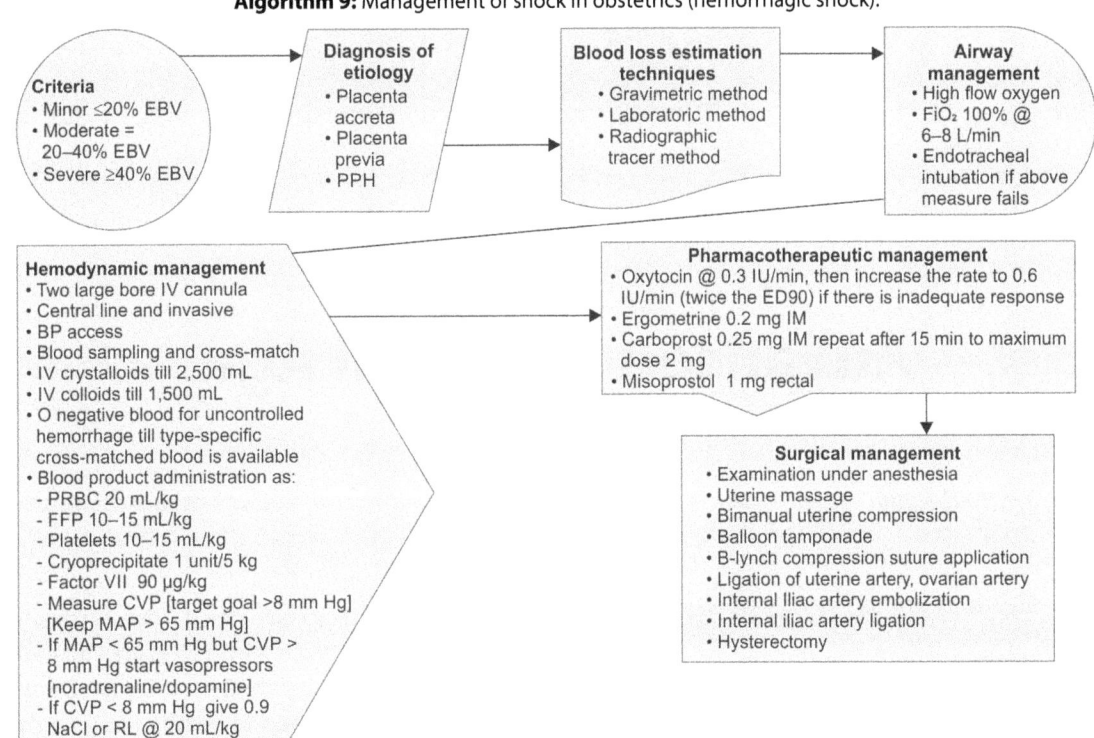

Algorithm 9: Management of shock in obstetrics (hemorrhagic shock).

- Use of albumin with crystalloids for initial resuscitation and subsequent maintenance is advocated.
- Use pulse pressure variation and stroke volume variation index to decide whether the patient's hypotension is responding to fluid or to vasopressor.
- *Norepinephrine:* 0.02–3 µg/kg/min is the first choice.
- *Epinephrine:* 0.01–0.1 µg/kg/min is added when an additional agent is being required to maintain the blood pressure.
- *Vasopressin:* 0.03 units/min can be added to norepinephrine to increase MAP.
- Dopamine is used only if the patient develops bradycardia.
- Phenylepinephrine is not recommended in septic shock.

REFERENCES

1. Micek ST, Welch EC, Khan J, et al. Emperic combination antibiotic therapy is associated with improved outcome against sepsis due to Gram-negative bacteria: a retrospective analysis. Antimicrob Agents Chemother. 2010;54:1742-8.
2. Axelrad A, Pandya P, Waqas M, et al. The significance of neurogenic shock and acute spinal cord injury (poster session). Critical Care Med. 2013;41(12):A49.
3. Bassingthwaighte JB, Holloway Jr. GA. Estimation of blood flow with radioactive tracers. Semin Nucl Med. 1976;6(2):141-61.
4. Habibi B, Seidl S. Recommendations from session 4. Vox Sanguinis. 1984;46(s1):64-5.
5. Hébert PC, Wells G, Blajchman MA, et al. A multicenter, randomized, controlled clinical trial of transfusion requirements in critical care. N Engl J Med. 1999;340:409-17.
6. American Society of Anesthesiologists Task Force on Perioperative Blood Management. Practice guidelines for perioperative blood management. An updated report by the American Society of Anesthesiologists Task Force on Perioperative Blood Management. Anesthesiology. 2015;122:241-75.
7. Stein DM, Dutton RP. Use of recombinant factor VII a in trauma. Curr Opin Crit Care. 2009;15:536-41.

Chapter 10

Advanced Maternal Age

Vidya Thobbi, Jyothi Goulay

INTRODUCTION

Improvements in women's general health have led to this term tending to be reserved for pregnancies in women at or over 40 years of age. Fertility clearly declines with advancing age, especially after the mid-30s, and women who conceive are at greater risk of pregnancy complications. With use of assisted reproductive technologies (ARTs), births have been reported in women as old as 66 years of age. The oldest woman to achieve a naturally conceived pregnancy was 57 years old.[1]

Pregnancy at advanced maternal age may be due to:
- Late marriage
- Long period of primary infertility
- Delayed childbearing **(Algorithm 1)**.

Are risks in pregnancy increased in women of advancing age?
- There is always some risk to the mother and baby in all pregnancies
- As age advances, these risks are more
- Younger women have lower risk during pregnancy compared to those who are 35 years and above[2]
- Pregnancy risks are higher in older women due to comorbid conditions **(Algorithm 2)**.

What are some of these increasing risks?
Some of these increasing risks are given in **Algorithm 3**.
- Chromosomal abnormalities—with advancing age, ova quality deteriorates leading to higher risk of chromosomal abnormalities.

Various characteristic changes of the fetus, mental changes, and altered life expectancies of the neonate are seen associated with these chromosomal abnormalities.

The incidence of Down syndrome among all newborns—1:800 **(Algorithm 4)**. For mothers age 35 years, the incidence is higher, i.e. 1:385, and for mothers age 45 years, the incidence is 1:33.

Because of increased genetic mutations, autosomal dominant disease rates such as Marfan syndrome are higher in children of fathers of advanced paternal age.[3,4]

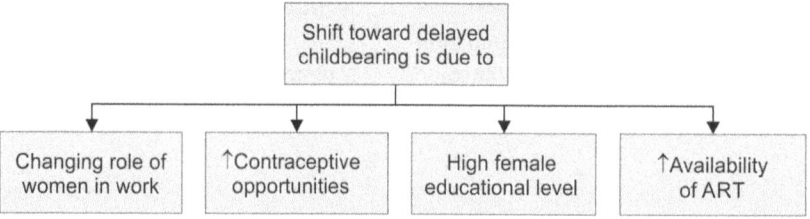

Algorithm 1: Factors causing shift toward delayed childbearing.

Algorithm 2: Adverse pregnancy outcomes.

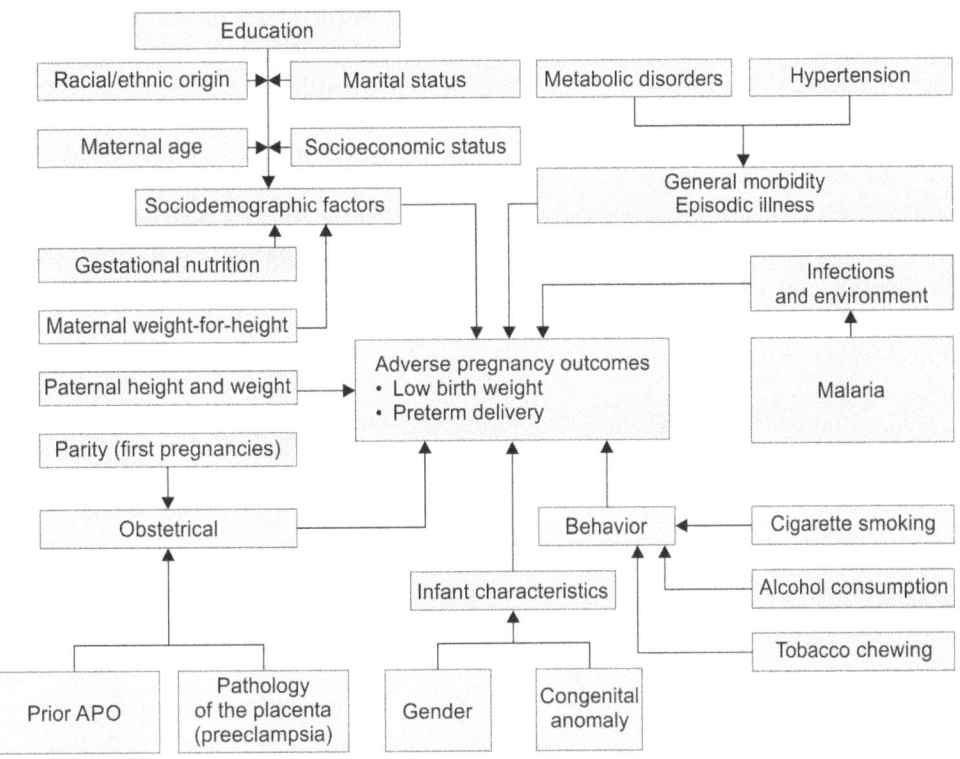

(APO: adverse pregnancy outcome)

Algorithm 3: Increasing risks of pregnancy.

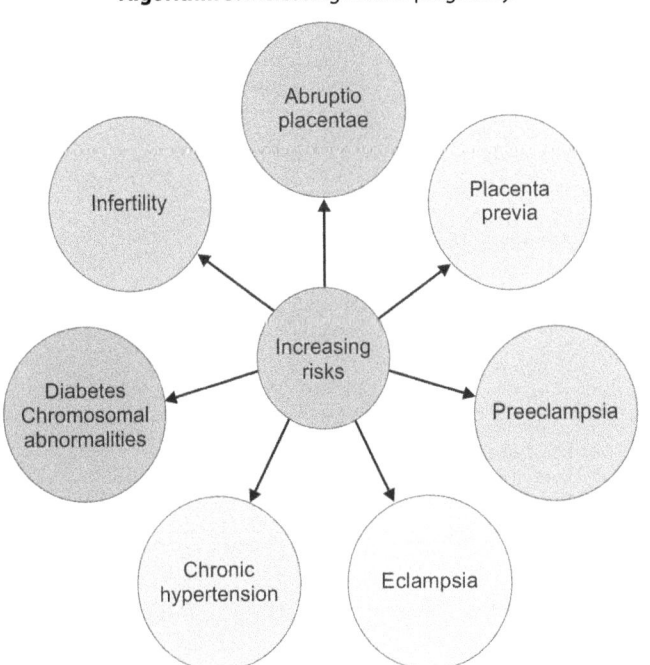

Algorithm 4: Characteristics of major syndromes.

- Down syndrome (trisomy 21)
- Edwards syndrome (trisomy 18)
- Klinefelter syndrome (sex chromosome)

Table 1: Estimated risk for trisomies in relation to maternal age at birth.

Age of mother	Risk of Down syndrome	Risk of trisomy 18	Risk of trisomy 13
20 years	1:1530	1:18 013	1:42 423
30 years	1:900	1:10 554	1:24 856
35 years	1:360	1:4202	1:9876
40 years	1:100	1:1139	1:3544
42 years	1:55	1:644	1:1516
44 years	1:30	No recent data	No recent data

Source: Fetal Medicine Foundation.[5]

- Infertility—premature ovarian failure, perimenopause and menopause, anovulation, anatomical defects, or a variety of other problems in the female are the various causes of infertility. It may also be due to abnormal spermatogenesis in the male.

PREGNANCY FOR FIRST BIRTHS, THE PROPORTION TO WOMEN

In the past quarter century, older women in the USA have accounted for an increasing proportion of total births. In 2005, 14% of all births were to women ≥35 years of age.[6,7]

For first births, the proportion to women:
- 30–34 years have increased threefold
- 35–39 years have increased sixfold, and
- ≥40 years have increased 15-fold **(Algorithm 5)**.

PRECONCEPTIONAL RISKS AND MANAGEMENT (ALGORITHM 6)

Congenital malformation rate:
- 3.5% in women 20–24 years of age
- 4.4% in women 35–39 years of age
- 5% in women ≥40 years of age.

Algorithm 5: Proportion to women in different years of pregnancy.

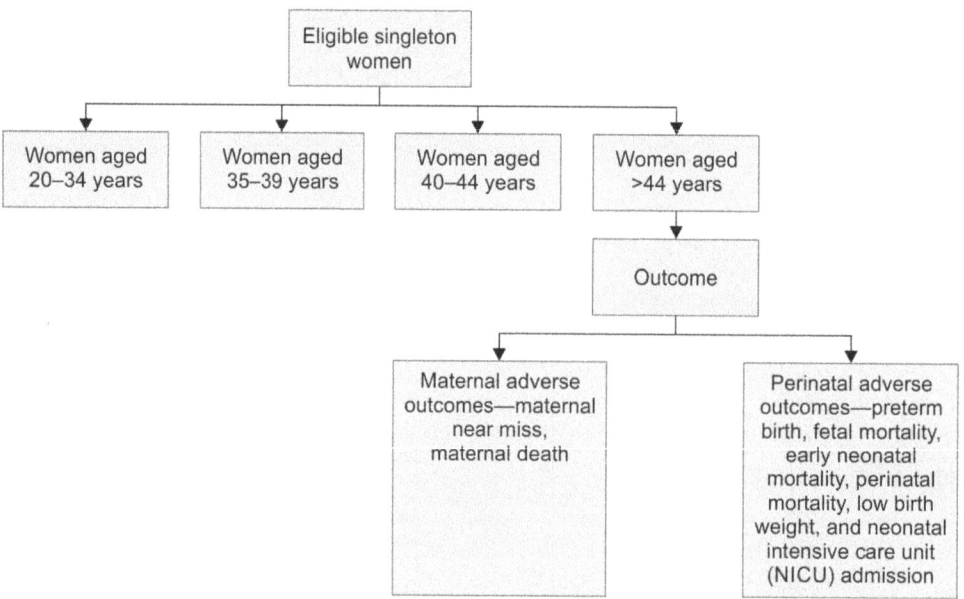

Algorithm 6: Preconceptional risks and management.

Chapter 10
Advanced Maternal Age

Algorithm 7: Early pregnancy issues.

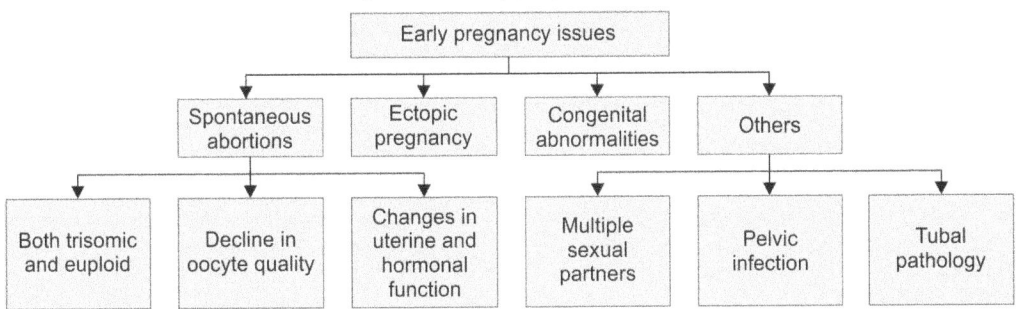

Algorithm 8: Late pregnancy issues.

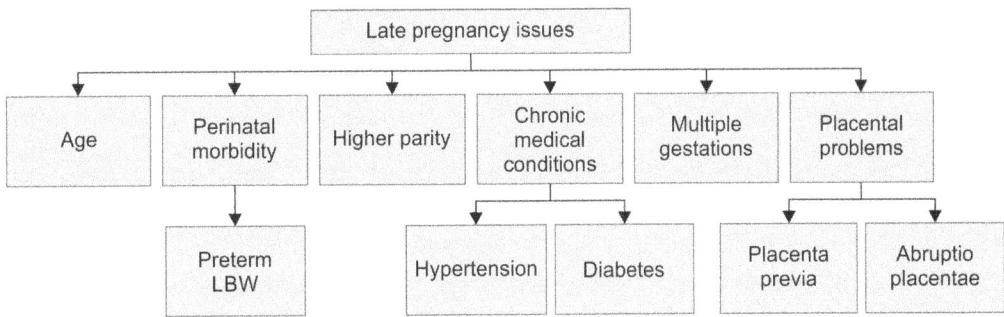

Algorithm 9: ANC visits in advanced maternal age.[7]

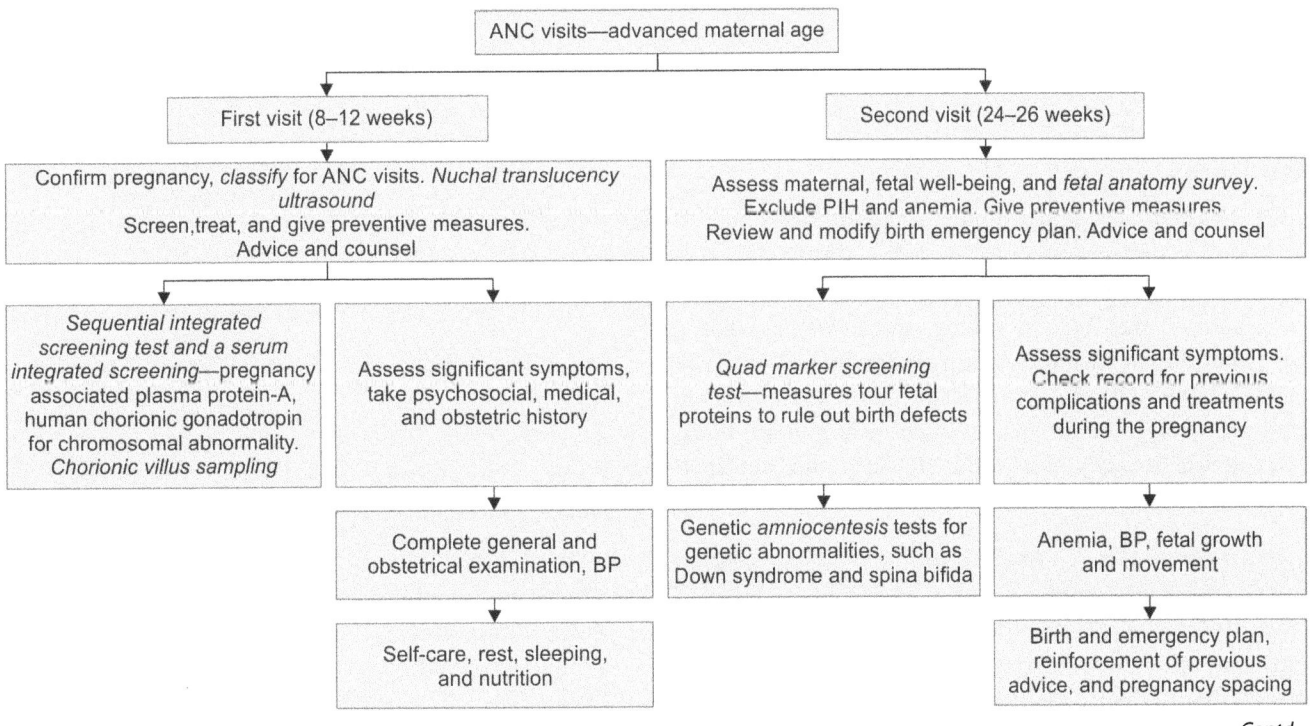

Contd...

Contd...

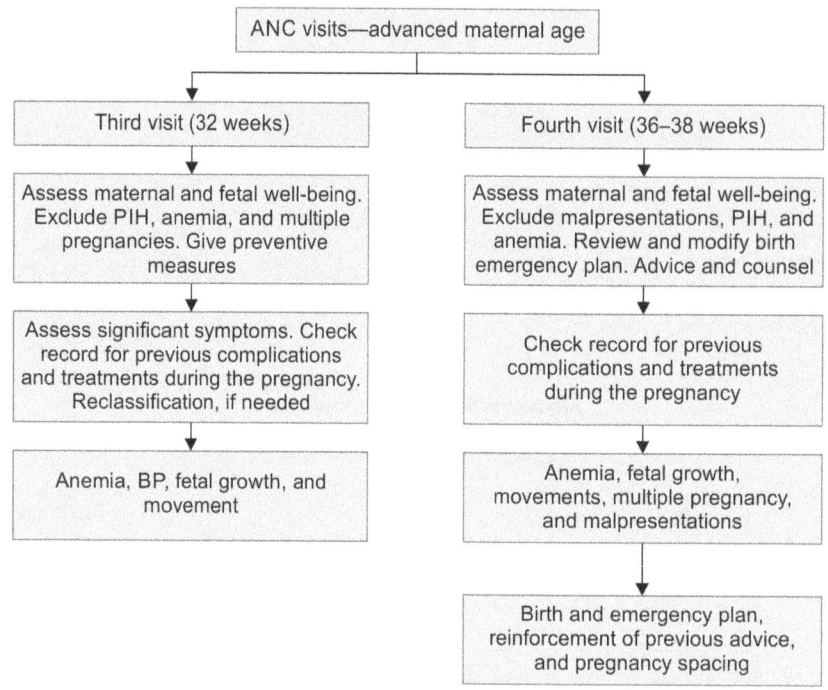

(ANC: antenatal care; BP: blood pressure; PIH: pregnancy-induced hypertension)

HYPERTENSION

Hypertension is the most common medical problem encountered in pregnancy and is particularly prevalent in older women. Chronic hypertension is two- to four-fold higher in women ≥35 years of age than in other women.

Incidence

- Thirty five percent in women over age 50 years
- About 5–10% in women over age 40 years
- General obstetric population is 3–4%.

Maternal and fetal morbidity and mortality related to hypertensive disorders during pregnancy can be reduced with careful monitoring and appropriately timed intervention, but with an increase in preterm birth, intrauterine growth restriction (IUGR), and cesarean delivery.

DIABETES MELLITUS

The prevalence of diabetes increases with maternal age. The rates of both preexisting diabetes mellitus and gestational diabetes increase fold in women ≥40 years compared with other women **(Algorithm 10)**.

Algorithm 10: Incidence of gestational diabetes.

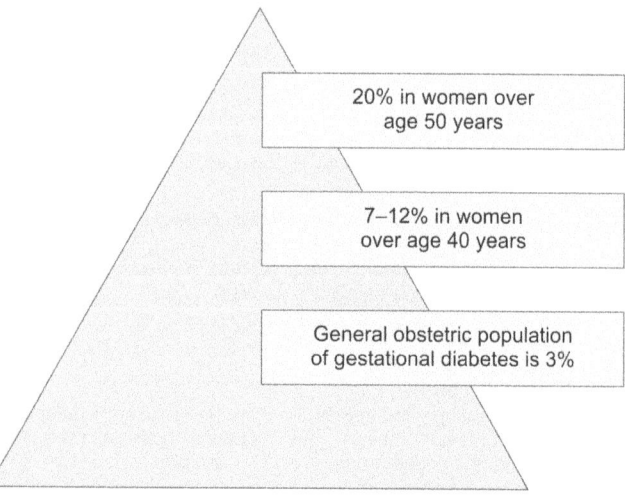

Incidence: 20% in advanced maternal age.

Preexisting diabetes is associated with increased risks of:
- Congenital anomalies
- Perinatal mortality
- Perinatal morbidity.

The major complication of gestational diabetes is macrosomia and its sequelae.

During Labor

Pre-existing diabetes during labor is described in **Algorithm 11**.

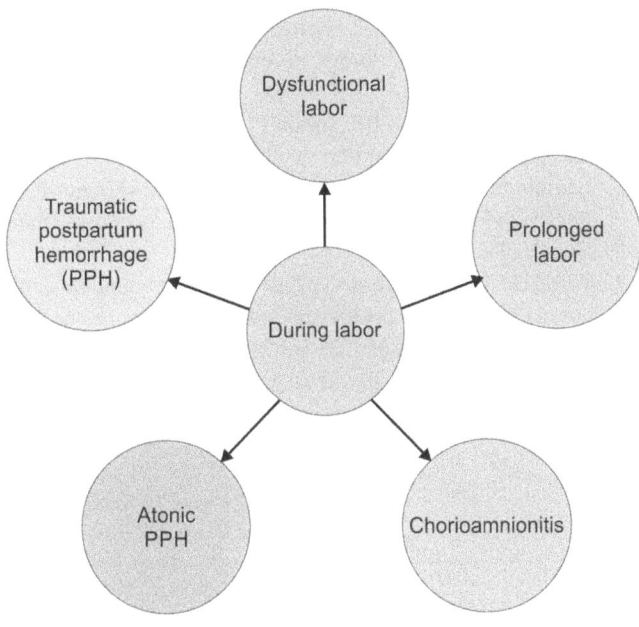

Algorithm 11: Pre-existing diabetes during labor.

During Puerperium

- Subinvolution of the uterus
- Puerperal sepsis.

The reasons for the high rate of operative delivery in older women are given in **Algorithm 12**.

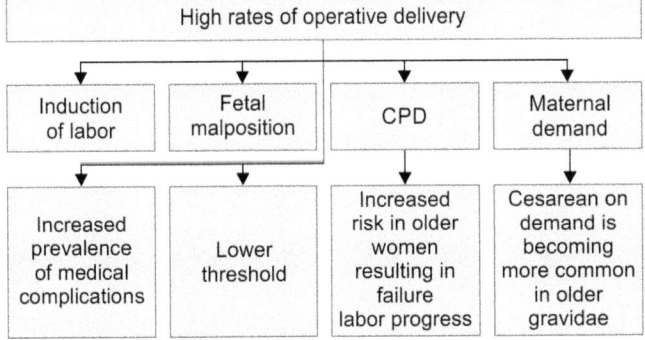

Algorithm 12: Reasons for the high rate of operative delivery in older women.

How can you counsel your patients?
- Prenatal vitamins and folic acid and maintaining a healthy diet.
- Moderate exercise—various complications like preeclampsia, thromboembolism, C-section, wound infection, and anesthesia complications are seen in women with body mass index (BMI) of >29 kg/m^2.
- Avoiding drinking, smoking, and drugs.
- Counseling regarding importance and obtaining prenatal care.
- Comorbidities—Education of patients regarding lifestyle modifications. It is vital to motivate them to get their conditions under control before becoming pregnant.
- Medications—educate patients about their medications [Rx, over-the-counter (OTC), and supplements]. Determination of pregnancy categories and risk versus benefit. The decision to change or stop medications is essential.
- Genetic counseling—counsel and collect information from your patient, assessment of the risk of the mother developing disease or conceiving an infant with congenital abnormalities, give vital information regarding screening and diagnostic tests which are available, and also to discuss alternative reproductive options, if necessary. All the queries should be answered in an easily understood language to the satisfaction of the patient. Aim of counseling is to be informative and supportive to the patient, but free of personal opinion.

INFORMATION GATHERING AND WOMEN'S PREPARATION FOR PREGNANCY

Being well-prepared for pregnancy—both mentally and physically. Preparation often means losing weight, going on diets, and taking exercise. Visiting specialist doctors to discuss existing health issues, such as blood pressure, choosing hospitals, and birth care options. Awareness of the high risks associated with the age, value the availability of emergency services at hospitals. Marital status, economic status, smoking, parity, BMI, preexisting diagnoses, history of using medications before conception, and previous adverse prenatal outcome are confounding factors whose influence on patients must be considered. It is of utmost importance that each woman of AMA should be treated as an individual, and not simply as a member of a certain group. Awareness of the various experiences of older pregnant women can help doctors and other healthcare providers to understand the needs of these women better. Healthcare providers should consider their own, personal, and individual way of approaching older pregnant women, along with being updated and well-informed of all the risks related to AMA in order to be successful.

OTHER FACE OF THE COIN

The older age groups are often:
- Better educated
- Financially more secure
- Emotionally better prepared for pregnancy.

Several factors may influence women's perception of pregnancy risk including medical risk, psychological elements, characteristics of the risk, stage of pregnancy, and healthcare provider's opinion. Understanding these influential factors may help health professionals who care for pregnant women of AMA to gain insight into their perspectives on pregnancy risk and improve the effectiveness of risk communication strategies.[4]

REFERENCES

1. Odibo AO, Nelson D, Stamilio DM, et al. Advanced maternal age is an independent risk factor for intrauterine growth restriction. Am J Perinatol. 2006;23:325-8.
2. Salihu HM, Shumpert N, Slay M, et al. Childbearing beyond maternal age 50 and fetal outcomes in the United States. Obstet Gynecol. 2003;102:1006-14.
3. Ozalp S, Tanir HM, Sener T, et al. Health risks for early (< or =19) and late (> or =35) childbearing. Arch Gynecol Obstet. 2003;268:172-4.
4. Maheshwari A, Porter M, Shetty A, et al. Women's awareness and perceptions of delay in childbearing. Fertil Steril. 2008;90:1036-42.
5. Martin JA, Hamilton BE, Sutton PD, et al. Births: final data for 2004. Natl Vital Stat Rep. 2006;55:1-101.
6. Lampinen R, Vehviläinen-Julkunen K, Kankkunen P. A Review of Pregnancy in Women Over 35 Years of Age. Open Nurs J. 2009;3:33-8.
7. World Health Organization (WHO). (2016). New guidelines on antenatal care for a positive pregnancy experience. [online] Available from https://www.who.int/reproductivehealth/news/antenatal-care/en/. [Last accessed October, 2019].

Rh Isoimmunization

Meenakshi Barsaul Chauhan, Vani Malhotra

HISTORY

Landsteiner and Weiner discovered Rhesus factor in 1940. Anti-D was developed for maternal prophylaxis by Fin et al. in 1961 from the United Kingdom and Freda et al. in 1963 from the United States. The incidence of alloimmunization varies greatly among the populations. The overall incidence of alloimmunization has declined dramatically since last 1990s owing in part to immunoprophylaxis and smaller families. **Table 1** depicts the antigens responsible for alloimmunization.

Table 1: Antigens causing fetal hemolytic disease.

Common	Uncommon
Rhesus family: D, C, E, c, e Kell	JK (Kidd) Fy (Duffy) Kp S

PATHOPHYSIOLOGY AND RISKS

Rh isoimmunization occurs when the mother is Rh-negative and father is Rh-positive and the fetus is Rh-positive. Some fetal RBCs enter circulation of mother and IgM antibodies are produced but they cannot cross the placenta. IgGs are produced in 6 months, cross the placenta, bind to fetal red cells antigen, and cause hemolysis in Rh-positive fetus. Sensitization is more common during the third trimester and during childbirth. Fetal effects may be hemolytic anemia, erythroblastosis fetalis, hydrops fetalis, and kernicterus. **Algorithm 1** depicts the pathophysiology of Rh isoimmunization.

INVESTIGATIONS

The investigations and management of potential fetal hemolytic disease can be done by employing various methods, which detect antibodies either in maternal serum or are bound to fetal red blood cells (RBCs) as shown in **Algorithm 2**.

MANAGEMENT OF A NONSENSITIZED RH-NEGATIVE MOTHER

All the women attending the antenatal clinic should be checked for ABO Rh blood typing at the first antenatal visit and if found to be Rh-negative, indirect Coombs testing (ICT) is done at 18–20 weeks. If ICT test is negative, they are labeled as nonsensitized and if found to be positive, they are labeled as sensitized and managed accordingly. **Algorithm 3** depicts the management of a nonsensitized Rh-negative mother.

Management of Sensitized Rh-negative Women

Once an all-immunized woman is identified, the medical practitioner caring for antenatal women should estimate the risk of fetal hemolytic disease by noninvasive and invasive evaluation. The magnitude of fetal and neonatal disease typically progresses from one pregnancy to

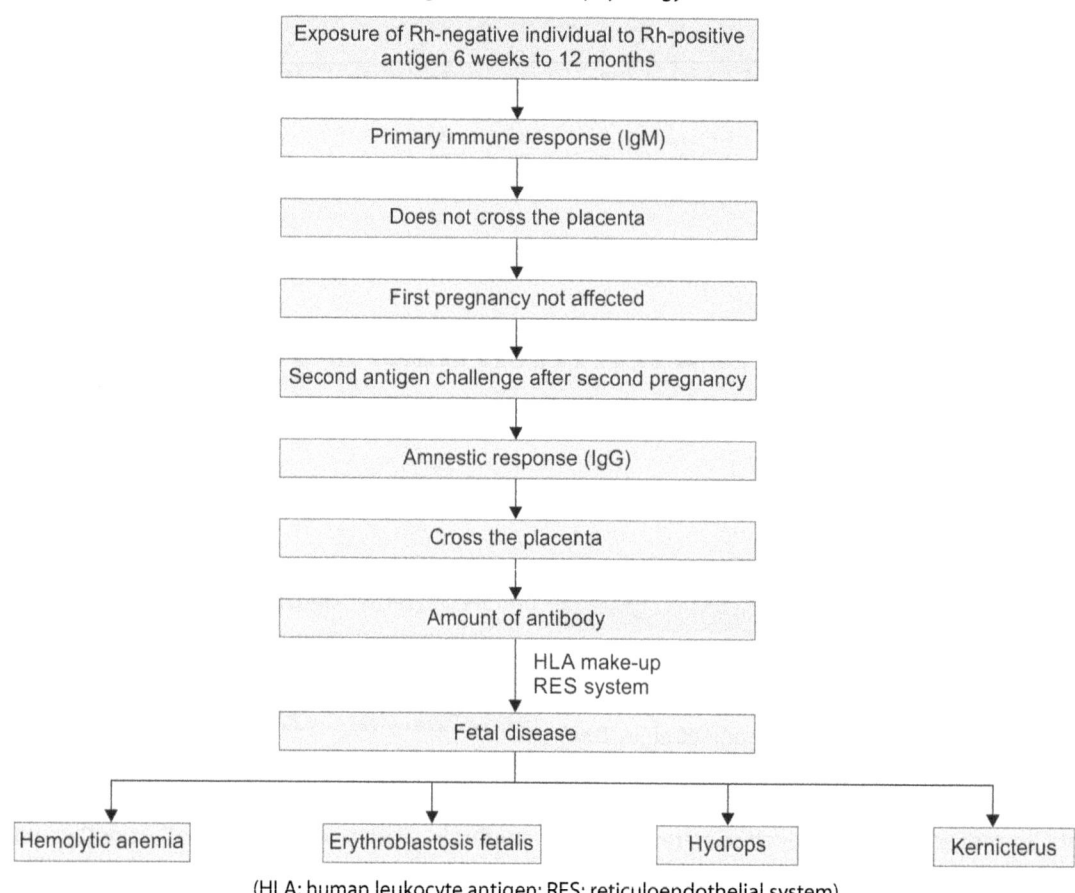

(HLA: human leukocyte antigen; RES: reticuloendothelial system)

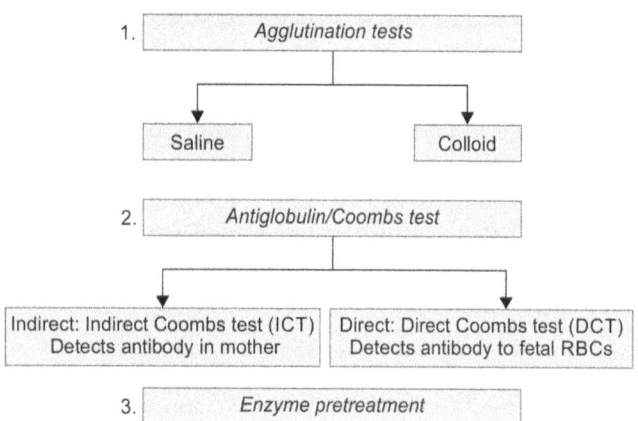

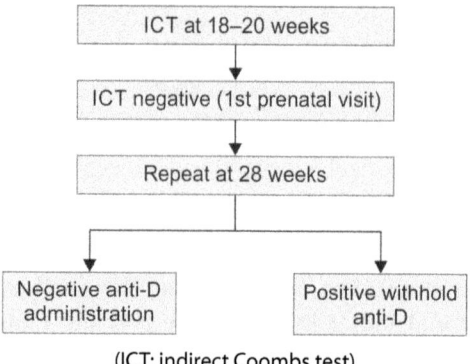

another. Management of a sensitized woman is shown in **Algorithm 4**. **Table 2** shows the indications for referral to a fetal medicine unit.

NONINVASIVE EVALUATION

Measurement of middle cerebral artery peak velocities is an excellent noninvasive tool for the monitoring of fetal

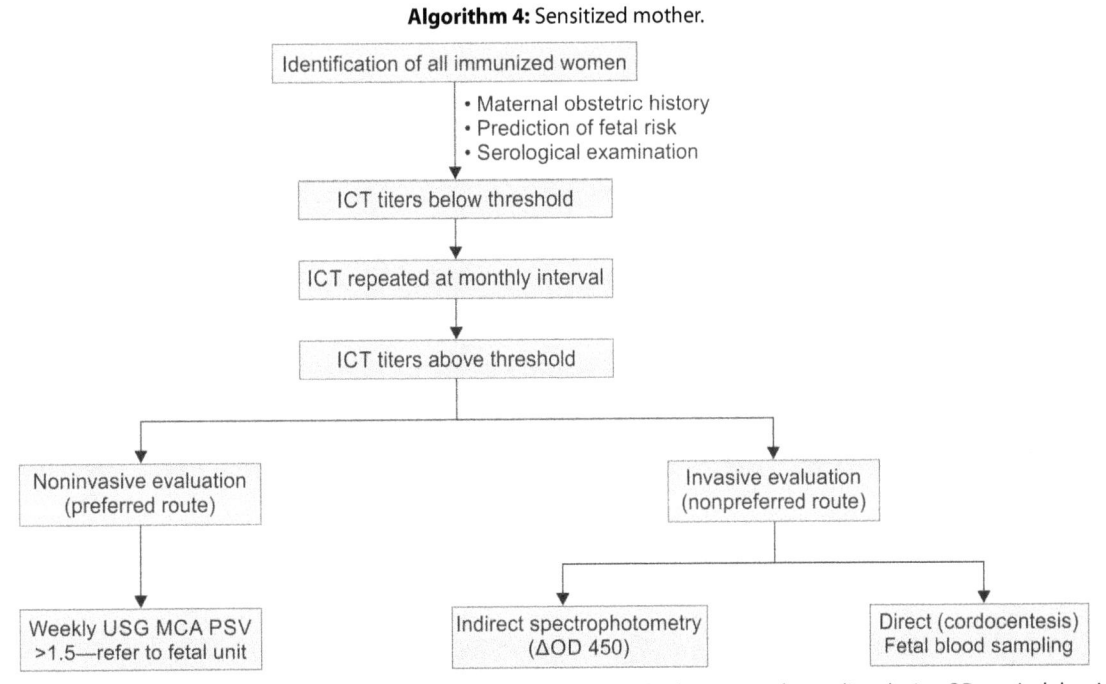

Algorithm 4: Sensitized mother.

(ICT: indirect Coombs test; USG: ultrasonography; MCA-PSV: middle cerebral artery-peak systolic velocity; OD: optical density)

Table 2: Indications for referral unit.

Refer to fetal unit	Referral to fetal unit
• Anti-D > 4 IU/mL • Anti-c > 7.5 IU/mL • Anti k—once detected • Anti E—once detected • Ab other that anti-d, anti-e, anti-k • >1.5 MoM	• Indirect Coombs testing titers above threshold • Rising antibody titers • USG features of fetal anemia • H/o unexplained severe neonatal jaundice/anemia requiring transfusion or exchange transfusion

(MoM: multiples of the median)

anemia and determines the timing of invasive fetal testing. Middle cerebral artery (MCA), peak systolic velocity (PSV) testing is predictive of moderate or severe fetal anemia with 100% sensitivity and a false-positive rate of 12%.[1] **Algorithms 5 and 6** show noninvasive evaluation and invasive evaluation, respectively, of a sensitized pregnancy which is the preferred route.

INDIRECT SPECTROPHOTOMETRY

The fetus with hemolytic anemia has elevated bilirubin levels and William Liley standardized the approach to utilize it for the management of fetal hemolytic disease.[2] He measured optical density of amniotic fluid obtained

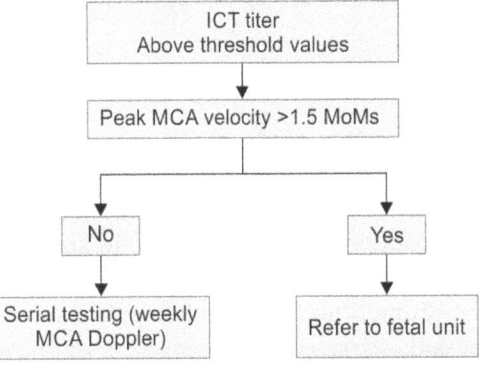

Algorithm 5: Noninvasive evaluation.

(ICT: indirect Coombs test; MCA: middle cerebral artery; MoM: multiples of the median)

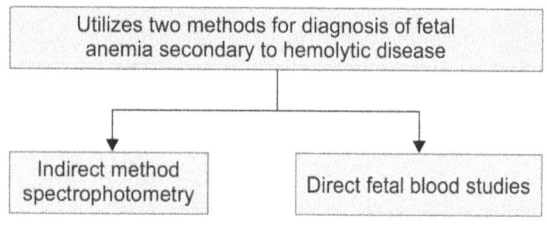

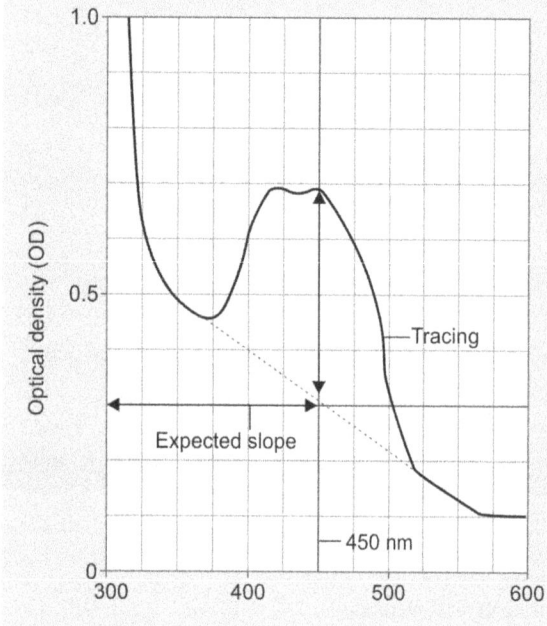

Fig. 1: Spectrophotometric analysis of amniotic fluid showing optical density difference at 450 nm wavelength with "deviation bulge" in Rh hemolytic disease.

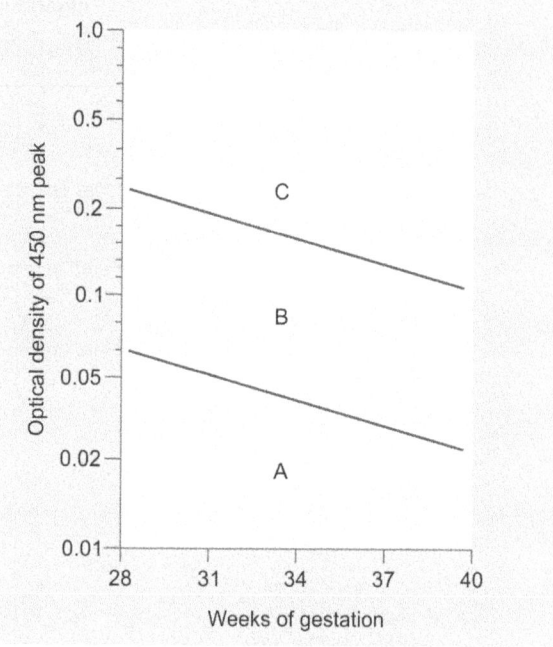

Fig. 2: Liley's graph to show severity of fetal hemolysis in Rh isoimmunization.

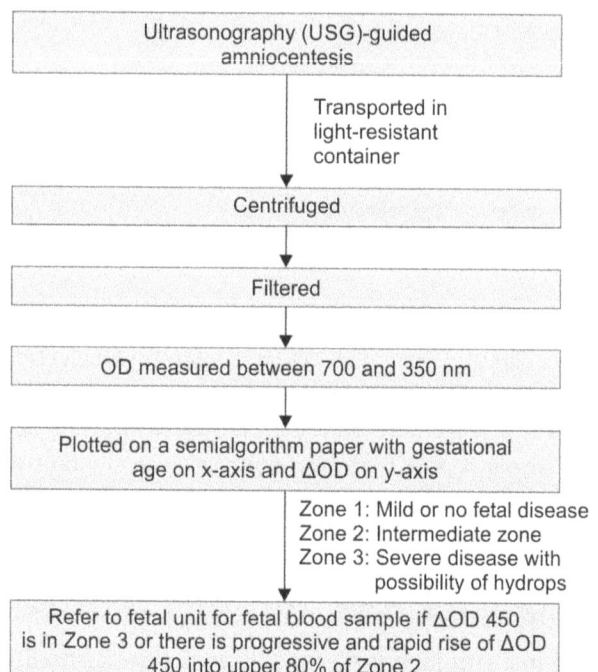

by amniocentesis, plotted it on a graph, and graded fetal hemolytic disease accordingly **(Figs. 1 and 2)**. **Algorithm 7** depicts this.

Direct Fetal Blood Studies

Fetal blood sampling is indicated when peak MCA velocity is >1.5 MoM or Liley chart shows an affected baby. It is only once the fetal anemia is detected that the fetal transfusion therapy should be employed, that too in an experienced center. **Algorithm 8** explains this mechanism. **Table 3** shows the formula for intravascular transfusion according to the gestational age.

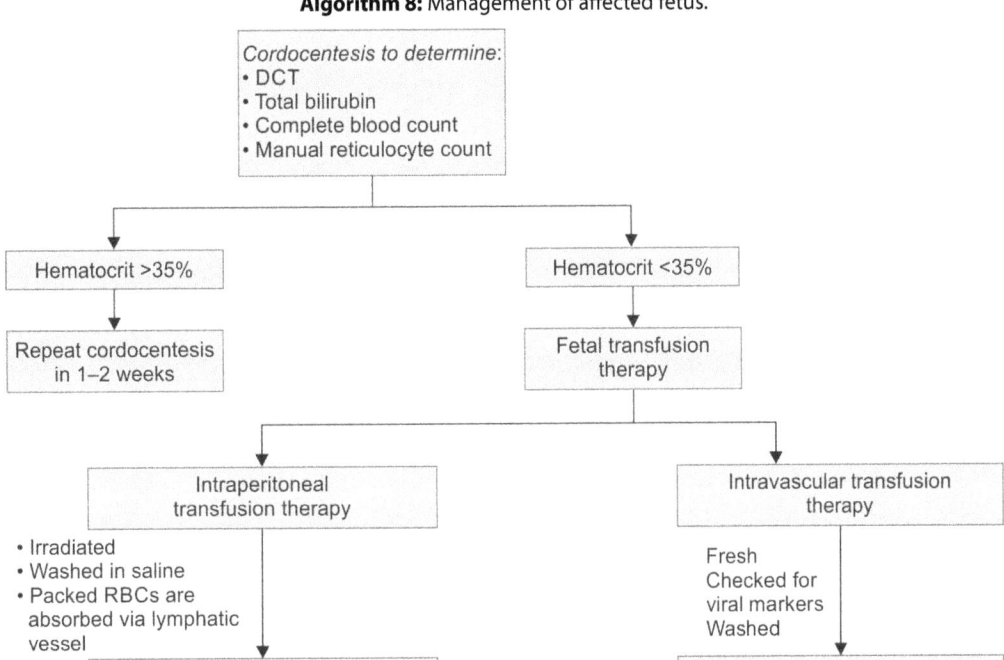

Algorithm 8: Management of affected fetus.

| Table 3: Intravascular transfusion according to gestational age.[5] ||
Gestational week	Volume of blood (mL)
<23	25–40
23–28	45–65
28–32	75–90
>32	100–120

Drawbacks

- Slow correction
- Risk of reducing cardiac return if intra-abdominal pressure high.

Timing of Delivery

Gestational age for delivery is decided after taking factors such as ICT titers, ΔOD 450, MCA values and hematocrit values into account. **Algorithm 9** depicts the timing of delivery.

PRECAUTIONS DURING DELIVERY

- Prophylactic ergometrine should be withheld after delivery.
- Early cord clamping of the umbilical cord.
- Length of the umbilical cord should be kept long.
- Manual removal of the placenta should be avoided.
- Avoid spillage of blood into peritoneal cavity.

Anti-D Immunoglobulin

- It has a half-life of 24 days, and a standard dose of 300 μg provides protection up to 12 weeks against exposure of 30 mL blood/15 mL of RBCs.
- Postpartum anti-D (PPAD) administration within 72 hours reduces the incidence of immunization by 90%.
- Routine antenatal anti-D prophylaxis (RAADP) at 28 weeks further reduces the incidence.[3]
- Also administered after chorionic villus sampling, amniocentesis, external cephalic version, abdominal trauma, antepartum hemorrhage.[4]

Algorithm 9: Plan of termination of pregnancy.

```
Timing of delivery
      ↓
   ICT titers
   ↙        ↘
Below critical value    Above critical value
   ↓                           ↓
Repeat titers           Do serial MCA Doppler
   ↓                    amniocentesis (ΔOD 450)
Remain below critical level        ↓
   ↓                    ┌──────────┴──────────┐
Delivery at term    Peak MCA >1.5 MoM    ΔOD 450 in affected zone
                     ↙      ↘              ↙      ↘
                    No      Yes           Yes      No
                               ↓           ↓        ↓
                          Cordocentesis   Continue monitoring
                            ↙       ↘
                   Hematocrit <30%  Fetal hematocrit >30%
```

Weekly MCA: MCA <1.5 MoM → Delivered at 38 weeks

IU transfusion
Repeat till 34 weeks
MCA >1.5 MoM 34 weeks
↓
Amniocentesis for ΔOD in lung maturity

- Mature ΔOD 450 not in affected zone → Induce delivery at 38 weeks
- Mature ΔOD 450 in affected zone → Induced
- Immature ΔOD 450 not in affected zone → Repeat amnio in 10–14 days
- Immature ΔOD 450 in affected zone → Steroids

(ICT: indirect Coombs test; MCA: middle cerebral artery; MoM: multiples of the median; OD: optical density)

- Anti-D is not required after spontaneous abortions.
- Recommended after induced and ectopic pregnancy.
- Withheld if the father is RH negative, paternity not disputed, and last administration was <21 days.

NEONATAL MANAGEMENT

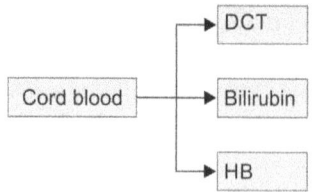

- Clinical assessment of neurobehavioral state
- Regular assessment of bilirubin and Hb levels till discharge
- Regular breastfeeding
- Look for signs of dehydration.
- Consider for phototherapy/exchange transfusion.

LONG-TERM FUTURE RISK

- Referral for early assessment of fetal medicine unit
- No maternal risk of adverse health consequences
- Anemia persisting for a few weeks
- Late anemia.

PREPREGNANCY

- Routine screening not indicated
- Women with clinically significant red cell antibodies informed about maternal and fetal complications.

RECENT DEVELOPMENT

Detection of fetal RhD status by using a free fetal DNA in maternal blood can be used as a new noninvasive marker.[6]

REFERENCES

1. Mari G, Deter RL, Carpenter RL, et al. Noninvasive diagnosis by Doppler ultrasonography of fetal anemia due to maternal red-cell alloimmunisation. Collaborative Group for Doppler Assessment of the Blood Velocity in Anemic Fetuses. N Engl J Med. 2000;342:9-14.
2. Liley AW. Errors in the assessment of hematolytic disease from amniotic fluid. Am J Obstet Gynecol. 1963;86:485-94.
3. American College of Obstetricians and Gynecologists. Prevention of Rh-D Cell Immunisation. Clinical Management Guideline no 4, May 1999. Washington, US: American College of Obstetricians and Gynecologists.
4. NICE. Routine Antenatal Anti-D Prophylaxis for Women who are Rhesus D Negative: NIC Technology Appraisal Guidance. London, UK: NICE; 2008.
5. Weiner CP, Pelzer CD, Heilskov J, et al. The effect of intravascular transfusion on umbilical venous pressure in anaemic fetuses with and without hydrops. Am J Obstet Gynecol. 1989;161:149E.
6. Gonec G, Isci H, Yigiter AB, et al. Non-invasive prenatal diagnosis of fetal RhD by using free fetal DNA. Clin Exp Obstet Gynaecol. 2015;42:344-6.

Chapter 12

H1N1 Infection in Pregnancy

Suparna Grover, Ajay Chhabra

INTRODUCTION

Influenza is a viral infection of the lungs that commonly presents as a seasonal epidemic and every few decades as a pandemic.

Pregnant women are not only at more risk of being infected by influenza virus but they are—four to five times more prone to suffering significant morbidity as well.[1,2] For the fetus also, adverse pregnancy outcomes such as abortions, preterm labor, and fetal distress are more common in those suffering from severe influenza infection during pregnancy.[1,3]

EPIDEMIOLOGY OF H1N1 INFECTION

Influenza viruses are mainly of three types based on their M capsid protein and the nucleoprotein. Among them, type A and type B are the ones responsible for most of the influenza epidemics in human population while type C is less common in humans and only causes sporadic cases of mild respiratory infection. Type A influenza viruses are further classified in many subtypes based on the surface glycoproteins hemagglutinin [H] and neuraminidase [N], and they tend to undergo mutations.

The last pandemic in 2009 was caused by H1N1 virus and was called swine flu because the virus was believed to have originated in pigs containing genes from different avian, swine, and human influenza strains causing a genetic re-assortment that created a new virus to which human population had no pre-existent immunity. This virus attacked younger population and had the potential to cause serious lower respiratory infection although a mild-to-moderate respiratory infection was the most common manifestation. The pandemic was declared over in 2010 and presently this virus persists globally as a causative agent for seasonal epidemics as well as sporadic cases. H1N1 infection in pregnancy is significant as epidemiological evidence gathered during pandemics has established that there is significantly higher morbidity as well as mortality in pregnant women infected by this virus, more so in the third trimester.[2,3] Pregnancies complicated by severe infection are also associated with a higher incidence of adverse pregnancy outcomes.[2,3] The epidemiologic characteristics of influenza virus are described in **Table 1**.

Table 1: Epidemiology of influenza infection.

| Causative agent: *Orthomyxoviridae influenza virus* | Type A | • Infects man, pigs, and birds
• Serotypes based on hemagglutinin [H] and neuraminidase [N]
• Undergoes mutations frequently
• *Antigenic drift*: Mutation within genome leading to new seasonal strain
• *Antigenic shift*: Re-assortment among genetic material of different subtypes leading to a new virus capable of causing pandemic |

Contd...

Contd...

	Type B	• Infects humans • No serotypes • Infrequent mutations • Causes epidemics and seasonal influenza
	Type C	• Mild respiratory disease • No mutations
Transmission		• Droplets from infected person • Fomites • Close contact like hand shaking
Incubation period		1–4 days
Communicability		• From onset of clinical disease up to 7 days • Children and immunocompromised patients may spread the virus longer
Seasonality		• Tropics/subtropics: rainy season • Temperate zones: winters

RISK FACTORS IN PREGNANCY

- Third trimester[2]
- Maternal smoking
- Chronic lung diseases such as asthma, chronic obstructive pulmonary disease (COPD), cystic fibrosis
- Immunodeficiency disorders, hemoglobinopathies
- Diabetes mellitus, renal disease, malignancy.

PATHOLOGY

Both influenza strains, i.e. type A and type B, have two surface glycoproteins—hemagglutinin and neuraminidase—that play a critical role in its pathogenesis (**Fig. 1**). The former attaches the virus to sialic acid receptors on host cell membrane and has a tropism for cells lining the respiratory tract and the later has a role in viral penetration as well as in the release of virus from infected cells once the virus has utilized cell machinery for replication of its genetic material.

Once the new virions leave the host cells, it leads to apoptosis of the host cell as well as an innate inflammatory response in order to check the spread of virus. This inflammatory response may be so exaggerated that it itself leads to damage of host cells lining the respiratory tract as well as widespread endothelial damage. Widespread alveolar damage, pulmonary edema, and acute respiratory

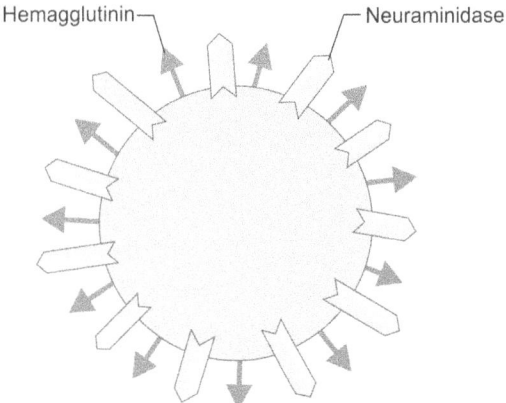

Fig. 1: Structure of H1N1 virus.

distress syndrome are the pathological findings in those suffering the most severe disease (**Fig. 2**). In mild-to-moderate cases, there may be mild bronchiolitis and alveolitis that start healing once the virus is cleared by innate and humoral immune response but during this recovery period, the respiratory tract remains prone to secondary bacterial infections.

CAUSES OF DEATH

- Respiratory failure
- Refractory shock
- Multiple organ dysfunction.

CLINICAL PRESENTATION

The characteristic feature of influenza virus is the rapid, almost sudden onset of symptoms (**Table 2**).[1]

CATEGORIZATION OF INFLUENZA[4]

Pregnant state automatically categorizes the patient into category B or above, i.e. category C (**Table 3**).

INVESTIGATIONS

- *Routine investigations:* Biochemical, hematological, microbiological, and radiological tests as dictated by the patient's general condition.
- *Confirmation:*
  - Real-time RT-PCR or
  - Isolation in a viral culture, or
  - Four times increase in virus-specific antibodies.

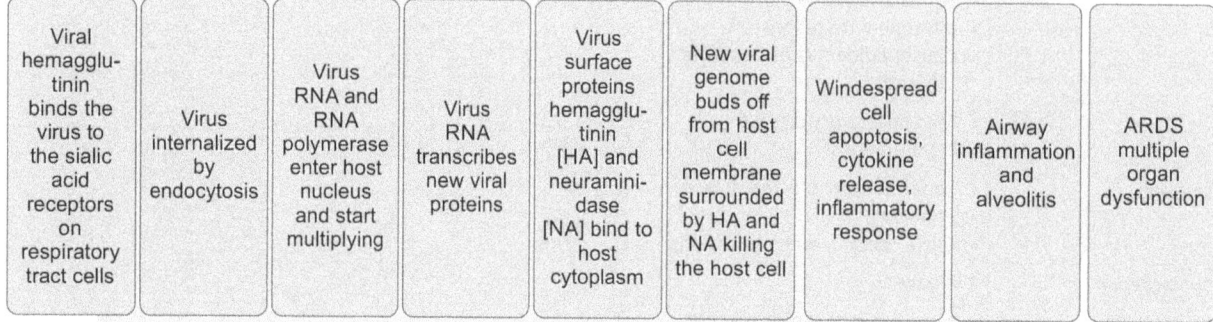

Fig. 2: Pathogenesis of H1N1 virus.

Table 2: Symptoms of influenza virus.

Influenza-like illness (ILI)	Gastrointestinal symptoms	Severe respiratory disease
• Fever • Cough • Sore throat • Coryza • Myalgia • Headache	• Vomiting • Diarrhea	• Breathlessness • Chest pain • Tachypnea • Sputum mixed with blood • Drowsiness • Hypotension • Cyanosis

Table 3: Categorization of H1N1 infection.[4]

Category A	Category B	Category C

Mild fever plus cough/sore throat with or without bodyache, headache, diarrhea and vomiting	• Signs and symptoms mentioned under Category-A plus high grade fever and severe sore throat
	• Signs and symptoms mentioned under Category-A individuals having one or more of the following high-risk conditions
	  – Children with predisposing risk factors
	  – Pregnant women
	  – Persons aged 65 years or older
	  – Patients with lung diseases, heart disease, liver disease, kidney disease, blood disorders, diabetes, neurological disorders, cancer and HIV/AIDS
	  – Patients on long-term cortisone therapy
		• Signs and symptoms mentioned under Category-A and B plus any of the following:
		  – Breathlessness, chest pain, drowsiness, fall in blood pressure, sputum mixed with blood, bluish discoloration of nails
		  – Children with influenza like illness who had a severe disease as manifested by the red flag signs (Somnolence, high and persistent fever, inability to feed well, convulsions, shortness of breath, difficulty in breathing, etc.)
		  – Worsening of underlying chronic conditions

- *Clinical specimens:* Respiratory secretions such as throat swab, nasopharyngeal swab, and tracheal secretions (in patients who are intubated). The specimen should be collected by technically trained personnel only and transported to central laboratories assigned by government with proper clinical record of the patient.

MANAGEMENT OF INFLUENZA IN PREGNANCY

There are three important aspects in the management of influenza in pregnancy **(Algorithm 1)**.

Prevention

Considering the serious risk to both maternal and fetal well-being, the role of prevention, especially during seasonal outbreak or pandemic, cannot be overstressed.

- *Vaccination:* Trivalent inactivated seasonal influenza vaccine is universally recommended for all pregnant women, irrespective of the period of gestation, as it provides protection not only to the women during pregnancy but also to their newborns up to 6 months. The Indian Government has recommended the following influenza vaccine for the period 2017–2018[5]:
  - An A/Michigan/45/2015 (H1N1) pdm09-like virus;
  - An A/Hong Kong/4801/2014 (H3N2)-like virus; and
  - A B/Brisbane/60/2008-like virus.
- *Timing of vaccination:*
  - One month before the start of the influenza season
  - The usual season of influenza in most parts of India is the monsoon season. In Central and Northern India, the peak incidence is in winter months (January to March).

WHO has recommended the following composition for tetravalent influenza vaccines for use in the northern hemisphere in 2018–2019[6]:
- An A/Michigan/45/2015 (H1N1) pdm09-like virus,
- An A/Singapore/INFIMH-16-0019/2016 (H3N2)-like virus,
- A B/Colorado/06/2017-like virus, and
- A B/Phuket/3073/2013-like virus.

It is recommended that trivalent vaccines should contain the B/Colorado/06/2017-like virus, of the B/Victoria/2/87-lineage.

The Government of India (GoI) is yet to issue an update on the same.

- *General measures:* Even after adequate matching, vaccine efficacy is not more than 80%[5] and considering the risk involved, all pregnant women should take the following precautions:
  - Pregnant women should avoid:
    - Crowded places, especially during community epidemics
    - Providing care for those with suspected influenza infection
    - Touching mouth and nose.

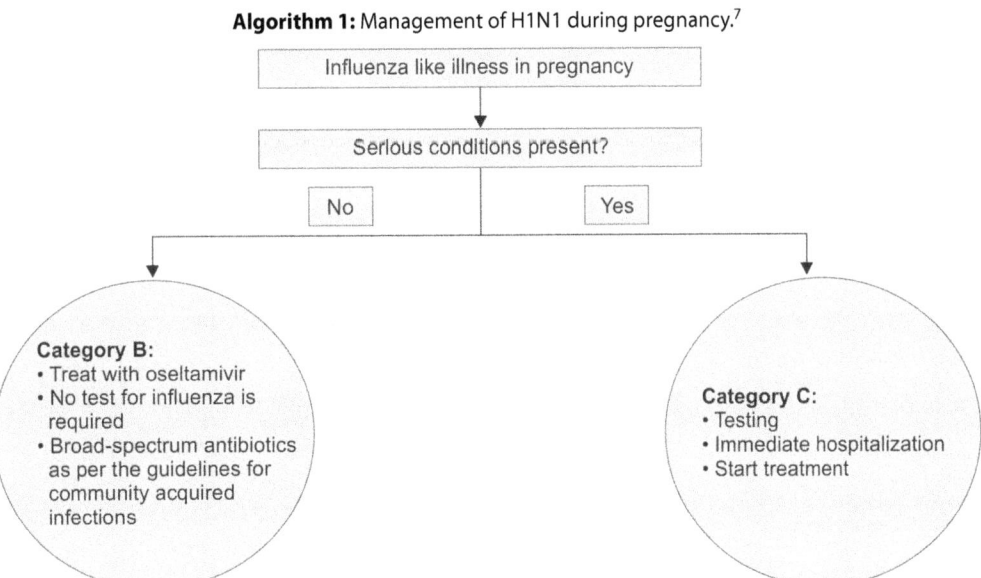

Algorithm 1: Management of H1N1 during pregnancy.[7]

- Washing hands with water and soap or alcohol-based hand sanitizer frequently.
- Soiled surfaces should be cleaned/disinfected to keep the environment free from the virus.
- Not involving any person with respiratory symptoms in care for a pregnant woman or a mother and newborn baby.
- Breastfeeding should be started within an hour of childbirth and it should be done exclusively and frequently.

Timely Diagnosis, Classification and Treatment

The clinical course and prognosis depend a lot on timely starting the pharmaceutical management on clinical suspicion without waiting for confirmatory tests.

- In the absence of symptoms of a severe disease, the patient is considered category B and oseltamivir is started in a dose of 75 mg twice a day for 5 days without confirming the diagnosis (**Algorithm 2**).
- In category C cases, immediate hospitalization, starting oseltamivir and supportive therapy is required. Oseltamivir may need to be continued for longer than 5 days in these patients (**Algorithm 3**).

If women have not been vaccinated, vaccination should be recommended soon after they have recovered, to protect them against the other strains that are circulating.[7]

Management during Labor and Prevention of Spread of Infection

Management during labor and prevention of spread of infection to newborn, healthcare providers, and community require strict adherence to infection control practices (**Table 4**).

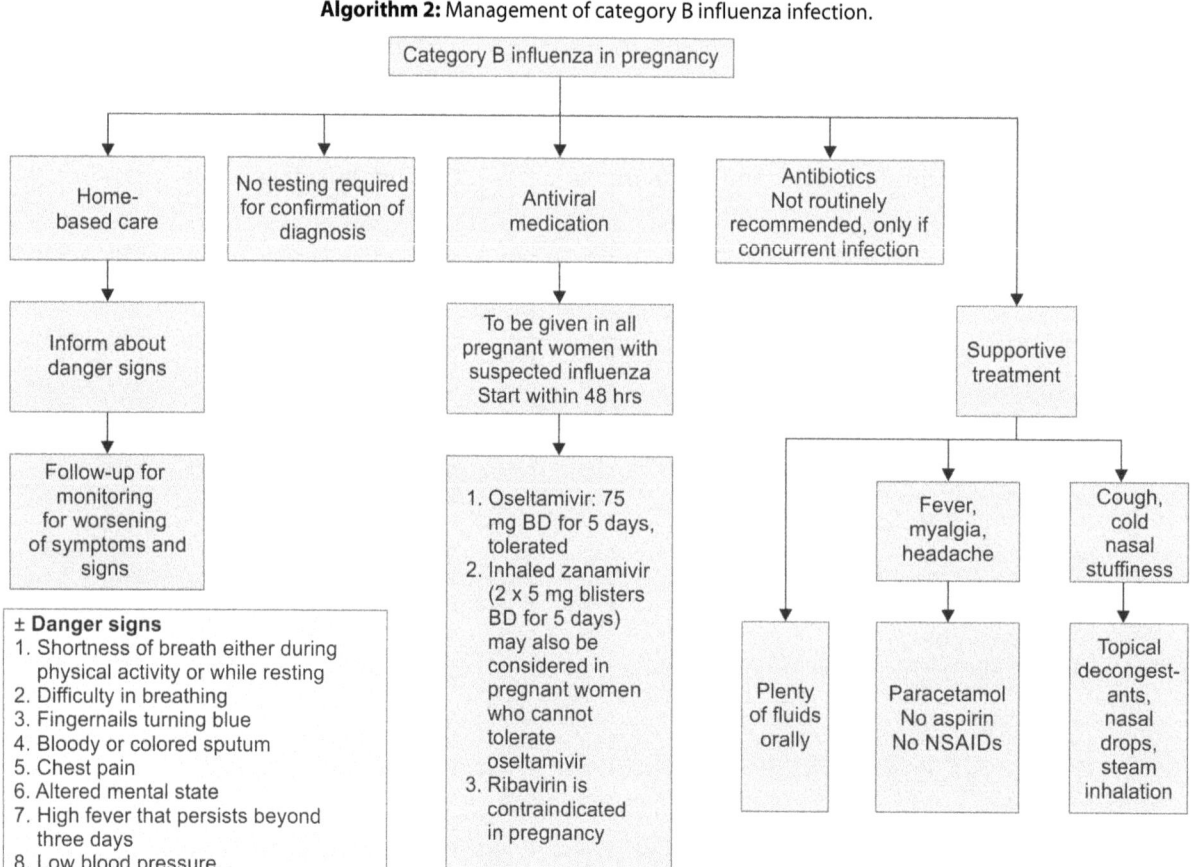

Algorithm 2: Management of category B influenza infection.

Algorithm 3: Management of category C infection.

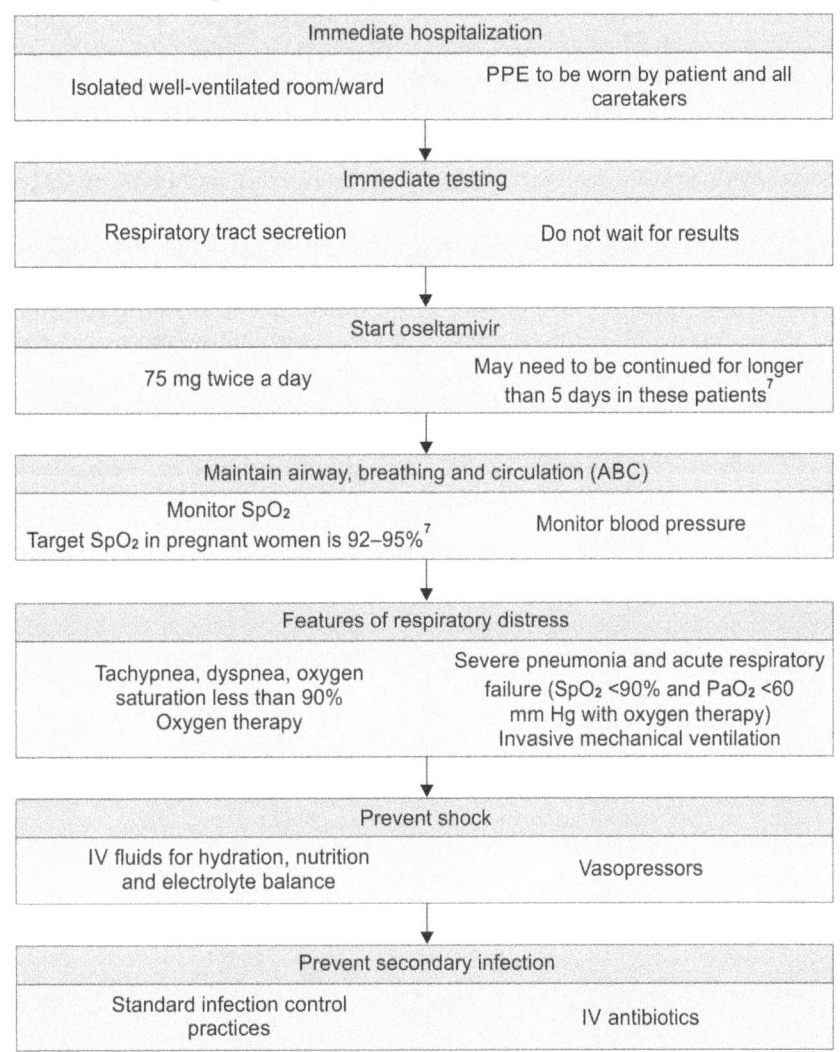

Table 4: Management during labor for a pregnant woman infected with influenza.

Obstetric care	Prevention of spread of infection
• Delivery in an isolated, well-ventilated room • Both patient and healthcare providers to wear masks • In case of preterm labor, corticosteroids for fetal lung maturation can be given in routine doses • Tocolytics causing hypotension should be used in a very guarded manner • Risk of fetal distress and operative interference is higher • In a severely sick patient, decision for lower segment cesarean section (LSCS) should be taken in discussion with anesthetist and intensivist *Prevention of the newborn* Rooming-in of the newborn with the mother and early and exclusive breastfeeding is recommended when all of the following criteria are met[8]: • The mother has received antiviral drugs for at least 2 days • The mother is afebrile for 24 hours without using paracetamol • The mother understands and follows respiratory hygiene	• Admission and delivery in an isolated room • Restricted entry in the room • Reinforce standard infection control precautions • Both patient and healthcare providers to wear masks • Triple-layer surgical masks are to be worn by all personnel involved in transport, care, and delivery of the patient. N 95 Respirator[9] masks are required for collection of respiratory samples and for performing aerosol producing procedures such as nebulization or bronchoscopy • Strict adherence to respiratory etiquette, i.e. covering their nose and mouth when sneezing and coughing. A disposable tissue paper should be preferred over cloth. Hands must be washed after disposal of tissue in a covered bin • Personal protection equipment (triple-layered masks, eye covers, gowns, gloves, head-cap, and shoe cover) should be used during delivery • Standard biomedical waste disposal protocol should be strictly adhered to • Use of HEPA filters[7] on expiratory ports of the ventilators helps reduce spread of infection • Antiviral prophylaxis to accidently exposed unvaccinated healthcare personnel

REFERENCES

1. World Health Organization. (2010). Pregnancy and pandemic influenza A (H1N1) 2009: Information for programme managers and clinicians. [online] Available from: https://www.google.co.in/url?sa=t&rct=j&q=&esrc=s&source=web&cd=1&cad=rja&uact=8&ved=0ahUKEwiBtN63y6XcAhWEvo8KHb-lDSsQFggnMAA&url=http%3A%2F%2Fwww.who.int%2Fcsr%2Fresources%2Fpublications%2Fswineflu%2Fh1n1_guidance_pregnancy.pdf&usg=AOvVaw0nWUOysgBp5vjkZ0vJVZth [Last accessed on September, 2019].
2. ANZIC Group. Critical illness due to 2009 A/H1N1 influenza in pregnant and postpartum women: population based cohort study. BMJ. 2010;340:c1279.
3. Creanga AA, Johnson TF, Graitcer SB, et al. Severity of 2009 pandemic influenza A (H1N1) virus infection in pregnant women. Obstet Gynecol. 2010;115:717-26.
4. Ministry of Health & Family Welfare. (2016). Seasonal Influenza Guidelines on categorization of Seasonal Influenza cases during screening for home isolation, testing, treatment and hospitalization [online]. Available from: https://mohfw.gov.in/media/disease-alerts/Seasonal-Influenza/technical-guidelines [Last accessed on November, 2019].
5. Ministry of Health and Family Welfare. (2017). Seasonal influenza: guidelines for vaccination with influenza vaccine. [online] Available from: https://mohfw.gov.in/media/disease-alerts/Seasonal-Influenza/technical-guidelines [Last accessed on November, 2019].
6. World Health Organization. (2018). Recommended composition of influenza virus vaccines for use in the 2018–2019 northern hemisphere influenza season. [online] Available from: http://www.who.int/influenza/vaccines/virus/recommendations/201802_recommendation.pdf?ua=1 [Last accessed on September, 2019].
7. Ministry of Health and Family Welfare. (2016). Clinical management protocol for seasonal influenza. [online] Available from:https://mohfw.gov.in/media/disease-alerts/Seasonal-Influenza/technical-guidelines [Last accessed on November, 2019].
8. Federation of Obstetrics and Gynaecological Societies of India. (2014). FOGSI consensus statement for H1N1 in pregnancy. [online] Available from: https://www.google.co.in/url?sa=t&rct=j&q=&esrc=s&source=web&cd=3&cad=rja&uact=8&ved=0ahUKEwiBtN63y6XcAhWEvo8KHb-lDSsQFgg6MAI&url=http%3A%2F%2Fwww.fogsi.org%2Fwp-content%2Fuploads%2F2015%2F11%2Fh1n1_in_pregnancy.pdf&usg=AOvVaw2LAQ-jKsl3edc-yRQdqxJQ [Last accessed on September, 2019].
9. Ministry of Health and Family Welfare. (2016). Seasonal influenza guidelines on use of masks for health care workers, patients and members of public. [online] Available from: http://164.100.158.44/showfile.php?lid=3092 [Last accessed on May, 2018].

Chapter 13

Zika Virus

Manishi Mittal

INTRODUCTION

The Zika virus (ZIKV) is an arbovirus that came into global prominence in 2015, after reports of microcephaly in babies born to infected mothers. It is a ribonucleic acid (RNA) virus (Flaviviridae family) related to the yellow fever, dengue, West Nile, and Japanese encephalitis viruses **(Fig. 1)**. The World Health Organization (WHO), declared ZIKV disease to be a Public Health Emergency of International Concern in 2016.

EPIDEMIOLOGY

Vector surveillance for ZIKV was started by the Indian Council of Medical Research (ICMR) in different areas from 2016 onward, but no positive results have yet been obtained. These findings show low level of transmission in India but the potential of spread is high **(Figs. 2 and 3)**.

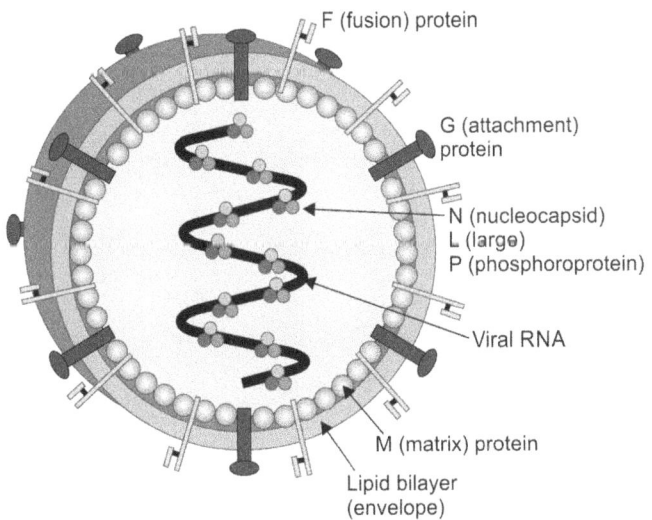

Fig. 1: Structure of Zika virus.

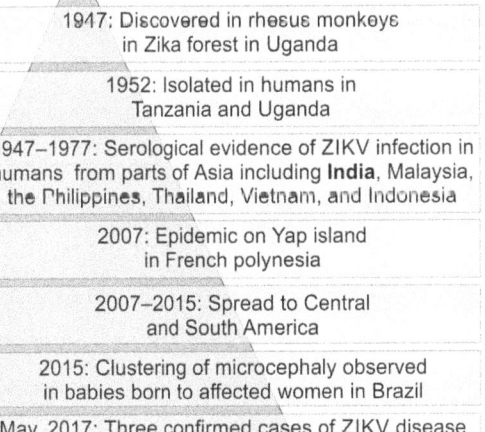

Fig. 2: Widening spread of Zika virus (ZIKV) infection.

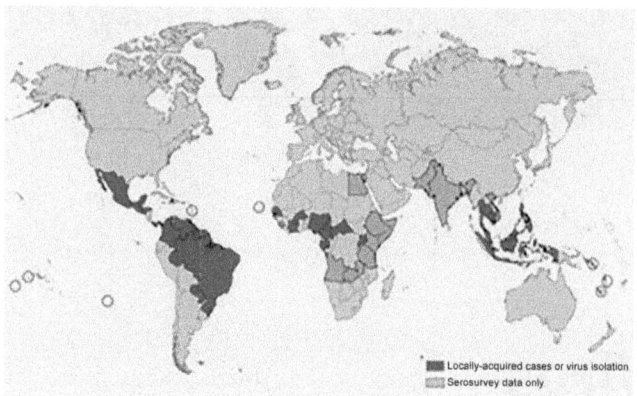

Fig. 3: Global spread of Zika virus (ZIKV) infection.

DYNAMICS OF TRANSMISSION

The Aedes group of mosquitoes is the vector for ZIKV; primarily *Aedes aegypti* and *Aedes albopictus* in Asia **(Fig. 4)**.[1]

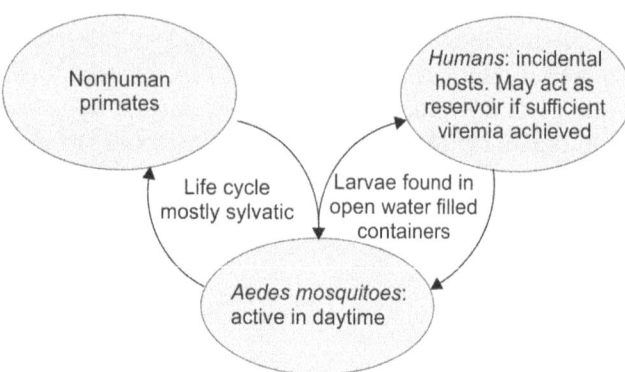

Fig. 4: Life cycle of Zika virus (ZIKV).[2]

Stipulated Modes of Transmission

- Bite of an affected mosquito (most common). Incubation period is around 3–12 days.
- *Maternal–fetal transmission*: Resulting in congenital anomalies.
- Blood transfusion and laboratory exposure.
- Sexual transmission.
- No reports of transmission from affected patients to healthcare workers or other patients during hospitalization, or due to organ and tissue transplantation.
- ZIKV detected in body fluids such as blood, amniotic fluid, urine, saliva, breast milk, and genital fluids. Whether these can act as a mode of spread is still unknown.

CLINICAL FEATURES

Infection with ZIKV usually goes undetected as only around 20% people show any signs, which are mostly mild and self-limiting **(Algorithm 1)**.[3] Confusion about the diagnosis may occur due to similarity with other diseases spread by *Aedes* mosquitoes like dengue and chikungunya. Few features can distinguish them **(Figs. 5 and 6, Table 1)**.

DIAGNOSIS

Zika virus disease can be easily missed in India due to widespread prevalence of dengue and chikungunya, leading to delayed clinical suspicion by clinicians. Moreover, confirmation can be done by only a few laboratories.

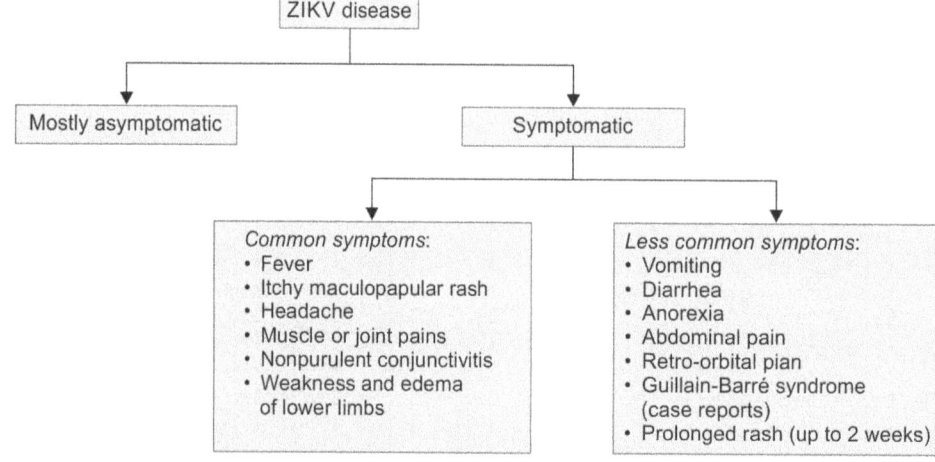

Algorithm 1: Clinical features of Zika virus (ZIKV) disease.

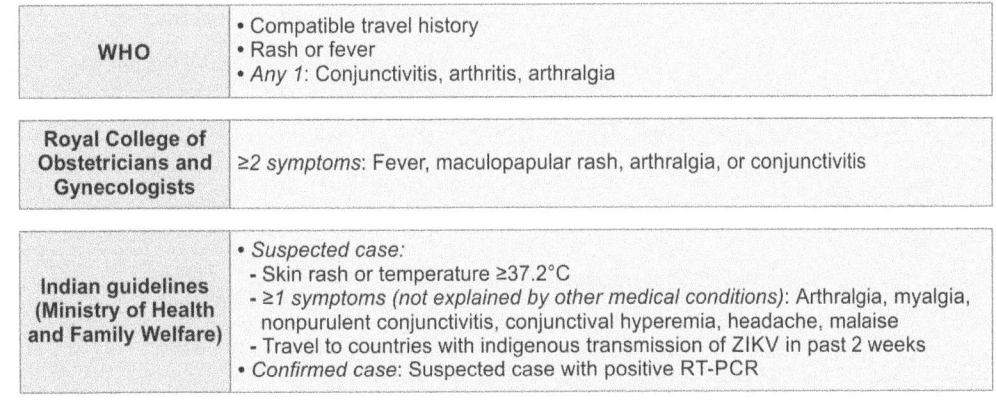

WHO	• Compatible travel history • Rash or fever • *Any 1*: Conjunctivitis, arthritis, arthralgia
Royal College of Obstetricians and Gynecologists	≥2 *symptoms*: Fever, maculopapular rash, arthralgia, or conjunctivitis

Indian guidelines (Ministry of Health and Family Welfare)	• *Suspected case:*
	  - Skin rash or temperature ≥37.2°C
	  - ≥1 symptoms *(not explained by other medical conditions)*: Arthralgia, myalgia, nonpurulent conjunctivitis, conjunctival hyperemia, headache, malaise
	  - Travel to countries with indigenous transmission of ZIKV in past 2 weeks
	• *Confirmed case*: Suspected case with positive RT-PCR

Fig. 5: Case definitions of Zika virus (ZIKV) disease.
(RT-PCR: reverse transcriptase polymerase chain reaction)

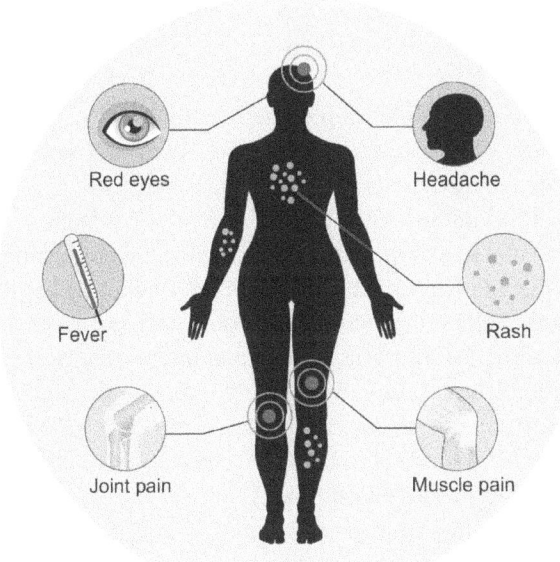

Fig. 6: Common symptoms of Zika virus (ZIKV) disease.

Table 1: Differentiation of clinical features of three common virus infections.[4]

Symptoms	Dengue	Chikungunya	Zika
Fever	++++	+++	+++
Muscle and joint pains	+++	++++	++
Limb edema	-	-	++
Maculopapular rash	++	++	+++
Retro-orbital pain	++	+	++
Conjunctival infection	-	+	+++
Lymph node enlargement	++	++	+
Hepatomegaly	-	+++	-
Fall in leukocyte and platelet count	+++	+++	-
Hemorrhage	+	-	-

However, diagnosis is important as seroprevalence of ZIKV antibody is high in Asian population. Furthermore, the distribution of the virus is gradually widening.

In India, the National Institute of Virology (NIV) at Pune and National Centre for Disease Control (NCDC) at Delhi are performing diagnosis of ZIKV infection. Further 25 laboratories have been trained **(Algorithm 2)**.

The reverse transcriptase-polymerase chain reaction (RT-PCR) is the most specific and validated test. It is done on acute-phase serum samples (within 1 week of onset of illness) to detect viral RNA. Additionally, it can be done using amniotic fluid and other fluid and tissues. As the virus may get cleared after a week of onset of symptoms, a negative RT-PCR after that time would not exclude ZIKV disease. The virus may stay in urine for few days longer than in serum.[5]

ZIKA VIRUS IN PREGNANCY

Zika virus has assumed prominence due to its potential to cause congenital malformations, especially microcephaly. Therefore, all clinicians should keep an open mind when an antenatal patient presents with ZIKV like illness. In regions endemic for the virus, around 1% of pregnant women getting infected in the first-trimester bear microcephalic babies. Moreover, roughly 20% of pregnancies may suffer from other malformations **(Algorithm 3)**. Vertical transmission of ZIKV has been documented in all three trimesters.[5]

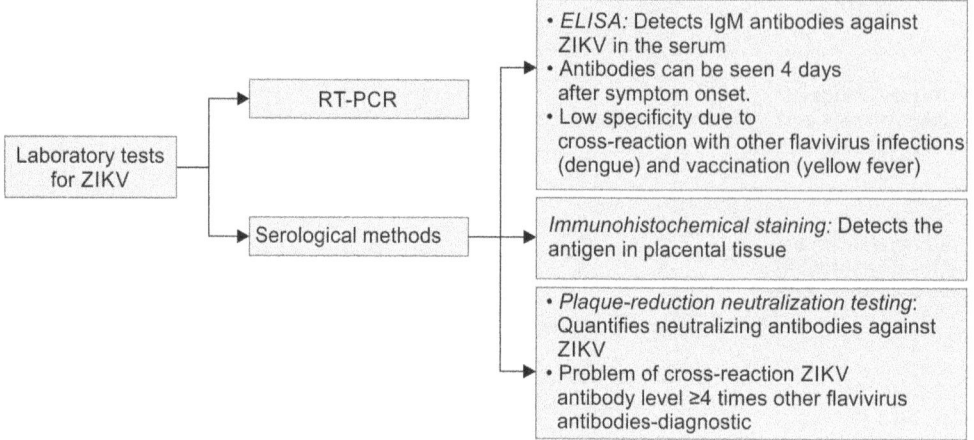

Algorithm 2: Different laboratory tests available for Zika virus (ZIKV) infection.

(IgM: immunoglobulin M; RT-PCR: reverse transcriptase polymerase chain reaction; ZIKV: Zika virus)

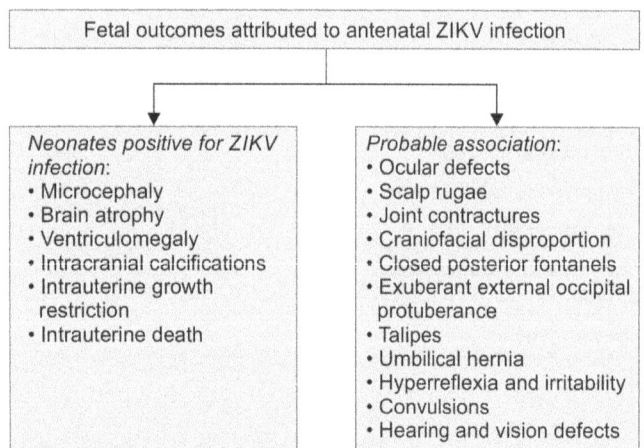

Algorithm 3: Abnormalities associated with Zika virus (ZIKV) infection.[6]

(ZIKV: Zika virus)

Unknown Factors for Congenital Zika Virus Infection

- Rate of transmission and the risk of malformation in infected fetus.
- Effect of immunodeficient state of pregnancy on susceptibility to infection or severity of the disease.
- Effect of viral load, or timing or severity of symptoms (risk may be highest in the first trimester).[7]

WHO (2016): "Causal relationship between ZIKV infection, birth defects, and neurological syndromes has not been established, but is strongly suspected."

- No standard definition of microcephaly.
- *Many other causes:* Genetic disorders and antenatal exposure to agents like alcohol and mercury.
- In the region with highest risk of ZIKV infection, the calculated absolute risk of having a malformed baby is 4 per 1,000 live births, that is, 99.6% of women in areas with high prevalence of ZIKV could have normal baby.[8]

Routine testing is not recommended in asymptomatic pregnant women. However, if ZIKV infection is suspected, diagnosis needs to be confirmed by RT-PCR of serum. Further testing needs to be done to see effect on the fetus **(Algorithms 4 and 5 and Box 1)**.

Centers for Disease Control (CDC), USA recommendations regarding which pregnant women to be tested:
- Symptomatic women with a history of possible exposure to ZIKV.
- Asymptomatic women with possible exposure to ZIKV (travel to endemic area or unprotected intercourse with an infected partner).
- Asymptomatic women with ongoing risk of ZIKV exposure.

The CDC recommendation for the management of women with suspected ZIKV infection has been discussed in **Algorithm 6**.

PREVENTION OF ZIKA VIRUS INFECTION

At present, there is no vaccine or medication available for prevention of infection with ZIKV. Guidelines available

Algorithm 4: Laboratory tests for congenital Zika virus (ZIKV) infection.

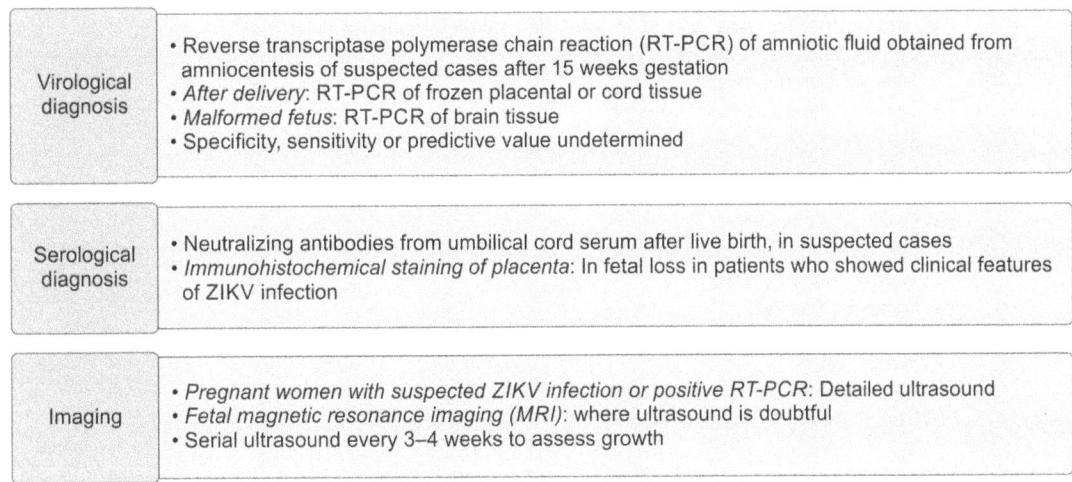

(RT-PCR: reverse transcriptase polymerase chain reaction; ZIKV: Zika virus)

Algorithm 5: Diagnosis of Zika virus (ZIKV) disease in pregnant women.

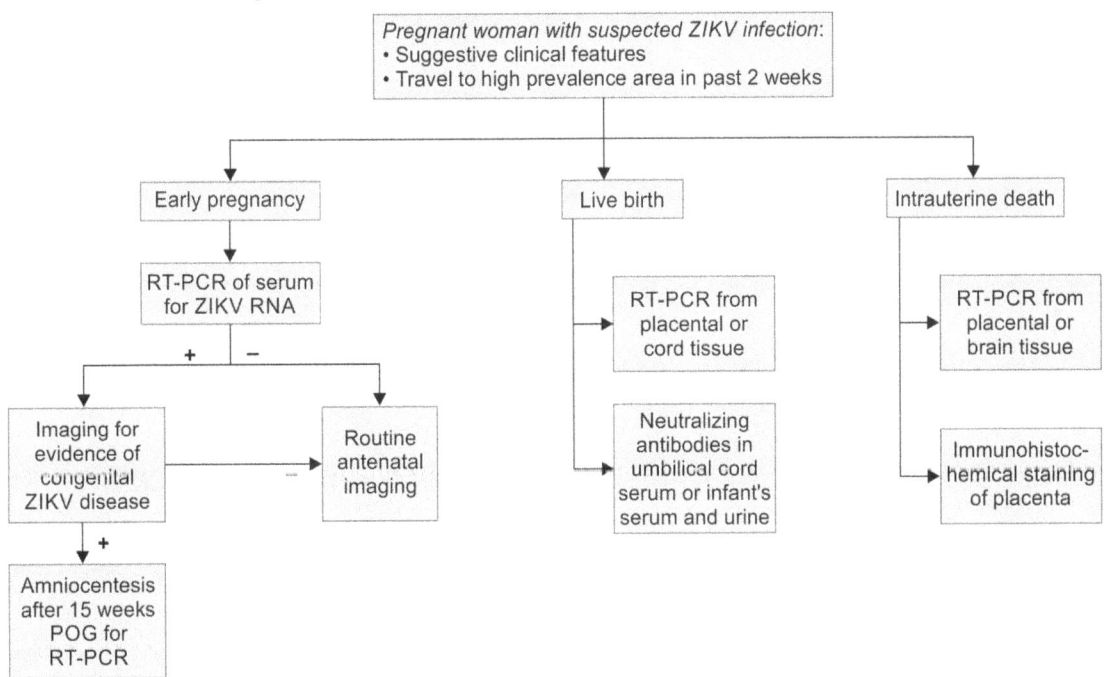

(POG: period of gestation; RNA: ribonucleic acid; RT-PCR: reverse transcriptase polymerase chain reaction; ZIKV: Zika virus)

are mainly for pregnant women and their partners **(Algorithm 7)**.

Different measures of vector control are discussed in **Algorithm 8**.

WHO Risk Assessment

- Circulation of ZIKV in South East Asia, with high risk of spread to areas having *Aedes* mosquito.
- No travel or trade restriction to India.

Box 1 | Imaging in congenital Zika virus (ZIKV) infection.

Various fetal abnormalities seen on imaging with probable association with ZIKV:
- Corpus callosal and vermian dysgenesis
- Enlarged cisterna magna
- Severe unilateral ventriculomegaly
- Agenesis of the thalami
- Cataracts and intraocular calcifications
- Cerebral and cerebellar atrophy
- Cerebral calcification
- Cortical white matter abnormalities like agyria, pachygyria, etc.
- Internal hydrocephalus
- Periventricular cysts
- Choroid plexus cysts
- Blake's cyst
- Brainstem and spinal cord degeneration

Algorithm 6: Centers for Disease Control (CDC) recommendation for the management of women with suspected Zika virus (ZIKV) infection.

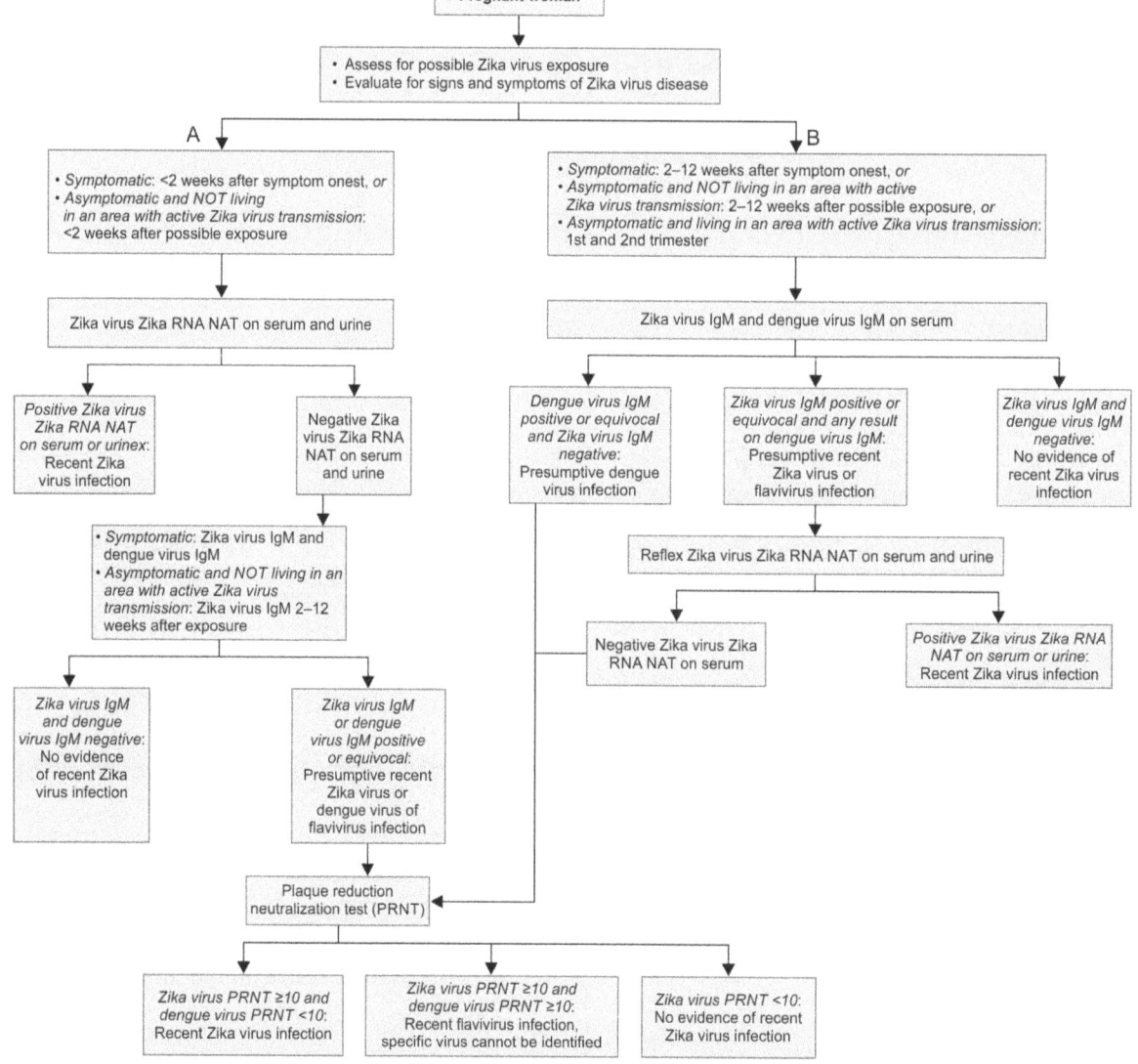

(IgM: immunoglobulin M; RNA NAT: RNA nucleic acid test)

Algorithm 7: Prevention of Zika virus (ZIKV) infection.

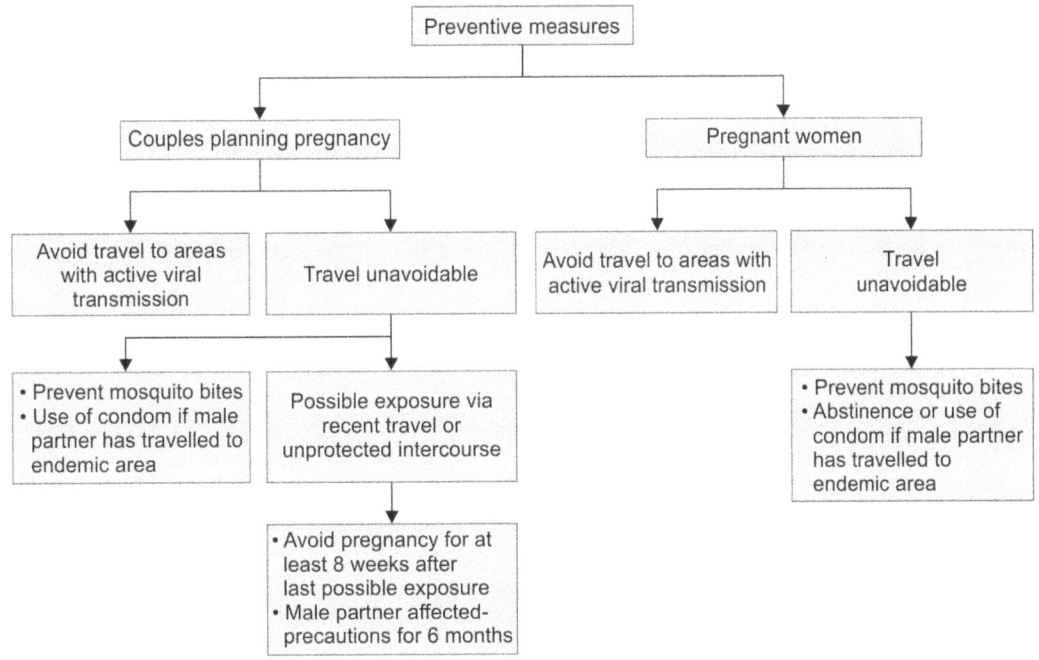

Algorithm 8: Measures for vector control.

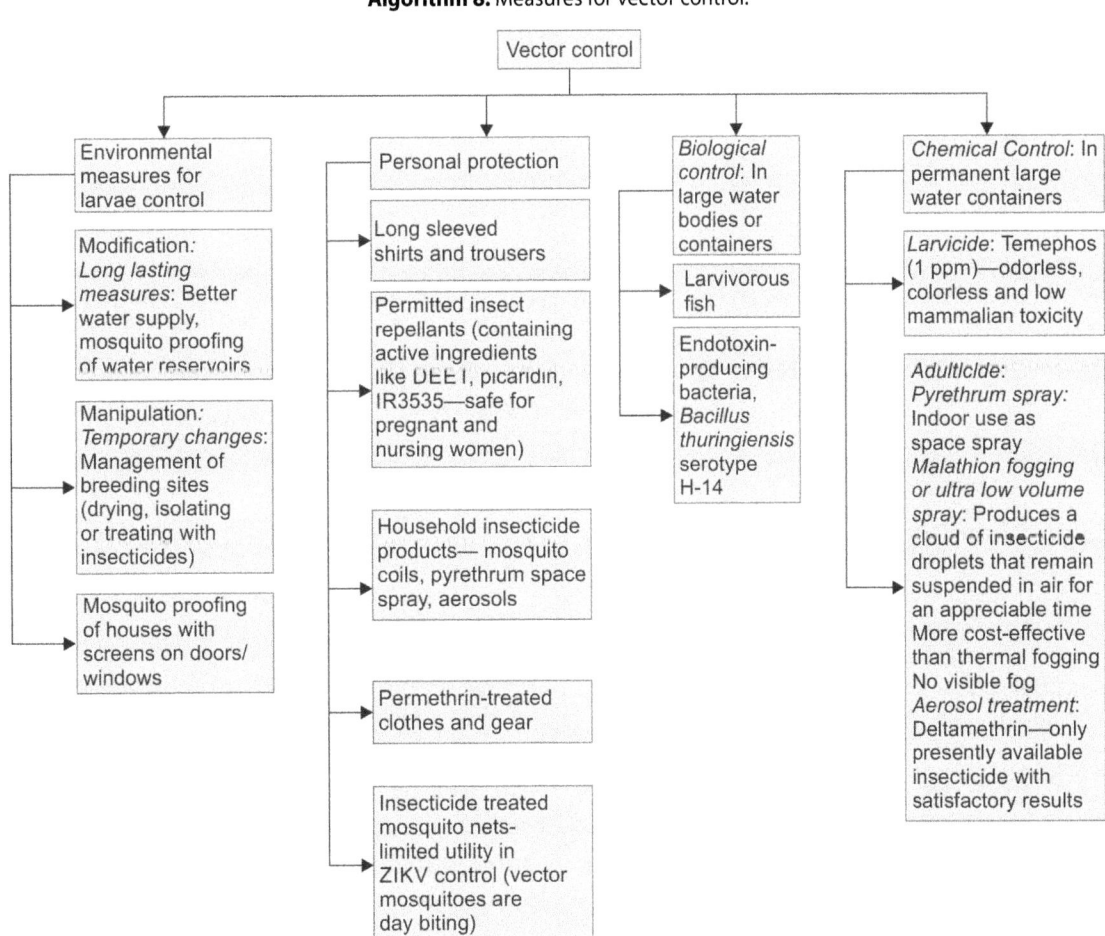

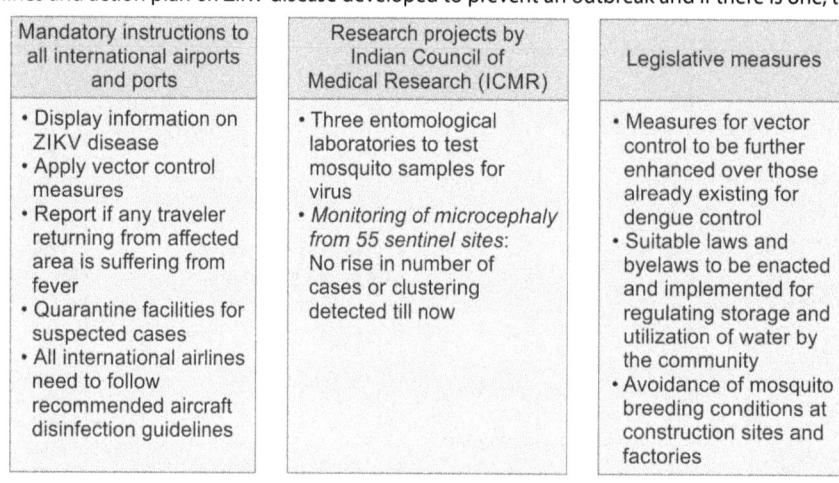

Algorithm 9: Measures taken by Government of India for control of Zika virus (ZIKV). (National guidelines and action plan on ZIKV disease developed to prevent an outbreak and if there is one, to contain the spread).

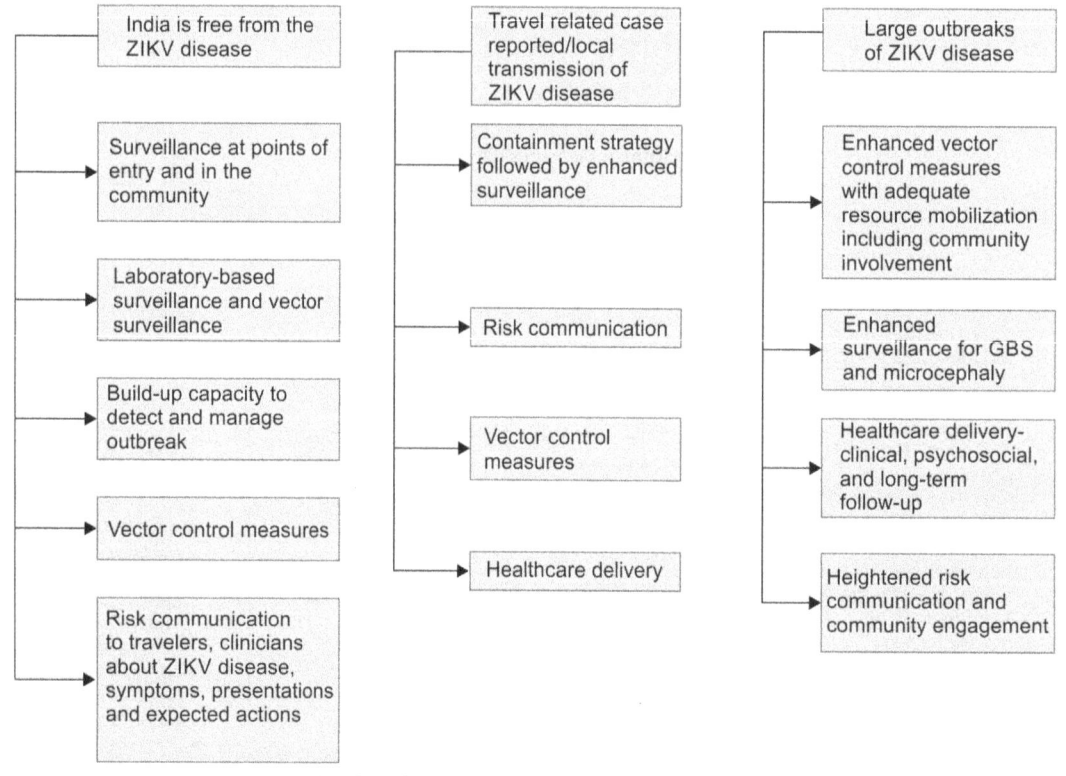

Algorithm 10: Scenario-based response to Zika virus (ZIKV) infection.

(GBS: Guillain-Barré syndrome; ZIKA: Zika virus)

The measures taken by Indian government for the control of ZIV are described in **Algorithm 9**.

TREATMENT

No specific antivirals are available for ZIKV disease. The symptoms are usually mild and taken care of by rest, fluids, analgesics, and antipyretics. Antipyretic preferred in pregnancy is paracetamol.

CONCLUSION

The ZIKV has shown wide transmission in the past few years, causing pandemics in previously naive areas in the Pacific region. Hence, there are high chances that it may spread to countries where *Aedes* mosquito is present like India. Therefore, high vigilance is required to prevent future pandemics **(Algorithm 10)**.

REFERENCES

1. Hayes EB. Zika virus outside Africa. Emerg Infect Dis. 2009;15(9):1347-50.
2. Duffy MR, Chen TH, Hancock WT, et al. Zika virus outbreak on Yap Island, Federated States of Micronesia. N Engl J Med. 2009;360:2536-43.
3. Dick GW. Zika virus. II. Pathogenicity and physical properties. Trans R Soc Trop Med Hyg. 1952;46:521-34.
4. Ioos S, Mallet HP, Leparc Goffart I, et al. Current Zika virus epidemiology and recent epidemics. Med Mal Infect. 2014;44(7):302-7.
5. Heang V, Yasuda CY, Sovann L, et al. Zika virus infection, Cambodia, 2010. Emerg Infect Dis. 2012;18(2):349-51.
6. Rani PR, Vishalakshi LA. Zika virus and pregnancy. Indian Obstet Gynaecol. 2017;7(2):22-5.
7. Schuler-Faccini L, Ribeiro EM, Feitosa IM, et al. Possible association between Zika virus infection and microcephaly—Brazil, 2015. Weekly/January 29. Morbidity Mortality Wkly Rep. 2016;65:59-62.
8. Lissauer D, Smit E, Kilby MD. Zika virus and pregnancy. BJOG. 2016;123(8):1258-63.

Chapter 14

Renal Disorders and Pregnancy

JB Sharma, Venus Dalal

INTRODUCTION

With advances in modern medicine, women with chronic medical disorders are experiencing increased life expectancy and willing to embark upon pregnancy, making this a contemporary issue in obstetrics.

PHYSIOLOGICAL CHANGES

Pregnancy presents a unique opportunity for medical evaluation of women (**Box 1**).

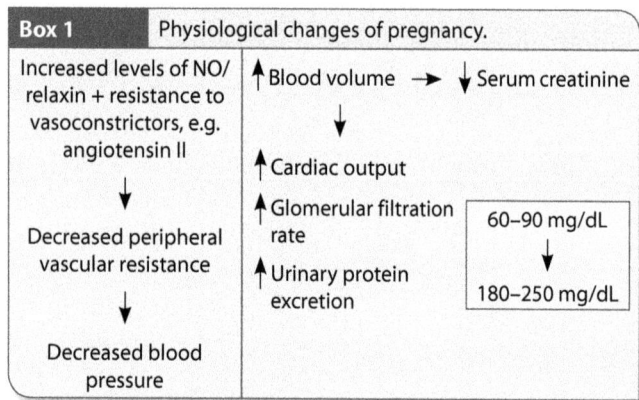

Box 1: Physiological changes of pregnancy.

The smooth muscle of the urinary system relaxes in response to effect of serum progesterone leading to physiological hydronephrosis. The compression by enlarging uterus compounds this effect.

Deciphering kidney function tests (KFTs)

Prepregnancy creatinine levels >0.87 mg/dL suggest a renal pathology in pregnancy.[1]

Some Practical Issues

How to measure glomerular filtration rate (GFR) in pregnancy?

24 hour creatinine clearance is the gold standard.

How to measure proteinuria in pregnancy?

Two indications:
- *Pre-existing proteinuric renal pathology*: Urinary protein to creatinine ratio (0.19–0.25)
- *PE*: Urinary protein to creatinine ratio followed by 24 hr protein (<300 mg/dL) if results are equivocal

Prognostic criteria:

Degree of renal insufficiency rather than underlying renal pathology

Effect of pregnancy on renal disease:
- With serum creatinine >2 mg/dL, 33% women experience deterioration in renal function during or immediately after pregnancy.
- Women with estimated GFR <40 mL/min/1.73 m^2 and proteinuria >1 g/d prepregnancy are prone to adverse renal events and should be discouraged from conception.

| Box 2 | Laboratory tests in renal disease. |

Urine:
- Urinalysis, urinary culture
- Creatinine clearance
- 24 h proteinuria (>300 mg)
- Spot protein/creatinine ratio

Blood/serum:
- Serum electrolytes (Na, K, Ca, P)
- Albumin
- Creatinine
- Urea
- Uric acid

ACUTE KIDNEY INJURY IN PREGNANCY

- *Predisposing factors (acute tubular necrosis)*: Sepsis, acute hemorrhage, hypertensive disorders of pregnancy, heart failure, acute fatty liver and thrombotic microangiopathy, atypical hemolytic uremic syndrome, sometimes hyperemesis gravidarum, and amniotic fluid embolism. Acute cortical necrosis is more frequently encountered with sudden hypotension.

Acute Kidney Injury Network defines acute kidney injury (AKI) as a rise of serum creatinine by more than 0.3 mg/dL over 48 hours or more than 1.5-fold rise. In pregnancy, a lower threshold may be safer.[2,3]

Encouraging decline in the rates of acute kidney injury in pregnancy (AKI-P) in the developing countries has been neutralized by reports of increase in AKI-P requiring dialysis in the developed regions. Management requires collaboration between nephrologist, obstetrician, and intensivist. Therapy is tailored to the underlying cause and renal status.

Stage chronic kidney disease	Glomerular filtration rate (mL/min/1.73 m^2)
1	>90
2	60–90
3a	45–60
3b	30–45
4	15–30
5	<15

CHRONIC KIDNEY DISEASE

The present definition of chronic kidney disease (CKD) includes all women with evidence of kidney disease irrespective of extent, thereby acknowledging that adverse outcomes are associated with the entire spectrum of disease though worsening is encountered with more severe forms and autoimmune disorders.[4]

Position Statement of the Italian Study Group on Kidney and Pregnancy Opines[5]

- Maternal mortality is low; more with systemic lupus erythematosus (SLE).
- With advancing stage of CKD, hypertension, worsening proteinuria (20–100%), and renal function (20–80%) are frequent (**Box 3**).
- Prematurity increases in both incidence as well as degree as the stage of CKD advances. This has implications since the final stages of maturation of glomerulus are achieved in the later gestation, translating into fewer nephrons and kidney disease in adulthood. Malformations are infrequent (exception, diabetic nephropathy). Perinatal mortality and small-for-gestational age (SGA) are a concern with immunologic and diabetic nephropathy.
- Multiple pregnancy compounds above risks (implication: ART).

Chronic Kidney Disease (CKD)/PE Differential Diagnosis[6]
- sFLT 1/PLGF; uteroplacental Doppler
  - *Normal*: CKD
  - *Abnormal*: PE
  - *Discordant*: Nephrology work-up—
    - *Positive*: CKD
    - *Negative*: Fetomaternal surveillance
- *Early pregnancy with deterioration*: Kidney biopsy (**Box 4**)
- *>34 weeks with deterioration*:
  - Early delivery under steroid cover
  - Follow with proteinuria assessment at 1 and 3 months:
    - Resolution indicates PE
    - Persistence/worsening indicates CKD

| Box 3 | Prenatal counseling: chronic kidney disease (CKD). |

S. creatinine	Fetomaternal outcome
<1.4 mg	Good
1.4–2.9 mg/dL	High risk for pregnancy complications
≥3.0 mg/dL	High risk of permanent loss of renal function

| Box 4 | Complications of renal biopsy in pregnancy.[7] |

- Hemorrhage requiring transfusion/embolization
- Severe obstetric complications
- Early preterm delivery
- Fetal death

Follow-up

- The aim is to identify complications, viz. anemia, hypertension, proteinuria, and coagulopathy; formulate a birth plan.
- Nephrology assessment should be 4–6 weekly without proteinuria/hypertension, pregnancies with Stage 1 CKD; weekly with proteinuria, hypertension, or advanced CKD **(Box 1)**.
- Both proteinuria and glomerular filtration rate (GFR) in pregnancy should be assessed using the 24-hour urine.
- Timely detection of proteinuria and urinary infection merit fortnightly to weekly urinalysis.

Hypertension in Chronic Kidney Disease

- Early identification improves outcome.
- Angiotensin-converting-enzyme inhibitor (ACE-I) and angiotensin receptor blockers (ARBs) should be substituted with step-up approach and drugs suitable in pregnancy.
- Overzealous control compromises uteroplacental flow. Hence is discouraged.

Lupus Nephritis

Women with connective tissue disease (CTD) on prenatal visit should be tested for antiphospholipid antibodies, ds DNA, anti-Ro/anti-La, and complement (C3, C4) besides kidney function tests (KFTs).

To distinguish lupus flare from worsening PE:
- *Lupus*: Proteinuria + red and white cells ± cellular casts
  PE: Isolated proteinuria.
- *Lupus*: Declining complement + rising titers of ds DNA
  PE: Escalating complement levels.
- *Lupus*: Isolated thrombocytopenia
  PE: Deranged liver function tests (LFTs) + KFTs, thrombocytopenia.
- *Lupus*: <20 weeks
  PE: >20 weeks (exceptions exist).

There is significant decline in live birth rates and increased likelihood of fetal growth restriction (FGR) and preterm birth.[8] With lupus flare or history thereof, pregnancy should be deferred until 6 months of remission.[9] Conversely despite encouraging birth experience, surveillance for postnatal flare is a must.

END-STAGE RENAL DISEASE

End-stage renal disease (ESRD) is associated with subfertility, secondary to disruption of hypothalamic-pituitary-ovarian (HPO) axis. Transplant aids conception.

Pregnancy with Renal Replacement Therapy (Box 5)[10]

- Owing to erratic ovulation and increase in serum human chorionic gonadotropin (hCG) in this group, pregnancy should be dated based on early viability scan.
- Timing of initiation of renal replacement therapy (RRT) is debatable. Proponents of "early" start at residual renal function of 20 mL/min while advocates of "delay" place the cut off at 10 mL/min.[6]
- Low protein diets help delay need for dialysis.
- In advanced pregnancy, dialysis versus early delivery (=34 weeks) must be considered.
- On dialysis, blood urea nitrogen (BUN) (target <50 mg/dL) is the most important parameter related to pregnancy outcome.
- The type of RRT [peritoneal dialysis (PD) versus hemodialysis (HD)] that best suits pregnancy is still debatable. Literature suggests preference toward hemodialysis.
- The diet/proteins should be unrestricted.
- Optimum weight gain should be 300 g/week in second and 300–500 g/week in the third trimester.
- Anemia is managed using erythropoietin stimulating agents and oral iron.
- Vitamin D and calcium supplements are indicated.
- Low serum magnesium levels may induce uterine contractions. Serum levels should be maintained at 5–7 mg/dL.
- Maternal mortality is low (0.4%).
- Prematurity is significantly higher with PD than with HD (66% vs. 31%).
- The risk of congenital malformations is not increased.

Box 5 | Complications of renal replacement therapy (RRT).

Maternal:
- Complications due to central venous access
- Hemorrhage secondary to anticoagulants
- Placental hypoperfusion secondary to diuretics
- Need for fistula placement

Fetal:
- Prematurity

Pregnancy in Renal Transplant

Since pregnancy itself is a sensitizing event, it is advisable to delay pregnancy by a year post-transplant. Immunosuppression should be suitably modified *(See section on Pharmacotherapy)*. Serum creatinine <1.5 mg/dL and stable immunosuppression regime are two prerequisites for a good outcome. While live birth rates and graft rejection rate match those of general population, PE (27%), gestational diabetes mellitus (GDM) (8%), and prematurity (45.6%) are higher.

Among *kidney donors*, the risk of PE is increased by nearly 2.5 times. Preterm or SGA risk is not appreciably increased.[11]

PHARMACOTHERAPY IN PREGNANCY

Antihypertensives

Alphamethyl dopa, labetalol, and nifedipine may be considered first-line drugs; beta-adrenergic blockers, clonidine, alpha-blockers, and diuretics second-line and short-acting nifedipine, ARBs, and ACE-I are contraindicated.[12]

Immunosuppressive Agents

European guidelines recommend azathioprine (AZA) (FDA Category D) to be safe in pregnancy since the fetal liver is unable to process the drug. They recommend switching over from mycophenolate to AZA preconceptionally.[13]

Calcineurin inhibitors, cyclosporine A and tacrolimus, have been permitted though caution should be exercised with respect to risks of maternal hypertension, nephrotoxicity and hyperglycemia, and fetal risks of preterm and SGA.

Short-acting steroids such as prednisone, prednisolone, and methylprednisolone as well as long-standing dexamethasone and betamethasone have been used safely despite known adverse effects on glucose homeostasis and premature rupture of membranes (PROM). The antimalarial hydroxychloroquine is safe despite transplacental transfer.

Women should avoid conception while on cyclophosphamide, mycophenolate, rituximab, and m-Tor inhibitors.

Antibiotics

While semisynthetic penicillin, clavulanic acid, cephalosporins, macrolides, nitrofurantoin, and fosfomycin (all FDA B) are safe, fluoroquinolones (FDA C) (adverse effect on cartilage), aminoglycosides (ototoxicity), tetracyclines, and sulfonamides (all FDA D) should be avoided.

Ceftriaxone is avoided close to delivery for fear of kernicterus as it competes with bilirubin for binding sites on albumin. Nitrofurantoin is contraindicated in women with G6PD deficiency and is avoided after 38 weeks for fear of neonatal hemolytic anemia.

Others

Aspirin (FDA not classified), low molecular weight heparin (LMWH), recombinant erythropoietin, and allopurinol (all FDA C) are safe.

REFERENCES

1. Wiles K, Bramham K, Seed PT, et al. Serum creatinine in pregnancy: a systematic review. Kidney Int Rep. 2018;4(3): 408-19.
2. Mehta R, Kellum J, Shah S, et al. Acute kidney injury network: report of an initiative to improve outcomes in acute kidney injury. Crit Care. 2007;11(2):R31.
3. Rao S, Jim B. Acute kidney injury in pregnancy: the changing landscape for the 21st century. Kidney Int Rep. 2018;3(2): 247-57.
4. Piccoli G, Zakharova E, Attini R, et al. Pregnancy in chronic kidney disease: need for higher awareness. A pragmatic review focused on what could be improved in the different CKD stages and phases. J Clin Med. 2018;7(11):415.
5. Cabiddu G, Castellino S, Gernone G, et al. A best practice position statement on pregnancy in chronic kidney disease: the Italian Study Group on Kidney and Pregnancy. J Nephrol. 2016;29(3):277-303.
6. Piccoli GB, Zakharova E, Attini R, et al. Acute kidney injury in pregnancy: the need for higher awareness. A pragmatic review focused on what could be improved in the prevention and care of pregnancy-related aki, in the year dedicated to women and kidney diseases. J Clin Med. 2018;7(10):318.
7. Piccoli G, Daidola G, Attini R, et al. Kidney biopsy in pregnancy: evidence for counselling? A systematic narrative review. BJOG. 2013;120(4):412-27.
8. Wu J, Ma J, Zhang W-H, et al. Management and outcomes of pregnancy with or without lupus nephritis: a systematic review and meta-analysis. Ther Clin Risk Manag. 2018;14: 885-901.

9. Wagner SJ, Craici I, Reed D, et al. Maternal and foetal outcomes in pregnant patients with active lupus nephritis. Lupus. 2009;18:342.
10. Cabiddu G, Castellino S, Gernone G, et al. Kidney and pregnancy study group of Italian Society of Nephrology. Best practices on pregnancy on dialysis: the Italian Study Group on Kidney and Pregnancy. J Nephrol. 2015;28(3):279-88.
11. Kidney Disease: Improving Global Outcomes Transplant Work Group. KDIGO clinical practice guideline for the care of kidney transplant recipients. Am J Transplant. 2009;9(Suppl 3):S1-155.
12. Magee LA, Pels A, Helewa M, et al. Canadian hypertensive diagnosis, evaluation, and management of the hypertensive disorders of pregnancy. Disorders of Pregnancy Working Group. Pregnancy Hypertens. 2014;4(2):105-45.
13. EBPG Expert Group on Renal Transplantation. Pregnancy in renal transplant recipients. Nephrol Dial Transplant 2002;17(Suppl 4):50-5.

APPENDIX 1: LIST OF ABBREVIATIONS

- *ACEi:* Angiotensin converting enzyme inhibitors
- *AKI:* Acute kidney injury
- *ARB:* Angiotensin receptor blockers
- *ART:* Artificial reproductive technology
- *AZA:* Azathioprine
- *BP:* Blood pressure
- *CKD:* Chronic kidney disease
- *CT:* Computerized tomography
- *CTD:* Connective tissue disease
- *ESRD:* End stage renal disease
- *FDA:* US Food and Drug Association
- *FGR:* Fetal growth restriction
- *GFR:* Glomerular filtration rate
- *LBW:* Low birth weight
- *LMWH:* Low molecular weight heparin
- *MRI:* Magnetic resonance imaging
- *NO:* Nitric oxide
- *PE:* Preeclampsia
- *PROM:* Premature rupture of membranes
- *SLE:* Systemic lupus erythematosus
- *SGA:* Small for gestational age

Chapter 14
Renal Disorders and Pregnancy

APPENDIX 2: SPECIFIC RENAL DISEASES IN PREGNANCY

Autosomal Dominant Polycystic Kidney Disease

- Increased risk of pyelonephritis/preeclampsia (PE)
- Cesarean only for obstetric indications
- Large cysts should be monitored for the presence of intracystic bleed immediately prior to and post delivery
- The role of preimplantation genetic testing currently, is inconclusive

IgA Nephropathy

- Pregnancy does not appear to worsen long-term renal prognosis although risk is significant with hypertension, proteinuria >1 g/d, pre-pregnancy eGFR <60 mL/min/1.73 m^2
- Risk of complications, viz. pregnancy loss (12%), PE/Eclampsia (7.3%), prematurity (8.5%), low-birth weight (LBW) (9.5%) is increased
- Immunosuppression is indicated only with active disease

Nephrolithiasis

- Incidence 1:1,500–3,000 despite several predisposing factors in pregnancy
- Associated with PE and preterm labor
- Presentation is with renal colic and gross hematuria; in a third of cases
- Transvaginal ultrasonography (USG) may be helpful in delineating stones in distal ureter
- MRI and CT can be offered in selected cases if USG is equivocal
- Symptomatic management with hydration and analgesics may aid spontaneous expulsion due to dilatation of urinary tract in pregnancy
- Ureteroscopy and laser may be reserved for rare unresponsive cases

Nephrotic syndrome	
Criteria	Magnitude
Massive proteinuria	Spot P/Cr >300–350 mg/mmol 24 hr urine protein > 3–3.5 g
Hypoalbuminemia	Serum albumin < 2.5 g/dL
Edema	Clinical
Hyperlipidemia	Optional
Nephrotic syndrome: Diagnostic criteria	

Diagnosis: In women meeting the above criteria presenting in early pregnancy it is easy to diagnose. In dubious cases renal biopsy aids confirmation.

Management:
- Restriction of sodium and fluids
- Diuretics to relieve edema
- Steroids in the setting of NS secondary to SLE
- Routine antibiotic prophylaxis, lipid lowering agents, thromboprohylaxis are not supported by current evidence

Complications: The incidence of PE, PROM, LBW, FGR is increased even if significant renal impairment or uncontrolled hypertension were not initially present.

Chapter 15

Thyroid Disorders

Reena Wani, Rashmi G Jalvee

INTRODUCTION

Pregnancy has a profound impact on the thyroid gland and thyroid function. Thyroid dysfunction during pregnancy can result in serious complications for both mother and infant, which can be prevented by optimal treatment of maternal overt thyroid dysfunction.

CHANGES IN THYROID FUNCTION IN PREGNANCY[1]

- Increase in serum thyroxine-binding globulin (TBG) concentration
- Stimulation of thyroid-stimulating hormone (TSH) receptor by human chorionic gonadotropin (hCG)
- Thyrotropic activity of hCG reduces the concentration of serum TSH.
- Both serum total thyroxine (T4) and triiodothyronine concentrations increase.
- Later in pregnancy, serum TSH concentration steadily returns to normal range and free T4 concentration declines.

RECOMMENDATIONS FOR THYROID SCREENING AND TREATMENT IN PREGNANCY[2,3]

- All pregnant and lactating women must ingest approximately 250 µg iodine daily.[4]
- Universal screening is not recommended in most countries due to scarcity of data, and most of the available guidelines recommend screening of high-risk pregnant women.
- However, the Indian Thyroid Society (ITS)[5] recommends screening of TSH levels in all pregnant women at the time of their first visit, ideally during pre-pregnancy evaluation or as soon as pregnancy is confirmed.
- Trimester-specific reference ranges for TSH, as defined in populations with optimal iodine intake, should be applied.
- If trimester-specific reference ranges for TSH are not available in the laboratory, certain reference ranges are recommended which are given in **Table 1**.

Table 1: Trimester-specific reference ranges for thyroid-stimulating hormone (TSH).

Trimester	TSH range (mIU/L)
First	0.1–2.5
Second	0.2–3.0
Third	0.3–3.0

HYPOTHYROIDISM IN PREGNANCY

Hypothyroidism is a very common endocrine disorder in pregnancy. In India, the prevalence of hypothyroidism during pregnancy ranges from 4.8% to 11%.[6]

Algorithm 1: Treatment algorithm in new-onset hypothyroidism in pregnancy.[2,3]

```
Administration of oral levothyroxine (LT4)
          ↓
Goal is to normalize serum TSH values within trimester-specific reference range
          ↓
Serum TSH should be monitored 4 weekly during first half of pregnancy
          ↓
Further LT4 dose adjustments may be required
          ↓
TSH should be checked at least once between 26 weeks' and 32 weeks' gestation
          ↓
Following delivery, LT4 can be discontinued especially when the dose required was 50 μg
          ↓
TSH testing should be performed at approximately 6 weeks' postpartum
```

Algorithm 2: Treatment in pre-existing hypothyroidism.[2,3]

```
Pregnant women with pre-existing hypothyroidism on LT4 should increase the dose of LT4 by ~25–30% once pregnancy is confirmed and notify caregiver promptly
          ↓
Dose of LT4 to increase from once-daily dosing to total of nine doses per week (29% increase)
          ↓
Goal is to normalize serum TSH values within trimester-specific reference range
          ↓
Serum TSH should be monitored 4 weekly during first half of pregnancy
          ↓
Further LT4 dose adjustments may be required
          ↓
TSH should be checked at least once between 26 weeks' and 32 weeks' gestation
          ↓
Following delivery, LT4 should be reduced to the preconception dose
          ↓
TSH testing should be performed at approximately 6 weeks' postpartum
```

Complications of Hypothyroidism in Pregnancy[7]

- *Maternal:*
    - Abortions
    - Gestational hypertension
    - Anemia
    - Abruptio placenta
    - Postpartum hemorrhage
- *Fetal:*
    - Preterm birth
    - Low birth weight
    - Respiratory distress
    - Risk of impairment in IQ scores and learning abilities
    - Neurocognitive developmental delay.

Treatment of new-onset hypothyroidism in pregnancy and pre-existing hypothyroidism is shown in **Algorithms 1 and 2**, respectively.

SUBCLINICAL HYPOTHYROIDISM

Subclinical hypothyroidism (SCH) is defined as increased TSH with normal concentrations of FT4 and FT3. Subclinical hypothyroidism has been associated with adverse maternal and fetal outcomes.

- Pregnant women with TSH concentrations > 2.5 mU/L should be evaluated for thyroid peroxidase antibody (TPO Ab) status.
- Subclinical hypothyroidism in pregnancy should be approached as follows: LT4 therapy is recommended for:
    - TPO Ab-positive women with a TSH greater than the pregnancy-specific reference range
    - TPO Ab negative women with a TSH greater than 10.0 mU/L
- Euthyroid women (not receiving LT4) who are TPO Ab or thyroglobulin antibody (TgAb) positive require monitoring for hypothyroidism during pregnancy. They should have measurement of serum TSH testing at time of pregnancy confirmation and every 4 weeks through mid-pregnancy and at least once between 26 weeks' and 32 weeks' gestation.

THYROTOXICOSIS IN PREGNANCY

Diagnosis of thyrotoxicosis in pregnancy is shown in **Algorithm 3**.

- Radioactive iodine (RAI) scanning or radioiodine uptake determination should not be performed in pregnancy.

Algorithm 3: Diagnosis of thyrotoxicosis in pregnancy.[2,3]

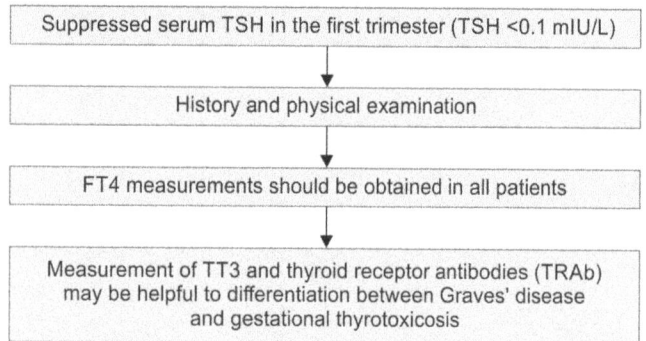

Algorithm 4: Treatment protocol for transient gestational thyrotoxicosis and/or hyperemesis gravidarum.[2,3]

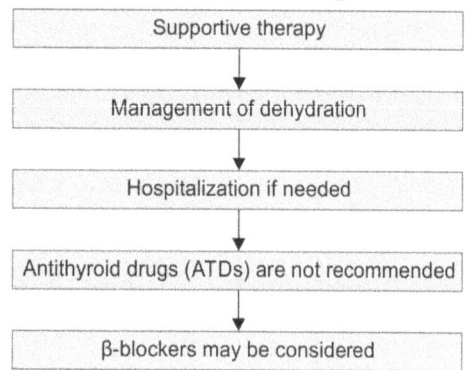

The ideal treatment for transient gestational thyrotoxicosis and/or hyperemesis gravidarum is shown in **Algorithm 4**.

The prevalence of fetal and neonatal hyperthyroidism is between 1 and 5% of all women with current or past history of Graves' hyperthyroidism and is associated with increased fetal and neonatal morbidity and mortality if unrecognized **(Algorithms 5 and 6)**.[8]

REFERENCES

1. Soldin OP, Tractenberg RE, Jonklaas J, et al. Trimester-specific changes in maternal thyroid hormone, thyrotropin, and thyroglobulin concentrations during gestation: trends and associations across trimesters in iodine sufficiency. Thyroid. 2004;14(12):1084-90.
2. American College of Obstetricians and Gynecologists. Practice Bulletin No. 148: thyroid disease in pregnancy. Obstet Gynecol. 2015;125:996-1005.
3. Alexander EK, Pearce EN, Brent GA, et al. 2017 Guidelines of the American Thyroid Association for the diagnosis and management of thyroid disease during pregnancy and the postpartum. Thyroid. 2017;27(3):315-89.

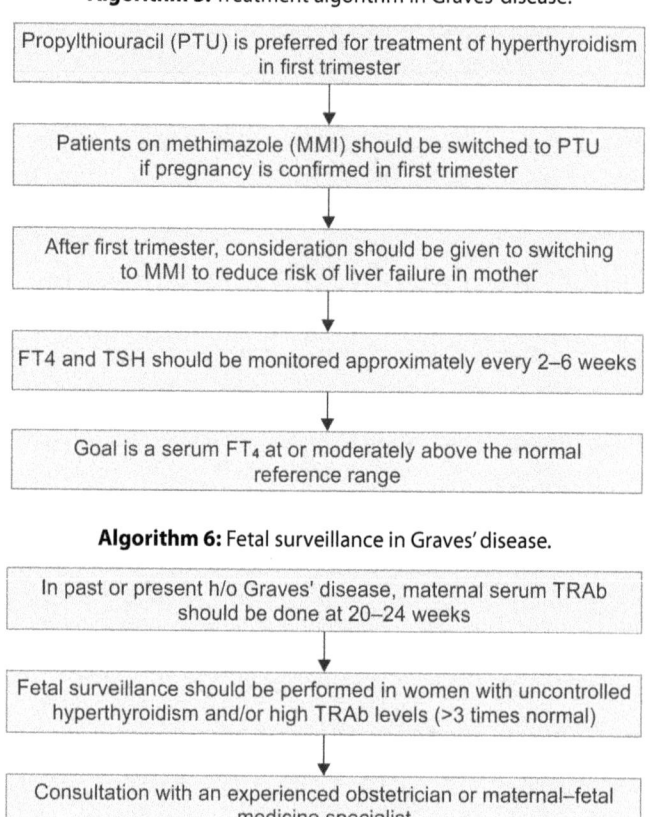

Algorithm 5: Treatment algorithm in Graves' disease.

Algorithm 6: Fetal surveillance in Graves' disease.

4. World Health Organization, UNICEF, ICCIDD. Assessment of Iodine Deficiency Disorders and Monitoring Their Elimination. A Guide for Programme Managers, 3rd edition. Geneva, Switzerland: World Health Organization; 2007.
5. Dave A, Maru L, Tripathi M. Importance of universal screening for thyroid disorders in first trimester of pregnancy. Indian J Endocrinol Metab. 2014;18(5):735-8.
6. Sahu MT, Das V, Mittal S, et al. Overt and subclinical thyroid dysfunction among Indian pregnant women and its effect on maternal and fetal outcome. Arch Gynecol Obstet. 2010;281(2):215-20.
7. Abalovich M, Gutierrez S, Alcaraz G, et al. Overt and subclinical hypothyroidism complicating pregnancy. Thyroid. 2002;12(1):63-8.
8. Zimmerman D. Fetal and neonatal hyperthyroidism. Thyroid. 1999;9(7):727-33.

Section 2

Antenatal Emergencies

- **Vomiting in Pregnancy**
  Sandeep Sharma

- **Abdominal Pain in Pregnancy**
  Abha Rani Sinha, Sneh Kiran

- **Bleeding in Early Pregnancy**
  Bhaskar Pal, Alpana V Chhetri

- **Bleeding in Late Pregnancy**
  Rashmi Bagga, Japleen Kaur

- **Preterm Labor**
  Madhu Nagpal

- **Prelabor Rupture of Membranes**
  Shyjus Puliyathinkal

- **Intrauterine Growth Restriction: An Evidence-based Approach**
  Minakshi Rohilla, Shivani Sharma

- **Multiple Gestations in Labor**
  Shailesh Kore, Pradnya Supe, Chaitra Thunga

- **Cervical Insufficiency**
  Neha Gupta

- **Reduced Fetal Movements**
  Geetha Balsarkar

- **Intrauterine Fetal Death**
  Savita Singhal, Shaveta Jain

- **Prolonged Pregnancy**
  Suman Thakur

- **Pregnancy after Lower Segment Cesarean Section**
  S Sampathkumari

- **Pregnancy after Infertility and Assisted Reproductive Technology**
  Shalini Gainder, Japleen Kaur

Chapter 16

Vomiting in Pregnancy

Sandeep Sharma

INTRODUCTION

Nausea and vomiting are common features seen in early pregnancy in up to 70% of pregnant women.[1] More often, it is physiological and related to the pregnant state. But we should be vigilant about other medical and surgical conditions which may be associated with pregnancy and cause vomiting.

Vomiting in pregnancy often occurs around 8–10 weeks and settles by 14–16 weeks and is thought mainly to be due to physiological hormone changes in pregnancy.[1] **Algorithm 1** shows the types of vomiting in pregnancy.

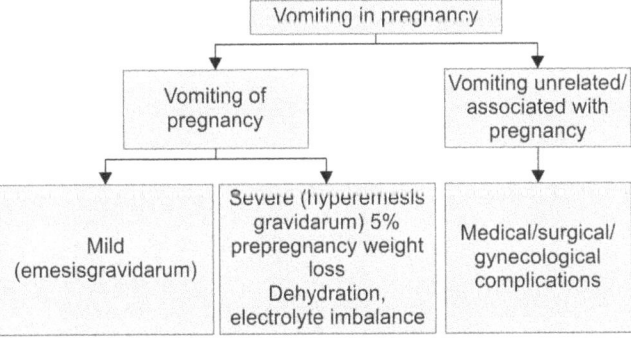

Algorithm 1: Vomiting in pregnancy and its types.

ETIOLOGY

The exact etiology is not known but thought to be due to:
- Excess human chorionic gonadotropin (hCG)
- High serum estrogen
- Progesterone excess.

The incidence increases in conditions associated with high hCG such as molar pregnancy and multiple pregnancies.

RISK FACTORS

- Young age
- Primigravida
- Multiple gestations
- Pregnancy with female fetus
- Low prepregnancy weight
- Low-to-middle socioeconomic status.
  Smoking and age more than 35 years decrease the risk.[2]

HYPEREMESIS GRAVIDARUM

It is a severe form of nausea and vomiting which produces weight loss, dehydration, ketosis, alkalosis, and hypokalemia.

Pathophysiology

The pathophysiology of hyperemesis gravidarum is controversial. Complex interaction of biological, psychological, and sociocultural factors is implicated. Several theories have been proposed for the basis of hyperemesis gravidarum.

Hormonal Changes

Women with hyperemesis gravidarum often have high hCG levels that cause transient hyperthyroidism. hCG can stimulate thyroid-stimulating hormone (TSH) receptor. hCG levels can peak in the first trimester. Some women with hyperemesis gravidarum appear to have clinical hyperthyroidism. Thyroid function, however, normalizes by the middle of the second trimester. A positive correlation between the s. hCG level and free T4 levels has been found and the severity of nausea appears to be related to the degree of thyroid stimulation.

Some studies link high estradiol levels to the severity of nausea and vomiting in pregnant women.

Previous intolerance to oral contraceptive is associated with nausea and vomiting in pregnancy. Thyroid dysfunction in hyperemesis is shown in **Algorithm 2**.

Algorithm 2: Thyroid dysfunction in hyperemesis gravidarum.

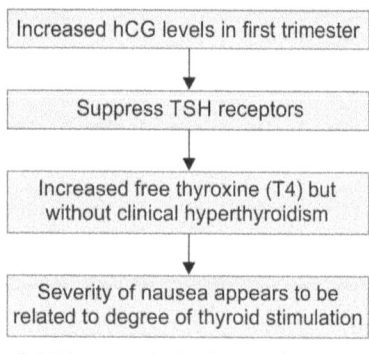

(hCG: human chorionic gonadotropin; TSH: thyroid stimulating hormone)

Gastrointestinal Dysfunction

Algorithm 3 shows gastrointestinal dysfunction.

Algorithm 3: Gastrointestinal dysfunction causing hyperemesis.

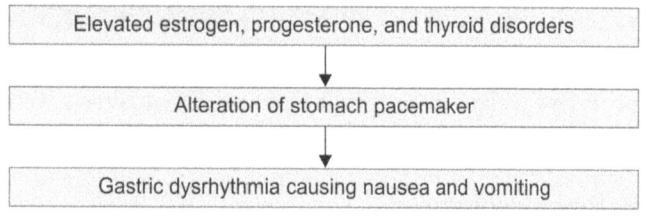

Hepatic Dysfunction

Algorithm 4 shows hepatic dysfunction in hyperemesis gravidarum.

Algorithm 4: Hepatic dysfunction in hyperemesis gravidarum.

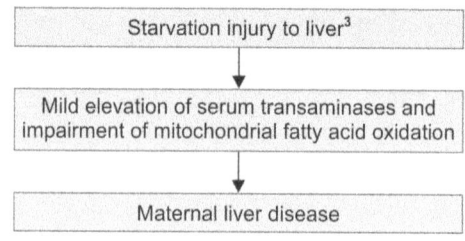

Lipid Alteration (Algorithm 5)

Algorithm 5: Lipid abnormalities in hyperemesis gravidarum.

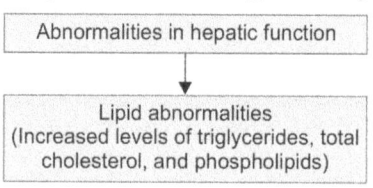

Genetic

Genetic predisposition also plays a role in the development of hyperemesis gravidarum (HG).

DIFFERENTIAL DIAGNOSIS

It is imperative to rule out conditions which are either unrelated to pregnancy or conditions that may be associated along with pregnancy which result in vomiting. **Algorithm 6** enumerates the differential diagnosis for vomiting in pregnancy.

Algorithm 6: Differential diagnosis for vomiting in pregnancy.

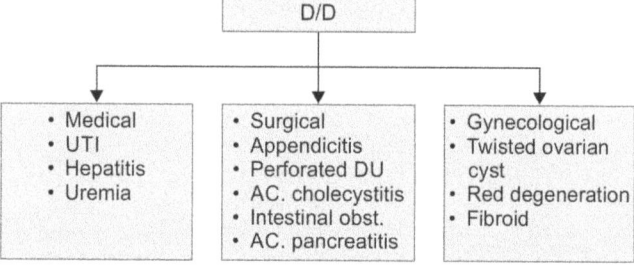

(AC: acute; D/D: differential diagnosis; DU: duodenal ulcer; UTI: urinary tract infection)

COMPLICATIONS

The complications arise as a result of continuous retching, dehydration, and starvation. The various complications are enumerated in **Algorithm 7**.

Algorithm 7: Complications in vomiting in pregnancy.

• Dehydration • Acute renal failure	• Cont. retching • Mallory Weiss tear • Pneumothorax • Pneumomediastinum • Diaphragm rupture • Boerhaave synd	• Starvation • Vitamin deficiency • Wernicke's encepha, pontine myelinosis, peripheral neuritis, korsakoff's psycho., coagulopathy • IC hemorrhage

(IC: intracerebral)

Management of Nausea Vomiting in Pregnancy

Algorithm 8 shows the investigations to be done in nausea vomiting in pregnancy (NVP).

Algorithm 8: Investigations in nausea vomiting in pregnancy (NVP).

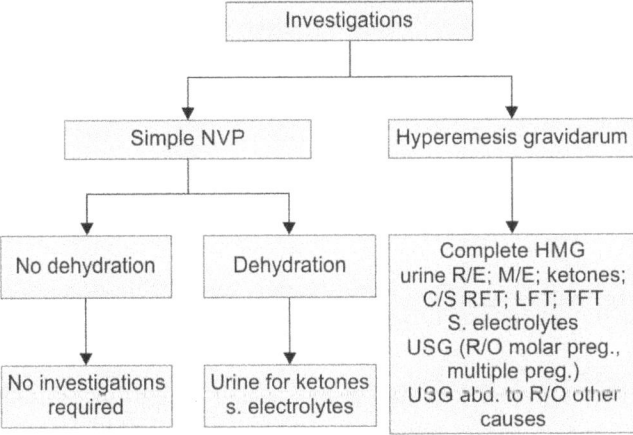

(abd.: abdominal; HMG: human menopausal gonadotropin; LFT: liver function test; R/O: rule out; TFT: thyroid function test; USG: ultrasonography)

Treatment of Nausea Vomiting in Pregnancy

Algorithms 9 and 10 show the treatment of NVP.

Algorithm 9: Treatment of nausea vomiting in pregnancy (NVP).

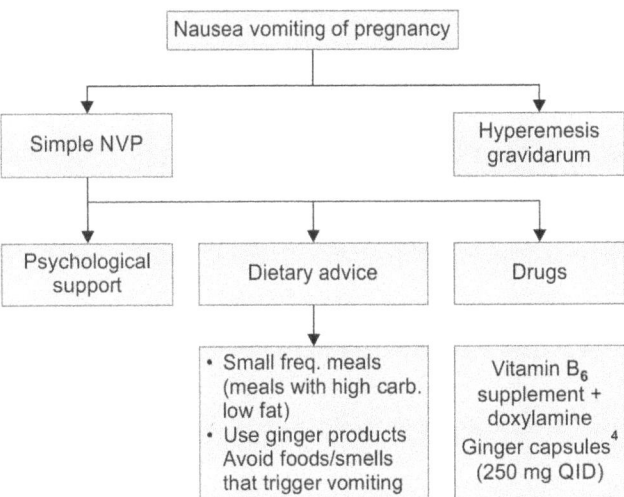

Algorithm 10: Treatment of nausea vomiting in pregnancy (NVP).

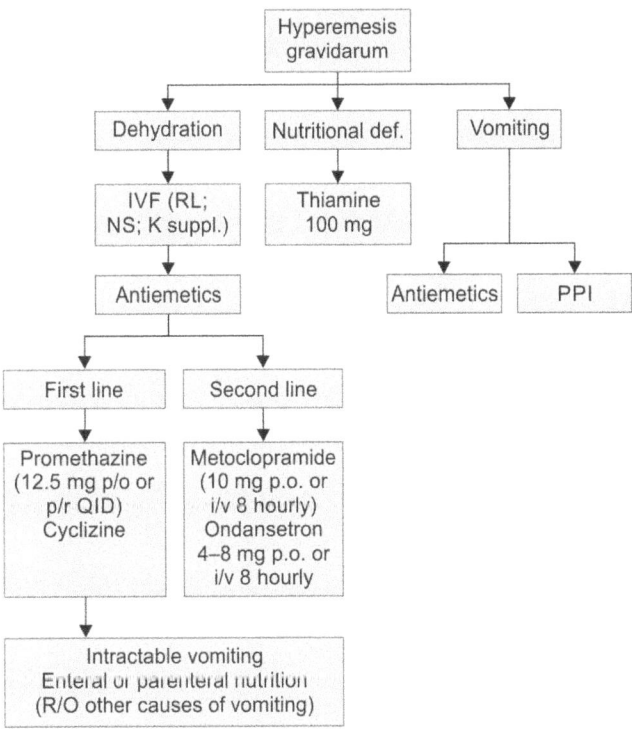

(IVF: in vitro fertilization; NS: normal salone; PPI: proton pump inhibitor; RL: ringer lactate; R/O: rule out)

REFERENCES

1. Gabbe S, Niebyl JR, Simpson JL, et al. Obstetrics: Normal and Problem Pregnancies, 6th edition. London, UK: Churchill-Livingstone; 2012.
2. Klebanoff MA, Koslowe PA, Kaslow R, et al. Epidemiology of vomiting in early pregnancy. Obstet Gynecol. 1985;66:612-6.
3. Adams RH, Gordon J, Combes B. Hyperemesis gravidarum. I. Evidence of hepatic dysfunction. Obstet Gynecol. 1968;31:659-64.
4. Borreli F, Capasso R, Aviello G, et al. Effectiveness and safety of ginger in the treatment of pregnancy-induced nausea and vomiting. Obstet Gynecol. 2005;105(4):849-56.

Chapter 17

Abdominal Pain in Pregnancy

Abha Rani Sinha, Sneh Kiran

INTRODUCTION

Abdominal pain in pregnancy is very common and usually obstetric in origin. Approximately 1 in 500–635 pregnant women will require nonobstetric abdominal surgery for acute pain abdomen during their pregnancies.[1] The initial goal is to identify patients who have a serious or even life-threatening etiology for their symptoms and require urgent intervention. Additional issues in pregnant women include consideration of the impact of physiologic changes related to pregnancy, causes of acute abdominal/pelvic pain that may be more common due to the pregnant state or related to obstetrical complications, and the impact of the disease process on the fetus. A general approach to abdominal pain in pregnancy is to manage these problems regardless of the pregnancy **(Algorithms 1 and 2)**.

DIFFERENTIAL DIAGNOSIS

- Early pregnancy
  - Miscarriage
  - Ectopic pregnancy
  - Ovarian hyperstimulation syndrome
- Late pregnancy
  - Preterm labor
  - Placental abruption
  - Chorioamnionitis
  - Uterine rupture
  - HELLP (hemolysis, elevated liver enzymes, low platelet count) syndrome
  - Acute fatty liver
- Gynecological
  - Adnexal mass
  - Ruptured ovarian cyst
  - Hemorrhagic ovarian cyst
  - Torsion of adnexa
  - *Uterine fibroids*: Red degeneration of myoma, torsion of pedunculated myoma
- Urological
  - Acute urinary retention due to retroverted gravid uterus
  - Acute cystitis
  - Acute pyelonephritis
  - Nephrolithiasis
  - Acute hydronephrosis
- Gastrointestinal
  - Appendicitis
  - Cholecystitis
  - Acute pancreatitis
  - Intestinal obstruction
- Traumatic
  - Splenic rupture
- Musculoskeletal
  - Rectus sheath hematoma.

EVALUATION OF ABDOMINAL PAIN IN PREGNANCY (ALGORITHM 3)

The following issues should be considered:
- Is the pain obstetric or nonobstetric?
- Is surgery indicated?
- What is the risk of anesthesia?

Algorithm 1: Management of abdominal pain in early pregnancy (obstetric causes).

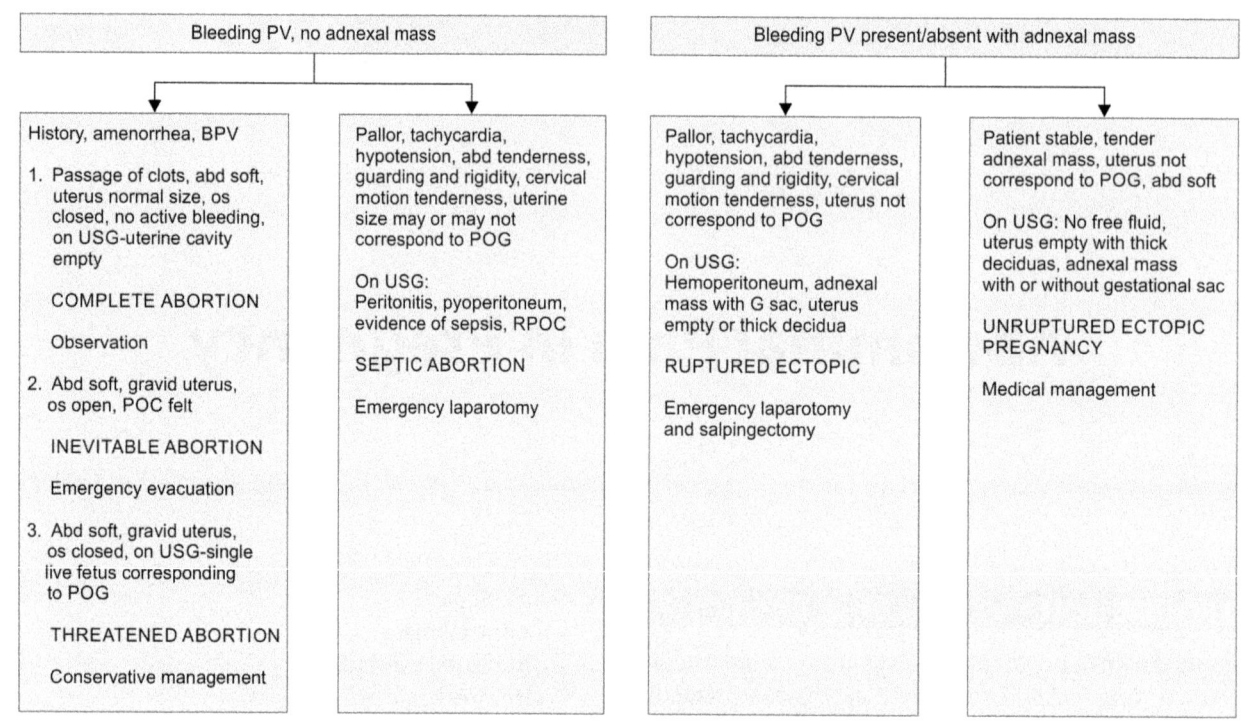

(G sac: gestational sac; POC: product of conception; POG: period of gestation; PV: per vaginum; RPOC: retained product of conception; USG: ultrasonography; Abd: abdominal)

Algorithm 2: Management of abdominal pain in early and late pregnancy (nonobstetric causes).

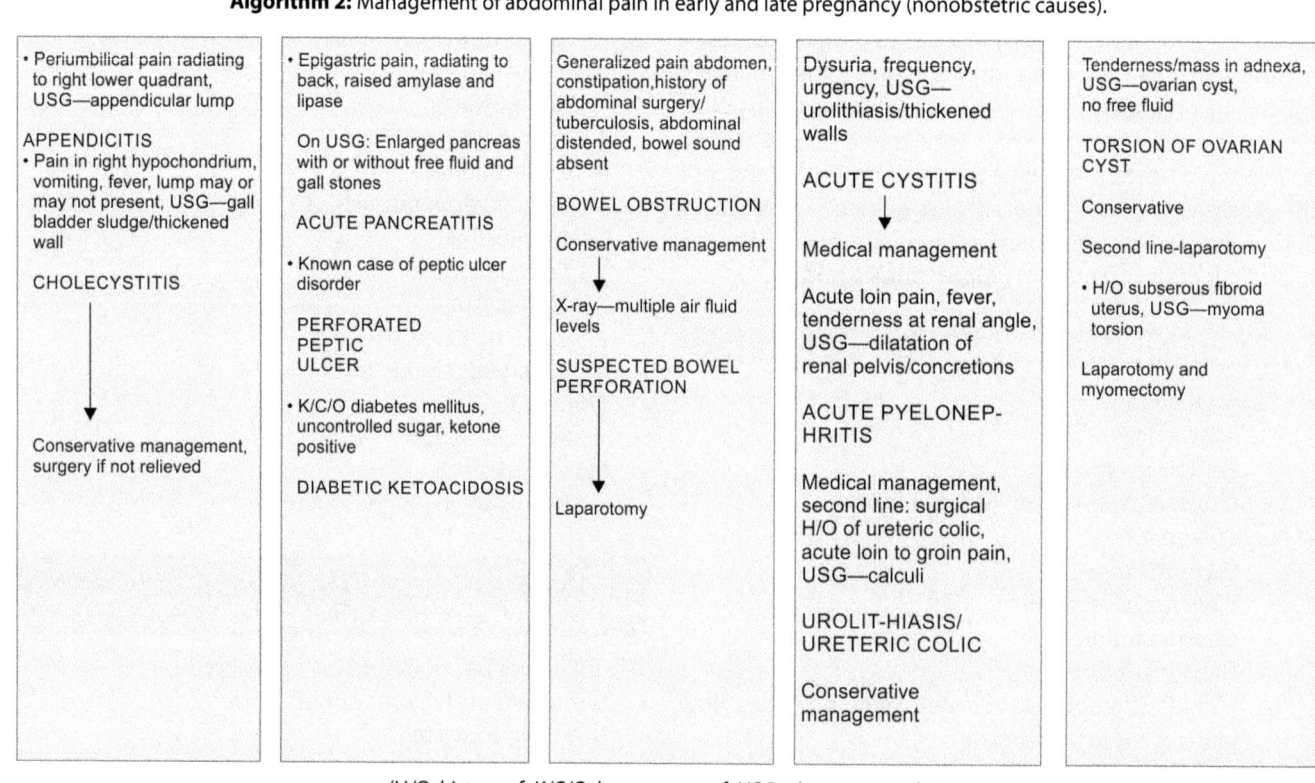

(H/O: history of; K/C/O: known case of; USG: ultrasonography)

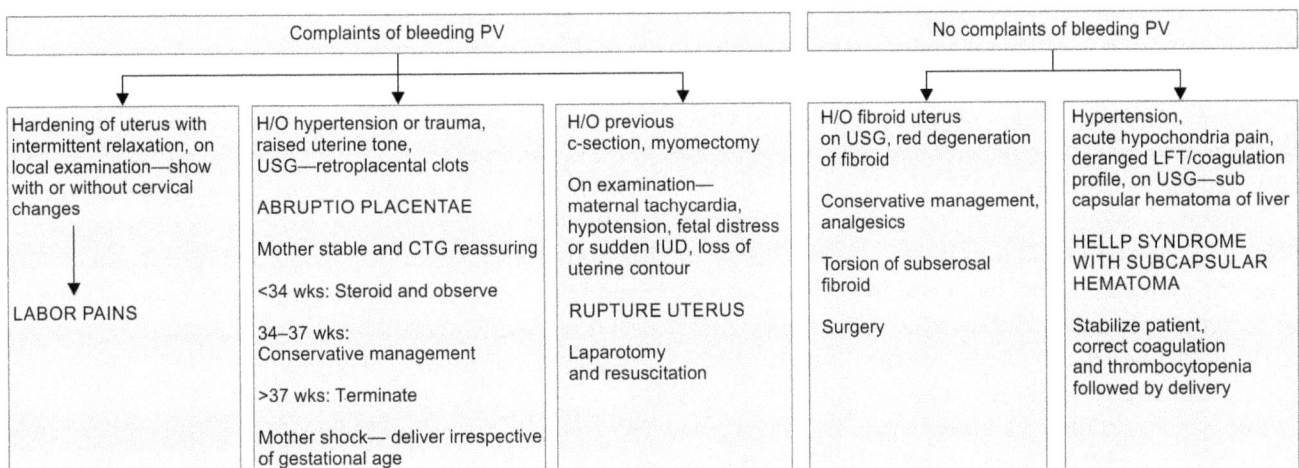

Algorithm 3: Evaluation of abdominal pain in late pregnancy.

(H/O: history of; HELLP: hemolysis, elevated liver enzymes, low platelet counts; IUD: intrauterine device; LFT: liver function test; PV: per vaginum; USG: ultrasonography)

- Are any investigations indicated?
- Will pregnancy effect result?
- What is the risk of investigation?

HISTORY

Detailed history should be taken regarding time of onset, duration, intensity, radiation, and character of the pain as well as associated symptoms. Danger signs are abrupt onset, localized, constant, or severe, or pain associated with nausea and vomiting, vaginal bleeding, syncopal attack, and fever.

Abdominal Examination

After recording the vital signs, abdominal examination should include assessment of symphysio-fundal height, consistency and tenderness of the uterus, position and engagement of the presenting part, and fetal heart rate. To differentiate between extra- and intrauterine tenderness, it is helpful to examine the patient in the right or left decubitus position by displacing the gravid uterus to one side. The location of some organs may vary according to the stage of pregnancy as the gravid uterus grows. In addition, the laxity of the anterior abdominal wall makes signs such as rebound tenderness and guarding nonspecific. This is particularly pronounced in multiparae due to a decrease in abdominal wall tone.

Pelvic Examination

In assessing early pregnancy conditions, such as ectopic pregnancy and miscarriage, it is essential to determine whether the pain originates from the uterus. Pelvic examination should be preceded by speculum insertion to visualize the cervix and take vaginal and cervical swabs if necessary. Digital evaluation should focus on the presence of cervical motion tenderness and thorough assessment of the adnexa.

Imaging

Abdominal/pelvic ultrasound is the most frequently used imaging modality for evaluating abdominal pain in pregnancy, largely due to its safety. It allows easy assessment of maternal gallbladder, pancreas, and kidneys and can exclude pancreatitis, pyelonephritis, nephrolithiasis, and cholelithiasis. In hemodynamically unstable patients, scanning should be performed expeditiously. Ultrasound remains the principal method of assessing the fetal gestational age, fetal heart activity, fetal activity, and amniotic fluid volume.

Transvaginal ultrasound is regarded as the imaging method of choice for patients who present with abdominal pain in early pregnancy, including diagnoses of miscarriage or ectopic pregnancy. Abdominal X-ray may be a necessary diagnostic tool in some rare cases (e.g. bowel obstruction, nephrolithiasis). The risks and benefits about exposing the fetus to radiation should be weighed against the morbidity and mortality that may result from a delayed diagnosis.

Computed tomography (CT) scan of the abdomen may be indicated in cases of severe necrotic pancreatitis or if the diagnosis of appendicitis or splenic rupture is unclear. As with plain film radiographs, such imaging techniques should only be considered if the risk of maternal morbidity and mortality outweighs the risk of fetal radiation exposure. This cautious approach has led to the development of evidence-based guidelines to support physicians in the evaluation of risks and benefits, which should always be considered and discussed with patients prior to their implementation.[2,3]

Magnetic resonance imaging (MRI) is expensive and time consuming and can be uncomfortable for pregnant patients. It may be of use in defining specific characteristics of an adnexal mass or aiding the diagnosis of nephrolithiasis. More recently, MRI has been considered the preferred test after inconclusive ultrasound scan in the evaluation of right lower quadrant (RLQ) pain, due to the lack of ionizing radiation.[4,5] However, it is not recommended during the first trimester, as the effect of MRI on fetal development is unclear.

LABORATORY INVESTIGATIONS

Early Pregnancy

Serum beta human chorionic gonadotropin (β-hCG) in combination with transvaginal ultrasound should be the initial test requested to all patients presenting with abdominal pain when <20 weeks pregnant. This also confirms or excludes the presence of an intrauterine pregnancy. Complete blood count (CBC) should also be included, particularly estimation of Hb, platelets, and hematocrit (if vaginal bleeding). If ovarian hyperstimulation syndrome (OHSS) is suspected, additional tests indicated include a serum electrolyte panel, liver function tests (LFTs), and coagulation screen.

Late Pregnancy

Complete blood count (particularly estimation of Hb, platelets, and hematocrit) is the initial investigation requested for all patients presenting with abdominal pain beyond 20 weeks pregnant. Serum electrolyte panel and LFTs and platelet count is indicated in HELLP syndrome, acute fatty liver of pregnancy and acute pancreatitis. A coagulation screen is indicated as clotting abnormalities may occur in placental abruption, uterine rupture, and HELLP syndrome.

Urinalysis is useful to assess the presence of urinary tract abnormalities, but the detection of protein in urine alerts the physician to the possibility of a serious underlying condition such as HELLP syndrome. Interpretation of all these results must take into account the effects of the physiologic changes of pregnancy.

CONCLUSION

In any patient with pregnancy, who presents with abdomen in the abdomen, the first obstetrical causes should be kept in mind. It is always good to follow protocols for emergency situations and if conservative management fails. Surgery should be considered timely to avoid complications.

REFERENCES

1. Kammerer WS. Nonobstetric surgery during pregnancy. The Medical Clinics of North America. 1979;63:1157-64.
2. Chen MM, Coakley FV, Kaimal A, et al. Guidelines for computed tomography and magnetic resonance imaging use during pregnancy and lactation. Obstet Gynecol. 2008;112:333-40.
3. Society of American Gastrointestinal and Endoscopic Surgeons. (2011). Guidelines for diagnosis, treatment, and use of laparoscopy for surgical problems during pregnancy. [online] http://www.sages.org/ [Last accessed on September 2019].
4. American College of Radiology (Revised 2018) ACR Appropriateness Criteria®; Right Lower Quadrant Pain-Suspected Appendicitis. http://www.acr.org/.
5. Long SS, Long C, Lai H, et al. Imaging strategies for right lower quadrant pain in pregnancy. Am J Roentgenol. 2011;196:4-12.

Bleeding in Early Pregnancy

Bhaskar Pal, Alpana V Chhetri

INTRODUCTION

Bleeding in pregnancy occurs in about 20–40% of clinically diagnosed pregnancy.[1] Bleeding during early pregnancy can be due to endometrial implantation. Approximately 15–20% of clinically recognized pregnancies will miscarry. When bleeding occurs in early pregnancy, 30% of them will have spontaneous abortions, 1–2% are due to ectopic pregnancy, and 0–2% are molar pregnancy. Around 60–70% pregnancies are carried beyond 20 weeks **(Algorithm 1)**.

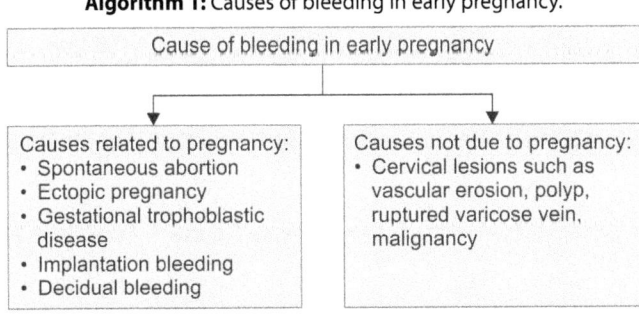

Algorithm 1: Causes of bleeding in early pregnancy.

ASSESSMENT AND DIAGNOSIS OF EARLY PREGNANCY BLEEDING

Assessment and diagnosis are made through a combination of history, physical examination, and clinical investigations. Initial assessment of hemodynamic stability is necessary.

History

- Menstrual history and last normal menstrual period (LMNP)
- Date of positive pregnancy test
- Previous pregnancies and outcome, e.g. miscarriage, ectopic
- Other significant gynecological history
- History of hormone intake or contraception
- Whether assisted conception
- Symptoms of early pregnancy
- Associated symptoms such as pain, vaginal bleeding, postural syncope, vomiting, and shoulder tip pain
- Passage of products of conception.

Physical Examination

- *Vital condition:* Pulse, blood pressure, temperature, heart rate, respiratory rate
- *Abdominal examination:* Tenderness, rigidity, distension
- Per vaginal blood loss on pad
- *Vaginal examination:*
  - Speculum examination to see the source and amount of bleeding or any evidence of product of conception
  - Bimanual examination for cervical motion tenderness, adnexal mass, and to assess size of the uterus; check if os is open or closed.

Investigations

- Urine for pregnancy test

- *Ultrasound scan:* Transvaginal scan (TVS) preferred over transabdominal scan (TAS)
- If TVS inconclusive, then serial beta-human chorionic gonadotropin (βhCG) monitoring
- Full blood count and group
- Midstream urine for RE, ME, and culture sensitivity if clinically indicated
- Screening for sexually transmitted infections.

VIABILITY AND LOCATION OF PREGNANCY

Interpreting Changes in Serum βhCG (Table 1)

Serum βhCG first becomes positive 9 days postconception. βhCG greater than 5 IU/L confirms pregnancy. A single βhCG does not differentiate between viable and nonviable pregnancy.[2] If βhCG shows more than 66% rise over 48 hours, then it is probably early viable intrauterine pregnancy (IUP):

- *If βhCG shows less than 66% rise:* Probably ectopic pregnancy or pregnancy of unknown location (PUL) or a nonviable pregnancy

Table 1: Interpretation of beta-human chorionic gonadotropin (βhCG) and transvaginal scan (TVS) findings.

βhCG/TVS in clinically stable women	Interpretation/recommendations
βhCG < 2,000 IU/L	Repeat TVS/βhCG after 48 hours
βhCG > 2,000 IU/L and TVS with no intrauterine pregnancy, complex adnexal mass, and/or free fluid in the pouch of Douglas	High probability of ectopic pregnancy
βhCG > 2,000 IU/L with no intrauterine pregnancy (IUP) and abnormal findings	Repeat βhCG in 48 hours/repeat TVS as appropriate
Declining or suboptimally rising βhCG levels	Indicating nonviable pregnancy (ectopic or intrauterine pregnancy)

- *βhCG falling:* Indicates failing pregnancy regardless of its location
- *βhCG static:* Active trophoblasts still present.

Discriminatory zone: The level of serum βhCG above which a gestational sac should be visible on transvaginal or a transabdominal scan if a viable intrauterine pregnancy is present.[3]

- 1500–1800 mIU/mL with transvaginal ultrasonography, but up to 2300 mIU/mL with multiple fetus
- 6000–6500 mIU/mL with abdominal ultrasonography

Intrauterine pregnancy is usually visible on TVS when the mean sac diameter (MSD) is greater than or equal to 3 mm size.

Serum Progesterone

In case of PUL, a single progesterone level may assist in identifying women with a low risk of having an ectopic pregnancy or persistent PUL.[4]

Ultrasound scan and serial βhCG monitoring helps in diagnosing location and viability of pregnancy.

Quantitative βhCG measurement along with TVS are often the only way to differentiate between early intrauterine pregnancy, ectopic pregnancy and pregnancy of unknown location **(Algorithm 2)**.

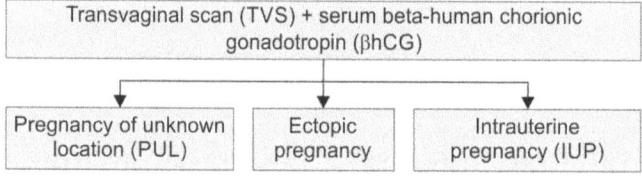

Algorithm 2: Assessment of location and viability in suspected pregnancy loss.

Pregnancy of unknown location or PUL is defined as a situation when the pregnancy test is positive but there are no signs of extrauterine or intrauterine pregnancy via TVS. To diagnose PUL, ultrasound along with serial βhCG measurement is essential to diagnose the location of pregnancy **(Algorithm 3)**.

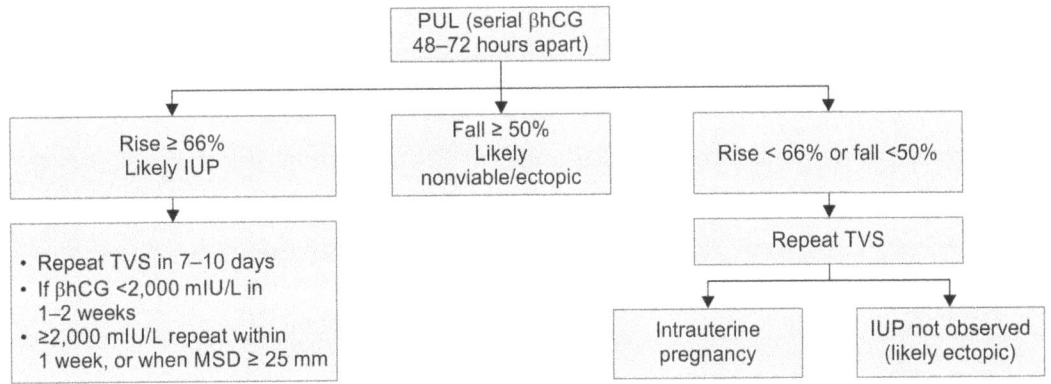

Algorithm 3: Pregnancy of unknown location (PUL).

(βhCG: beta-human chorionic gonadotropin; IUP: intrauterine pregnancy; MSD: mean sac diameter; PUL: pregnancy of unknown location; TAS: transabdominal scan; TVS: transvaginal scan)

Algorithm 4 shows USS diagnosis of intrauterine pregnancy (IUP) and assessment of fetal viability.

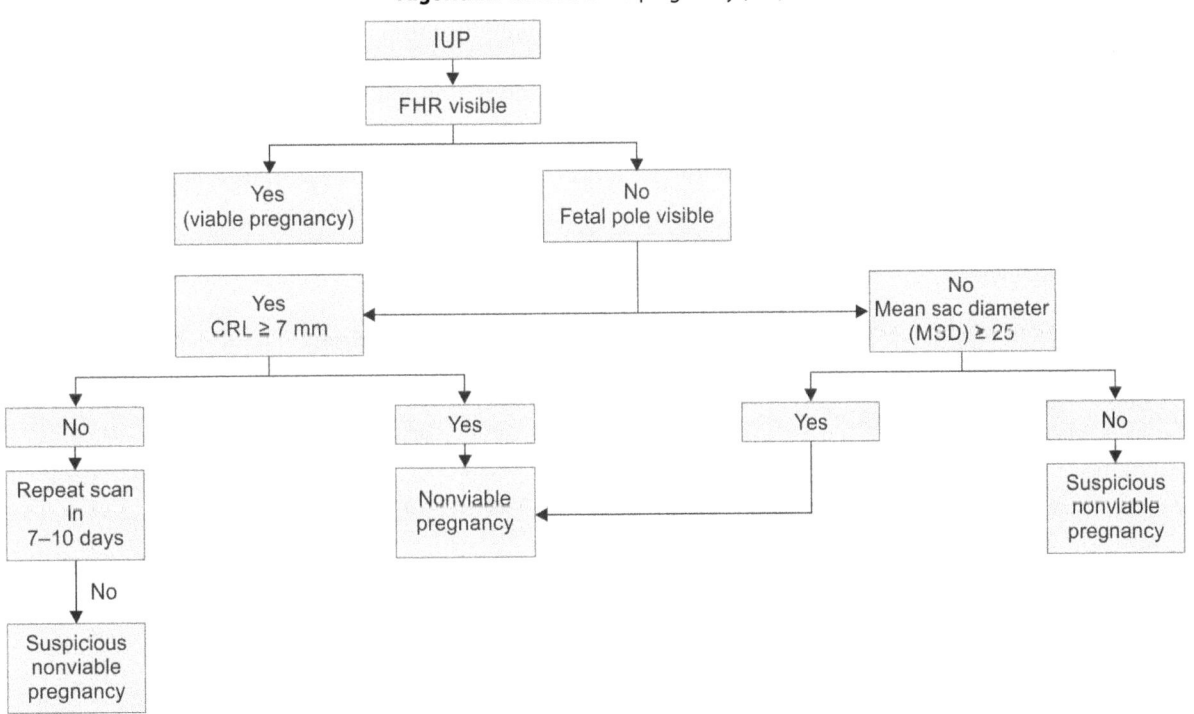

Algorithm 4: Intrauterine pregnancy (IUP).

(CRL: crown-rump length; FHR: fetal heart rate)

Ectopic pregnancy accounts for 2% of all pregnancies. TVS or serum βhCG, or both is needed to confirm diagnosis of ectopic pregnancy. **Algorithm 5** shows diagnosis and management of ectopic pregnancy respectively.

Algorithm 5: Ectopic pregnancy.

```
                Ectopic pregnancy
                        ↓
            Initial assessment vitals
                   UPT/βhCG
                   ↓         ↓
     Hemodynamically    Hemodynamically
         stable             unstable
            ↓                  ↓
      • βhCG            Presumptive ruptured
      • TVS                  ectopic
      • TAS (If TVS              ↓
        not available)    Immediate surgical
            ↓                 treatment
      • Empty uterine cavity
      • Noncystic adnexal mass
      • No specific endometrial sign
      • Free fluid in POD is not
        diagnostic
            ↓
      Management of ectopic
           pregnancy
        ↓     ↓      ↓
   Expectant Medical Surgical
```

(βhCG: beta-human chorionic gonadotropin; POD: pouch of Douglas; TAS: transabdominal scan; TVS: transvaginal scan; UPT: urine pregnancy test)

Expectant Management

Indications

- Hemodynamically stable
- No evidence of rupture
- Low and falling serum βhCG (<1,500 IU/L at initial presentation)
- Minimal/no fluid in pelvis on USS
- Tubal mass < 3 cm
- Pain free
- Woman understands the need for follow-up and can access medical services.

Ongoing Management

- Serial βhCG for 8 days
- If resolution occurring, then weekly βhCG until negative
- USS if clinically indicated
- Avoid conception until sonographic resolution.

Medical Management

Indications

- Hemodynamically stable
- No evidence of rupture
- No signs of active bleeding
- Normal FBC, electrolytes, and liver function tests.

Contraindications

- Allergy to methotrexate
- Potential noncompliance
- Presence of medical conditions (review on individual basis)
- Breastfeeding caution
- Baseline βhCG > 5,000 IU/L
- Ectopic >3 cm on TVS
- Fetal heart motion present.

Methotrexate Regimen

Single dose 50 mg/m^2 on day 0 and βhCG monitoring on days 0, 4, and 7. βhCG declines 15% between day 4 and day 7. Second dose on day 7 if βhCG does not decline 15%.

Regimen requires complete blood count, renal function test, and liver function tests at baseline.

Ongoing Management

- Early pregnancy assessment unit
- Serial βhCG as per methotrexate protocol
- USS if clinically indicated
- Avoid conception for 4 months due to potential teratogenicity.

Surgical Management

Indications

- Woman's preference
- Unsuccessful expectant or medical management
- Hemodynamically unstable
- Persistent excess bleeding
- Evidence of infected POC
- Suspected gestational trophoblastic disease
- Baseline βhCG> 5,000 IU/L
- Ectopic > 3 cm on TVS
- Fetal heart motion present.

Type of Surgery

Laparoscopic surgery should be performed whenever possible. A salpingectomy is usually performed unless the contralateral tube is damaged. A salpingostomy may result in a need for further treatment.[5]

General management of miscarriage—refer **Algorithm 6**.
Medical management of miscarriage—refer **Algorithm 7**.

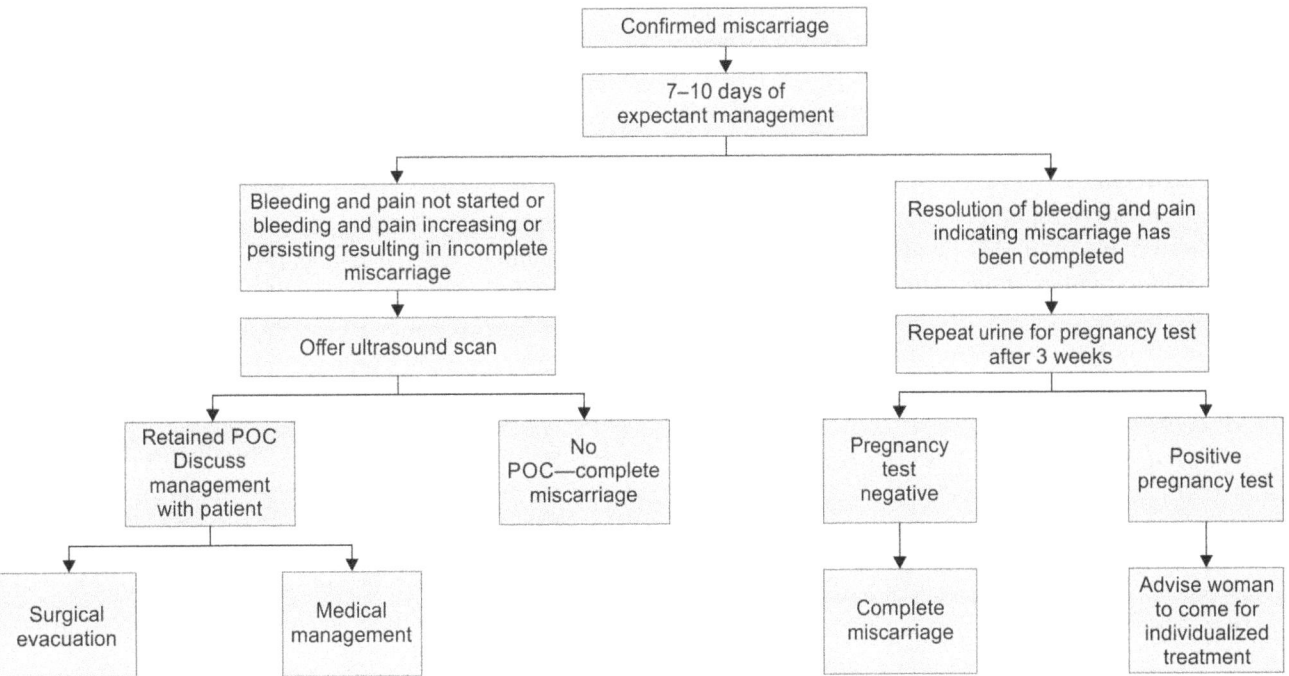

Algorithm 6: Management of miscarriage.

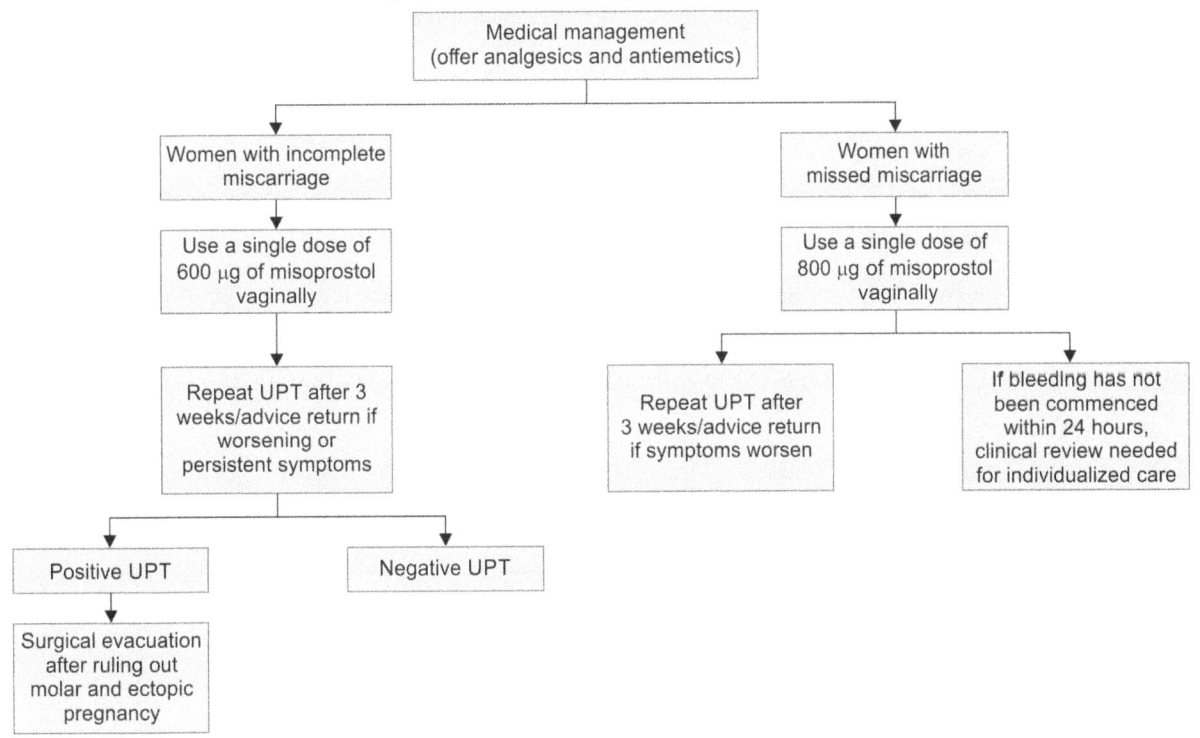

Algorithm 7: Medical management of miscarriage.

ANTI-D PROPHYLAXIS

Anti-D globulin should be given to all nonsensitive Rh-negative women in the following circumstances:
- *<12 weeks:* 250 IU, intramuscularly in case of uterine evacuation (medical and surgical) and ectopic pregnancies.
- *>12 weeks:* In all women with bleeding per vagina with 250 IU itramuscular before 20 weeks and with 500 IU after 20 weeks.

The diagnosis of molar pregnancy, the most common form of gestational trophoblastic disease (GTD) should be suspected by a number of signs and symptoms:

- Abnormal vaginal bleeding, hyperemesis, excessive uterine enlargement, and early failed pregnancy is the classical feature of molar pregnancy.
- USS shows characteristic features and histopathological examination of the products is the definitive diagnosis.

Figure 1 summarizes the clinical features, diagnosis, intervention and follow-up of molar pregnancies.

CONCLUSION

Early pregnancy bleeding causes great anxiety and stress to the women and her family. It is important to deal with the situation with great care and support, especially when a nonviable pregnancy is present. Reassurance and follow-up in early pregnancy unit are necessary.

REFERENCES

1. Queensland Clinical Guidelines. Maternity and Neonatal Clinical Guidelines. Early Pregnancy Loss. Brisbane: Queensland Health; 2011.
2. Kadar N, Caldwell BV, Romero R. A method of screening for ectopic pregnancy and its indications. Obstet Gynecol. 1981;58(2):162-6.
3. Barnhart KT, Sammel MD, Rinauds PF, et al. Symptomatic patients with an early viable intrauterine pregnancy: hCG curves redefined. Obstet Gynecol. 2004;104(1):50-5.
4. Van Calster B, Bobdiwala S, Guha S, et al. Managing pregnancy of unknown location based on initial progesterone and serum βhCG levels: development and validation of a two step triage protocol. Ultrasound Obstet Gynecol. 2016;48/5:642-9.
5. Hajenius PJ, Mol F, Mol BW, et al. Intervention for tubal ectopic pregnancy. Cochrane Database Syst Rev. 2007;(1):CD000324.

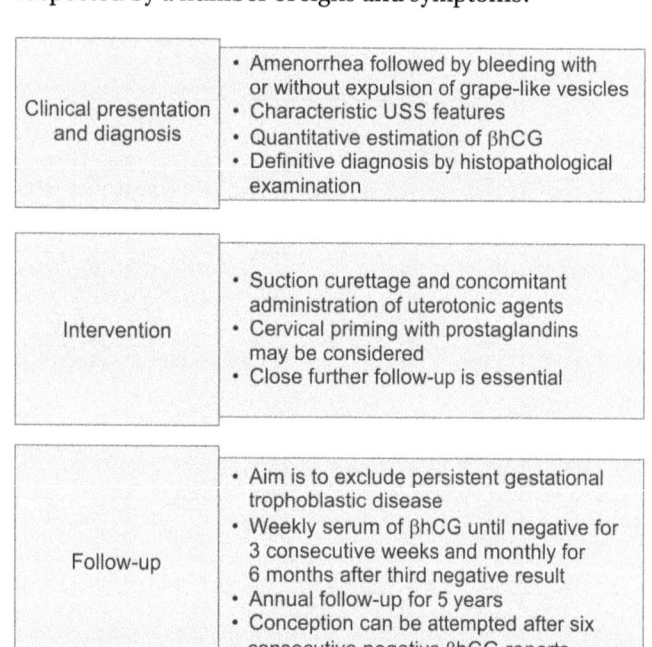

Fig. 1: Molar pregnancy.

Chapter 19

Bleeding in Late Pregnancy

Rashmi Bagga, Japleen Kaur

DEFINITIONS

Bleeding in late pregnancy or antepartum hemorrhage (as it is more popularly known as) is defined as bleeding from or into the genital tract after 24 weeks and before the birth of baby.[1] Two significant causes of antepartum hemorrhage are placental abruption and placenta previa, respectively **(Algorithm 1)**.

Abruptio placentae or placental abruption is defined as partial or complete premature separation of normally situated placenta from the uterine wall, before delivery of the baby. Placenta previa is defined as implantation of the placenta in the lower segment of the uterus, such that it presents ahead of the fetal presenting part.

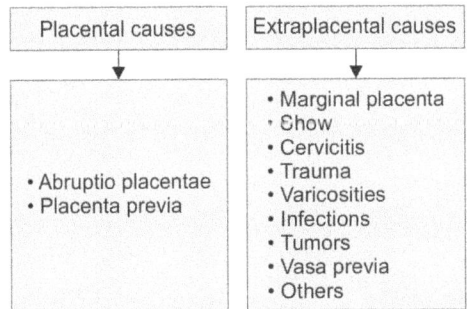

Algorithm 1: Causes of antepartum hemorrhage.

CLINICAL IMPORTANCE

Complicating about 3–5% of pregnancies, obstetric hemorrhage is an important cause of maternal mortality worldwide. The incidence of placental abruption is about 0.2–1.0%, whereas placenta previa complicates almost 1 in 300 pregnancies. Perinatal mortality rate attributed to abruption is approximately 12%, whereas 4–8% cases of placenta previa or vasa previa can lead to fetal or neonatal mortality.[2,3] The risk factors for the two major causes of antepartum hemorrhage are given in **Table 1**. The classification of antepartum hemorrhage is shown in **Algorithm 2**.

Table 1: Risk factors and associations of the two major causes of antepartum hemorrhage.

Placental abruption	Placenta previa
Previous abruption	Previous placenta previa
Pre-eclampsia	Previous cesarean
Fetal growth restriction	Advanced maternal age
Thrombophilias	Multiparity
Polyhydramnios	Previous curettage
Advanced maternal age	Manual removal of placenta
Multiparity	Multiple pregnancy
Trauma	Smoking
Smoking and drug abuse (cocaine)	
Preterm rupture of membranes	

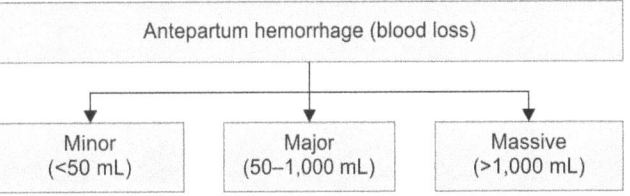

Algorithm 2: Classification of antepartum hemorrhage (based on estimated blood loss).

CLASSIFICATION OF PLACENTA PREVIA (RCOG)

- *Major placenta previa:* Placenta lies partly or wholly over the internal os.
- *Minor placenta previa:* The leading edge of the placenta is in the lower uterine segment but not covering the cervical os.

MANAGEMENT OF BLEEDING IN LATE PREGNANCY (ALGORITHM 3)

Management depends on the hemodynamic stability of the mother, period of gestation (in relation to period of viability), cause/severity of hemorrhage, and condition of the fetus **(Algorithms 4 to 6)**. General principles of management include intravenous access, infusion of crystalloids, arranging adequate blood and blood products, and involving a senior obstetrician in the process of decision making. Use of anti-D immunoglobulin is recommended in a rhesus negative mother.[4]

ELABORATION OF MACAFEE AND JOHNSON REGIMEN[5]

Premise
Minor previa presenting early may resolve by term during expectant management. Most episodes of bleeding are small and self-limiting and unlikely to be lethal to the mother or the fetus.

Aim
The aim of the regimen is to prolong pregnancy in order to decrease perinatal morbidity and mortality.

Components
- Informed consent, explaining the purpose, possible benefits, and risks
- Admission in hospital and bed rest
- Transfusion support to maintain hemoglobin above 10 g/dL
- Antenatal corticosteroid for fetal lung maturity

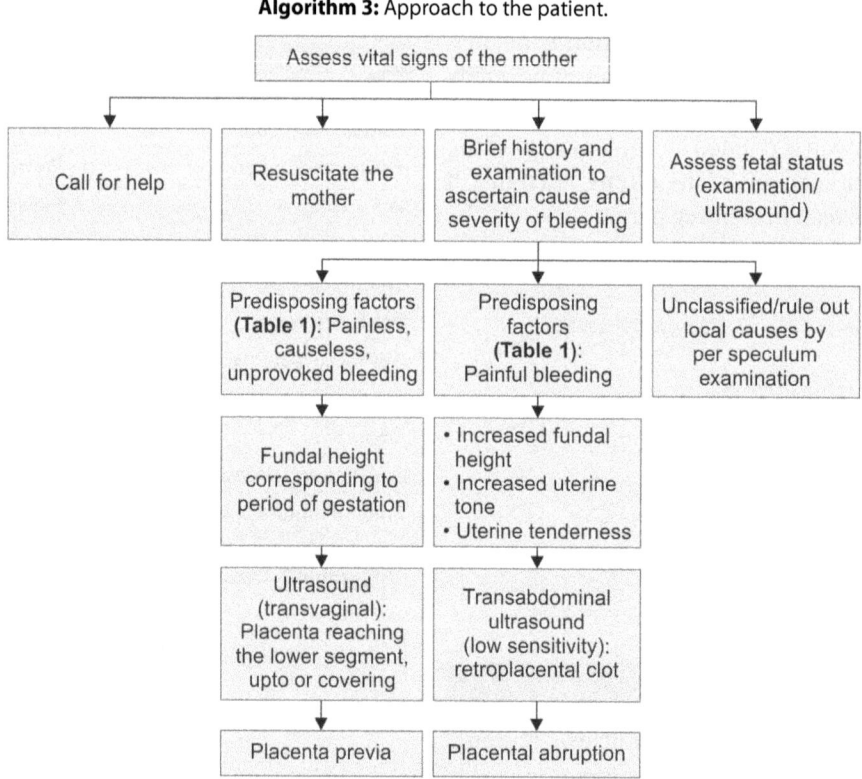

Algorithm 3: Approach to the patient.

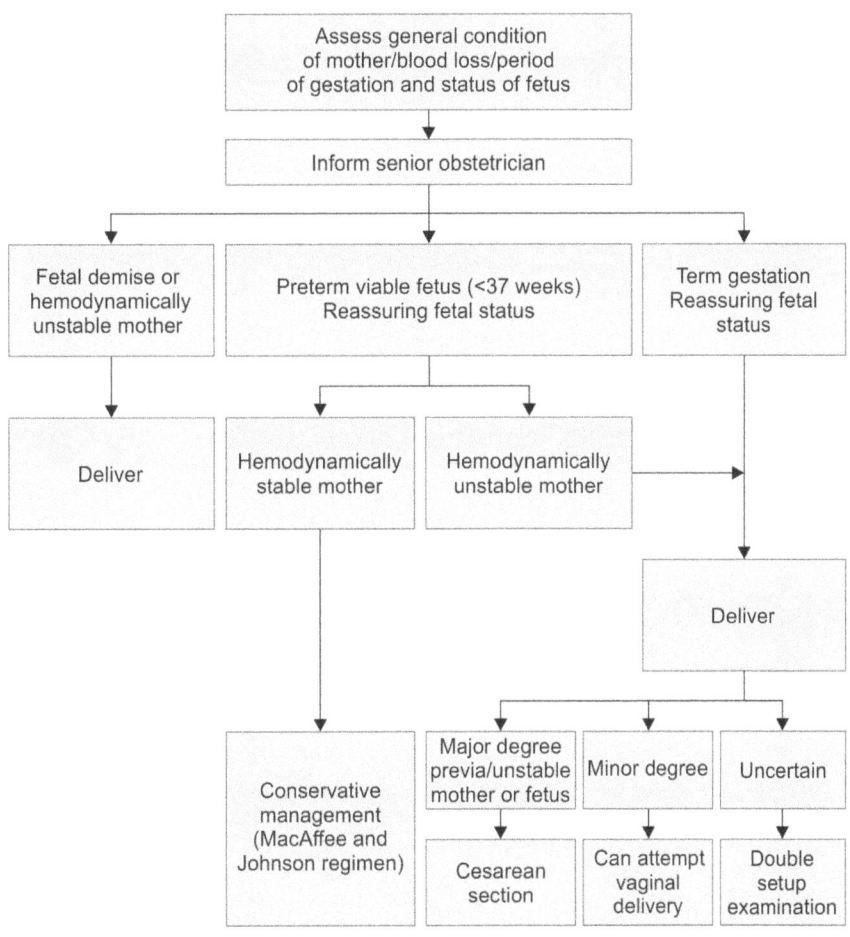

Algorithm 4: Management of bleeding due to placenta previa.

- Close maternal and fetal monitoring
- Involvement of neonatologist.

Contraindications include fetal demise, malformation, profuse bleeding, hemodynamic instability, and preterm labor.

ROLE OF TOCOLYTICS

Tocolysis for treatment of bleeding due to placenta previa may be useful in selected cases. However, beta-mimetics which have been used in most studies are known to be associated with significant adverse effects. Therefore, the agent and optimum regime are still debatable and further research is required for making a recommendation.[4]

PLACENTA ACCRETA

Placenta accreta is abnormally adherent placenta, which is generally associated with low-lying placenta (although it may be rarely seen in upper segment placentae also). There is a defect in the decidua basalis, which leads to invasive implantation of the placenta. Risk factors include placenta previa, especially with history of previous cesarean section, previous uterine surgery, previous curettage, and submucous fibroids. Management includes inpatient management and well-planned elective cesarean delivery (unless there is active bleeding at any time). Meticulous preoperative preparation includes informed consent for classical cesarean and peripartum hysterectomy with blood transfusion, arranging adequate blood and blood products, involving a senior anesthetist, and arrangement of postoperative intensive care. Conservative procedures such as leaving the placenta in situ, with uterine artery embolization or postpartum administration of antibiotics and methotrexate, have been tried in order to conserve fertility, but there is no definite consensus on this line of management.

Algorithm 5: Management of bleeding due to placental abruption (term and preterm fetus).

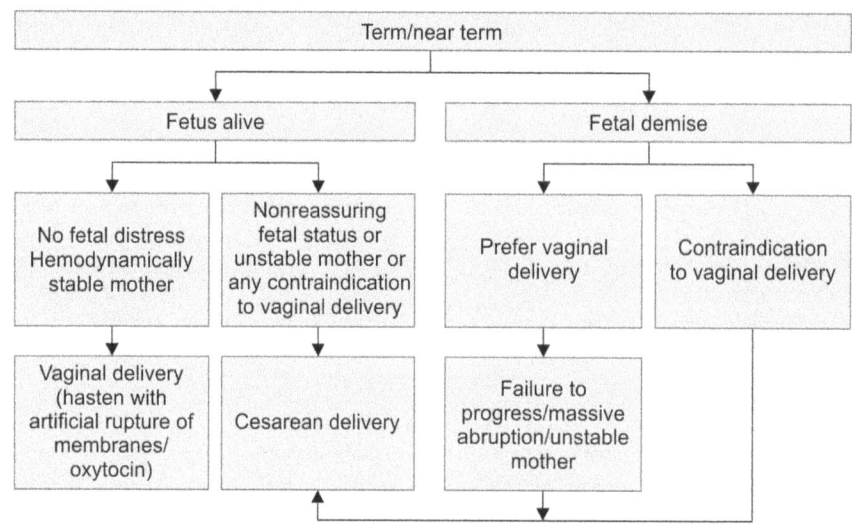

Algorithm 6: Management of bleeding due to placental abruption (preterm fetus).

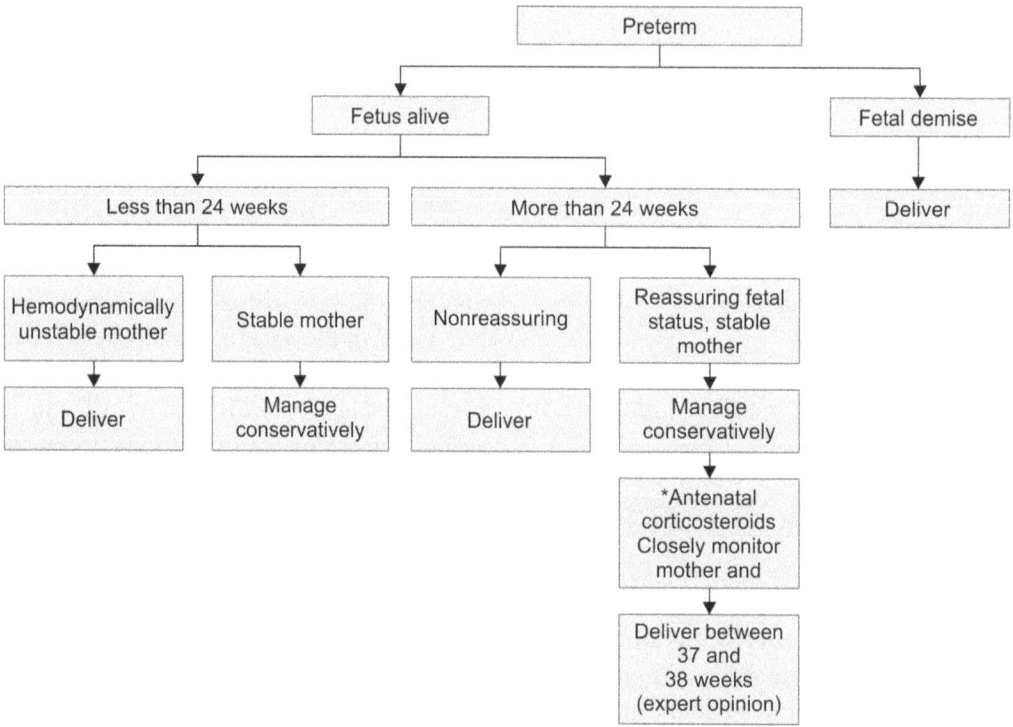

*Recent guidelines issued by the Society of Maternal-Fetal Medicine, on management of patients presenting with bleeding in late preterm period (34–36 weeks, 6 days), recommend administration of corticosteroids for this period of gestation also, if not previously given, in a stable patient not actively hemorrhaging.[6]

REFERENCES

1. Royal College of Obstetricians and Gynaecologists. Greentop Guideline No. 63. Antepartum Hemorrhage. London, UK: Royal College of Obstetricians and Gynaecologists; 2011.
2. Tikkanen M, Luukkaala T, Gissler M, et al. Decreasing perinatal mortality in placental abruption. Acta Obstet Gynecol Scand. 2013;92:298-305.
3. Lam M, Wong SF, Chow KM, et al. Women with placenta praevia and antepartum hemorrhage have a worse outcome than those who do not bleed before delivery. J Obstet Gynaecol. 2000;20:27-31.
4. Royal College of Obstetricians and Gynaecologists. Greentop Guideline No. 27. Placenta Previa, Placenta Accreta and Vasa Previa: Diagnosis and Management. London, UK: Royal College of Obstetricians and Gynaecologists; 2011.
5. MacAfee CH, Millar WG, Harley G. Maternal and fotal mortality in placenta praevia. J Obstet Gynaecol Br Emp. 1962;69:203-12.
6. Gyamfi-Bannerman C, Society for Maternal-Fetal Medicine (SMFM). Society for Maternal-Fetal Medicine (SMFM) Consult Series# 44: Management of bleeding in the late preterm period. Am J Obstet Gynecol. 2018;218(1):B2-8.

Chapter 20

Preterm Labor

Madhu Nagpal

Defined as: Labor after 20 completed weeks and before 37 completed weeks (259 days) since day 1 of last menstrual period.

National/global impact: Births/deaths in preterm
- About 5–18% incidence of preterm births (PTB) globally, 13% in India
- In India, 3.5 million are born preterm every year
- India ranks 1 with 1 million deaths/year (2010 data)

Neonatal death (NND)
Lower the gestation age—higher is NND rate:
- 0.2% at 37–40 weeks
- 18% at 32–36 weeks
- 21.8% at 24–31 weeks

Classified as:
- Very early preterm: <28 weeks
- Early preterm: <32 weeks
- Late preterm: <37 weeks

(Subclassified till 34 and 37 weeks)
The fragmented weeks are not rounded off for classification.

Preterm birth impact: Twenty-eight percent NND other than congenital anomalies.
Survivors suffer from:
- Cerebral palsy
- Delayed development
- Visual/hearing impairment
- Chronic lung disease
- Atherosclerosis
- Cardiovascular disease
- Hypertension in adulthood

Categorized as:
- Spontaneous: 60–70%
- Iatrogenic: 30–40%

Spontaneous as with:
- Preterm premature rupture of the membranes (PPROM): chorioamnionitis
- Congenital uterine anomalies
- Congenitally/surgically short cervix
- Cervical incompetence, dysfunction
- Multifetal gestation
- Polyhydramnios infections like bacterial vaginosis
- Asymptomatic/symptomatic urinary tract infection (UTI)
- Smoking, stress, strenuous lifestyle

Iatrogenic as with:
- Subclinical/clinical chorioamnionitis
- Severe pregnancy-induced hypertension (PIH)/eclampsia
- Antepartum hemorrhage
- Intrauterine fetal growth restriction
- Amputated, traumatized, short cervix
- External cephalic version
- Miscalculated gestational age
- Premature labor induction
- Obstetrical reasons for termination

Issues related to preterm labor:
Prediction of preterm labor : for primary prevention
Prevention of preterm labor } : for secondary prevention
Prophylaxis for threatened preterm
Management of premature labor } : for tertiary prevention
Care of preterm newborn

Prediction/identifying risk factors:
- Why predict?
- Aim is to prevent

Historical factors:
- **Previous preterm birth: strongest risk marker**
  - Risk 1.5–2 fold with one previous preterm labor (PTL)
  - Risk 28% with previous two PTL
- If medically indicated PTL—then know indication, recurrence of disease, and necessity to repeat termination
- Poor socioeconomic status, smoking, tobacco, and alcohol use
- Low maternal body mass index (BMI), poor weight gain during pregnancy
- Young and advanced age
- More common with male fetuses (55%)[1]
- Bleeding in early pregnancy, placenta previa, abruptio placentae
- Macrosomia, multiple pregnancy, polyhydramnios
- Fibroids, previous cervical surgeries
- *Infections:* Asymptomatic bacteriuria, periodontal disease
- Bacterial vaginosis
- *Iatrogenic:* Indicated group for termination
  - Wrong dates
  - Unintended PTB

Understanding pathophysiology for preterm:
Four pathways explain the pathology and measures used to test at specified gestational ages as below:
- *Inflammatory, infective:* Liberating cytokines and prostaglandin cascade, affecting matrix metalloproteinases
  - At <32 weeks—as in reproductive tract infection (RTI), bacterial vaginosis, urinary infection—do screening, detection
- *Decidual hemorrhage, thrombosis:* Initiating thrombin cascade—any gestational age—as in antepartum bleeding, antiphospholipid antibodies—test for thrombin cascade
- *HP adrenal axis:* Activation at 32–34 weeks—as in stress—do salivary estriol—fetal fibronectin,[2] home uterine activity monitoring (HUAM)
- *Uterine overdistension:* Expression of gap junction proteins, prostaglandins, oxytocin receptors >28 weeks
  - As in multiple gestation, polyhydramnios, big baby, uterine anomaly
  - Do cervical ultrasonography (USG)

Several genetic, metabolic, endocrine, physiological, environmental, and idiopathic phenomenon may coexist.

Role of proinflammatory cytokines:

Cytokines	Mechanism of action	Effect of cytokines
Interleukins-1, 6, 8, TNF-α	Degradation of collagen fibers	Results in cervical ripening
Interleukins-1, TNF-α	Induce matrix metalloproteinases	Results in membrane rupture
Interleukins-1, 2, 6, TNF-α	Increase PGE2, PGF2α	Results in uterine contractions
PGE: prostaglandin E; TNF: tumor necrosis factor		

Proinflammatory response:
Common effect of all pathways is by evoking maternal fetal inflammatory response syndrome with release of proinflammatory cytokines, corticotropin releasing hormone, proteases, and matrix metalloproteinases which bring myometrial contractile and cervical changes initiating preterm labor

Genetic causes:
Attribute to idiopathic group mainly.
Single gene polymorphisms of cytokines in mother and fetus both may be the cause.
Polymorphisms in TNFα-308, IL-1β, and IL-6 are invariably seen in spontaneous PTL.

Based on pathophysiology, preventive measures are:
- Clinical markers: Accurate dating
- Uterine contraction monitoring
- Cervical length measurement
- *Laboratory markers:*
  - Fibronectin assessment
  - Other biochemical tests

Clinical markers related to accurate dating and maturity for avoiding iatrogenic reasons

Parameter	Accuracy	Details	Availability, feasibility	Limitations of method
D-1 (LMP) last menstrual period	=/+/- 14 days	Definite, sure	Widely used	Poor recalling, irregular periods
USG in early pregnancy	±5 d in 1st trimester ±7 d after 1st trimester	CRL, BPD, FL between 6 weeks and 18 weeks	Usually available	Less accurate in fetal malformation, FGR, obesity
Fundal height	=/+/- 3 weeks	Metric measurement	Low cost, feasible	LMP needs to be accurate
Birth weight as surrogate of gestational age	More Ss/Sp at lower gestational age < 1,500 g weight as preterm		Standard parameters available	Need scales, skills
Newborn examination	=/+/- 13 ds for Dubowitz, higher range for all others	GPE, neurological exam	Needs skills, more accurate with neurological scores	Observer based
Best obstetrical estimate	Around ±10 days between USG and newborn examination	Serial observations		Algorithms not standardized
(BPD: biparietal diameter; CRL: crown-rump length; FGR: fetal growth rate; FL: femur length; GPE: general physical examination; USG: ultrasonography)				

Clinical markers: Clinical features, uterine activity monitoring, cervical changes

Clinical features of threatened preterm labor
- Low abdominal pain
- Low backache
- Crampy feeling
- Increased wetness per vaginum
- Discharge/bleeding/show p/vag
- Contractions: Periodical, ill sustained

Home uterine activity monitoring
- Data collected by tocodynamometer twice a day for 1 hour while performing routine activities
- If contractions are 4/hour, the woman monitors for additional 1 hour lying down with additional hydration
- If situation persists—evaluate in hospital

HUAM benefits debated as a preventive measure
Prophylactic use in multiple pregnancy not recommended.

Clinical diagnostic criteria
Between 20 weeks and 37 weeks:
- Contractions are 6 or more/hr
- Cervical dilatation is 3 cm or more
- Effacement is 80% or more
- Ruptured membranes or bleeding p/v

ACOG criteria
Contractions are regular in nature, 4 in 20 minutes/8 in 60 minutes associated with progressive changes in cervix seen as cervical dilatation >1 cm and cervical effacement > 80%

Risk reduction strategies for iatrogenic reasons
- Early identification of disease
- Optimizing management of disease
- Identifying other risk factors for PTB
- Cervical length screening from 24 weeks onward
- Clinical/biochemical markers evaluation periodically
- Use of progesterone: IM, vaginal
- Use of antenatal steroids
- Interventions to prevent multifetal gestation on in vitro fertilization (IVF)
- Scrutiny of congenitally abnormal uterus, stress reduction

Clinical markers: Cervical dysfunction/changes

Cervical competency
- It depends on anatomical integrity and biological components of cervix
- Cervical effacement begins weeks before term labor—approximately 32 weeks in normal labor and from 16 weeks to 24 weeks

In PTL:
Cervical incompetency is thus early predictor of PTL

Ultrasonographic cervical length measurement methods
- *Transabdominal:* Inadequate as bladder expansion results in cervical lengthening and masks funneling. Cervix is obscured with fetal parts and is long away from probe
- *Translabial/transperineal:* Poor visualization due to bowel gas but has no problems as those with transabdominal ultrasound (TAS). Cervix is close to probe and 100% visible without entering vagina

Transvaginal: Best for cervical length
- From external to internal os with fine recording in millimeter when whole length is visible
- With anterior lip to canal equidistant as posterior lip to canal
- Shortest length out of three measurements is recorded

Ultrasonographic transcervical length measurement
- Clinically useful to identify signs of effacement (funneling) and cervical length (CL)
- Assessment of the cervix can be done at rest with application of transfundal/abdominal pressure. Transfundal pressure is more effective than standing position in eliciting cervical changes
- CL measured when anterior cervical and posterior cervical lengths are equal on TVS probing with gentle pressure and shortest of the three readings recorded

Laboratory marker: Fetal fibronectin

Fetal fibronectin
- An extracellular matrix glycoprotein localized at maternal fetal interface of amniotic membranes between chorion and decidua where it is concentrated in area between decidua and trophoblast in normal conditions
- Found in significant levels in cervicovaginal secretions before 20 weeks and after 37 weeks
- Its presence after 24 weeks suggests disruption of chorioamnion to underlying decidua, hence may be a marker of inflammation of fetal membrane/decidual interface with/without infection–may herald onset of PTL
- Levels >50 ng/mL at or after 22 weeks are associated with increased risk of PTL—so used for high-risk women selection
- Concentration >50 ng/mL between 22-37 weeks gest (3% and 4% respectively) as against 93.8% with PPROM and 50.4% in PTL with intact membranes : Ss 81.7% and Sp 82.5%
- Meta-analysis of studies revealed high –ive. P value for fFN in predicting onset of labor pains within next 3 weeks. Specificity was 89% within 1–2 weeks and 92% within 3 weeks
- Sensitivity was low 71% and 59% within 1 week and 3 weeks—Leitich H, 2003
- fFN more useful for prediction of early PTL <28 weeks than late <35 weeks and more for prediction within 1 or 2 weeks after testing than remote
- *Risk of 65% PTL*: If cervical length is <25 mm and fFN is +ive and risk is 25% if fFN is –ive, so useful as predictor of PTL.

Preventive screening: specific situations, markers

Bacterial vaginosis (BV) screening
- *Lactobacillus* produces lactic acid from glycogen and produces low pH, ensures availability of hydrogen peroxide in genital environment
- In normal pregnancy, *Lactobacillus* increases as pregnancy advances
- In BV, abnormality of bacterial flora is characterized by decreased lactobacilli number, increased pH, and increase in pathogenic bacteria including *Gardnerella vaginosis* associated with increased risk of PTL
- Results of various studies are variable
- Overall BV doubles the risk of PTL
- Still unclear, if treatment of bacterial vaginosis with antibiotics decreases risk of PTL
- ACOG, SCOG, NICE 2008 recommends: No consensus to use as screening tool in general population in asymptomatic low risk women
- Women with increased risk for PTL may be benefitted by routine screening

Corticotropin level
- Corticotropin-releasing hormone (CRH) is produced in human placenta and fetal membranes maximally in last trimester.
- Rising fetal cortisol level stimulates expression of CRH by fetal membranes.
- This paradoxical effect attributes to the role of placenta in labor determining the gestational length.
- Studies are underway defining CRH levels as predictor of gestational age.
- At present, CRH screening is not recommended routinely.

Beta-hCG and alpha-fetoprotein
- Increased level in cervicovaginal fluid in early second trimester
- Is associated with adverse outcome including PTL
- A strong negative correlation exists in time from sampling of cervicovaginal human chorionic gonadotropin (hCG) and delivery
- At cut off value of >32 mIU/mL, positive p value is 89% and negative p value is 95% for delivery within 1 week
- Alpha fetoprotein level at 24 weeks is related to PTL

Other biochemical markers
- *C-reactive protein* in early second trimester, if raised is marker of preterm birth
- *Cervical interleukin-6* levels when high at 24 weeks, predict early preterm birth at <32 weeks
- *Cervical IGFBP-1* (Insulin-like growth factor binding protein-1) of unselected asymptomatic female in early and mid-pregnancy are associated with increased chance of PTL. It has Ss 73% and Sp 61% in predicting PTL[3]
- *Elevated cervical fluid pH* in first trimester was associated with enhanced risk of PTL
- *Estriol* level from maternal saliva which represents maternal circulatory levels, if raised (2.3 ng/mL) is related to PTL
- *Maternal serum AFP, serum alkaline phosphatase, granulocyte colony stimulating factors:*
  - All have cumulative Ss of 81% and Sp of 78% for prediction of PTL at 32 weeks' gestation and Ss of 60% and Sp of 73% at <35 weeks' gestation

Prediction summary
- In asymptomatic women: CL 25 mm predicts PTB within 7 days
- In symptomatic women: CL 15 mm predicts PTB in 7 days' time

Other predictors are:
- Absence of fetal breathing movements

So, start serial USG: CL and funneling measurement from 20 weeks to 24 weeks onward
- Do amniotic fluid interleukin-6
- Do serum CRP
- Do fFN at period <34–37 weeks

Basic preventive interventions
Global action report by WHO on "Babies born too soon" aims to reduce preterm births significantly: like—family planning, infection control, prenatal care are basic measures.
- *Primary prevention:* Preconceptional, prenatal risk elimination
- *Secondary prevention:* Prenatal interventions in asymptomatic subjects with high risk.
  - Prenatal interventions in threatened preterm subjects (symptomatic)
- *Tertiary prevention:*
  - Management of preterm birth
  - Management of preterm newborn

Primary intervention
Preconceptional risk reduction strategies are:
- *Minimize stress:* Physical, mental, environmental
- Avoid long-standing, exertion, long work hours, night shifts, job security
- *Reduce unwanted pregnancies:* Contraception use
- Keep interpregnancy interval 18–24 months
- *Plan early:* Avoid extreme of ages
- Care for nutrition, diet, exercise, normal BMI, folic acid intake
- *Prevent sexually transmitted infection (STI):* BV, trichomoniasis, chlamydia, gonorrhea
- *Avoid substance abuse:* Nicotine, tobacco, cocaine, etc.
- *Give vaccination:* For rubella

Do accurate dating: pregnancy test after missed period, dating USG

Primary preventive interventions in antenatal period
Global trends with Very High Human Developmental Index (VHHDI) specified with high quality evidence-based interventions have reported risk reduction by <5%
- Smoking cessation : 0.01%
- Single embryo transfer : 0.06%
- Cervical cerclage : 0.15%
- Progesterone use : 0.01%
- Avoiding unindicated IOL/CS : 0.29%

Secondary prevention in index pregnancy
In asymptomatic subjects: Aim is to prolong gestation
- Identify historical and antenatal risk factors
- Optimize obstetrical problem
- Do serial cervical length measurement
- Home uterine activity monitoring
- Biochemical testing: Fetal fibronectin
- Use of progesterone (medical cerclage)
- Use of long-term tocolysis
- Applying surgical encirclage

- Use of antibiotics especially with PPROM
- Use of pessary
- Use of antenatal steroids before 32 weeks
- Decision making for termination of pregnancy

Secondary prevention in index pregnancy
In threatened preterm labor/symptomatic subject:
- Identify historical/antenatal risk factors
- Optimize obstetrical problem
- Do preliminary clinical examination, p/v, p/s
- Do transabdominal/TVS for fetal maturity, cervical state
- Ascertain early onset of preterm labor
- Use of acute tocolysis
- Use of high dose progesterone
- Gaining time for antenatal steroids effect
- Maintenance tocolysis in quiescent uterus
- Applying rescue surgical encirclage
- Use of antibiotics
- Decision making for time/route of delivery

Cervical length alone for prediction
- CL >3 cm: Excludes diagnosis of PTL
- CL >2.5 cm: Negative p value is 97%
- CL <2.5 cm: Risk of PTL = 17.8%
- CL 1.5–2.5 cm: 35% risk of PTL
- CL <1.5 cm: 50% risk of PTL before 32 weeks and 90% before 34 weeks

Cervical length +fFn prediction together
- Negative fFN with TVS CL >20 mm: Low risk for delivery in next 7 days with irregular, infrequent contractions
- If positive fFN and/or cervical change, TVS CL <20 mm: Increased risk of delivery in next 7 days with painful and persistent uterine contractions for 2 hrs—give tocolysis
- Absence of fFN in cervical secretions is negative predictor of imminent birth negative p value for birth in next 7 days is 97–98%

Cervical length measurement for screening, confirming, follow-up
- Cervical length (TVS) in mid-gestation is single best prognosticator of PTB
- 61% prediction on CL vs. 4.4% on history features
- CL <25 mm predictive at <28 weeks in singleton pregnancy[4]
- Decrease in cervical length between the 24th and 28th weeks of gestation was associated with an increased risk of PTB (R.R. 2.03; 95% CI, 1.28–3.22)

Measures (at 24 weeks)	Relative risk
Cervical length ≤25th percentile (30 mm) as compared to >75th percentile	3.79 (95% CI, 2.32–6.19)
Cervical length ≤10th percentile (25 mm) as compared to >75th percentile	6.19 (95% CI, 3.84–9.97)

Risk of PTL with prior history of PTB with fetal fibronectin (fFN)

Estimated recurrence risk of PTB <35 weeks gestation		
	If fFN +ve	If fFN – ve
Cervical length ≤25 mm	65%	25%
Cervical length 26 to 35 mm	45%	14%
Cervical length > 35 mm	25%	7%

Progesterone
Action is of uterine relaxation in later half of pregnancy by limiting the prostaglandins production. The release of contraction associated protein genes/ion channels/oxytocin/PG receptors, and gap junctions within uterine musculature is inhibited.

Csapo et al. gave "See Saw theory"
- While high levels of progesterone hormones inhibit uterine contractions, the lower levels augment labor.
- Progesterone has anti-inflammatory action, decreases conduction of contractions, and spontaneous uterine activity.
- Progesterone helps in increasing threshold for stimulation of contractions and maintain cervical competency.
- Progesterone can be used prophylactically to *prevent* preterm labor. However, it may not inhibit established active preterm labor successfully. So, cannot be used as a uterine tocolytic.
- Progesterone is recommended in subjects at risk with short cervix for preventing spontaneous preterm delivery when given between 16 weeks and 20 weeks and continued till 36 completed weeks.

Progesterone antagonists: These are used to induce labor.
ACOG Committee Opinion:[5] Recommended in women with singleton pregnancy with previous spontaneous PTB due to PTL or preterm premature rupture of membrane (PPROM) and asymptomatic women with short CL (no. 419, 2008)
SOGC—Technical Update:[6] Recommended use
- Women with history of previous PTL: As 17 OHP-C 250 mg IM weekly till 36 weeks (Evi-level-IA)
- Women with short cervix (<15 mm): As micronized progesterone 200 mg daily vaginally (Evi-level-IA) (no. 202, Jan 2008)

- *Tocolytics*: Result in uterine quiescence and prevent preterm labor
- *Beta-2 agonists*: Result in relaxation of smooth muscles in uterus, bronchi, and vasculature, e.g.
  - Ritodrine
  - Terbutaline
  - Salbutamol
- *Beta-3 agonists*: BRL37344—possess equal potency but with milder cardiovascular s/e than ritodrine
- *Magnesium sulfate*: Acts by uterine muscle relaxation effect. It is given as loading dose of 4–6 g IV slowly over 20 minutes, followed by maintenance dose (1–4 grams/hour)
- *Calcium channel blockers*: Action is by reducing influx of calcium ions across the cell membrane which results in reduction of smooth muscles tonus.

- *Nifedipine:* It is usually used as 20 mg orally stat, repeated 20 mg after 30 minutes, then 20 mg orally every 3–8 hours over 48–72 hours. Maximum dose is 160 mg/day, provides acute tocolysis, thereafter chronic maintenance tocolysis is given.
- *Prostaglandin synthetase inhibitors* include drugs like indomethacin, aspirin, ibuprofen, sulindac.
- *Indomethacin:* It is used 100 mg rectally followed by 50 mg orally every 6 hours for 2 days. The fetal risk is that of oligohydramnios, premature closure of ductus, and necrotizing enterocolitis.
- *Atosiban:* Atosiban as oxytocin antagonist is used for treatment of preterm labor. Initially, a bolus dose of 6.75 mg is given over 1 minute, followed by an infusion of 18 mg/hr for next 3 hours, then 6 mg/hr for up to total 48 hours (maximum of 330 mg). If needed again, restart with bolus dose of 6.75 mg/mL followed by infusion. It is quickly effective in 10 minutes, brings uterine quiescence remaining for 12 hours and can delay preterm labor for a week.
- *Progesterone:* It has an accepted role in pregnancy maintenance.

Tertiary prevention in established labor and imminent preterm birth
- Acute tocolysis to gain time for antenatal steroids use
- Optimizing acute morbid condition
- Optimizing time of terminating pregnancy
- Decision for route of delivery, intrapartum care
- Neonatal care

Antenatal steroids
As per ACOG committee opinion (2016):[7]
- Early preterm <24 weeks: May be beneficial
- From 24 to 33, 6/7 weeks: Give single course of two doses
- From 34 to 36, 6/7 weeks: Give single course of two doses
- For PPROM <34 weeks: Give single course of two doses (no increased risk of maternal/neonatal infection observed)
- For multiple gestation with PTL: Give single course of two doses at gestation <34 weeks and at risk of delivery within 7 days
- For repeat course in case of pregnancy continuing beyond 7 days: Consider if >14 days have lapsed after first dose
- Rescue course can be given as early as 7 days after first dose if clinical condition warrants it—so decision is individualized

Dose:
- Two 12 mg doses of betamethasone IM 24 hours apart
- Four 6 mg doses of dexamethasone IM 12 hours apart

Accelerated dose schedule/frequent dosing in imminent delivery is not beneficial, so may not be considered.

Antibiotics
- Chorioamnionitis: Causes 20–30% of all PTL cases
- Indicated:
  - I/V Ampicillin/sulbactam 3 grams 8 hourly
  - I/V Cefoperazone/sulbactam 2 grams 8 hourly
  - Metronidazole 500 mg 8 hourly
- Urinary tract infection: Use nitrofurantoin
- *Asymptomatic bacteriuria:* Use urinary antibiotics
- *Respiratory tract infection:* Use appropriate antibiotics
- Long-term use of antibiotics is not recommended
- Use in PPROM also is not justified for longer duration

Cervical cerclage
- Reduces risk of PTB without significant reduction of PNM/NNM
- Higher rates of cesarean delivery recorded
- No trial comparing it with progesterone use in short cervix available
- Indirect results did not find much difference
- *Cochrane review:* Individualize each case on merits

Tertiary preventive measures
- *Use of tocolytics:* Justified to gain time for antenatal steroids and prolonging pregnancy
- The choice of use is decided on merits out of nifedipine, ritodrine, betamimetics, magnesium sulfate, cyclo-oxygenase inhibitors, oxytocin receptor antagonists, atosiban, prostaglandin synthetase inhibitors)
- Antibiotics given in PPROM (ORACLE TRIAL)[8]
- A lives saved tool analysis (LiST): Universal coverage of selected interventions claimed to have achieved 84% decline of preterm neonatal deaths annually when antenatal steroids and kangaroo mother care were given.

Intrapartum monitoring
- The risk of intraventricular hemorrhage increases with fetal hypoxia or acidosis.
- So, closely monitor for signs of hypoxia during labor, preferably by continuous electronic fetal monitoring.
- Give oxygen therapy at low flow rate to maintain saturation around 90%.
- Avoid hyperoxia (saturation > 95%) to minimize the risk of retinopathy.
- The major cause of mortality/morbidity is respiratory distress syndrome.
- Thus the treatment includes:
  - Antibiotic prophylaxis: Given where high incidence of group B streptococcal infection exists.
  - Delivery: Delivery must be conducted in the presence of expert pediatrician/neonatologist.
- Ventouse application is not indicated in preterm deliveries.
- The use of forceps for premature baby is protective against intracerebral trauma and worth considering

Care of newborn
- The preterm baby should be received by a neonatologist.
- Maintain euthermia and keep baby dry under radiant warmer.
- Avoid excessive extraneous stimuli.
- Maintain proper ventilation, oxygenation, circulation, as well as body temperature control.
- Exogenously surfactant may be instilled through endotracheal tube at about 100 mg/kg body weight if decided.
- Risk is of retinopathy in premature baby which can result in impaired vision. Its incidence is high (68%) in infants who weigh <1,251 g. In some babies, it may regress on its own but sometimes may progress to retinal detachment and blindness. Severe retinopathy of prematurity (ROP) should be treated by laser or cryotherapy.

Future avenues of concern
- The role of fetal genome in genetic predisposition to spontaneous PTB has been found in Finnish families. A preterm birth gene AR has been identified by linkage and association analysis of X chromosomal markers. [PLoS 2012]
- In mouse, uterine deletion of Trp 53 has been related to changes in decidua predisposing to PTB due to oxidative stress.[9]
- Progesterone and rapamycin have been reported to inhibit proteins in signaling pathway.
- Polymorphisms of genes in affected families have association with complement, coagulation, and oxytocin pathway related to PTB.
- The sequence variants in oxytocin pathway gene are under study.[10]
- The studies of gene environmental interactions are also under study.[11]
- The maternal coding variants in complement receptor 1 and idiopathic PTB are under research.[12,13]

Society of fetal medicine recommendations
May 2012[14]

In singleton pregnancy:
- No prior history of PTB
- Short CL ≤20 mm

At ≤24 weeks gestation, vaginal progesterone as 200 mg pessary or 90 mg gel is useful.
The evidence suggests lowering of perinatal morbidity and mortality, so can be offered.
SMFM AJOG May 2012

- Recommendation in singleton pregnancy with prior preterm birth between 20 and 36.6/7 weeks, is to give inj. 17 α hydroxyl progesterone caproate 250 mg IM weekly, starting at 16–20 weeks till 36 completed weeks
- Also recommend cervical encirclage in women with prior PTB, if the TVS CL is <25 mm at <24 weeks.

SMFM AJOG May 2012

- The current data does not report benefit or harm of use of transabdominal ultrasound screening of CL for prevention of PTB using progesterone or any other interventional therapy with short CL.
- The randomized data reports benefit from use of CL screening by transvaginal ultrasound using vaginal progesterone in women with short CL.

SMFM AJOG May 2012

- Progesterone has no benefit of use for prevention of PTB in women with multiple gestation and preterm labor/PROM
- The evidence of its use lacks in these women with or without short cervical length

SMFM AJOG May 2012

- Cervical length screening for prevention of PTB in singleton pregnancy without prior h/o PTB is still disputed as a universal screening method.
- It can be considered on individual basis if justified.

SMFM AJOG May 2012

REFERENCES

1. Zeitlin JA, Saurel-Cubizolles MJ, Ancel PY, et al. Marital status, cohabitation and risk of preterm birth in Europe where births outside marriage are common and uncommon. Paediatr Perinat Epidemiol. 2002;16(2):124-30.
2. Leitich H, Kaider A. Fetal fibronectin–how useful is it in the prediction of preterm birth. BJOG. 2003;110 (Suppl 20): 66-70.
3. Kurkinen-Räty M, Ruokonen A, Vuopala S, et al. Combination of cervical Interleukin-6 and -8, phosphorylated Insulin-like growth factor-binding protein-1 and transvaginal cervical ultrasonography in assessment of the risk of preterm birth. BJOG. 2001;108(8):875-81.
4. Berghella V, Roman A, Daskalakis C, et al. Gestational age at cervical length measurement and incidence of preterm birth. Obstet Gynaecol. 2007;110(2pt1):311-7.
5. Society for Maternal Fetal Medicine Publications Committee. ACOG Committee opinion no. 419-2008: Use of progesterone to reduce preterm birth. Obstet Gynaecol. 2008;12(4):963-5.
6. Farine D, Mundle WR, Dodd J. SOGC Technical update. The use of progesterone for prevention of preterm birth. J Obstet Gynaecol Can. 2008;30(1):67-71.
7. ACOG. ACOG –Opinion 617, Oct 2016. Antenatal corticoid therapy for fetal maturation. Replaced by No. 713. Aug 17 and reaffirmed in 2018. Obstet Gynaecol. 2017;130(2):e101-9.
8. Kenyon S, Taylor DJ, Tarnow-Mordi WO, et al. ORACLE-antibiotics for preterm prelabour rupture of the membranes: short-term and long-term outcomes. Acta Paediatr Suppl. 2002;91(937):12-5.
9. Kristin E, Hirota Y, Baker ES, et al. Uterine deletion of Trp 53 compromises anti oxidant response in mouse decidua. Endocrinology. 2012;153(9):4568-79.
10. Kim J, Stirling KJ, Cooper ME, et al. Sequence variants in oxytocin pathway genes and preterm birth: a candidate gene association study. BMC Med Genet. 2013;14:77.
11. Cha J, Bartos A, Egashira M, et al. Combinatory approaches prevent preterm birth profoundly exacerbated by gene-environment interactions. J Clin Invest. 2013;129(9):4063-75.
12. Plunkett J, Doniger S, Orabona G, et al. An evolutionary genomic approach to identify genes involved in human birth timing. PLoS Genet. 2011;7(4):e1001365.
13. McElroy JJ, Gutman CE, Shaffer CM, et al. Maternal coding variants in complement receptor 1 and spontaneous idiopathic preterm birth. Hum Genet. 2013;132(8):935-42.
14. Berghella V. Society of maternal fetal medicine publications committee. Am J Obstet Gynaecol. 2012;206(5):376-86.

Chapter 21

Prelabor Rupture of Membranes

Shyjus Puliyathinkal

INTRODUCTION

Prelabor rupture of membranes is defined as spontaneous rupture of membranes before the onset of labor. Preterm prelabor rupture of membranes is defined as prelabor rupture of membranes before 37 completed weeks of gestation. The incidence of term and preterm PLROM is approximately 8% and 3%, respectively.[1]

CAUSES AND RISK FACTORS (BOX 1)

Multiple etiologies are probably involved and operate along various pathways involving both mechanical and nonmechanical factors.
- Infection (genital tract/urinary tract) is the primary etiological factor in prelabor rupture of membranes (PROM), more so in preterm prelabor rupture of membranes (PPROM). Preterm labor and PPROM seem to be expressions of a more general process of intrauterine inflammation and thus share many antecedents. Group B *Streptococcus*, *Chlamydia trachomatis*, and bacterial vaginosis are the most common organisms implicated. Apart from the weakening of membranes due to the proteases released by these microorganisms, PROM can also occur due to an ill-fitting presenting part wherein the pressure from the hind waters gets directly transmitted to the forewaters.
- Abnormal presentations as in transverse lie/breech.
- Multifetal gestation/polyhydramnios.
- Following invasive procedures such as amniocentesis/fetoscopy/percutaneous umbilical blood sampling (PUBS).

Box 1	Risk Factors for preterm prelabor rupture of membranes (PPROM).
• History of preterm labor in a previous pregnancy • History of PPROM in a previous pregnancy • Cervical insufficiency • Present pregnancy with multifetal gestation/antepartum bleeding	

DIAGNOSIS (ALGORITHM 1)

The classic clinical presentation of PROM is a sudden gush of clear or pale yellow fluid from the vagina. However, many women complain of intermittent or continuous leaking of small amounts of fluid or just a sensation of wetness within the vagina.

Direct observation of amniotic fluid coming out of the cervical canal or pooling in the posterior fornix is pathognomonic of PROM. If there is no demonstrable leaking, the woman is asked to push on her fundus, perform Valsalva, or cough to elicit leakage. If the diagnosis is still uncertain, the fluid in the posterior fornix is subjected to certain special tests:
- *Nitrazine test:* Used to test the pH of the vaginal fluid. Amniotic fluid has a pH of 7.0–7.3 compared with the normal acidic pH of the vagina of 3.8–4.2 and of urine of

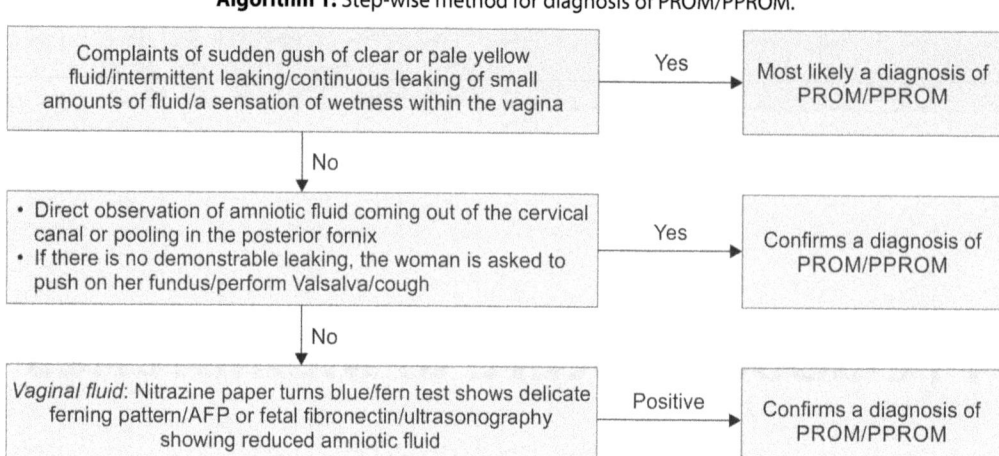

Algorithm 1: Step-wise method for diagnosis of PROM/PPROM.

(PPROM: preterm PROM; PROM: prelabor rupture of membranes)

5.0–6.0.[2] The color of the nitrazine paper changes from yellow to blue as pH changes from acidic to alkaline. False-positive results can be due to the presence of alkaline fluids such as blood, semen, or soap in the vagina.

- *Fern test:* The fluid from the fornix is swabbed onto a glass slide and allowed to dry for at least 10 minutes. Amniotic fluid produces delicate ferning pattern, in contrast to the thick and wide arborization pattern of dried cervical mucus.

Several other newer test kits are commercially available nowadays. These include placental alpha macroglobulin-1 protein assay (PAMG-1/amnisure) and insulin-like growth factor binding protein 1 assay (IGFBP-1/actim PROM).[3]

- *Fetal fibronectin in vaginal fluid:* A negative fetal fibronectin test strongly supports the absence of membrane rupture but a positive result only indicates disruption of the choriodecidual interface which can happen even with intact membranes.
- *Alpha-fetoprotein (AFP) in vaginal fluid:* A positive result suggests the presence of amniotic fluid.
- *Ultrasonography:* In equivocal cases, an ultrasound is performed to look for a reduction in amniotic fluid. A reduced amniotic fluid index (AFI) can help to confirm the diagnosis of PROM, although a normal AFI cannot rule out the possibility of a membrane rupture.

The pregnancy complications and outcomes in PROM/PPROM are shown in **Box 2**.

Box 2 Pregnancy complications and outcome in PROM/PPROM.

- Preterm birth (in PPROM)
- Maternal/fetal/neonatal infection (more in PPROM)
- Abruptio placenta
- Cord prolapse
- Retained placenta
- Need for classical cesarean section (in PPROM)
- Fetal/neonatal musculoskeletal deformities (only in PPROM)
- Pulmonary hypoplasia in the newborn
- Fetal/neonatal death

(PROM: prelabor rupture of membranes; PPROM: preterm prelabor rupture of membranes)

MANAGEMENT (ALGORITHM 2)

Term PROM: In this situation, a vaginal examination is first done to rule out a cord presentation or a cord prolapse. Expectant management for up to 24 hours is an option, if the patient wishes, with the hope of a spontaneous labor setting in, once the indications for an emergency delivery are ruled out. Otherwise it is induction with oxytocin infusion if the cervix is favorable, or cervical ripening with PGE1/PGE2 followed by oxytocin infusion, if cervix is unfavorable. Antibiotics are not routinely indicated in case of a term PROM unless significant time has elapsed (more than 12–18 hours) from the time of membrane rupture to the time of induction.

Preterm PROM: The key to decision making in PPROM is about balancing the risks of infectious complications

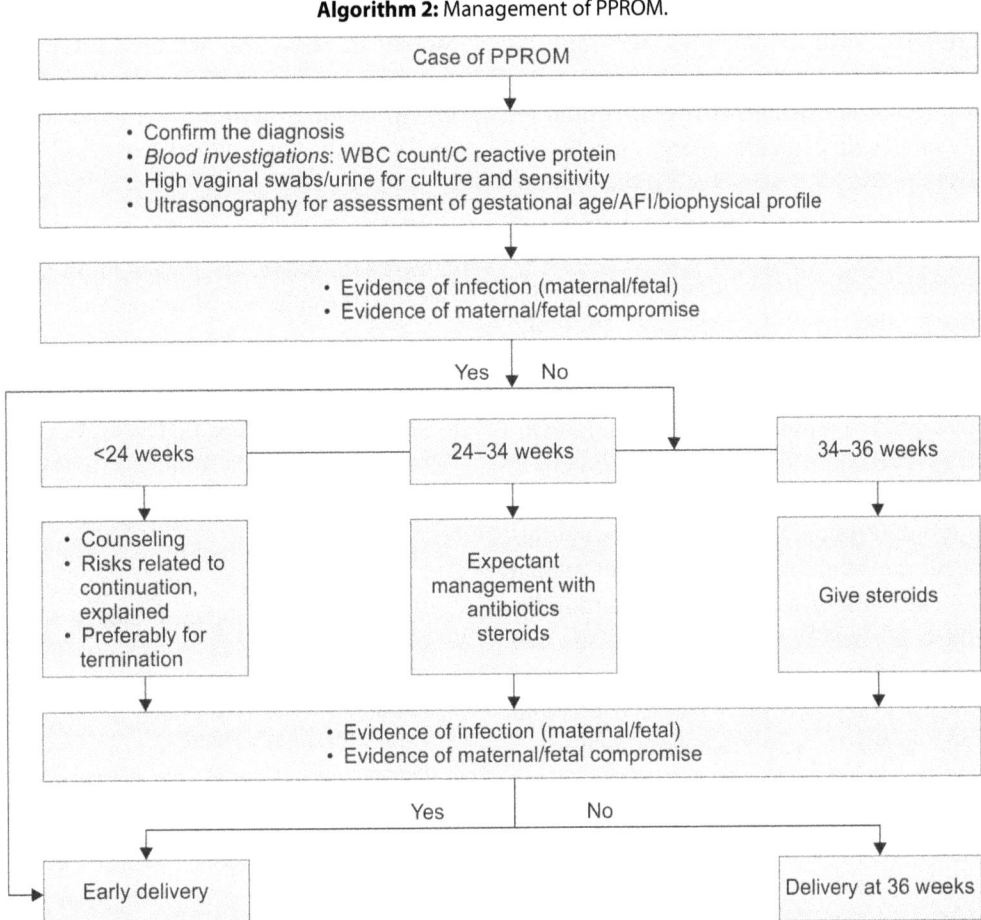

Algorithm 2: Management of PPROM.

(PPROM: preterm prelabor rupture of membranes)

of expectant management with the risks of prematurity associated with immediate delivery **(Boxes 3 and 4)**.

Gestational age <24 weeks: Continuation of pregnancy poses significant risks of chorioamnionitis and sepsis for the mother. Fetal complications such as pulmonary hypoplasia and postural deformities are also seen commonly. Hence, the parents are counseled regarding these risks and termination of pregnancy is advised. Steroids are not recommended at this gestational age.

Gestational age between 24 weeks and 34 weeks: In general, expectant management is the norm, unless there are signs of infection. A speculum examination is performed to confirm the rupture, exclude cord prolapse, and to take a high vaginal swab for culture and sensitivity. Antibiotics are routinely indicated in this subset of patients.

| Box 3 | Decision-making factors in preterm prelabor rupture of membranes. |

- Gestational age
- Presence/absence of maternal/fetal infection
- Presence/absence of labor
- Fetal presentation
- Fetal well-being
- Fetal lung maturity
- Cervical status (by visual inspection)
- Availability of neonatal intensive care

| Box 4 | Investigations at admission in preterm prelabor rupture of membranes. |

- Ultrasonography for assessment of gestational age/amniotic fluid index (AFI)/biophysical profile
- *Blood investigations*: White blood cells (WBCs) count/C-reactive protein
- High vaginal swab/urine for culture and sensitivity

There is no clear-cut consensus on the ideal regimen. One amongst the preferred regimes includes azithromycin 1 g orally plus ampicillin 2 grams IV every 6 hours for 48 hours, followed by oral amoxicillin 500 mg thrice daily for another 5 days. Women with penicillin allergy but with low risk of anaphylaxis can use intravenous cefazolin followed by oral cephalexin. Those with high risk of anaphylaxis can use intravenous clindamycin plus gentamicin followed by oral clindamycin plus single dose of oral azithromycin.[4] Labor and delivery also need to have the antibiotic cover. Chemoprophylaxis for Group B *Streptococcus* is used for those who are GBS positive or when status is unknown and delivery is imminent. Injecting ampicillin 2 g intravenously every 6 hours for 48 hours and switching over to a combination of oral amoxicillin + azithromycin for the next 5 days is the regime. Maternal fever, maternal/fetal tachycardia, uterine tenderness, and purulent vaginal discharge are the clinical indicators of chorioamnionitis. Leukocytosis and a positive C reactive protein are the laboratory indicators. Ultrasonography for liquor volume and nonstress test (NST) are done twice weekly. Antenatal corticosteroids are given to accelerate lung maturity.[5] The only contraindication for steroids is frank infection, in which case, expectant management is given up. When these patients go into labor, a continuous fetal heart rate (FHR) monitoring with cardiotocography (CTG) is indicated, in view of the possibility of cord compression due to oligohydramnios.

Gestational age between 34 and 36 weeks: In most hospitals in India, the neonatal survival rates are pretty good at or beyond 34 weeks. Steroids are given for these women. Labor is induced if spontaneous labor does not set in, once she has reached 36 weeks.

Mode of delivery: Cesarean delivery is performed only for obstetric indications. With a favorable cervix, labor is induced with oxytocin. In case of an unfavorable cervix, PGE1/PGE2 can be used for ripening.

REFERENCES

1. Scorza WE, Lockwood CJ. (2018). Management of prelabor rupture of the fetal membranes at term. [online] Available from https://www.uptodate.com/contents/management-of-prelabor-rupture-of-the-fetal-membranes-at-term [Last accesed September, 2019].
2. Seeds AE, Hellegers AE. Acid-base determinations in human amniotic fluid throughout pregnancy. Am J Obstet Gynecol. 1968;101:257.
3. Ramsauer B, Vidaeff AC, Hösli I, et al. The diagnosis of rupture of fetal membranes (ROM): a meta-analysis. J Perinat Med. 2013;41:233.
4. Pierson RC, Gordon SS, Haas DM. A retrospective comparison of antibiotic regimens for preterm premature rupture of membranes. Obstet Gynecol. 2014;124:515.
5. Roberts D, Brown J, Medley N, et al. Antenatal corticosteroids for accelerating fetal lung maturation for women at risk of preterm birth. Cochrane Database Syst Rev. 2017;3:CD004454.

Chapter 22

Intrauterine Growth Restriction: An Evidence-based Approach

Minakshi Rohilla, Shivani Sharma

INTRODUCTION

Intrauterine growth restriction (IUGR) is the term applied to a fetus when estimated fetal weight is less than 10th percentile for that period of gestation or abdominal circumference on ultrasound is less than 10th percentile.[1] However, approximately 50–70% fetuses are constitutionally small and their weight is appropriate for their maternal height, weight, parity, and ethnicity and may be appropriately termed as small for gestational age (SGA) without any etiologically relevant growth restriction **(Table 1 and Algorithm 1)**.[2] True growth restriction is a pathological entity wherein a fetus fails to achieve its expected growth potential irrespective of its genetic constitution.

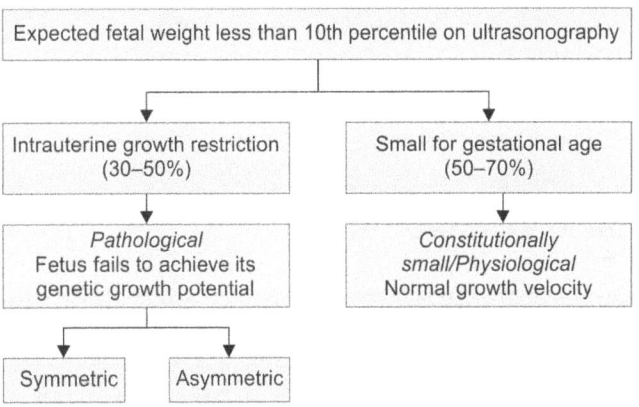

Algorithm 1: Categorization of intrauterine growth restriction (IUGR).

ETIOLOGY

Different etiological factors are described in **Table 2**.

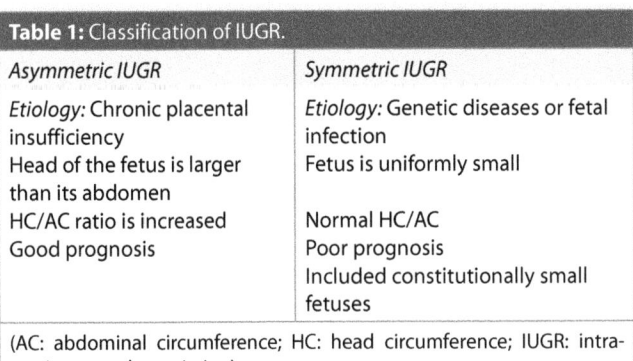

Table 1: Classification of IUGR.

Asymmetric IUGR	Symmetric IUGR
Etiology: Chronic placental insufficiency	*Etiology:* Genetic diseases or fetal infection
Head of the fetus is larger than its abdomen	Fetus is uniformly small
HC/AC ratio is increased	Normal HC/AC
Good prognosis	Poor prognosis
	Included constitutionally small fetuses
(AC: abdominal circumference; HC: head circumference; IUGR: intrauterine growth restriction)	

Table 2: Causes of IUGR.[3]

Placental	Maternal	Fetal
• Abruption	• Hypertensive disorders	• Chromosomal abnormalities
• Infarction	• Pregestational diabetes	• Structural malformations
• Circumvallate	• Renal diseases	• Multiple gestation
• Hemangioma	• Autoimmune diseases	
• Chorioangioma	• Multiple gestation	
• Abnormal cord insertion	• Exposure to teratogens	
• Single umbilical artery	• APLA	
	• Substance abuse	
	• Infectious diseases	
(APLA: antiphospholipid antibody; IUGR: intrauterine growth restriction)		

SCREENING

It involves careful assessment of pregnancies with the potential risk of fetal growth restriction. Critical review of medical and obstetric history to screen for factors which have predictive effect on outcome of present pregnancy is required **(Table 3)**. It also involves use of biochemical parameters like pregnancy-associated plasma protein A (PAPP-A) in current pregnancy to further judge for the possibility of occurrence of IUGR **(Table 4)**.

Table 3: Risk factors for IUGR.[4]

Minor risk factors (Odds ratio 1–2)	Major risk factors (Odds ratio >2)
• Maternal age more than 35 years • Nulliparity • Smoker less than 10 cigarettes/day • IVF pregnancy • Prepregnancy fruit intake was low • History of preeclampsia • Pregnancy interval less 6 months or more than 60 months	• Maternal age more than 40 years • Smoker more than 11 cigarettes/day • Cocaine abuse • Previous IUGR baby • History of stillbirth • Maternal/Paternal SGA • Chronic hypertension • Diabetes with vasculopathy • Chronic kidney disease • Antiphospholipid syndrome

(IUGR: intrauterine growth restriction; IVF: in vitro fertilization; SGA: small for gestational age)

Table 4: Risk factors for IUGR in present pregnancy.[4]

Minor risk factors (Odds ratio 1–2)	Major risk factors (Odds ratio >2)
• Mild preeclampsia • Placental abruption • Caffeine intake >300 mg/day in 3rd trimester	• Threatened miscarriage • Fetal anomaly scan showing echogenic bowel • Preeclampsia • Pregnancy-induced hypertension with severe features • Unexplained antepartum hemorrhage • Inadequate maternal weight gain • Maternal infections, e.g. tuberculosis, syphilis, malaria • PAPP-A < 0.4 MoMs (multiple of medians)

(PAPP-A: pregnancy-associated plasma protein-A)

Measurement of Uterine Fundal Height

Measurement of symphysis fundal height (SFH)/uterine fundal height is an excellent screening tool for assessment of IUGR after 24–26 weeks of gestation. Discrepancy of more than 3 cm is indicative of probable growth restriction and calls for further evaluation.[5] In women with body mass index (BMI) >35, large fibroids, hydramnios, and multiple gestation, SFH measurement alone is inaccurate and serial assessment of fetal size using ultrasound is recommended.

Role of Uterine Artery Doppler in Screening of IUGR

Uterine artery Doppler is recommended if more than three minor risk factors for IUGR are present.[4] With the advancement of gestational age, uterine artery diastolic flow falls due to invasion of spiral arteries by trophoblast cells. This results in loss of diastolic notch by 18–22 weeks of gestation **(Figs. 1A and B)**. Pulsatility index (PI) >95th percentile or notch in uterine artery Doppler is suggestive of uteroplacental insufficiency. Abnormal flow warrants umbilical artery Doppler studies at 26–28 weeks of gestation onward **(Algorithm 2)**.

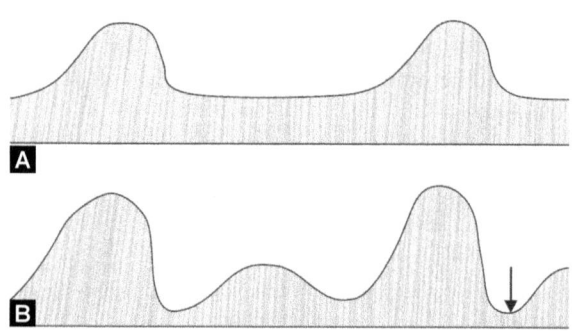

Figs. 1A and B: Doppler waveform of uterine artery blood flow. (A) Normal in late second and third trimester; (B) In preeclampsia after 24 weeks period of gestation (POG) with diastolic notch (arrow).

Algorithm 2: Screening of IUGR fetuses.[4]

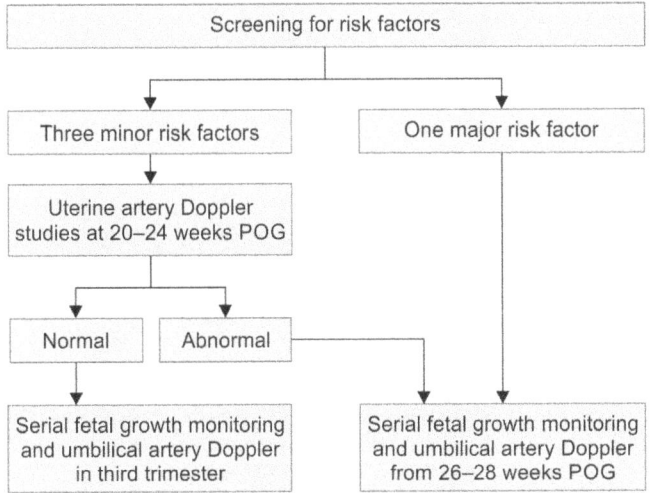

(IUGR: intrauterine growth restriction; POG: period of gestation)

COMPLICATIONS ASSOCIATED WITH IUGR

Several complications associated with IUGR are listed in **Table 5**.

Table 5: Early and late complications associated with IUGR.[6]

Adult	Fetal	Neonatal
• Type 2 diabetes mellitus • Risk of hypertension • Atherosclerosis	• Prematurity • Increased rate of stillbirth • Birth asphyxia	• Meconium aspiration syndrome • Seizures, Sepsis • Neonatal hypoglycemia • Hyperbilirubinemia • Hypothermia • Respiratory distress Syndrome • Intraventricular hemorrhage • Necrotizing enterocolitis • Neonatal death

(IUGR: intrauterine growth restriction)

PREVENTION

Prevention of growth restriction is possible if modifiable risk factors like optimization of maternal health and nutrition, avoiding drugs causing IUGR, cessation of smoking, and decreasing caffeine intake are identified and appropriate measures and should preferably be taken before conception. Low dose aspirin is recommended for prophylaxis of IUGR before 16 weeks of gestation if a woman is at high risk for preeclampsia.[4] Use of multivitamins, calcium supplements, progesterone, bed rest, or dietary modifications is not recommended.

INVESTIGATIONS

Box 1 lists the investigations for IUGR.

Box 1	Investigations for severe IUGR detected in early pregnancy.[4]

- Level II ultrasonography for detailed fetal anatomic survey at 18–20 weeks
- Testing for malaria and syphilis in a population who is at high risk for these infections
- Screening for CMV, toxoplasmosis by serological examination
- Karyotyping in fetuses with severe IUGR, especially when uterine artery Doppler and amniotic fluid is normal

(CMV: cytomegalovirus; IUGR: intrauterine growth restriction)

DIAGNOSIS AND MANAGEMENT OF FETAL GROWTH RESTRICTION (ALGORITHMS 3 AND 4)

Sonographic Measurement of Fetal Size

Objective fetal growth estimation using various fetal biometric measurements is recommended from 26 weeks of gestation onward. This includes combined head, abdomen, and femur measurements to estimate fetal growth velocity and prediction of growth restriction using customized fetal weight reference charts. Customized charts are specific for a race, ethnicity, height, weight, and parity and fetuses with weight <3rd percentile of reference has severe growth restriction and is associated with poor obstetrical outcomes.

Amniotic Fluid Volume Measurement

Approximately 10% of the pregnancies with oligohydramnios are associated with fetal growth restriction probably due to chronic hypoxia and reduced fetal renal perfusion.[7] Estimation of single deepest vertical pocket (SDVP) has been found to be more specific than measurement of amniotic fluid index.[4]

Role of Doppler Studies

Doppler study is used along with nonstress tests and biophysical profiles in management of growth-restricted fetuses. It can predict the perinatal mortality in IUGR fetuses associated with absent or reversed end-diastolic

Algorithm 3: Management of growth restricted fetus at less than 34 weeks POG.[4,8]

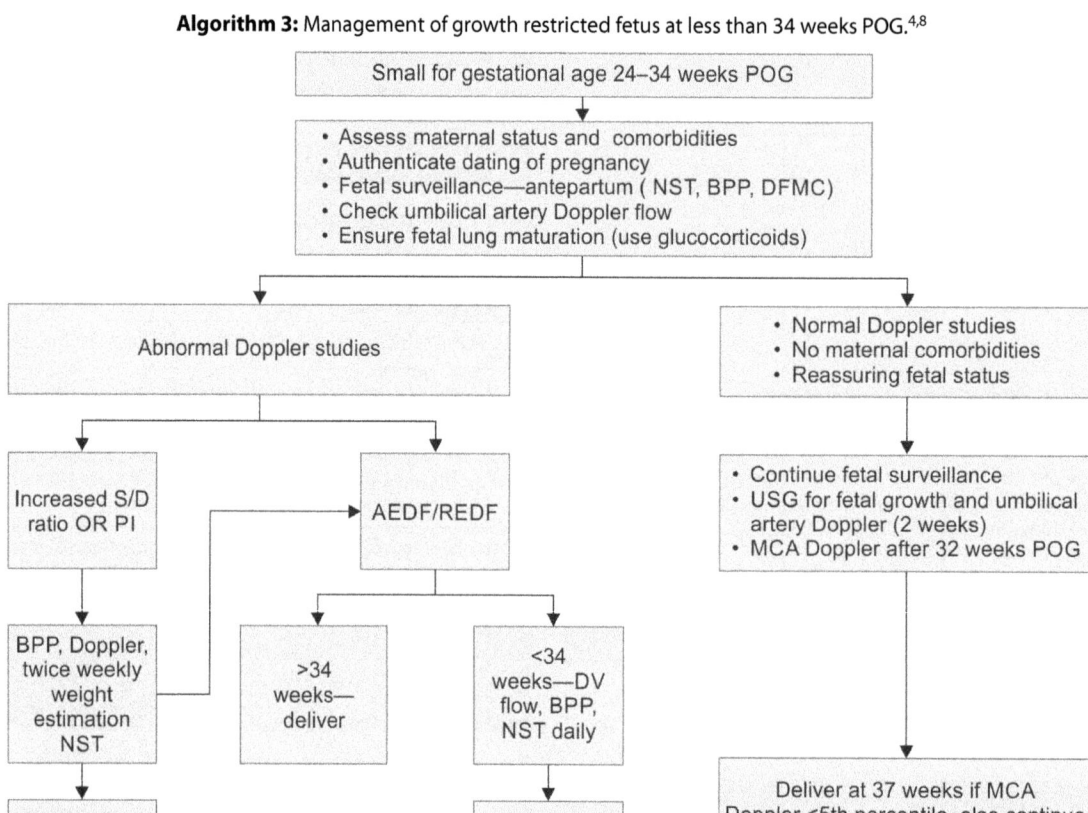

(AEDF: absent end-diastolic flow; BPP: biophysical profile; DFMC: daily fetal movement count; DV: ductus venosus; MCA: middle cerebral artery; NST: nonstress test; PI: pulsatility index; POG: period of gestation; REDF: reversed end-diastolic flow; S/D: systolic diastolic ratio; USG: ultrasonography)

Algorithm 4: Management of growth restricted fetus at more than 34 weeks POG.[4,8]

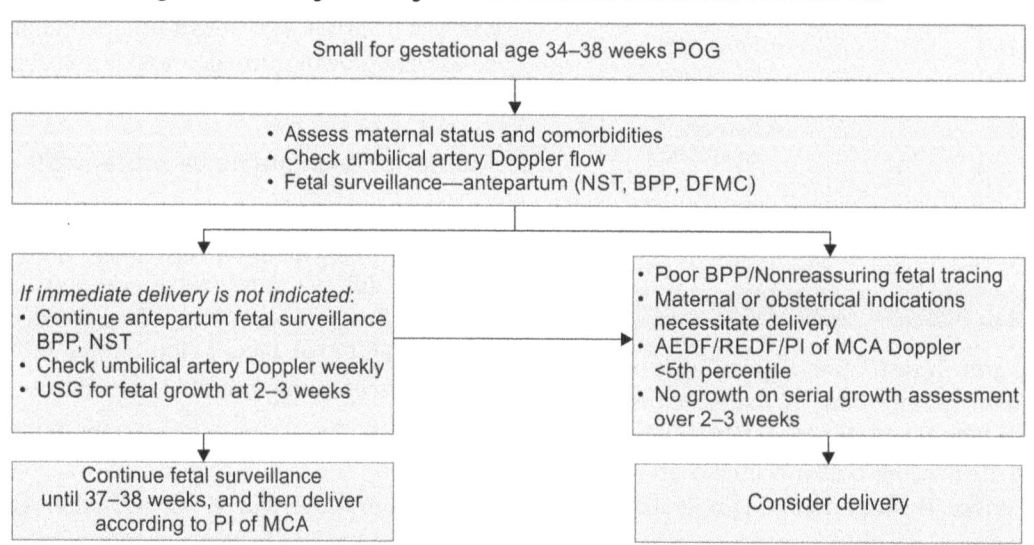

(AEDF: absent end-diastolic flow; BPP: biophysical profile; DFMC: daily fetal movement count; DV: ductus venosus; MCA: middle cerebral artery; NST: nonstress test; PI: pulsatility index; POG: period of gestation; REDF: reversed end-diastolic flow; S/D: systolic diastolic ratio)

flow (AREDF) and aids in decision regarding timing of termination of pregnancy **(Fig. 2)**.
- S-D Ratio: Systolic diastolic ratio
- (S-D)/S: Resistance index (RI)
- (S-D)/Mean: Pulsatility index (PI)

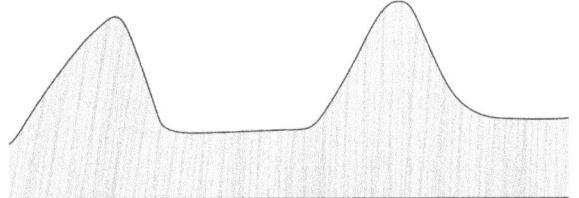

Fig. 2: Normal Doppler flow velocity of umbilical artery.

Umbilical Artery Doppler

Normal mean value of umbilical artery S/D ratio decreases from 3.6 to 2.5 as the gestation advances. IUGR fetuses with placental insufficiency may have increase PI (more than 2 standard deviation) for gestational age in umbilical artery, which may worsen to AREDF subsequently **(Figs. 3 to 5)**.

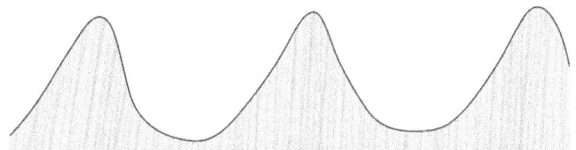

Fig. 3: High pulsatility index (raised SD ratio) of umbilical artery.

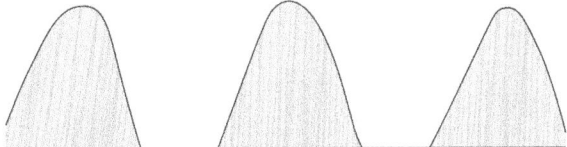

Fig. 4: Absent end-diastolic flow of umbilical artery.

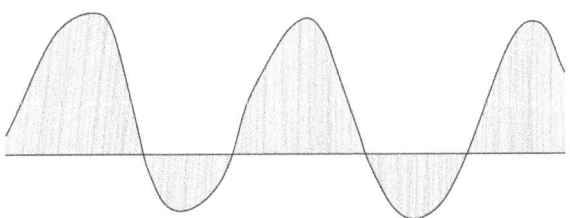

Fig. 5: Reversed end-diastolic flow of umbilical artery.

Fetal Middle Cerebral Artery Doppler

In case of abnormal umbilical artery Doppler, middle cerebral artery (MCA) Doppler is done. Physiological basis behind Doppler changes in MCA is that in cases with placental insufficiency, blood supply to essential organs like brain is maintained which is also known as the "brain sparing effect." PI less than 5th percentile suggests fetal acidosis in IUGR fetus.

Ductus Venosus and Umbilical Vein Doppler

Ductus venosus (DV) Doppler should be used in surveillance of IUGR fetuses, which have abnormal umbilical artery Doppler. It has importance in deciding the timing of delivery. Absence or reversal of *a* wave in DV suggests fetal hypoxia and delivery is recommended **(Figs. 6 to 8)**. Pulsatility in umbilical vein suggests fetal cardiac compromise and urgent delivery is suggested.

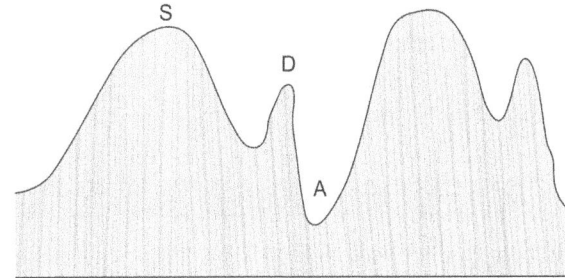

Fig. 6: Normal Doppler flow velocity of ductus venosus. (S-Ventricular systolic flow, D-Early diastolic flow, A-Atrial contraction)

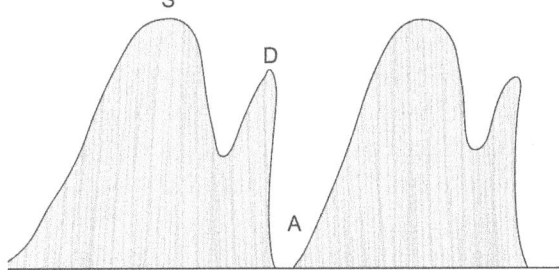

Fig. 7: Abnormal Doppler flow velocity of ductus venosus—absent a wave.

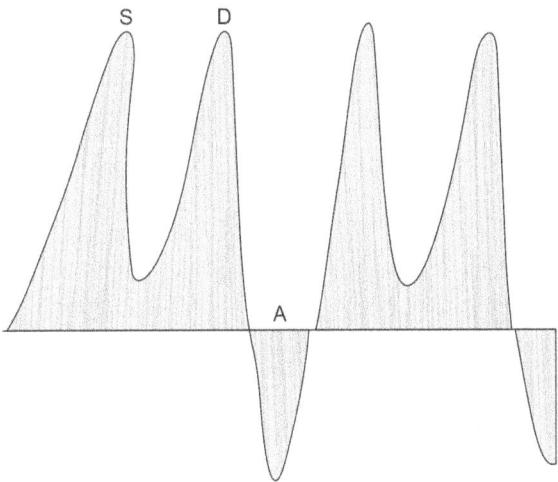

Fig. 8: Abnormal Doppler flow velocity of ductus venosus—reversed a wave.

In IUGR fetuses with normal umbilical artery Doppler, fetal surveillance at 2 weeks interval is reasonable, while in case of abnormal Doppler studies twice weekly and daily in AREDF is mandatory.

Mode of Delivery

In IUGR fetuses with umbilical artery AREDF, cesarean section is recommended. However, in fetuses with abnormal umbilical artery Doppler, induction of labor may be offered with anticipated high risk of emergency cesarean section. Continuous fetal cardiotocography (CTG) is recommended as soon as uterine contractions begin. Computerized interpretation of cardiotocograph based on short-term variability is better predictor of fetal compromise or ongoing hypoxia.[4]

CONCLUSION

Intrauterine growth restriction is an important obstetric condition which is best prevented, careful screening of at risk pregnancies, early objective diagnosis, and diligent monitoring, are the cornerstone of its management. In majority, the etiology remains obscure and warrants vigilant surveillance. Early supervision and careful monitoring of pregnancy along with well-timed delivery can reduce perinatal morbidity and mortality. Judicious use of modern techniques of fetal and maternal Doppler studies, biophysical profile, and computed CTG has changed the outlook of management of IUGR recently.

REFERENCES

1. Ii Chang TC, Robson SC, Boys RJ, et al. Prediction of the small for gestational age infant: which ultrasonic measurement is best? Obstet Gynecol. 1992;80:1030-8.
2. Alberry M, Soothill P. Management of fetal growth restriction. Arch Dis Child Fetal Neonatal Ed. 2007;92:62-7.
3. American College of Obstetricians and Gynecologists. ACOG Practice Bulletin No. 134: fetal growth restriction. Obstet Gynecol. 2013;121:1122-33.
4. Royal College of Obstetricians and Gynecologists. The Investigation and Management of the Small for Gestational Age Fetus. Green-Top Guideline No. 31, 2nd edition. London: Royal College of Obstetricians and Gynecologists; 2013.
5. Figueras F, Gardosi J. Intrauterine growth restriction: new concepts in antenatal surveillance, diagnosis, and management. Am J Obstet Gynecol. 2011;204(4):288-300.
6. McIntire DD, Bloom SL, Casey BM, et al. Birth weight in relation to morbidity and mortality among newborn infants. N Engl J Med. 1999;340:1234-8.
7. Chauhan SP, Taylor M, Sheilds D, et al. Intrauterine growth restriction and oligohydramnios among high risk patients. Am J Perinatol. 2007;24(4):215-21.
8. Cunningham FG. Fetal growth disorders. In: Leveno KJ, Bloom SL, Spong CY, Dashe JS, Hoffman BL, et al (Eds). Williams Obstetrics, 24th edition. New York: McGraw-Hill Education Medical; 2014. pp. 872-90.

Chapter 23

Multiple Gestations in Labor

Shailesh Kore, Pradnya Supe, Chaitra Thunga

INTRODUCTION

The term multiple gestation is defined as two or more fetuses developing in utero simultaneously. These may be twins, triplets, quadruplets, and so on. The incidence of multiple gestations has been rising due to increase in maternal age, parity, geographic factors, race, use of artificial reproductive techniques, and thereby, is increasing the risk of complications associated with pregnancy, delivery, and neonatal issues. Due to lack of well-designed clinical trials, there still exists a controversy regarding the intrapartum management of multiple gestations. The scope of this chapter is to outline the strategy to be followed in the management of various scenarios in the labor and delivery of multiple gestations.

AIMS OF MANAGEMENT

Optimal gestational age for the delivery of twin pregnancy is an issue, which is highly debatable. However, a study conducted by Ahmad F Bakr et al. concluded that in the absence of significant maternal complications, it is advisable to deliver twins only at 38 completed weeks' gestation or later to avoid neonatal complications.[1] Also several observational studies report that there are lesser chances of fetal and neonatal complications when elective birth is planned at 36 weeks in monochorionic twins and 35 weeks in triplet pregnancies.[2] Current practice is to deliver monoamniotic twins by planned cesarean section at 34 weeks because of the increased risk of cord complications.[3] Further studies are needed to determine the optimal timing for delivering multiple gestations **(Algorithms 1 and 2)**.

American College of Obstetrics and Gynecologists (ACOG) recommends that "the route of delivery for twins should be determined by the position of the fetuses, the ease of fetal heart rate monitoring, and the maternal and fetal status".[4]

In Canadian Guidelines, Consensus statement 20 and 21 give recommendations for the route of delivery in twin pregnancy as "Delivery of cephalic twin A/noncephalic twin B: Estimated weight 1,500–4,000 g. Vaginal delivery is indicated as long as the obstetrician is comfortable with and skilled in vaginal breech delivery."[5]

"Delivery of cephalic twin A/noncephalic twin B: Estimated weight 500–1,500 g, there is no consistent evidence to support either cesarean section or the vaginal route for delivery." [5]

Algorithm 1: Algorithm on aims of management of a patient with multiple gestations.

- Identify high risk factors
- Determine optimum time and mode of delivery
- Prevent perinatal asphyxia in all fetuses
- Predict and prevent birth injuries

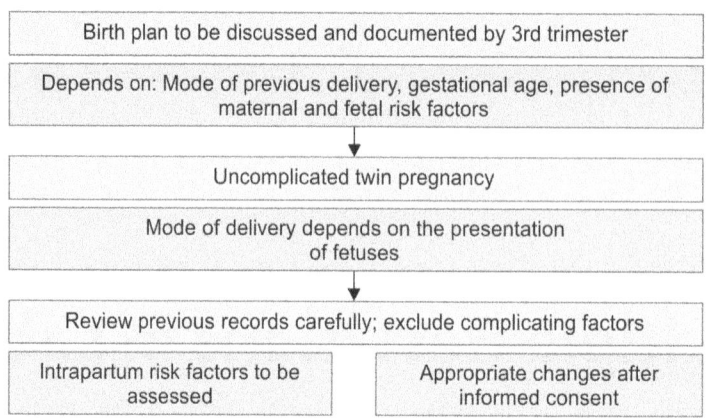

Algorithm 2: Algorithm on management of a patient with twin gestation.

The Cochrane Database reviewed one randomized trial on mode of delivery for twins and concluded that cesarean delivery should not be universally adapted as the route of delivery for twins.[6]

MANAGEMENT IN LABOR

First Stage of Labor

Management of twin pregnancy during first stage of labor is shown in **Algorithms 3 and 4**.

Second Stage of Labor

Delivery of Twin A

Managed entirely as for a singleton but with monitoring of the cotwin throughout. If there are any concerns for the monitoring of twin B, expedite the delivery of both twins by cesarean section.

In case of diamniotic twins, delivery of the first twin is similar to singleton except that the umbilical cords should be marked with progressive numbers of clamps (e.g. one for the first twin birth, two for the second twin birth). *In monochorionic twins*, signs of acute peripartum twin-twin transfusion syndrome may include bradycardia or a sinusoidal fetal heart rate pattern, and may necessitate urgent delivery.[7] Also, in *monochorionic diamniotic twins*, the umbilical cord must be clamped after delivery of first twin because the cotwin could develop hypovolemic shock from exsanguinating into the placenta and out of the unclamped cord of the first twin. Avoid uterotonics (e.g. methylergometrine) at the time of delivery of anterior shoulder of first twin. Avoid obtaining cord blood of first

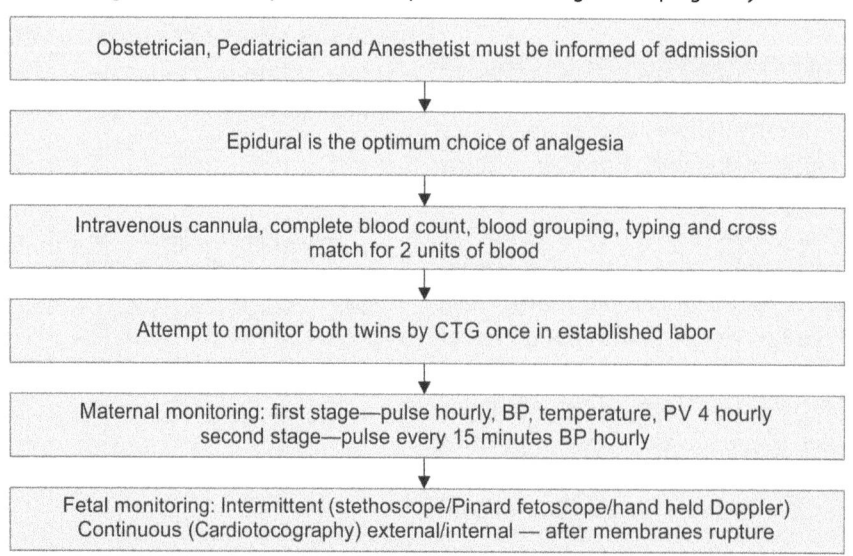

Algorithm 3: Prerequisites for intrapartum monitoring of twin pregnancy.

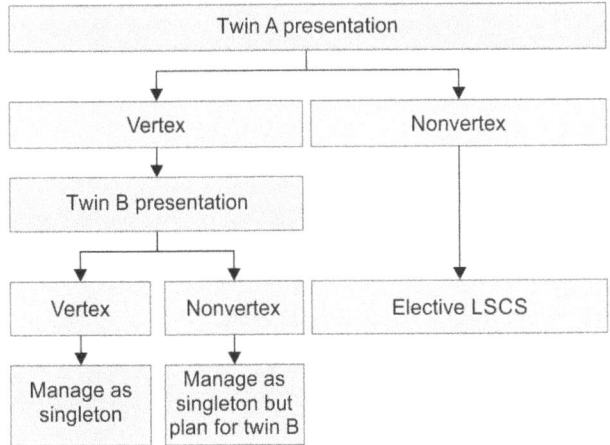

Algorithm 4: Labor management depending on presentation of fetuses.

twin before delivery of the second twin. In majority of the cases, twin B delivers by 30 minutes.

Delivery of Twin B (Algorithm 5)

Soon after the delivery of first twin, determine the lie and presentation of the second twin and whenever possible, confirm by ultrasound. If the lie is longitudinal, oxytocin infusion may be started to ensure adequate uterine contractions. A team of experienced obstetricians, nurses, anesthetists, and neonatologists should be in attendance during the delivery.[8-10]

Twin B with vertex presentation: The procedure for delivery of twin B with vertex presentation is shown in **Algorithm 6**.

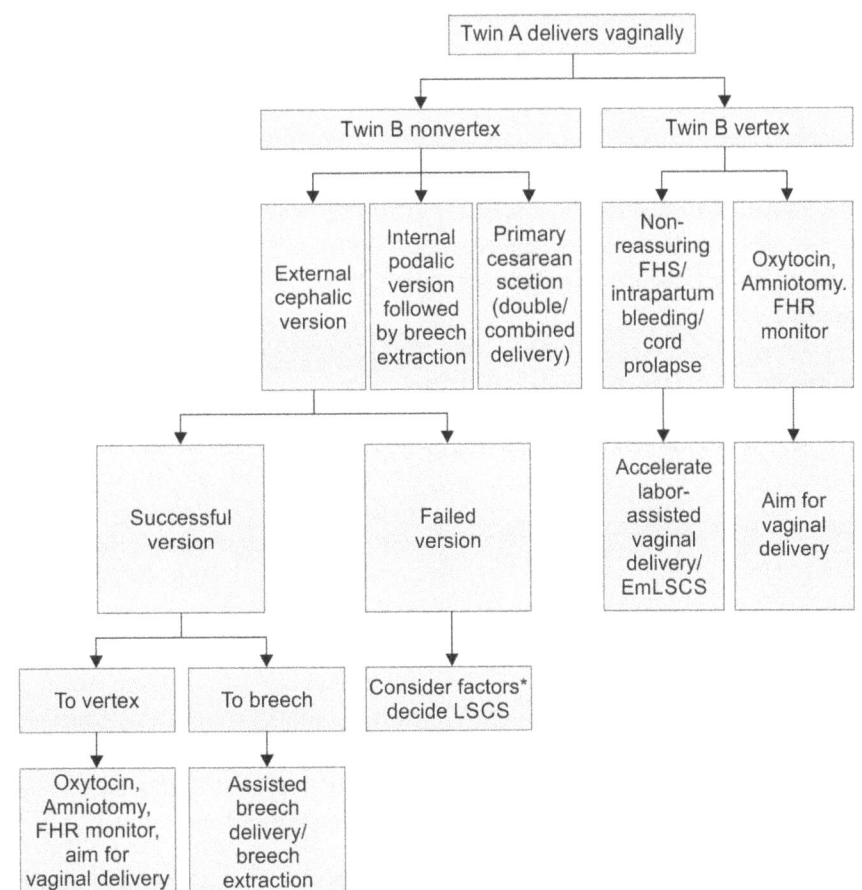

Algorithm 5: Flowchart showing management of labor after delivery of first twin.

(factors* = available skill, weight discrepancy in A and B, B more than 25% of A, weight extremes <1,500 g/>3,500 g, age, parity, fertility).

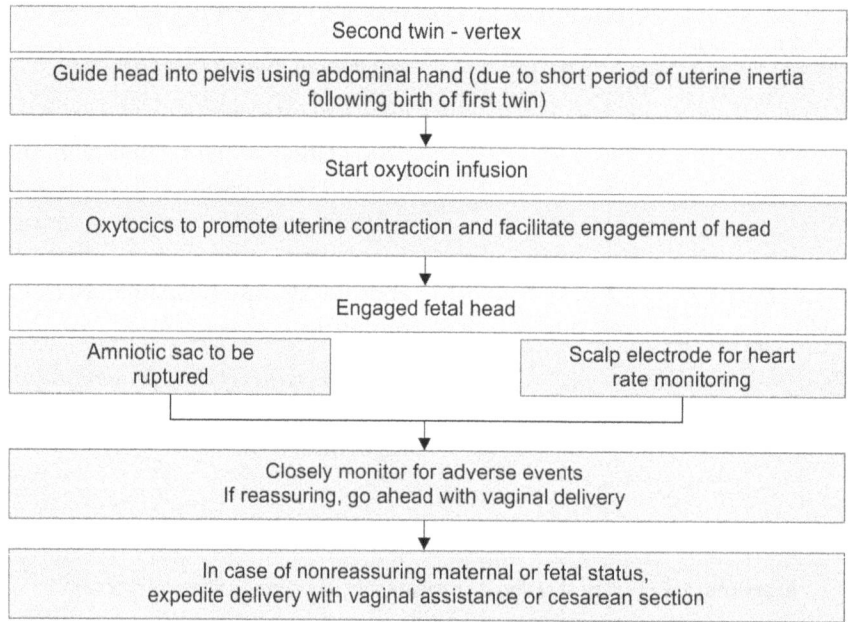

Algorithm 6: Delivery of second twin with vertex presentation.

Twin B with nonvertex presentation: Expertise of the obstetrician is crucial in this situation. When the second twin is nonvertex, the obstetrician may choose one of the following three options depending on the clinical circumstances, his/her knowledge, skill, and expertise. These options include external cephalic version or internal podalic version followed by breech extraction or primary cesarean section **(Algorithm 5)**.

Third Stage Management

Management of third stage of labor after twin delivery is shown in **Algorithm 7**.

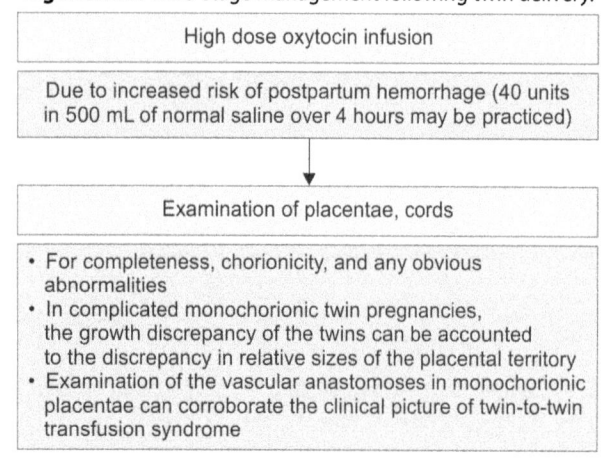

Algorithm 7: Third-stage management following twin delivery.

DOCUMENTATION

Documentation of all aspects of labor and delivery should be clear, contemporaneous, and consistent among all involved healthcare providers. The birth order of the newborns should be clearly identified on their respective charts.

SUMMARY

Considering all the above-discussed conditions, it becomes clear that there is no single best method to manage multiple gestation during labor. Clinical skill of the obstetrician to predict the outcome, judge the circumstance, and take an informed decision stands to be the crucial step. Counseling the patient and relatives and documentation of events are considered to be of utmost importance in this era of ethics and litigations. However, the availability of adequate nursing staff, well-equipped delivery suite, anesthetists, functional operation theater, and neonatologists with a good neonatal care are the requirements, which add on to obstetrician's success in managing multiple gestation.

REFERENCES

1. Bakr AF, Karkour T. What is the optimal gestational age for twin delivery. BMC Pregnancy Childbirth. 2006;6:3.

2. National Institute of Health and Clinical Excellence. (2011). Clinical Guideline Number 129. Multiple pregnancy: antenatal care for twin and triplet pregnancies. [Online] Available from: https://www.nice.org.uk/guidance/cg129 [Last accessed October, 2019].
3. Bajoria R, WeeL Y, Anwar S, et al. Outcome of twin pregnancies complicated by single intrauterine death in relation to vascular anatomy of the monochorionic placenta. Hum Reprod. 1999;14(8):2124-30.
4. American College of Obstetricians and Gynecologists Committee on Practice Bulletins-Obstetrics; Society for Maternal-Fetal Medicine; ACOG Joint Editorial Committee. ACOG Practice Bulletin #56: Multiple gestation: complicated twin, triplet, and high-order multifetal pregnancy. Obstet Gynecol. 2004;104(4):869-83.
5. Barrett J, Bocking A. The SOGC Consensus Statement: management of twin pregnancies. SOGC. 2000;91:5-15.
6. Crowther CA. Caesarean delivery for the second twin. Cochrane Database Syst Rev. 2000;(2):CD000047.
7. Christopher D, Robinson BL, Peaceman AM. An evidence-based approach to determining route of delivery for twin gestations. Rev Obstet Gynecol. 2011;4(3-4):109-16.
8. Rayburn WF, Lavin JP Jr, Miodovnik M, et al. Multiple gestation: time interval between delivery of the first and second twins. Obstet Gynecol. 1984;63(4):502-6.
9. Rydhstrom H, Ingemarsson I. Interval between birth of the first and the second twin and its impact on second twin perinatal mortality. J Perinat Med. 1990;18(6):449-53.
10. Brown HL, Miller JM Jr, Neumann DE, et al. Umbilical cord blood gas assessment of twins. Obstet Gynecol. 1990;75(5):826-9.

Chapter 24: Cervical Insufficiency

Neha Gupta

INTRODUCTION

Cervical insufficiency, also called as cervical incompetence, has no established definition. As American College of Obstetricians and Gynecologists (ACOG) states, it is the inability of the uterine cervix to hold the pregnancy in its place during the second trimester in the absence of signs and symptoms of contractions or labor.[1] It involves painless uterine contractions without any provocative factor-like bleeding per vaginam, infection, or ruptured membranes **(Algorithm 1)**.

INCIDENCE

It is estimated to be occurring in 1% of obstetric population[2] and about 8% in those with recurrent mid-trimester miscarriages.[3]

RISK FACTORS

Women who are at risk for cervical insufficiency are difficult to identify. Some at-risk may be identified by means of their previous history or by history of some cervical disease. Largely remains unknown.

The risk factors can be:
- Congenital **(Algorithm 2)**
- Acquired **(Algorithm 3)**
- *Obstetrical history:*
    - Previous one or more mid-trimester losses with no unknown cause
    - Previous medical termination of pregnancy
    - Previous preterm birth/premature rupture of membranes
    - History of smoking
    - Multiple gestations
    - Polyhydramnios
    - Sonographic findings of short cervical length (<25 mm), cervical dilatation, and funneling.
- *Surgical causes:*
    - Forced dilatation during medical termination of pregnancy (MTP) and dilatation and curettage (D&C)

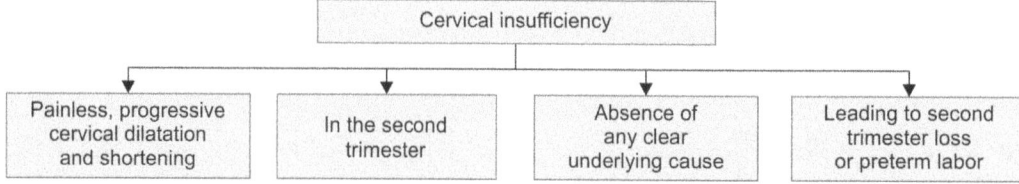

Algorithm 1: Characteristics to define cervical insufficiency.

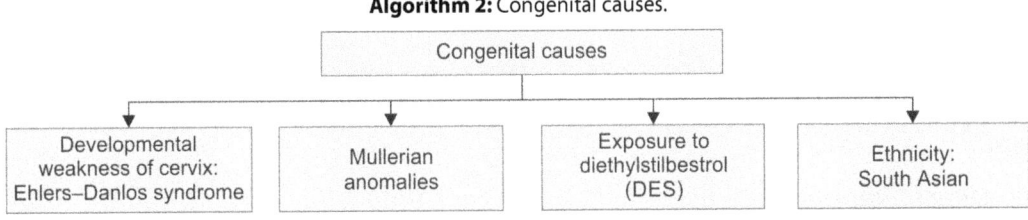

Algorithm 2: Congenital causes.

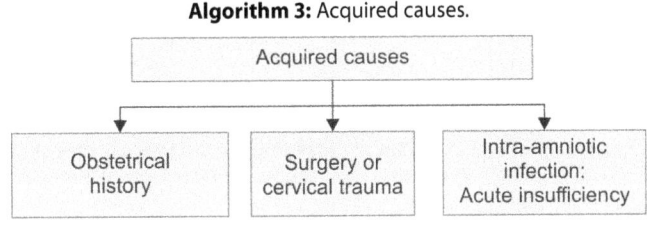

Algorithm 3: Acquired causes.

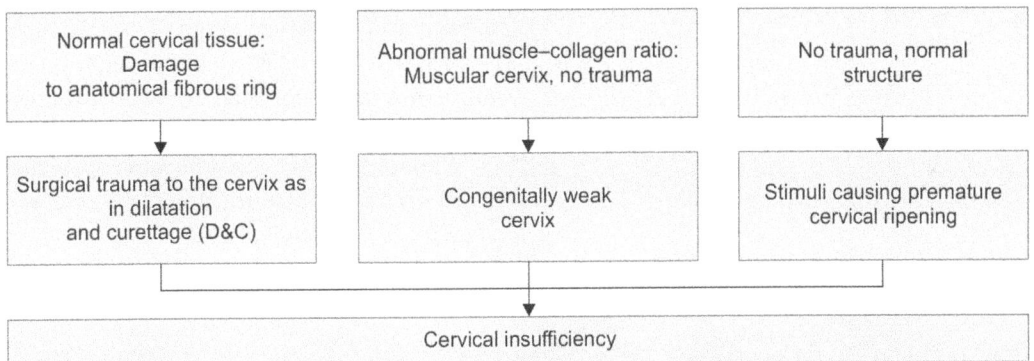

Algorithm 4: Pathophysiology of cervical insufficiency.

- Cervical conization: Loop electrosurgical excision procedure (LEEP)
- Cervical amputation during Fothergill operation
- Cauterization of cervix.

PATHOPHYSIOLOGY (ALGORITHM 4)

Cervix is integral to the maintenance of pregnancy. Any change in its anatomic or biologic function can affect the length of pregnancy. It is mainly composed of fibrous tissue, which provides main support to the pregnancy.

An important thing to consider is that cervical insufficiency arises due to defects in the cervix or external factors. This is essential to decide the optimal modality of treatment.

SCREENING

Women with cervical insufficiency are difficult to identify. In the majority, no cause is identified. Some are identified on the basis of history. So whom to screen?

Universal versus Selective Screening

The issue of universal cervical length screening of singleton gestations without prior preterm birth (PTB) for the prevention of PTB remains an object of debate. Cervical length screening in singleton gestations without prior PTB cannot yet be universally mandated. Nonetheless, the implementation of such a screening strategy can be

viewed as reasonable and can be considered by individual practitioners, following strict guidelines.[4]
- Duration of surveillance: 16–24 weeks.

How to Screen?

Screening by Means of Transvaginal Cervical Length Assessment

The protocol as laid down by Fetal Medicine Foundation is shown in **Algorithm 5** (Available at https://fetalmedicine.org).

Algorithm 5: Screening by means of transvaginal cervical length assessment.

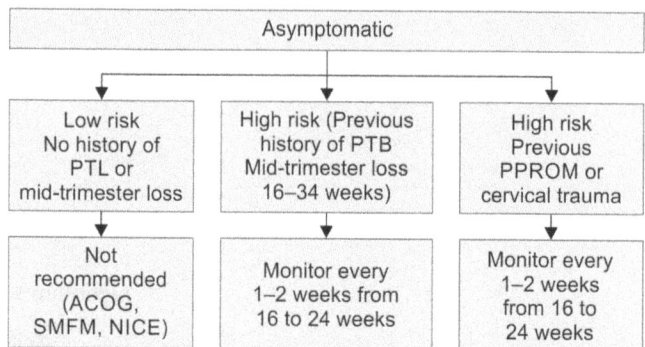

Algorithm 6: Whom to screen for cervical insufficiency?

(ACOG: American College of Obstetricians and Gynecologists; NICE: National Institute for Health and Care Excellence; PPROM: preterm premature rupture of the membranes; PTB: preterm birth; PTL: preterm labor; SMFM: Society of Maternal-Fetal Medicine)

MANAGEMENT

The avoidance of risk factors ranging like surgical trauma to the cervix, smoking cessation, reduction of physical activity and work, cessation of sexual activity and the prophylactic use of cervical cerclage, progesterone, and antibiotics are beneficial to what extent, still remains unclear.

Whenever cervical insufficiency is suspected, whether based on history or ultrasound, the options described in **Algorithm 7**, are considered.

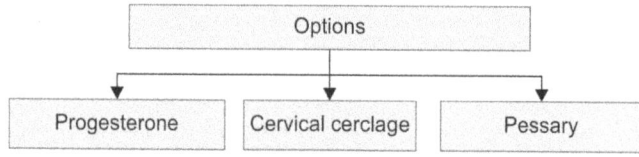

Algorithm 7: Management options.

Progesterone (Algorithm 8)

It is responsible for maintaining myometrial quiescence during pregnancy. Cochrane review[7] suggests reduction in the risk of preterm labor (PTL) when given progesterone.

Which progesterone to use?
Evidence exists for these common types of progesterone, as described in **Algorithm 9**.

No evidence of benefit exists for the addition of an alternative form to the current form of progesterone. Also, there is no evidence of benefit exists from shifting from one modality of progesterone to the other in case of cervical insufficiency is identified.

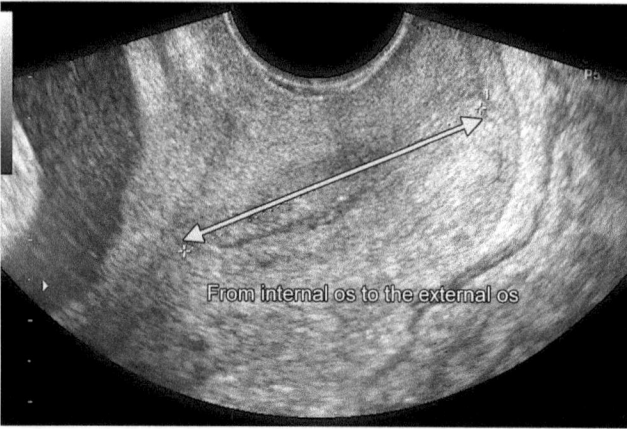

Fig. 1: Cervical length measurement—distance from the internal os to the external os.

Selective Screening

As laid down by NICE 2015[5] and SMFM 2016,[6] it is summarized in **Algorithm 6**.

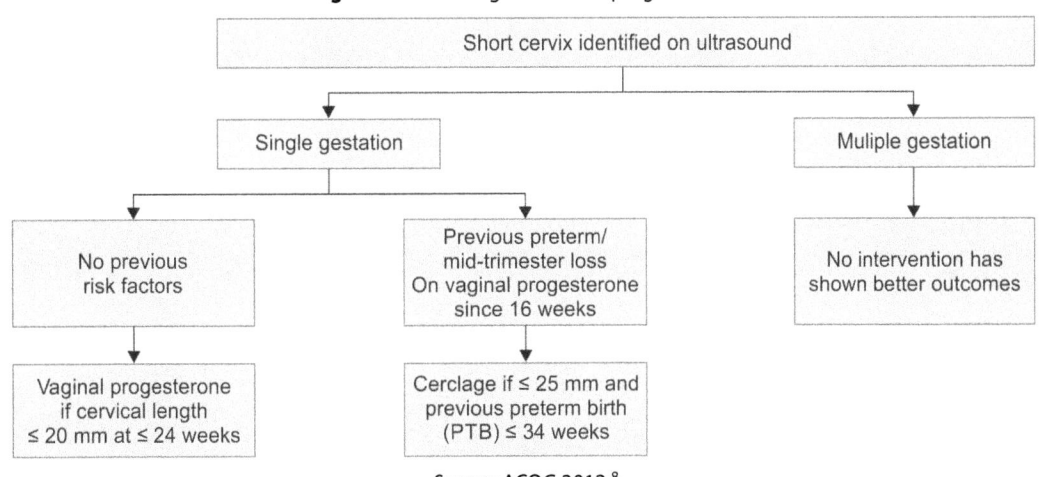

Algorithm 8: Management with progesterone.

Source: ACOG 2012.[8]

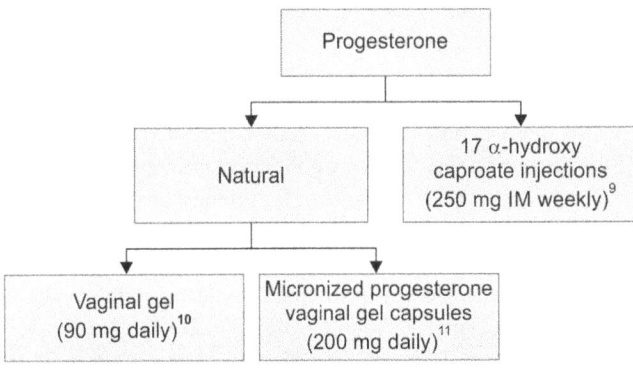

Algorithm 9: Types of progesterone.

Cerclage[12]

Types (Algorithm 10)

Techniques
- McDonald
- Shirodhkar.

Prerequisites

1	• Viability and combined first trimester screening • Early anomaly scan if planned in second trimester
2	• Urine culture and sensitivity • Vaginal swabs especially for bacterial vaginosis

Contraindications

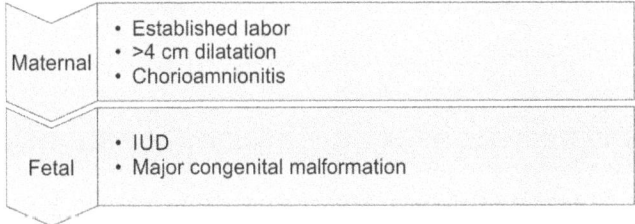

Postcerclage follow-up: Not recommended yet.

Removal of cerclage **(Algorithm 11)**.

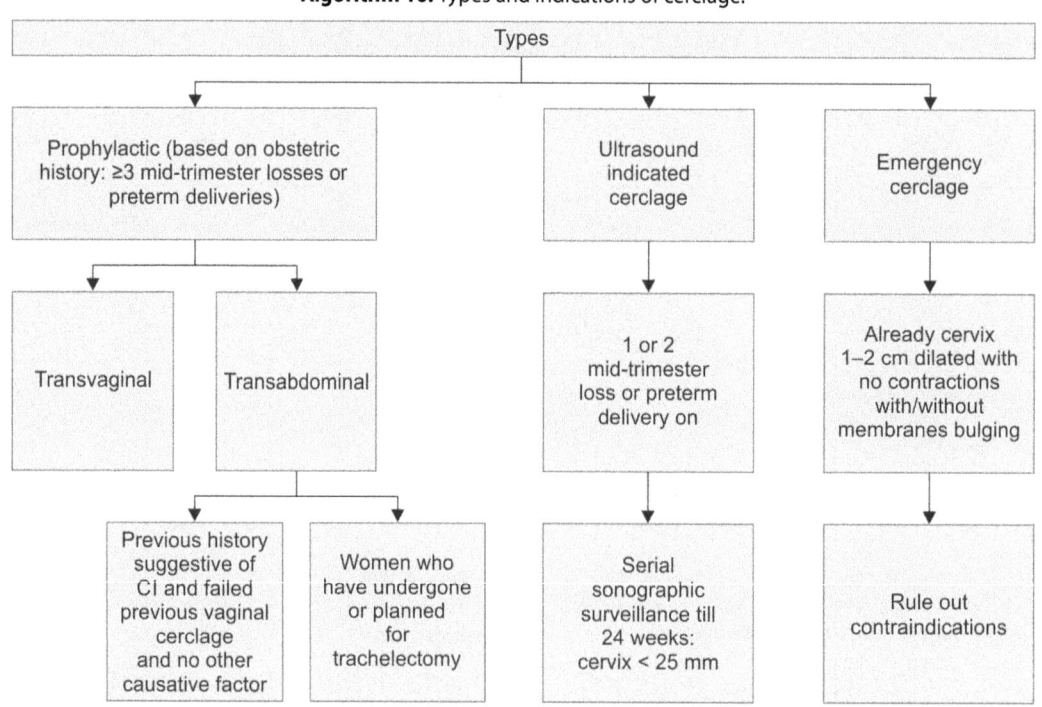

Algorithm 10: Types and indications of cerclage.

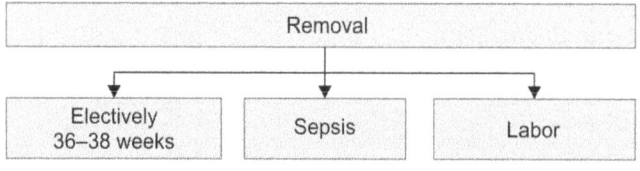

Algorithm 11: Removal of cerclage.

REFERENCES

1. American College of Obstetricians and Gynecologists. ACOG Practice Bulletin No.142: Cerclage for the management of cervical insufficiency. Obstet Gynecol. 2014;123(2 Pt 1):372-9.
2. Rand L, Norwitz ER. Current controversies in cervical cerclage. Semin Perinatol. 2003;27:73-85.
3. Drakeley AJ, Roberts D, Alfirevic Z. Cervical stitch (cerclage) for preventing pregnancy loss in women. Cochrane Database Syst Rev. 2003;(1):CD003253.
4. Society for Maternal-Fetal Medicine Publications Committee, with assistance of Vincenzo Berghella. Progesterone and preterm birth prevention: translating clinical trials data into clinical practice. Am J Obstet Gynecol. 2012;206(5): 376-86.
5. National Institute for Health and Care Excellence. Preterm Labour and Birth, NICE Guideline. London, UK: National Institute for Health and Care Excellence (UK); 2015.
6. Society for Maternal-Fetal Medicine (SMFM), McIntosh J, Feltovich H, et al. Role of routine cervical length screening in high risk and low risk women for preterm birth prevention. Am J Obstet Gynecol. 2016;215(3):B2-7.
7. Dodd JM, Flenady V, Cincotta R, et al. Prenatal administration of progesterone for preventing preterm birth (review). Cochrane Database Syst Rev. 2006;(1):CD004947.
8. American College of Obstetricians and, Gynecologists. ACOG Practice Bulletin No. 130: prediction and prevention of preterm birth. Obstet Gynecol. 2012;120:964-73.
9. Meis PJ, Klebanoff M, Thom E, et al. Prevention of recurrent preterm delivery by 17 α hydroxyprogesterone caproate. NEJM. 2003;348:2379-85.
10. Hassan SS, Romero R, Vidyadhari D, et al. Vaginal progesterone reduces the rate of preterm birth in women with sonographic short cervix: a multicenter, randomized double blind, placebo controlled trial. PREGNANT trial. Ultrasound Obstet Gynecol. 2011;38:18-31.
11. Fonseca EB, Celik E, Parra M, et al. Progesterone and risk of preterm birth among women with a short cervix. Fetal Medicine Foundation Second Trimester Screening Group. NEJM. 2007;357:462-9.
12. SOGC Clinical Practical Guideline. Cervical insufficiency and cervical cerclage. J Obstet Gynaecol Can. 2013;35(12): 1115-27.

Chapter 25

Reduced Fetal Movements

Geetha Balsarkar

INTRODUCTION

Maternal perception of fetal movement is one of the first signs of fetal life and is regarded as a manifestation of fetal well-being and growth. Movements are first felt by the mother between 18 weeks and 20 weeks of gestation and rapidly acquire a regular pattern. In multigravidas, the perception is slightly earlier as they remember the movements from previous pregnancy. Although it varies from woman to woman, fetal movements have been defined as any kick, roll, slush, or flutter felt by the mother.[1,2]

The pregnant mother complaining of reduced fetal movements (RFMs) near term is a common presentation in obstetric emergency ward. It is perceived as a state of suboptimal fetal condition by the mother and often presents clinical dilemma. Most of the times, after a certain time period, the patient is able to perceive movements again, and the anxiety of the mother is relieved.

One of the greatest challenges in management of such patients is the lack of consensus among clinicians on what is a "normal" number of fetal movements and at what gestational age. Fetal movements vary from 4 per hours to 100 per hours and so definitions of RFM based on counting less than 10 movements in 2 hours, 12 hours, or 24 hours are not helpful to the clinician.[3]

Reduced or absent fetal movements may be a warning sign of chronic placental insufficiency and impending fetal death. RFM is thought to be a symptom of nutrient or oxygen restriction and is related to changes in improper placental structure and function. The perception of RFM affects up to 15% of all pregnancies. Studies of fetal physiology using ultrasound have demonstrated an association between RFM and poor perinatal outcome. The majority of women (55%) experiencing a stillbirth perceived a reduction in fetal movements prior to diagnosis of absent fetal heart.[4]

Lack of prompt management in RFM has been recognized as a main contributing factor for stillbirth. Other factors were lack of awareness and hence failure of mothers to report RFM, and a failure of the doctor to explain the importance of reporting changes in movements.[5]

Clinicians should be themselves aware and should advise women that although fetal movements tend to plateau at 32 weeks of gestation, there is no reduction in the frequency of fetal movements in the late third trimester, even in the first stage of labor. As the fetus advances in the gestational age, the neurological maturity is reflected by changes in number and nature of the fetal movements. Though movements have been described by 16 weeks, by 20 weeks, the fetus shows diurnal variation. The movements improve during the day and peak during the afternoon and evening. Absent fetal movements have been noticed during the fetal "sleep cycles" occurring at regular intervals as the day progresses and persists even during night lasting for 20–40 minutes. In a normal healthy fetus growing well, the sleep cycles usually do not exceed 90 minutes.

Fetal movements should be assessed by subjective maternal perception of fetal movements. 85% of women will be concerned about the reduction of fetal movements and therefore RFM must be managed meticulously to avoid an adverse perinatal outcome.[6,7]

Fetal activity is influenced by many factors. When the mother is lying down in left lateral position, the movements are maximum. It reduces when they are sitting and working. It is least when the mothers are standing. When patients complain of reduced fetal movements, they should be advised to observe fetal movements while lying down in left lateral position in a quiet room after a meal. In primigravidas with good abdominal tone and an anteriorly placed placenta, movements could be perceived as late as 28 weeks.[8,9]

Sedating drugs taken by the mother, which cross the placental barrier such as alcohol, benzodiazepines, methadone, and other opioids can have a transient effect on fetal movements. There could be an increase in fetal movements following the elevation of glucose concentration in maternal blood, especially after eating.[10] From 30 weeks of gestation onward, the level of carbon dioxide in maternal blood influences fetal respiratory movements, and hence cigarette smoking is associated with a decrease in fetal activity.

Fetuses with major structural malformations are generally more likely to demonstrate reduced fetal activity. However, normal or excessive fetal activity has been reported in anencephalic fetuses. A lack of vigorous motion may relate to abnormalities of the central nervous system, muscular dysfunction, or skeletal abnormalities (**Box 1**).[11]

Box 1 | Common causes of reduced fetal movements.

- Maternal causes—position—most movements are felt in the left lateral supine position, fewest on standing
  - Busy daily lifestyle in a working mother
  - Diurnal variation of fetal awake and sleep cycles
  - Very good abdominal tone and obese mother
  - When the mother is put on certain drugs that sedate her, it sedates baby too
  - When there is increased or reduced liquor
  - Certain maternal diseases like hypothyroidism, anemia
- Fetal—certain fetal neurological, muscular, and skeletal defects
- Placental causes—insufficiency in any form like intrauterine growth restriction (IUGR)

DIAGNOSIS

Count to 10 fetal movements and kick count charts are very popular among patients and clinicians to keep track of fetal movement. However, there is not enough evidence that formally counting fetal movements over a specified time everyday is better than relying on maternal general perception of RFM after 28 weeks of gestation. Therefore, if a mother expresses concern over RFM, she should be advised to lie on their left side and focus on movements for 2 hours in a quiet dark room, so that she can focus on fetal movements.[12]

If she does not feel 10 or more movements over this time, she should contact her clinician or be directed to the nearest maternity unit without delay. If movements are felt, then the mother should be reassured and asked to remain mindful of her baby's individual movement pattern. If this changes and there is further concern, she should not hesitate to seek medical advice again.

INVESTIGATIONS

Before 24 weeks of gestation, fetal heart assessment should be performed with a handheld Doppler and if no fetal movements have been felt at all ever by this time, a detailed ultrasonography should be made to exclude structural abnormalities and oligohydramnios. Doppler confirms the presence of fetal heart and therefore reassures the mother, when she hears it.

For women who have high-risk factors as baseline risk, when associated with reduced fetal movement, maternal blood pressure (BP), pulse and temperature, and urinalysis should be performed at every possible contact. Palpation of abdomen and measurement of symphysial fundal height (SFH) to exclude small for gestational age (SGA) and oligohydramnios should be done.

If there are no risk factors for stillbirth, the fetal heart is heard on auscultation, and examination findings are normal, the woman can be reassured and advised to see her clinician within the next week for further evaluation.

If the mother is not reassured, is very anxious, concerns are raised by the clinician, there are risk factors for stillbirth, or the RFM occurred suddenly then the woman should be admitted to maternity unit for further investigations.

General advice, including adequate diet and hydration, smoking cessation, and drug/alcohol reduction/cessation, should be given and also documented.

MANAGEMENT

Currently, there are many options for interventions for RFM after the initial basic assessment. These antepartum testing techniques should be individualized depending on the patient's history and complaints. These include nonstress test (NST) for detecting fetal compromise, ultrasound scan including biophysical profiling, umbilical artery Doppler assessment, estimated fetal weight and liquor volume, and kick charts.

By and large, reassurance that 70% of normal pregnancies with a single episode of reduced fetal movements do not affect the outcome works wonders for the confidence of these mothers. In addition, as of today, we do not have any data to support that daily kick counts help those with normal investigations and hence should not be recommended. If these women present with a second episode of such complaints, they should be admitted and observed for the cause. Recurrent episodes have poor perinatal outcome.

The delivery would be done in tertiary care centers only if the woman presents with a subsequent episode of RFM (with or without other risk factors). Also, there should be a backup of neonatal unit in such cases.

The Royal College of Obstetricians and Gynaecologists (RCOG) guidelines recommend use of NST only if gestation is beyond 28 weeks (age of viability) and only if fetal auscultation is unsatisfactory. The fetal heart rate normally accelerates with 92–97% of all gross body movements felt by the mother. NST should be performed for 20 minutes to assess fetal well-being.[13]

ULTRASOUND SCAN

Ultrasonography is only recommended in addition to NST when there are combination of factors involved. At the least, a limited scan for amniotic fluid index should be done. Umbilical artery Doppler should be added on if growth restriction is present.[14]

PROGNOSIS

About 70% of patients with single episode of reduced fetal movements have normal outcome, only 3–5% will have recurrent episodes, which will have poor outcome.[15]

Each patient should have proper review of case history every time they present with reduced fetal movements to arrive at a decision whether to continue pregnancy, undergo induction, or cesarean section.

CONCLUSION

Since it is on the perception of the mother and the accurate history taken by the clinician, which decides which way the pregnancy continues or needs to be terminated, good record keeping goes a long way to aid decision making. There should be a standardized approach to these women, excluding the risk factors for better outcome.[16,17]

ONGOING TRIALS

Reduced Fetal Movement Intervention Trial-2 (ReMIT-2) is an ongoing randomized control trial to determine placental function in RFM patients using blood investigations going on in Nottingham, UK since 15th October, 2017.

REFERENCES

1. Rayburn WF. Fetal body movement monitoring. Obstet Gynecol Clin North Am. 1990;17:95-110.
2. Neldam S. Fetal movements as an indicator of fetal well-being. Dan Med Bull. 1983;30:274-8
3. D'Elia A, Pighetti M, Moccia G, et al. Spontaneous motor activity in normal fetuses. Early Hum Dev. 2001;65:139-47.
4. Harrington K, Thompson O, Jordan L, et al. Obstetric outcome in women who present with a reduction in fetal movements in the third trimester of pregnancy. J Perinat Med. 1998;26:77-82.
5. Sanfilippo JS, Smith RP. Primary Care in Obstetrics and Gynecology: A Handbook for Clinicians, 2nd edition. New York: Springer-Verlag; 2007.
6. Efkarpidis S, Alexopoulos E, Kean L, et al. Case-control study of factors associated with intrauterine fetal deaths. MedGenMed. 2004;6:53.
7. Patrick J, Campbell K, Carmichael L, et al. Patterns of gross fetal body movements over 24-hour observation intervals during the last 10 weeks of pregnancy. Am J Obstet Gynecol. 1982;142:363-71.
8. Johnson TR, Jordan ET, Paine LL. Doppler recordings of fetal movement: II. Comparison with maternal perception. Obstet Gynecol. 1990;76:42-3.
9. Johnson TR. Maternal perception and Doppler detection of fetal movement. Clin Perinatol. 1994;21:765-77.
10. Robertson SS, Dierker LJ. Fetal cyclic motor activity in diabetic pregnancies: sensitivity to maternal blood glucose. Dev Psychobiol. 2003;42:9-16.
11. Tveit JV, Saastad E, Stray-Pedersen B, et al. Reduction of late stillbirth with the introduction of fetal movement information and guidelines—a clinical quality improvement. BMC Pregnancy Childbirth. 2009;9:32.
12. Unterscheider J, Horgan R, O'Donoghue K, et al. Reduced fetal movements. Obstet Gynaecol. 2009;11:245-51.
13. Dayal AK, Manning FA, Berck DJ, et al. Fetal death after normal biophysical profile score: An eighteen-year experience. Am J Obstet Gynecol. 1999;181:1231-6.
14. Heazell AE, Sumathi GM, Bhatti NR. What investigation is appropriate following maternal perception of reduced fetal movements? J Obstet Gynaecol. 2005;25:648-50.
15. Sinha D, Sharma A, Nallaswamy V, et al. Obstetric outcome in women complaining of reduced fetal movements. J Obstet Gynaecol. 2007;27:41-3.
16. O'Sullivan O, Stephen G, Martindale E, et al. Predicting poor perinatal outcome in women who present with decreased fetal movements. J Obstet Gynaecol. 2009;29:705-10.
17. Hofmeyr GJ, Novikova N. Management of reported decreased fetal movements for improving pregnancy outcomes. Cochrane Database Syst Rev. 2012;4:CD009148.

Intrauterine Fetal Death

Savita Singhal, Shaveta Jain

INTRODUCTION

Fetal death is one of the common adverse pregnancy outcomes and great psychological trauma for the parents. Stillbirth is the preferred term over fetal death and is defined as when a baby is delivered with no signs of life. There is no uniformity with regards to birth weight and gestational age criteria for defining stillbirth, as per Royal College of Obstetricians and Gynaecologists (RCOG)[1] (2010) stillbirth is defined as death of fetus after 24 weeks of gestation, and as per American College of Obstetricians and Gynecologists (ACOG)[2] (2009), fetal death at ≥20 weeks of gestation or weight ≥350 g if gestational age is not known.

INCIDENCE

Stillbirth complicates about 1:160 deliveries and varies from 5 to 32 per 1,000 live birth in different countries and being more in developing countries.[3]

RISK FACTORS

Various risk factors for stillbirth are as follows:[4]
- Nonhispanic blacks
- Obesity (fivefold increased risk)
- Advanced maternal age
- Low educational status
- Nulliparity
- Multiple gestations (fourfold increased risk)
- Diabetes mellitus
- Hypertensive disorders
- Previous history of preterm delivery, pre-eclampsia, growth restriction, and stillbirth
- Personal or family history of thrombophilia or thromboembolism
- Smoking, drugs, alcohol use.

CAUSES OF STILLBIRTH

- About 15–20% of all stillborn have major malformations and 20% have dysmorphic features.
- Abnormal karyotype is seen in 8–13% of all stillbirths. Common abnormalities seen are trisomy 21, 18, 13, and monosomy X.[5]
- Causes of stillbirth are mentioned in **Algorithms 1 to 4**.
- 19% of stillbirth at <28 weeks and 2% at term are associated with infections.[6] Common infections are parvovirus, cytomegalovirus, listeria, and syphilis.

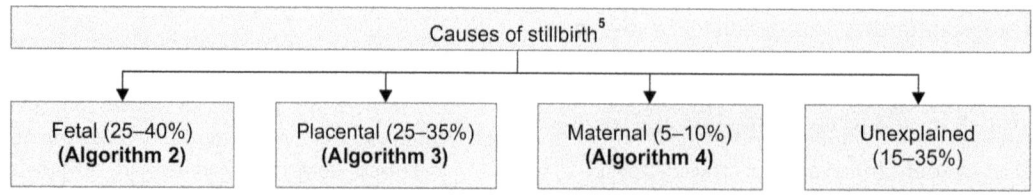

Algorithm 1: Causes of stillbirth[5]

Chapter 26
Intrauterine Fetal Death

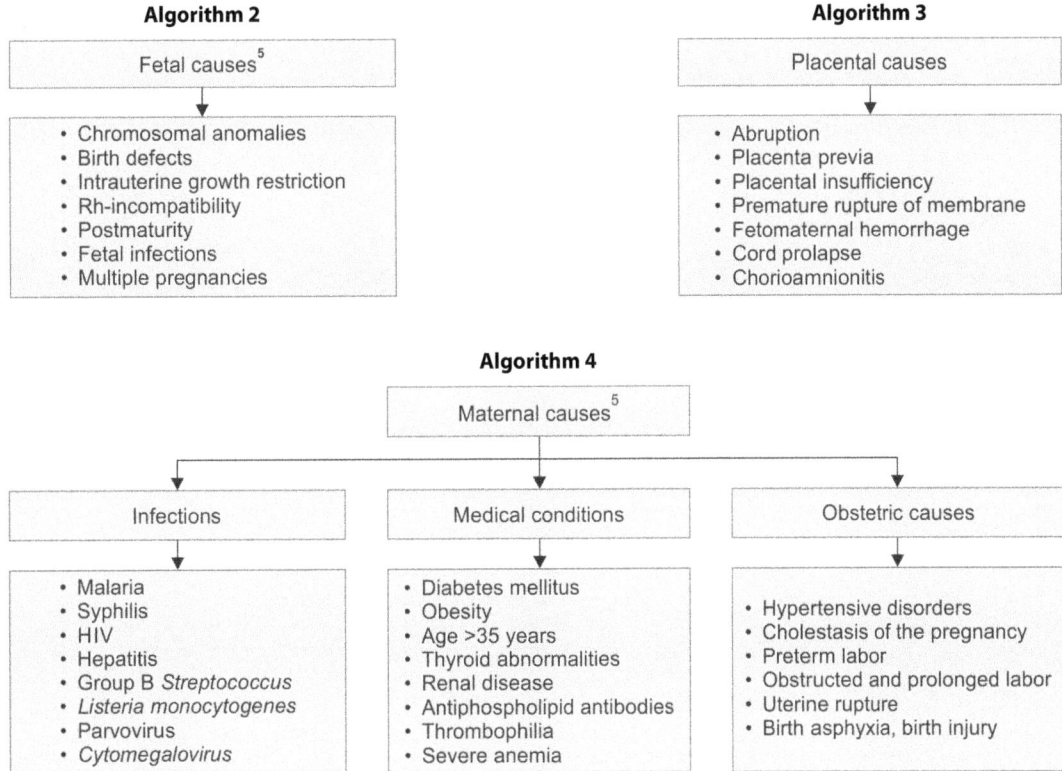

- In developing countries, maternal infections with malaria, tuberculosis, and hepatitis are common.
- In multiple pregnancies, especially monochorionic twins are at increased risk of stillbirth due to twin-to-twin transfusion syndrome.

DIAGNOSIS OF STILLBIRTH

Real-time ultrasonography is the gold standard for accurate diagnosis of stillbirth. On ultrasound, following findings are suggestive of stillbirth:
- Absent fetal heart
- Absent fetal movements
- Overlapping of skull bones (Spalding sign)
- Gross distortion of fetal anatomy (maceration)
- Gas shadow in the fetal heart (Robert sign) is suggestive of stillbirth.
- Various investigations done for late stillbirth as mentioned in **Algorithm 5**.

MATERNAL EVALUATION

- A thorough maternal history and examination should be carried out, looking for known conditions or symptoms that are suggestive of stillbirth.
- Relevant medical records and documentation should be obtained.
- Clinical examination, especially with regards to pre-eclampsia, chorioamnionitis, and placental abruption, is suggested.
- Test for coagulation should be advised twice weekly if fetus is retained in utero for more than 48 hours.
- Maternal evaluation done for stillbirth are mentioned in **Algorithm 6**.

TIMING OF DELIVERY

- Empathetic approach should be used while discussing with parents about stillborn fetus.
- Fetal death is a tragic event for the woman and her family and if the interval between diagnosis of fetal death and induction of labor increases then it further aggravates stress.
- Time of delivery is not critical, prolonged retention is associated with coagulopathy. Mother preference should be taken into consideration and most of the parents prefer early delivery.
- Urgent delivery is indicated in:
  - Sepsis
  - Pre-eclampsia

Section 2
Antenatal Emergencies

Algorithm 5

Investigations

- Complete blood count, blood group, LFT, RFT, CRP, coagulation profile
- Kleihauer–Betke test (if Rh incompatibility)
- Lupus anticoagulant
- Anticardiolipin antibodies
- Maternal bacteriology[7]
  - Blood cultures
  - Midstream urine
  - Vaginal swabs
  - Cervical swabs
- Maternal serology
  - Viral screen
  - Syphilis
- Blood sugar, HbA1c, thyroid function test, thrombophilia screen, anti-Ro, anti-La antibodies, parental karyotyping

Algorithm 6

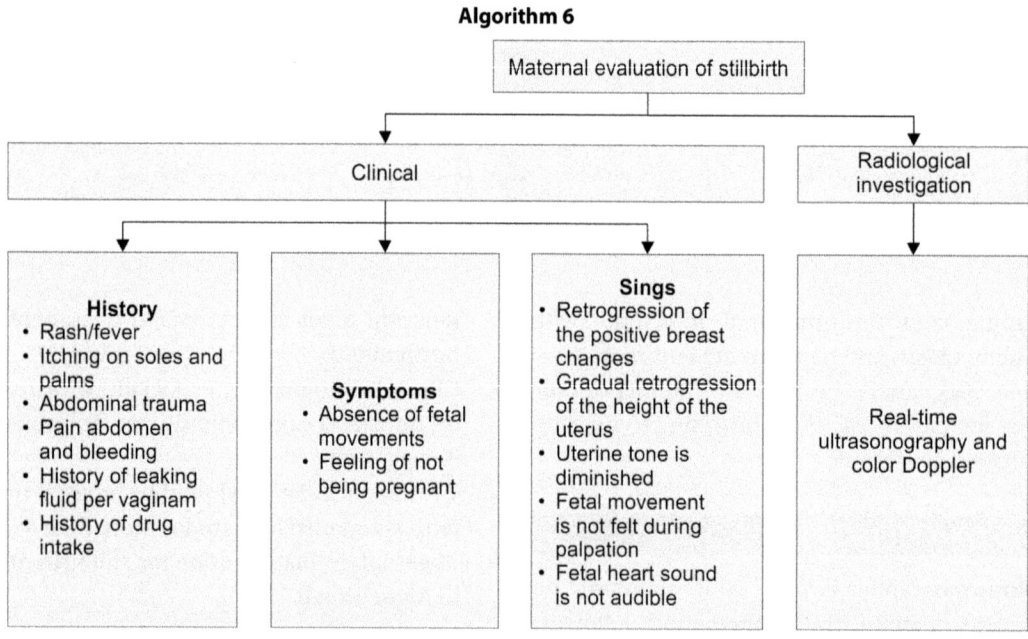

Maternal evaluation of stillbirth

Clinical / Radiological investigation

History
- Rash/fever
- Itching on soles and palms
- Abdominal trauma
- Pain abdomen and bleeding
- History of leaking fluid per vaginam
- History of drug intake

Symptoms
- Absence of fetal movements
- Feeling of not being pregnant

Sings
- Retrogression of the positive breast changes
- Gradual retrogression of the height of the uterus
- Uterine tone is diminished
- Fetal movement is not felt during palpation
- Fetal heart sound is not audible

Real-time ultrasonography and color Doppler

Algorithm 7

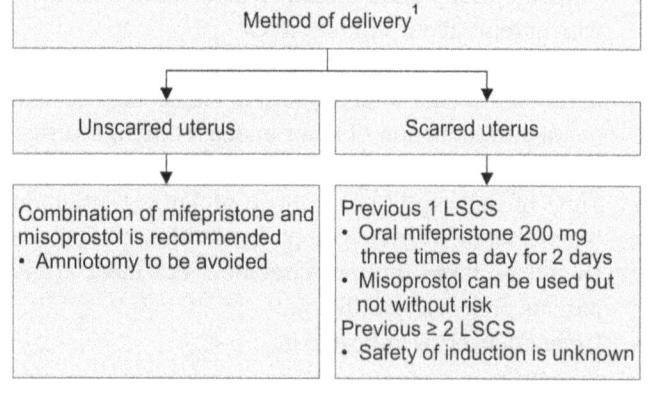

Method of delivery[1]

Unscarred uterus:
- Combination of mifepristone and misoprostol is recommended
- Amniotomy to be avoided

Scarred uterus:
- Previous 1 LSCS
  - Oral mifepristone 200 mg three times a day for 2 days
  - Misoprostol can be used but not without risk
- Previous ≥ 2 LSCS
  - Safety of induction is unknown

- Placental abruption
- Coagulation disorder
- Membrane rupture.
- Intravenous broad-spectrum antibiotic therapy should not be advised prophylactically and is recommended only in women with sepsis.

METHOD OF DELIVERY

- The method of delivery depends on:[1]
  - The gestational age
  - On the maternal history of previous uterine scar.

Dilatation and evacuation can be advised in second trimester by experienced doctor after counseling but it limits efficacy of autopsy for detecting macroscopic fetal abnormalities.
- Before 28 weeks of gestation, vaginal misoprostol is the most efficient method of induction.[8]
- Addition of mifepristone decreases induction–delivery interval.
- Usual obstetric protocol for induction of labor can be followed after 28 weeks of gestation.

PROTOCOL AFTER DELIVERY OF STILLBORN

- Complete perinatal and family history to be taken.
- Consent for fetal autopsy, cytological and histo-pathological specimens must be taken.
- Parents to be counseled that results of these will be useful in planning future pregnancy.
- The general examination of stillborn fetus and gross and microscopic examination of placenta is recommended.
- Whole-body photograph and close-up photograph of specific abnormality are vital for subsequent review and for managing future pregnancy.
- Full radiograph (fetogram) helps in identifying skeleton abnormalities.
- Karyotype analysis to be performed in all cases of stillbirth. If the fetus shows dysmorphic features, growth restriction, hydrops, it is of great value.
- Most viable tissue for karyotyping is the placenta or segment of umbilical cord closest to the placenta

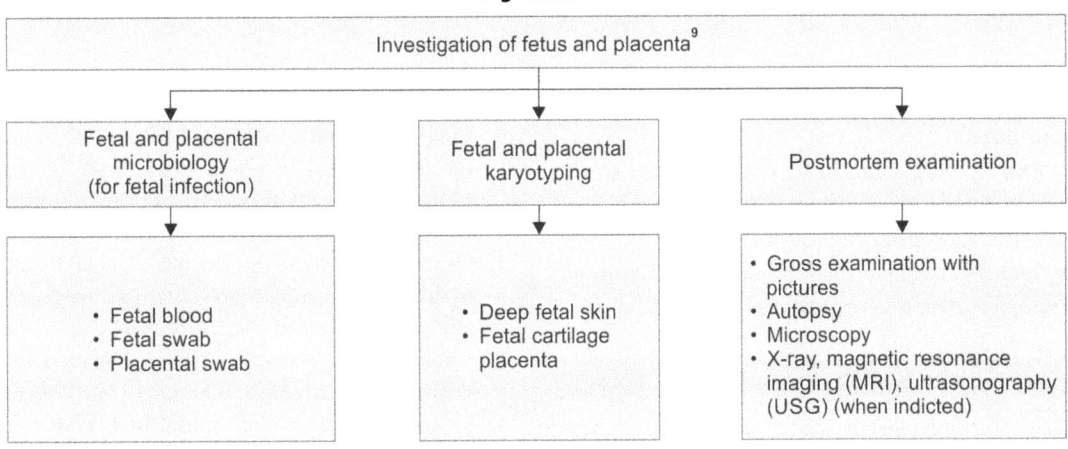

Algorithm 8

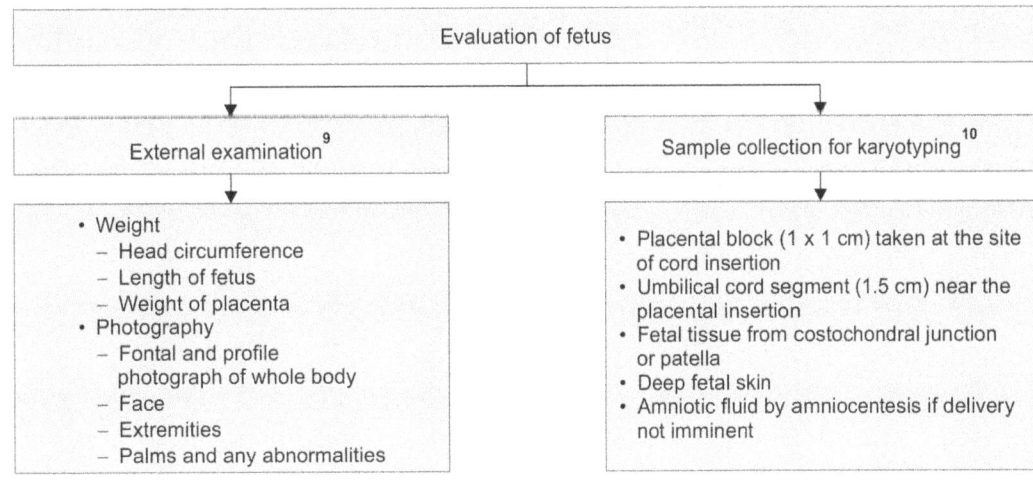

Algorithm 9

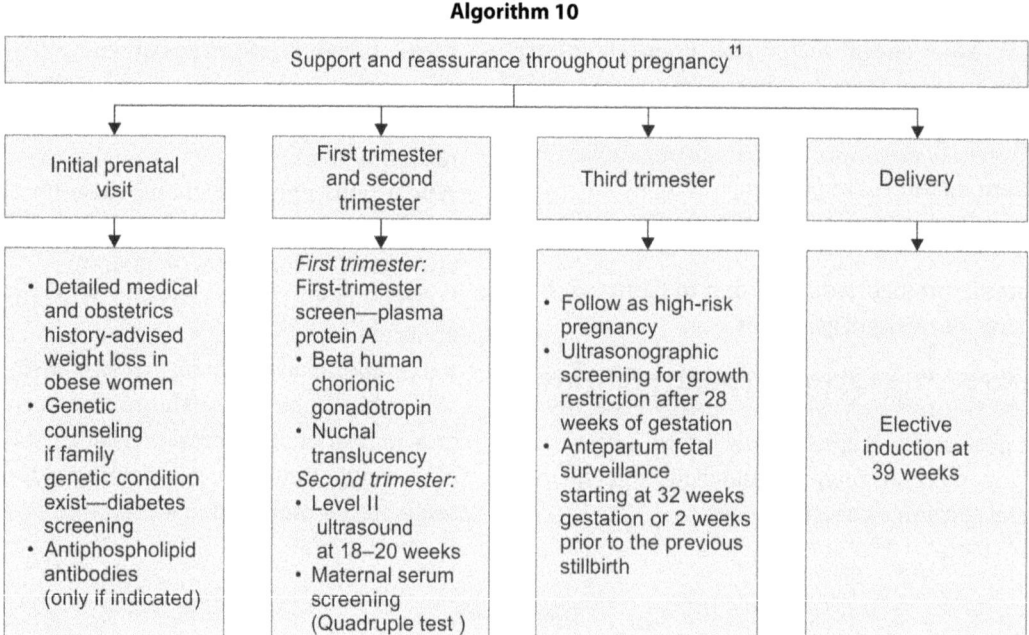

followed by fetal cartilage obtained from costochondral junction or patella.[9]
- Specimen for cytology should be collected in a sterile tissue culture medium of ringer lactate solution and keep it at room temperature.
- If family declines consent for fetal autopsy, histologic study of the placenta is acceptable alternative.

REFERENCES

1. Royal College of Obstetricians and Gynaecologists. (2010). Late intrauterine fetal death and stillbirth. [online] Available from: https://www.rcog.org.uk/globalassets/documents/guidelines/gtg_55.pdf [Last accessed September, 2019].
2. ACOG Practice Bulletin No. 102: management of stillbirth. Obstet Gynecol. 2009;113(3):748-61.
3. MacDorman MF, Munson ML, Kirmeyer S. Fetal and perinatal mortality, United States, 2004. Natl Vital Stat Rep. 2007;56:1-19.
4. Fretts R. Etiology and prevention of stillbirth. Am J Obstet Gynecol. 2005;193:1923-35.
5. Silver RM. Fetal death. Obstet Gynecol. 2007;109:153.
6. Copper RL, Goldenberg RL, DuBard MB, et al. Risk factors for fetal death in white, black, and Hispanic women. Collaborative Group on Preterm Birth Prevention. Obstet Gynecol. 1994;84:490-5.
7. Osman NB, Folgosa E, Gonzales C, et al. Genital infections in the aetiology of late fetal death: an incident case referent study. J Trop Pediatr. 1995;41:258-66.
8. Dickinson JE, Evans SF. The optimization of intravaginal misoprostol dosing schedules in second-trimester pregnancy termination [published erratum appears in Am J Obstet Gynecol 2005;193:597]. Am J Obstet Gynecol. 2002;186:470-4.
9. Reed GB, Claireaux AE, Cockburn F (Eds). Diseases of the Fetus and Newborn: Pathology, Imaging, Genetics and Management. London, UK: Chapman & Hall Medical; 1995.
10. Valdes-Depena M, Huff DS. Perinatal Autopsy Manual. Washington, DC: Armed Forces Institute of Pathology; 1983.
11. Reddy UM. Prediction and prevention of recurrent stillbirth. Obstet Gynecol. 2007;110:1151-64.

Chapter 27

Prolonged Pregnancy

Suman Thakur

INTRODUCTION

Prolonged pregnancy is a cause of concern among pregnant women as well as obstetrician because of a small but significant increased risk in perinatal mortality and morbidity.

DEFINITION

- *Post-term pregnancy*: Gestation that has completed or gone beyond 42 weeks or 294 days from first day of last menstrual period (LMP) (ACOG, WHO).[1]
- Postmature, postdate, prolonged, and post-term have been used leading to confusion regarding proper definition.
- The term "Term" should be replaced with designations like:
  - Early term (37-0/7 till 38-6/7 gestation)
  - Full term (39-0/7 till 40-6/7 gestation)
  - Late term (41-6/7 till 42-0/7 gestation)
- Factors like race and ethnicity affect duration of pregnancy. Asians and African American have short duration.[2]

INCIDENCE

About 2–13%.

ETIOLOGY

- Unknown
- Error in dating
- Estimated date of delivery (EDD) based on LMP: Unreliable
- Dysregulation of hypothalamic-pituitary-adrenal (HPA) axis may play a role
- Placental sulfatase deficiency (X-linked recessive disorder), absence of enzyme steroid sulfatase
- Risk factors:
  - Primigravida
  - Previous prolonged pregnancy
  - Male fetus
  - Obesity
  - Genetic predisposition.

DIAGNOSIS

- Accurate gestational dating.
- *Based on*: LMP, timing of intercourse, and first-trimester ultrasound.
- *EDD only based on LMP is inaccurate*: Ovulation may vary among individuals and individual menstrual cycle.
- Ultrasound in first trimester is superior to use LMP alone.

PERINATAL MORBIDITY AND MORTALITY

- Risk of perinatal mortality increases as gestational age advances beyond EDD.
- Increased frequency of neonatal convulsions, meconium aspiration syndrome, APGAR <4 at 5 minutes (Clausson and colleague evaluated a large Swedish database).
- Intrauterine death (IUD)-rate increases beyond 41 weeks.

COMPLICATIONS

- Mortality, abnormal antepartum, and intrapartum fetal heart rate (FHR) abnormalities.
- *Fetal growth*: Macrosomia (twofold increased risk).
- *Postmaturity*: About 10–20%, decreased subcutaneous fat, lack lanugo, and vernix.
- *Meconium-stained fluid*: Meconium aspiration, a serious condition that causes chemical pneumonitis, decreased lung compliance, and abnormal production of surfactant.

MATERNAL COMPLICATIONS

- Anxiety
- Perineal laceration
- Chorioamnionitis
- Endomyometritis
- Postpartum hemorrhage
- Cesarean section.

MANAGEMENT[3,4]

- Accurate assessment of gestational age.
- Antenatal surveillance:
  - Nonstress test (NST)-modified biophysical profile (BPP), BPP initiated at 41 weeks of gestation (no modality is superior to another).
  - Amniotic fluid volume assessment is important as oligohydramnios is associated with cord compression, abnormal fetal heart tracing, and meconium-stained fluid (ACOG).
  - Umbilical artery Doppler measurement: Not useful.

EXPECTANT MANAGEMENT OR INDUCTION OF LABOR

- The gestational age at which expectant management is no longer recommended is not defined.
- Delivery by 42 completed weeks is indicated because of small but increased risk of perinatal mortality and morbidity.
- Gestational age that requires clinical concern—41 weeks.
- PGE1 or PGE2 can be used for induction.

MULTIPLE GESTATIONS

No defined gestational age cutoff to define prolonged pregnancy in twins, triplets or higher-order multiples.

Indians have a tendency toward constitutionally small baby and a tendency toward early maturity, study in south Indian women on duration of pregnancy has shown higher rate of meconium aspiration beyond 40 weeks and two and half times more beyond 41 weeks, thus in our set of population, induction should be done at 40 weeks of gestation. Conservative management beyond 40 weeks will not be cost-effective because of increase in the number of patients admitted for monitoring and increased cesarean section rate for meconium-stained liquor.[5]

REFERENCES

1. Definition of term pregnancy. ACOG Committee opinion no. 579 November 2013, Reaffirmed 2019.
2. Drysdale H, Ranasinha S, Kendall A, et al. Ethnicity and the risk of late pregnancy stillbirth. Med J Aust. 2012;197(5):278-81.
3. Antenatal care, Routine care for the healthy Pregnant Women. NICE (2008 updated 2017).
4. Management of late term and post term pregnancies. ACOG Practice Bulletin No. 146. August 2014, Reaffirmed 2016. American College of Obstetricians and Gynaecologists.
5. Davies-Tuck ML, Davey MA, Wallace EM. Maternal region of birth and stillbirth in Victoria Australia 2000-2011: A Retrospective cohort study of Victorian perinatal data. PLoS One. 2007;12(6):e0178727.

Chapter 28

Pregnancy after Lower Segment Cesarean Section

S Sampathkumari

INTRODUCTION

Pregnancy after cesarean section (CS) incidence is now increased because of the increased incidence of primary section due to lifestyle changes and overdiagnosis.

Pregnancy after lower segment cesarean section (LSCS) is a high-risk pregnancy. For such patients, obtain information regarding labor pain duration of previous pregnancy, transportation duration, drugs for induction and duration, previous cesarean indication, scar type, and postoperative complication. Effects of previous pregnancy are mentioned as per **Algorithm 1**. Early detection of medical problems and routine investigations are to be done. Two doses of Inj. tetanus toxoid (TT), iron, and folic acid to be given.

Planning for a vaginal birth after cesarean (VBAC) or choosing an elective repeat cesarean section (ERCS) have different benefits and risks. It depends on the history, indication, type of incision, and complications.

Algorithm 1: Effects of previous pregnancy.

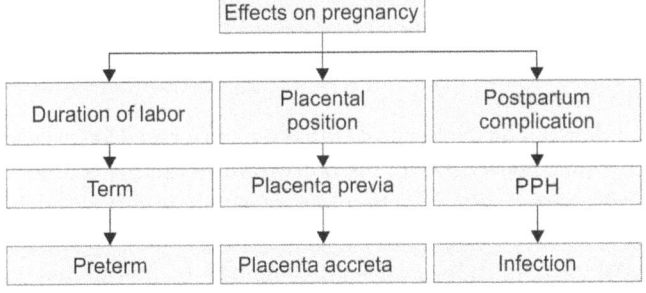

(PPH: postpartum hemorrhage)

The cesarean, if done for recurrent or nonrecurrent indication, is essential as mentioned in **Algorithm 2**.

Recurrent indication cases are always taken up for ERCS. ERCS is done at completion of 39 weeks. Antibiotics should be given at theater before surgery. If surgery is done before 39 weeks, neonatal respiratory complication is increased. To avoid this complication, antenatal corticosteroids are given. Inj. Dexamethasone 8 mg (four doses)—6 hourly.[1] If done for nonrecurrent indication, the type of cesarean, classical or lower segment, plays a role in decision in this pregnancy.

ACOG RECOMMENDATIONS FOR ERCS

- All elective cesareans to be planned at 39 completed weeks.
- Recommends one course of antenatal corticosteroids for all cesarean done till 38 weeks + 6 days.

ACOG CRITERIA FOR LUNG MATURITY

- Fetal heart sound documented for 20 weeks by nonelectronic fetoscope or 30 weeks by Doppler.
- 36 weeks since positive serum human chorionic gonadotropin (hCG) test.
- Sonographic measurement between 6 weeks and 11 weeks.

Risk again depends on the type of scar and is comparatively higher with classical rather than lower segment as mentioned in **Table 1**.

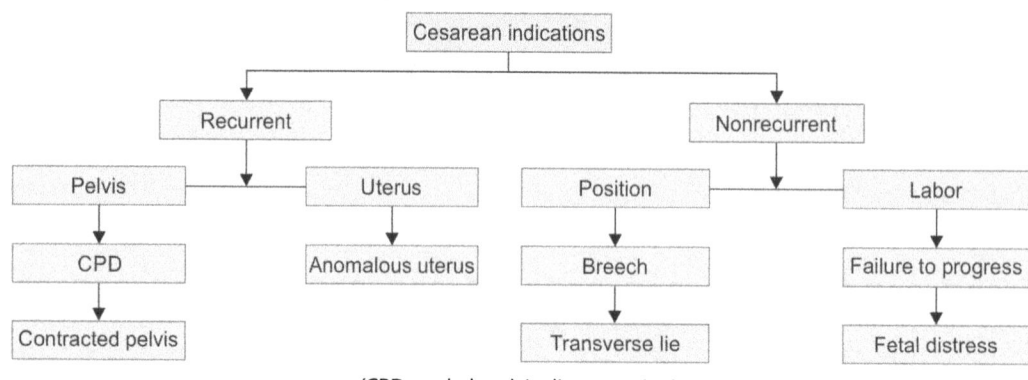

Algorithm 2: Cesarean indications.

(CPD: cephalopelvic disproportion)

Table 1: Risks associated.

	Classical	Lower segment
Apposition	Difficult	Perfect
Uterus during healing	Contracting and retracting	Inert
Stretching	At right angles	Along line of scar
Placenta	Scar implantation more common	Scar implantation less common
Rupture	4–9%	0.2–1.5%
Mortality	More	Less

Beyond the site of scar, the immediate postoperative period has a role in the health of scar. Infection and defective wound healing due to anemic or vitamin deficiency can result in weak scar.

Scar dehiscence is earlier stage of scar rupture. Identification of both and baby complications are as mentioned in **Table 2**. Successful VBAC occurs in 72–80% with risk of rupture depending on type of the previous incision. The background risk for rupture during VBAC is 1%.[2]

Table 2: Complications.

	Dehiscence	Rupture
Feature	Separation along scar, serosa intact	Unscarred tissue also involved, serosa ruptured
Fetus	Tachycardia, distress	Mortality

Scar dehiscence can be identified by ultrasonography (USG). Sonogram-transvaginal ultrasound (TVS) is better than transabdominal ultrasound (TAS) for assessment for scar integrity. Measurement of lower uterine segment (LUS) thickness or myometrial thickness will help to decide the mode of delivery in this pregnancy.

Safe threshold of:
- LUS thickness   2.0–3.5 mm
- Myometrial thickness 1.4–2 mm

If LUS thickness <2 mm and myometrial thickness <1.4 mm, risk of rupture increased by fivefold. Prior scar rupture increases the rate to 9–32%.[3]

Lower segment cesarean section audit should be conducted in all hospitals. Indications should be analyzed as per Robson's classification as in **Algorithm 3**.

Indication comes under which category should be analyzed and corrected to reduce the CS rate.

Cesarean causes prolonged hospital stay, immobilization, increased blood loss, possibility of hysterectomy in conditions of adherent placenta, neonatal intensive care unit (NICU) admission, and bladder injuries. Success of VBAC increases with previous normal vaginal deliveries.[4]

Patient of previous LSCS with cephalic presentation, single scar in uterus—only should be allowed for VBAC. Hospital set-up should have theater staff, blood component, pediatrician, obstetrician, cardiotocographic (CTG) monitoring, and intensive care facility available all 24 hours. Patient and attender should be informed about the risks as possibility of emergency LSCS, exploration of uterus if bleeding present, rupture uterus, and peripartum hysterectomy.

Vaginal birth after cesarean is not performed in cases of previous classical scar, previous rupture uterus, obstetric indications such as complete placenta previa, breech, and transverse lie. Success of VBAC depends on previous type of scar, indication, and prognosis as mentioned in **Algorithm 4**.

Algorithm 3: Robson's classification.

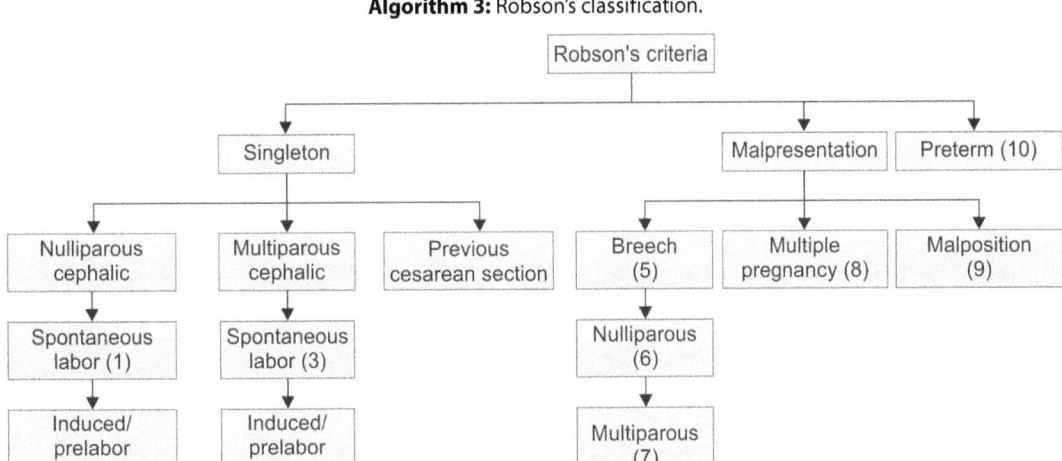

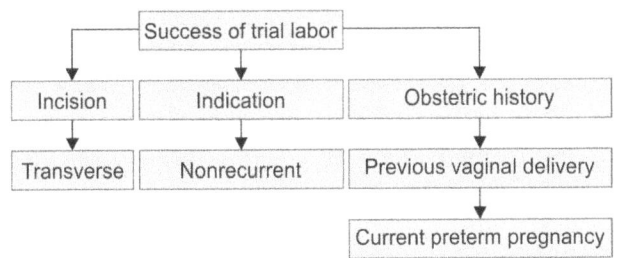

Algorithm 4: Success of trial labor.

Induction of labor is not contraindicated but with low success rate. Oxytocin is used with caution. Misoprostol contraindicated and dinoprostone is not recommended.[5]

LABOR MANAGEMENT IN PREVIOUS LSCS

Written and informed consent about the risks and benefits of VBAC should be obtained.
- *First stage:* Keep the patient in nil oral, secure IV line, anesthetist and neonatologist to be kept informed. Continuous FH/CTG monitoring, partogram, judicious use of oxytocin for augmentation, watch for signs and symptoms of scar dehiscence and impending rupture.
  - *Signs:* Nonreassuring fetal heart rate (FHR) pattern, scar tenderness, unexplained tachycardia, hypotension, and shortness of breath.
  - *Symptoms:* Suprapubic pain, slight vaginal bleeding, loss of station of presenting part, uterine contour changed, bladder tenesmus, and frank hematuria.

- *Second stage:* This stage should not be prolonged, bladder emptied, liberal episiotomy given, outlet forceps or vacuum applied in appropriate cases with caution.
- *Third stage:* Do not explore uterine scar unless there is heavy bleeding. Follow active management of the third stage of labor (AMSTL).[6]

Benefits of VBAC over repeat cesarean section are short hospital stay, early ambulation and resumption to work, less chance of bleeding and infection, reduced scar, and surgery-related complications.[7] 90% ruptures occur during labor. Signs and symptoms of rupture uterus are:
- Severe abdominal pain, especially if persisting between contractions
- Acute onset scar tenderness and cessation of previously efficient uterine activity
- Abnormal vaginal bleeding
- Hematuria
- Maternal tachycardia
- Hypotension, fainting, or shock
- Loss of station of the presenting part
- Change in abdominal contour and inability to pick up FHR
- Postnatally patient should be followed with contraceptive methods such as postpartum intrauterine contraceptive device (PPIUCD)/oral contraceptive (OC) pills/sterilization depending on mother and baby condition.

To summarize, when patient presents with previous cesarean section:[8]
- Confirm correct gestational age
- Confirm fetal well-being, fetal weight, amniotic fluid index (AFI)
- Rule out risks associated with surgery and anesthesia
- Counsel patient regarding risks and benefits of trial of labor after cesarean (TOLAC) and ERCS
- Patient denies VBAC, history of previous classical cesarean—repeat CS beyond 37 weeks
- Patient denies VABC, history of previous LSCS–ERCS at 39 weeks
- Patient willing for VBAC, informed consent regarding risks of rupture, await spontaneous onset or induction if required, continuous fetal monitoring, with facilities for emergency LSCS as and when required.

CONCLUSION

Pregnancy after LSCS should be carefully examined with previous history, type and indication of surgery, and decided for VBAC or ERCS. Patient should be counseled about merits and demerits of both modes of delivery and also about emergency surgery if any complication presents during the process of VBAC. Reducing the incidence of primary LSCS is the only way to reduce LSCS incidence.

REFERENCES

1. Royal College of Obstetricians and Gynaecologists. Green Top Guideline 45: Birth after Previous Cesarean. London: Royal College of Obstetricians and Gynaecologists; 2015.
2. Crosby DA, Ramphaul M, Murphy DJ. Antenatal discussion of risks and benefits of ERCS and VBAC. BJOG. 2014;121(11):1440-1.
3. Queenan JT, Spong CY, Lockwood CJ. Protocols for High-Risk Pregnancies: An Evidence-Based Approach, 6th edition. New Jersey, USA: Wiley Blackwell; 2015.
4. Cunningham FG, Leveno KJ. Williams Obstetrics. New York, USA: McGraw-Hill Education; 2014.
5. Arias F, Bhide A, Kaizad AS, Daftary DS (Eds). Arias Practical Guide to High-Risk Pregnancy and Delivery: A South Asian Perspective, 4th edition. Netherlands: Elsevier; 2015.
6. Norwitz ER, Saade GR, Miller H, Davidson CM (Eds). Obstetric Clinical Algorithms, 2nd edition. New Jersey, USA: Wiley Blackwell; 2016.
7. Royal College of Obstetricians and Gynaecologists. NICE Clinical Guideline 132: Cesarean Section London: Royal College of Obstetricians and Gynaecologists; 2011.
8. American College of Obstetricians and Gynecologists. ACOG recommendations on deciding trial of labour after cesarean. Washington, USA: American College of Obstetricians and Gynecologists.

Chapter 29

Pregnancy after Infertility and Assisted Reproductive Technology

Shalini Gainder, Japleen Kaur

INTRODUCTION

Infertility is of significant personal as well as social concern in our society. Educational, employment, and career prospects contribute to stress and delayed parenthood and consequently age-related decline in fertility.[1] On one hand, the advent of assisted reproductive technology (ART) has been a solution for various causes of infertility, on the other hand, it has also given rise to certain specific concerns. A major problem faced by obstetricians and gynecologists worldwide is the unique challenge of management of pregnancy after infertility and ART.

According to CDC, ART includes all fertility treatments which involve handling of oocytes and embryos.

Box 1 and Table 1 summarize the patient risk factors and anticipated obstetric and perinatal complications in patients conceiving with ART, respectively.

Preconceptional counseling has been outlined in **Algorithm 1.**

Table 1: In vitro fertilization/intracytoplasmic sperm injection (IVF/ICSI) pregnancies are at higher risk of following obstetric and perinatal complications when compared with spontaneous conceptions.[2]

Obstetric complications	Perinatal complications
Hypertensive disorders of pregnancy	Multiple pregnancy
Gestational diabetes	Miscarriage/preterm delivery
Antepartum hemorrhage	Low birth weight
Prelabor rupture of membranes	Small for gestational age
Induction of labor	Congenital anomalies
Cesarean section	Perinatal mortality

MANAGEMENT OF PREGNANCIES CONCEIVED AFTER ART

Although there is a lack of specific guidelines, most experts believe that ART pregnancies are different and should be managed as high-risk pregnancies by experienced obstetricians. Management of ART pregnancy in first trimester has been outlined in **Algorithm 2**.

Special Conditions

- *Role of thromboprophylaxis:* IVF has been shown to double the risk of venous thromboembolism when compared to spontaneous conception. Therefore, RCOG recommends that women with IVF pregnancy and three other risk factors (detailed in **Box 2**), should

Box 1	Associated problems with infertility and assisted reproductive technology (ART).

Patient risk factors
- Older age
- Obesity
- Polycystic ovarian syndrome (PCOS)
- Fibroids
- Uterine anomalies
- Medical comorbidities (hypertension, diabetes)

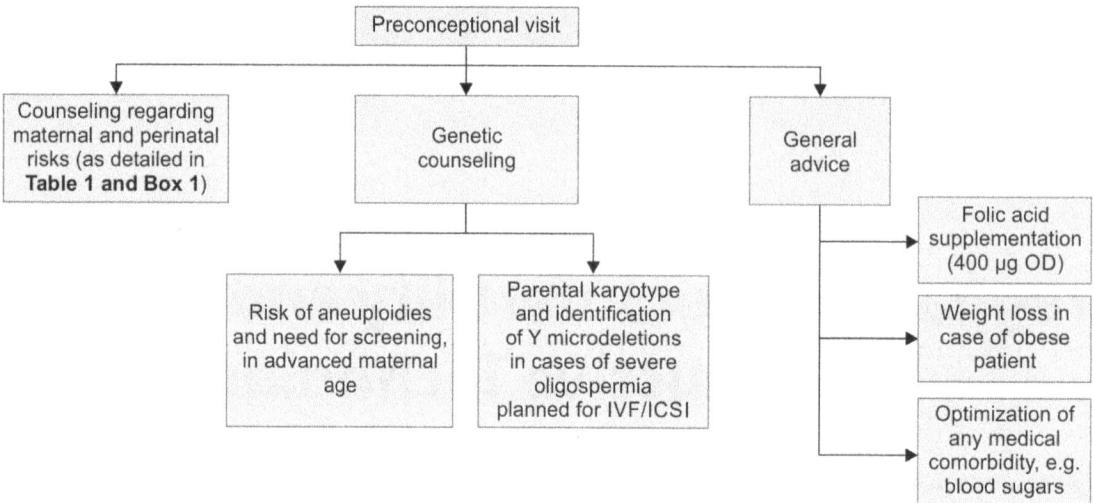

Algorithm 1: Preconceptional counseling.[3]

(ICSI: intracytoplasmic sperm injection; IVF: in vitro fertilization)

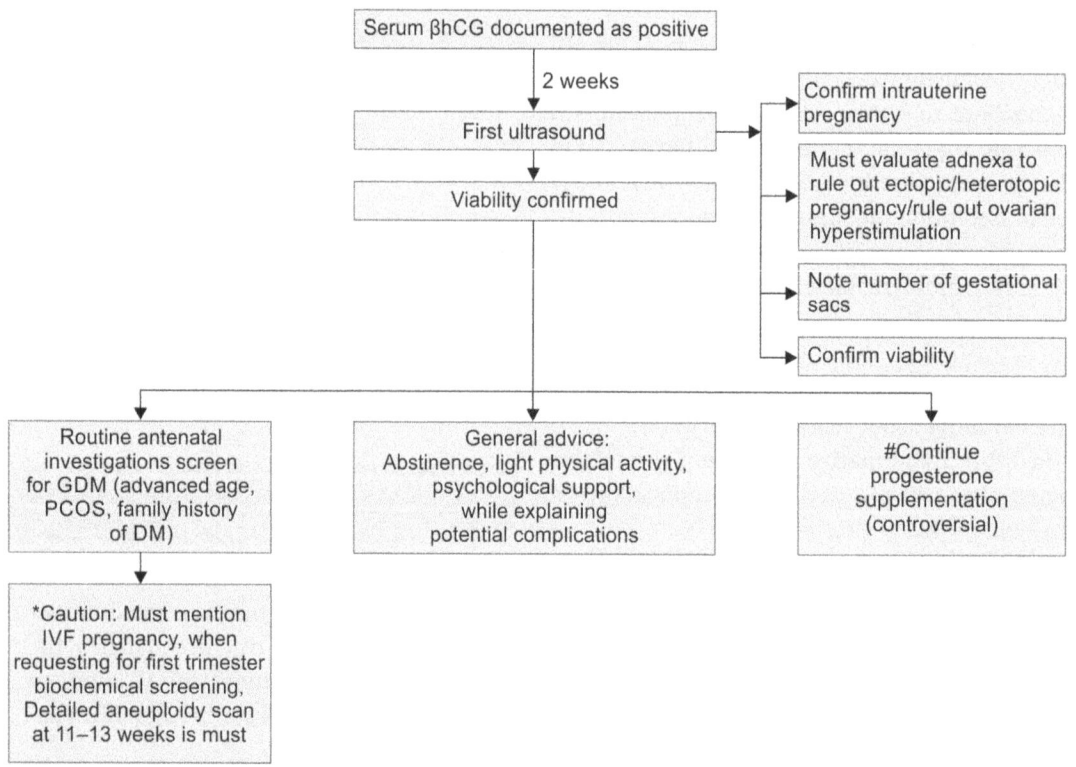

Algorithm 2: Outline of management of ART pregnancy in first trimester.

* First-trimester biochemical screen which includes serum pregnancy-associated plasma protein-A (PAPP-A) and serum β-human chorionic gonadotropin (β-hCG), has higher false-positive rates in the ART pregnancies compared from age-matched controls. Serum PAPP-A multiples of median value has been shown to be decreased in case of fresh cycles of in vitro fertilization/intracytoplasmic sperm injection (IVF/ICSI) pregnancies when compared with spontaneous conceptions, whereas no difference has been documented with frozen embryo transfers.[4]

Duration of progesterone supplementation in ART pregnancies has been an issue of debate. Even though the benefit of progesterone supplementation beyond the positive βhCG result has not been proven, majority IVF experts continue it till 12 weeks (when the uteroplacental switch has been established), or at least till documentation of fetal cardiac activity (approximately 6–8 weeks).[5]

(β-hCG: beta-human chorionic gonadotropin; GDM: gestational diabetes mellitus; IVF: in vitro fertilization; PCOS: polycystic ovarian syndrome)

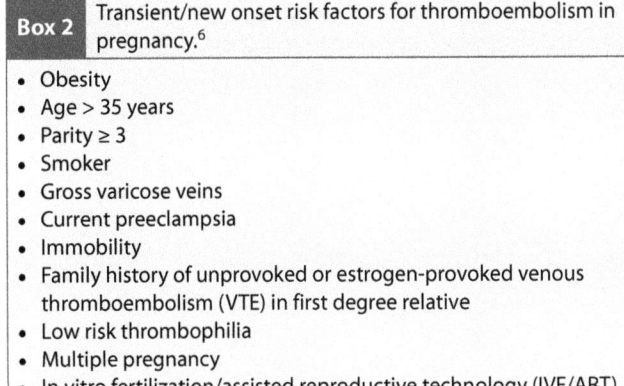

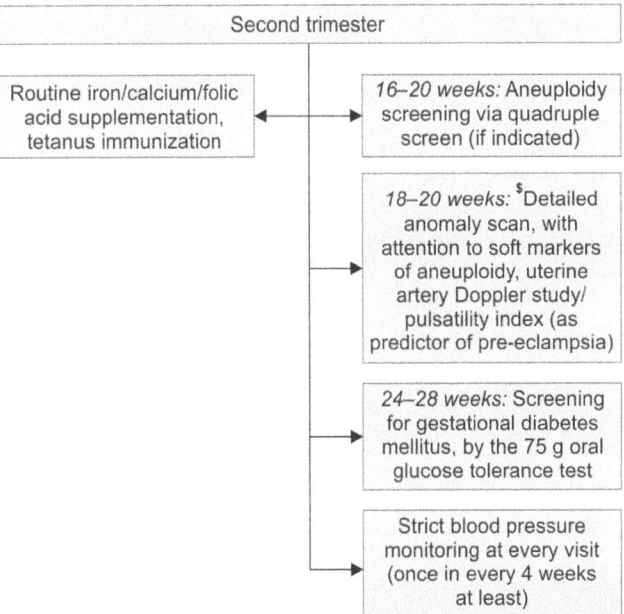

Algorithm 3: Outline of management in second trimester.

be given due consideration for thromboprophylaxis with low molecular weight heparin, commencing from the first trimester (Grade C recommendation).[6] In case of severe or critical ovarian hyperstimulation syndrome, a complication quite unique to IVF/ART, it is recommended to give thromboprophylaxis in first trimester.

- *Selective fetal reduction:* The incidence of multiple pregnancy is higher in IVF/ART. Multiple pregnancy is also one of the most significant factors for adverse maternal and perinatal outcomes after IVF/ART. Therefore, nondirective patient counseling explaining the pros and cons of the procedure should be offered to women with higher multifetal gestation.[7]
- *Metformin in women with PCOS:* Recent meta-analysis has concluded that continuation of metformin in pregnancy, in women with PCOS has beneficial effects like decrease in early pregnancy losses, preterm delivery, and decreased incidence of gestational diabetes and pregnancy-induced hypertension.[8]

Management of ART pregnancy in second trimester has been outlined in **Algorithm 3**.

Management of Third Trimester

A higher incidence of pre-eclampsia, gestational diabetes, antepartum hemorrhage, fetal growth restriction, prematurity, and preterm labor has been attributed to ART pregnancies.[2] Therefore, these pregnancies are to be treated like high-risk pregnancies and increased surveillance is warranted compared from spontaneous conceptions **(Algorithm 4)**.

$ *Assisted reproductive technology pregnancies and congenital anomalies:* Large cohort studies have concluded that IVF/ICSI pregnancies have a higher relative risk of major congenital malformations (almost twice as spontaneous conceptions). Some factors responsible may be higher incidence of advanced maternal age, damaged spermatozoa (severe oligo/azoospermia), underlying diabetes mellitus and multiple gestations, rather than the ART procedure itself. An association has been found between ART and imprinting syndromes like Beckwith Wiedemann syndrome, Angelman syndrome, and maternal hypomethylation syndrome. Hypospadias, cleft lip palate, esophageal/anal atresia, and septal heart defects have been associated with ART, in isolation or as part of VACTERL (Vertebral defects, Anal atresia, Cardiac defects, Tracheo-Esophageal fistula, Renal malformations and Limb defects) association.[9]

Labor and Delivery

Planned elective cesarean delivery can be considered based on above factors. If patient undergoes labor (spontaneous or induced), intrapartum electronic fetal monitoring should be offered.

Specific Postpartum Management

Contraceptive advice must be given to patients, taking into consideration the indication for ART. Contraception is unwarranted in cases like blocked/removed fallopian tubes or if there is irreversible azoospermia.

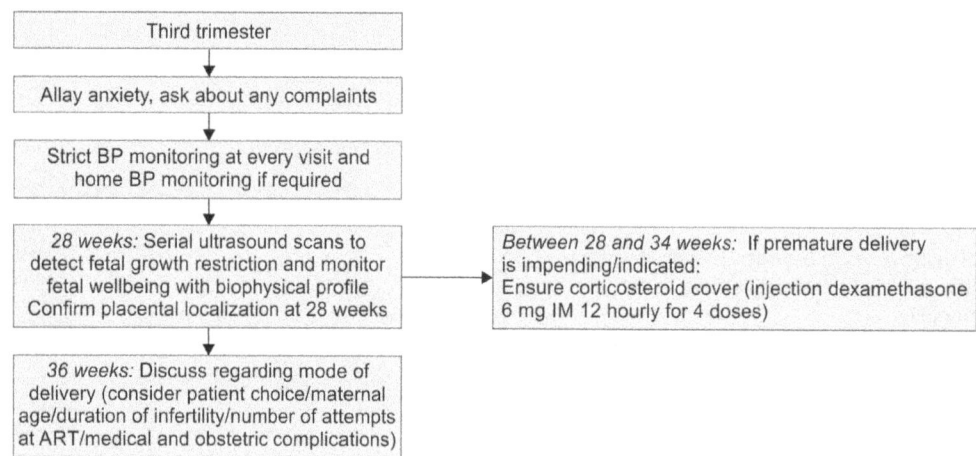

Algorithm 4: Salient points in management of third trimester.

(ART: assisted reproductive technology; BP: blood pressure; IM: intramuscular)

PREGNANCY OUTCOMES FOLLOWING SPECIFIC ART PROCEDURES

- Use of donor oocytes has been associated with increased risk of low birth weight and preterm birth.[10]
- *Blastocyst culture:* Potential negative effects like higher risk of monozygotic twinning, preterm birth, and congenital malformations have been reported in few human studies, while certain animal studies have been associated with imprinting disorders and behavioral abnormalities.[11,12]

PROPOSED STRATEGIES FOR REDUCTION OF COMPLICATIONS

- Incidence of multiple gestations can be reduced with use of softer stimulation protocols, selective single embryo transfer (balance with reduction in pregnancy rates), and elective embryo reduction.
- Screening for pre-eclampsia and fetal growth restriction, with early pregnancy biochemical markers like PAPP-A and uterine artery Doppler studies and use of low-dose aspirin for prevention of the same.
- Cervical length monitoring and prophylactic cerclage. No definite consensus on the routine cervical length monitoring in IVF pregnancies, without any other risk factors of preterm delivery. Some authors have challenged the role of cervical length monitoring and prophylactic cerclage in IVF pregnancies, especially multiple gestations.[13] But there have been case reports of successful pregnancy outcomes after rescue cerclage in IVF pregnancies.[14] Therefore, the decision for cerclage should be individualized after assessing the risk–benefit ratio and include counseling regarding the possible side effects of infection, vaginal bleeding, and preterm rupture of membranes.

CONCLUSION

Assisted reproductive technology pregnancies need expert care and special attention throughout antenatal period as they are associated with increased risk of adverse maternal and fetal outcomes. Whether this increased risk is attributable to ART itself or to the underlying high-risk factors like advanced age, medical comorbidities, or subfertility, is not established. Continued research is warranted to find novel methods of reducing these complications.

REFERENCES

1. Mills M, Rindfuss RR, McDonald P, et al. Why do people postpone parenthood? Reasons and social policy incentives. Hum Reprod Update. 2011;17:848-60.
2. Pandey S, Shetty A, Hamilton M, et al. Obstetric and perinatal outcomes in singleton pregnancies resulting from IVF/ICSI: a systematic review and meta-analysis. Hum Reprod Update. 2012;18:485-503.
3. Nekuei N, Esfahani MH, Kazemi A. Preconception counseling in couples undergoing fertility treatment. Int J Fertil Steril. 2012;6:79.

4. Ashiru DA, Lee R, Benton J, et al. Published online in Wiley InterScience. [online] Available from: www.interscience.wiley.com [Last accessed September, 2019].
5. Liu XR, Mu HQ, Shi Q, et al. The optimal duration of progesterone supplementation in pregnant women after IVF/ICSI: a meta-analysis. Reprod Biol Endocrinol. 2012;10:107.
6. Royal College of Obstetricians and Gynaecologists. RCOG Greentop Guideline 37a Reducing the Risk of Venous Thromboembolism during Pregnancy and the Puerperium. London, UK: Royal College of Obstetricians and Gynaecologists; 2015.
7. American College of Obstetricians and Gynecologists. Committee Opinion No. 719. Multifetal pregnancy reduction. Obstet Gynecol. 2017;130:e158-63.
8. Zeng XL, Zhang YF, Tian Q, et al. Effects of metformin on pregnancy outcomes in women with polycystic ovary syndrome: a meta-analysis. Medicine. 2016;95(36):e4526.
9. Reefhuis J, Honein MA, Schieve LA, et al. Assisted reproductive technology and major structural birth defects in the United States. Hum Reprod. 2009;24:360-6.
10. Nakashima A, Araki R, Tani H, et al. Implications of assisted reproductive technologies on term singleton birth weight: an analysis of 25,777 children in the national assisted reproduction registry of Japan. Fertil Steril. 2013;99:450-5.
11. Fernández-Gonzalez R, Moreira P, Bilbao A, et al. Long-term effect of in vitro culture of mouse embryos with serum on mRNA expression of imprinting genes, development, and behavior. Proc Natl Acad Sci USA. 2004;101:5880-5.
12. Källén B, Finnström O, Lindam A, et al. Blastocyst versus cleavage stage transfer in in vitro fertilization: differences in neonatal outcome? Fertil Steril. 2010;94:1680-3.
13. Jorgensen AL, Alfirevic Z, Tudur Smith C, et al. Cervical stitch (cerclage) for preventing pregnancy loss: individual patient data meta-analysis. BJOG. 2007;114:1460-76.
14. Kumbak B, Attar R, Yıldırım G, et al. Rescue cerclage in IVF pregnancies with second trimester cervical dilatation: case report and literature review. J Turk Ger Gynecol Assoc. 2009;10:244.

Section 3

Labor

- **Decision and Induction of Labor**
  Dilpreet Kaur Pandher, Shikha Rani

- **Augmentation and Management of Labor**
  Leena Wadhwa, Sanjita

- **Fetal Surveillance during Labor**
  Monika Gupta, Namrata Verma

- **Pain Relief in Labor**
  Kartik Syal, Geetika Syal

- **Meconium**
  Anshuja Singla, Charu Yadav

- **Placental Adhesive Disorders**
  Taruna Sharma, Bindiya Gupta

Chapter 30

Decision and Induction of Labor

Dilpreet Kaur Pandher, Shikha Rani

INTRODUCTION

Spontaneous onset of labor is an anticipated natural process in every pregnant female, still, data shows that around 25% of them are undergoing through artificial induction of labor (IOL) in the developed countries as well as many developing countries either due to non-initiation of spontaneous labor or due to medical reasons.[1]

Induction of labor is the process of initiating labor by artificial means. Augmentation of labor is the process of enhancing labor, which has begun spontaneously. Labor induction should be done only if there are clear cut indications to terminate the pregnancy and certainly after ruling out any contraindication to the vaginal birth.

Clinical assessment prior to induction of labor:

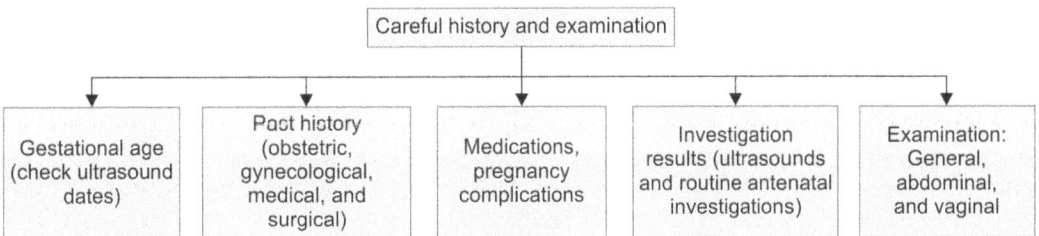

For elective induction, confirmation of fetal maturity and evaluation of cervical status by modified Bishop scoring is mandatory. World Health Organization (WHO) recommends IOL at 41 weeks period of gestation with certainty.

CONFIRMATION OF FETAL MATURITY

The recommendations regarding the method for estimating gestational age and due date are as follows:[2]

- Ultrasound measurement of the embryo/fetus in the first trimester (up to 14 weeks of gestation) is the most accurate method to establish or confirm gestational age.
- According to the date of embryo transfer in in-vitro fertilization (IVF) pregnancies.
- Dating with no ultrasound confirmation before 22 + 0/7 weeks of gestational age is regarded as suboptimal.

Modified Bishop Score (Calder Score)[3]

Cervical findings	Scoring			
	0	1	2	3
Dilatation (cm)	<1	1–2	2–4	>4
Length of cervix (cm)	>4	2–4	1–2	<1
Station (cm relative to ischial spines)	−3	−2	−1 to 0	+1 to +2
Consistency	Firm	Average	Soft	–
Position	Posterior	Mid	Anterior	–

Modifiers of the Bishop Score[4]

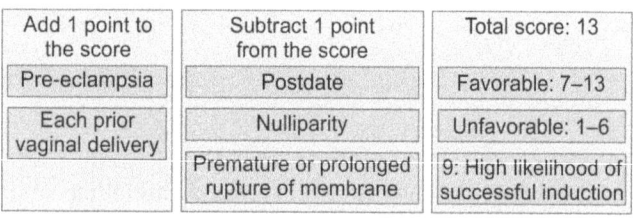

For medically indicated labor induction, risks of continuation of pregnancy to the mother and/or the fetus must outweigh the benefits of the continuation of pregnancy and the risks of initiating labor and the subsequent vaginal birth. Woman must be informed about the reason for IOL, mode of IOL, risk/benefit of the procedure, further plan in case of unsuccessful attempt, and must be given adequate time to make her decision. Informed written consent must be obtained which should be signed by the treating obstetrician.

MEDICAL INDICATIONS OF INDUCTION OF LABOR

Common medical indications of induction of labor are as follows:

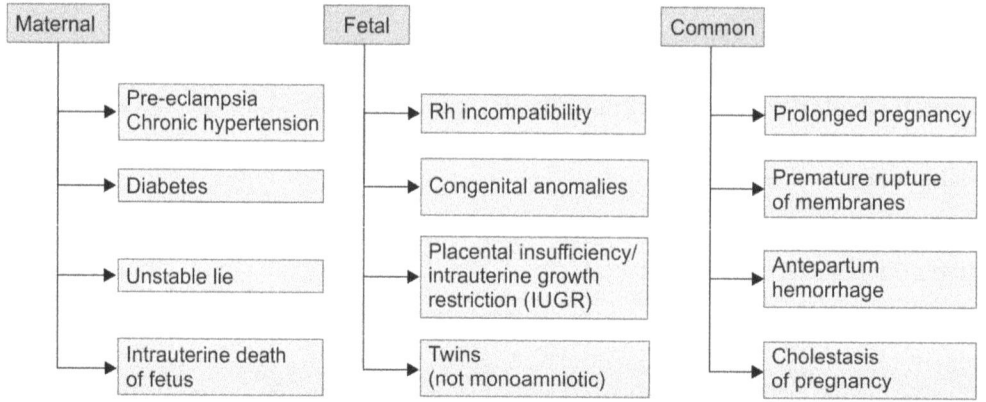

TIMING OF INDUCTION[1,5-9]

Indication	Timing of induction	
	Queensland	American College of Obstetricians and Gynecologists (ACOG)
Low-risk pregnancy	41–42 weeks	At 39 weeks or later
Previous stillbirth	To be individualized	
Premature rupture of membranes (PROM)	24–33 weeks: Conservative	Preterm: 34–35 weeks
	34 weeks or beyond: Individualize the case	Term: At the time of diagnosis
Oligohydramnios		36–38 weeks
Polyhydramnios		39–40 weeks
Growth restriction	Umbilical artery, middle cerebral, and ductus venosus Doppler, severity of affection decides timing and mode of birth	Normal Doppler: 38–40 weeks
		Raised UA S/D: 37–38 weeks
		AE/REDF UA: 32–35 weeks

Contd...

Contd...

Indication	Timing of induction	
	Queensland	American College of Obstetricians and Gynecologists (ACOG)
Fetal macrosomia	Induction of labor (IOL) after 38 weeks if estimated fetal weight (EFW)>: o 3,500 g at 36 weeks o 3,700 g at 37 weeks o 3,900 g at 38 weeks	
Uncomplicated twin pregnancy	Monochorionic or dichorionic: After 37 weeks	Dichorionic diamniotic (DCDA): 38–39 weeks
		Monochorionic diamniotic (MCDA): 34–38 weeks
Intrahepatic cholestasis of pregnancy	37–38 weeks	
Hypertensive disorders of pregnancy	No maternal risk: Beyond 37 weeks	Chronic HT controlled on medications: 37–40 weeks
	Moderate maternal risk: 34–37 weeks	Gestational hypertension (HT)/pre-eclampsia: 37–38 weeks
	Hemolysis, Elevated Liver enzymes, and Low Platelet count syndrome (HELLP): As soon as feasible	Gestational HT/preeclampsia with severe features: 34–35 weeks
		Eclampsia/pre-eclampsia with HELLP: soon after maternal stabilization
Diabetes	Well-controlled on medical nutrition therapy (MNT), no fetal macrosomia: wait for spontaneous labor	Overt: 36–39 weeks
	Suspected fetal macrosomia/other complication: 38–39 weeks	Gestational well controlled on diet and MNT: 39–41
	EFW 4,500 g or more: Consider cesarean delivery	Gestational; well controlled on medication: 39–40 weeks
		Gestational; poorly controlled: Individualized
Maternal request	Consider IOL at term based on exceptional circumstances of the woman and her family	
Advanced maternal age, 40 years or over	Offer IOL at 39–40 weeks	

CONTRAINDICATIONS FOR THE INDUCTION OF LABOR

Contraindications for the induction of labor are as follows:[10]

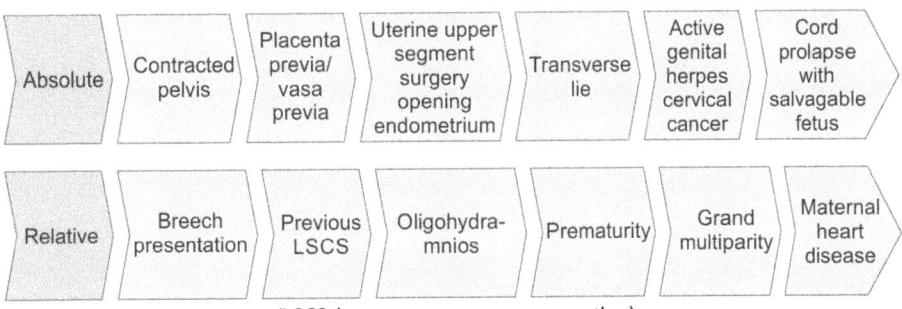

(LSCS: lower segment cesarean section)

COMPLICATIONS OF INDUCTION OF LABOR

Inducing labor predisposes mother to more physical and psychological stress as compared to the spontaneous labor and fetus to iatrogenic prematurity. Few of the common problems arising due to IOL are as enumerated below:

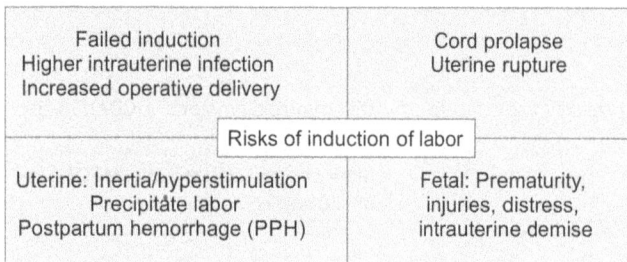

Uterine Hyperstimulation

- Uterine tachysystole or hypertonus [without fetal heart rate (FHR) abnormalities]
- Uterine hyperstimulation (with FHR abnormalities)[1,11,12]
- The incidence varies from 1% to 5%
- Contraction frequency more than five in 10 minutes (for at least 20 minutes) or contractions exceeding 2 minutes in duration.
- Hyperstimulation is more likely with prostaglandins in the presence of premature rupture of membranes (PROM).

Management[1,3,11]

- Remove dinoprostone gel or pessary if still in situ
- Stop oxytocin infusion
- Position left lateral with oxygen inhalation
- Check maternal vitals: Pulse rate (PR), blood pressure (BP)
- Start intravenous (IV) fluids via new administration set for hydration
- *Per abdomen and vaginal examination:* Assess for cervical dilation and exclude cord prolapse
- If persists, consider use of tocolytic:
  - Terbutaline: 250 µg subcutaneously or
  - Terbutaline: 250 µg in 5 mL dilution IV over 5 minutes
  - Salbutamol: 100 µg by slow IV injection
  - Sublingual glyceryl trinitrate (GTN) spray 400 µg
- Excessive uterine activity in the absence of evidence of fetal compromise is not in itself an indication for tocolysis
- If clinically indicated, prepare for instrumental birth or cesarean section (CS) (e.g. FHR does not return to normal).

METHODS OF INDUCTION

- Sweeping membranes are recommended for reducing formal IOL.[1]
- *Balloon catheter:*

Procedure	Indications	Contraindications	Cautions in
• Lithotomy position • 26G Foley's catheter • Balloon passed through cervical canal • Inflated with 30–80 mL sterile water or 0.9% sodium chloride, withdraw catheter • Proximal end tied to thigh for traction • If discomfort: Remove 10 mL of volume	• Modified Bishop Score (MBS) ≤6 • Previous cesarean section (CS) • Following dinoprostone, if no/minimal effect on cervical ripening and artificial rupture of membranes (ARM) not technically possible	• Ruptured membranes • Undiagnosed bleeding • Simultaneous use of prostaglandins • Low lying placenta • Polyhydramnios • Abnormal fetal heart rate (FHR)	• Antepartum bleeding • Lower tract genital infection • Fetal head not engaged (4/5 or 5/5 above pelvic brim)

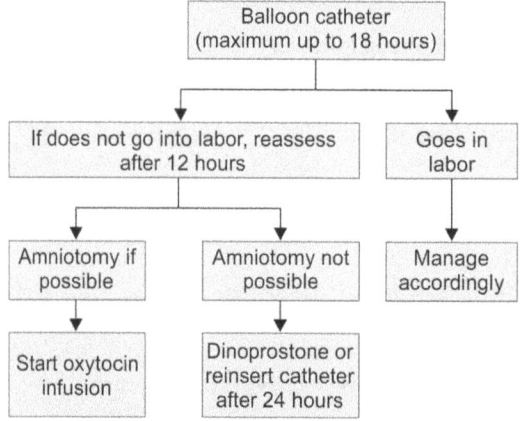

- *Prostaglandin E_1 (misoprostol):* WHO recommendations[1]

Dose and route	Contraindication
Oral misoprostol (25 μg, 2-hourly) Vaginal misoprostol (25 μg, 6-hourly)	Women with previous cesarean section

- *Prostaglandin E_2 (dinoprostone):*

Dose and route	Indications	Contraindications	Cautions
Dinoprostone gel - Nulliparous: 2 mg PV - Multiparous: 1 mg PV	Unfavorable cervix (MBS ≤ 6)	- Known hypersensitivity - Ruptured membranes	Multiple pregnancies
- Insert high into posterior fornix - Wait at least 6 hours after insertion then reassess modified Bishop score (MBS) - May repeat to maximum of three doses at least 6 hours apart **Dinoprostone pessary** - 10 mg PV - Position transversely in posterior fornix - Wait at least 12 hours after insertion then reassess MBS - If need to repeat, give one dose of dinoprostone GEL	Following balloon catheter, if no/minimal effect on cervical ripening and ARM not technically possible **Pessary removal** - Onset of regular, uterine contractions, every 3 minutes regardless of cervical change - Ruptured membranes - Fetal distress - Uterine hyperstimulation - Maternal systemic adverse effects (e.g. nausea, vomiting, hypotension, tachycardia)	- Multiparity ≥ 5 - Previous cesarean section (CS) or uterine surgery - Malpresentation/high presenting part - Undiagnosed PV bleeding - Abnormal cardiotocographic (CTG)/fetal compromise	- Asthma, chronic obstructive pulmonary disease: may cause bronchospasm - Epilepsy - Cardiovascular disease - Raised intraocular pressure, glaucoma - Avoid concurrent oxytocin use
On timed assessment, if artificial rupture of membranes (ARM) is possible and done, start oxytocin infusion.			
If failed induction with dinoprostone, consider balloon catheter.			

- *Amniotomy/artificial rupture of membranes (ARM):*

Preprocedure evaluation	Preprocedure evaluation	Indications	Contraindications
- Complete pre-induction of labor (IOL) assessment since it is irreversible - Encourage to empty bladder	Document: - Abdominal palpation - Vaginal examination (VE) findings	- After cervical ripening method - Favorable cervix (MBS ≥ 7)	- Poor application of the presenting part/unstable lie - Fetal head not engaged (risk of cord prolapse)

- Abdominal palpation to determine:
  – Descent
  – Position
  – Presentation
Vaginal examination for:
- Stage of labor
- Modified Bishop Score (MBS)
- Presentation
- Position and descent
- Membranes
	- Fetal heart rate (FHR)
	- Uterine activity
	- Vaginal loss (liquor amount, color, consistency)
		Before starting oxytocin infusion	Hepatitis B, hepatitis C, herpes simplex virus (HSV) and human immunodeficiency virus (HIV) infection (in order to minimize the hazards to the fetus of ascending infection).[13]

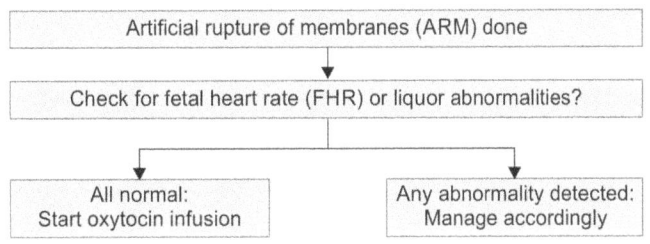

- *Oxytocin:*

Indications	Side effects	Caution

• Induction of labor (IOL) with ruptured membranes
• Favorable Modified Bishop Score (MBS)
Dosage
Oxytocin Infusion: oxytocin 30 IU in 500 mL,
1 milliunit/minute = 1 mL/hour
• Aim for contractions:
  – 3–4 in a 10-minute period
  – Duration of 40–60 seconds
  – Resting period of at least 60 seconds
• Titrate against uterine contractions
• Increase at 30 minutes or longer intervals
• Obstetric review required:
  – Prior to exceeding 20 milliunits/minute
  – At 32 milliunits/minute if labor has not commenced
  – If infusion ceased then prior to recommencing
	• Uterine hyperstimulation
	• Nausea and vomiting
	• Water intoxication or hyponatremia with prolonged infusion (rare with isotonic infusion)
	• Primary postpartum hemorrhage
	• If planned vaginal birth after cesarean section (VBAC): uterine dehiscence and rupture
	• Rarely (<0.1%) arrhythmias, electrocardiogram (ECG) changes, anaphylaxis, tetanic contractions, transient hypotension, reflex tachycardia
		• Do not commence oxytocin within:
		  – 6 hours of dinoprostone gel
		  – 30 minutes of removal of dinoprostone pessary
		• Review decision, if:
		  – Previous uterine surgery (e.g. cesarean section)]
		  – Multiple pregnancy
		  – More than four previous births
		  – Cardiovascular disease

REFERENCES

1. World Health Organization. WHO Recommendations on Induction of Labour at or Beyond Term. Geneva: World Health Organization; 2018.
2. Committee on Obstetric Practice, the American Institute of Ultrasound in Medicine, and the Society for Maternal-Fetal Medicine. ACOG Committee opinion, no. 700. Methods for estimating the due date. Obstet Gynecol. 2017;129(5): e150-4.
3. Royal College of Obstetricians and Gynaecologists. RCOG Clinical Effectiveness Support Unit. Induction of Labour. Evidence-based Clinical Guideline Number 9. London: RCOG Press; 2001.
4. Frye A. Holistic Midwifery: A Comprehensive Textbook for Midwives in Homebirth Practice, vol 1. Care during Pregnancy. Portland, OR: Labrys Press; 1995. p. 1184.
5. ACOG Committee opinion, number 764. Late-preterm and early-preterm deliveries. Obstet Gynaecol. 2019;133(2): e156-63.
6. Queensland Health. (2017). Queensland clinical guidelines. Induction of labour guideline no. MN17.22-V6-R22. [online] Available from: http://www.health.qld.gov.au/qcg [Last accessed September, 2019].
7. Queensland Health. (2015). Queensland Clinical Guidelines. Hypertensive disorders of pregnancy Guideline No. MN15.13-V7-R20. [online]. Available from: http://www.health.qld.gov.au/qcg [Last accessed September, 2019].
8. Queensland Health. (2015). Queensland Clinical Guidelines. Gestational diabetes mellitus. Guideline No. MN15.33-V1-R20. [online]. Available from: http://www.health.qld.gov.au/qcg [Last accessed September, 2019].
9. Queensland Health. (2016). Queensland Clinical Guidelines. Early onset Group B Streptococcal disease. Guideline No. MN16.20-V3-R21. [online]. Available from: http://www.health.qld.gov.au/qcg [Last accessed September, 2019].
10. ACOG Committee on practice bulletins—Obstetrics. ACOG practice bulletin no. 107: Induction of labor. Obstet Gynecol. 2009;114:386-97.
11. The Royal Australian and New Zealand College of Obstetricians and Gynaecologists. (2014). Intrapartum fetal surveillance clinical guideline-third edition. [online]. Available from: http://www.ranzcog.edu.au/ [Last accessed September, 2019].
12. Northern Devon Healthcare NHS Trust. Induction and Augmentation of Labour Guideline. Devon, UK: NHS Trust; 2018.
13. Royal Australian and New Zealand College of Obstetricians and Gynaecologists. Provision of Routine Intrapartum Care in the Absence of Pregnancy Complications. Melbourne, Australia; RANZCOG; 2017.

Chapter 31

Augmentation and Management of Labor

Leena Wadhwa, Sanjita

LABOR

It can be defined as the series of events that take place in the genital tract for the expulsion of viable products of conception out of womb through vagina into the outer world.

The mechanism of labor has been outlined in **Algorithm 1**.

The process of labor and delivery has been divided into various stages **(Algorithm 2)**.

Each stage carries particular risks to the mother and child so it is necessary to monitor each stage closely and to take necessary action at the earliest.

AUGMENTATION OF LABOR (ALGORITHMS 3 AND 4)

Augmentation of labor is the process of stimulating the uterus to increase the frequency, duration, and intensity of contractions after the onset of spontaneous labor. It is used for delayed labor in which the cause is commonly inadequate uterine contractions.

Augmentation is done when there is slow progress of labor characterized by various definitions:
- When cervical dilatation crosses the alert line
- WHO partograph with 4 hours delay between alert line and action line
- No change in dilatation or station within 2 hours[1]
- <2 cm change in dilatation during 4 hours[2]
- Slow progress in the first stage active phase:[1]
  - <1.2 cm/hr in nulliparous women
  - <1.5 cm/hr in multiparous women.

WHO practices for the management and augmentation of labor:[3]
Recommended:
- Active phase partograph with a 4-hour action line to monitor labor progress

Algorithm 1: Mechanism of normal labor.

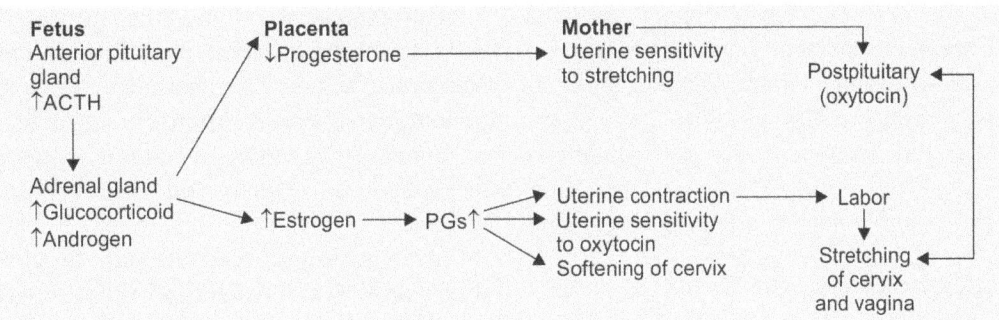

(ACTH: adrenocorticotropic hormone)

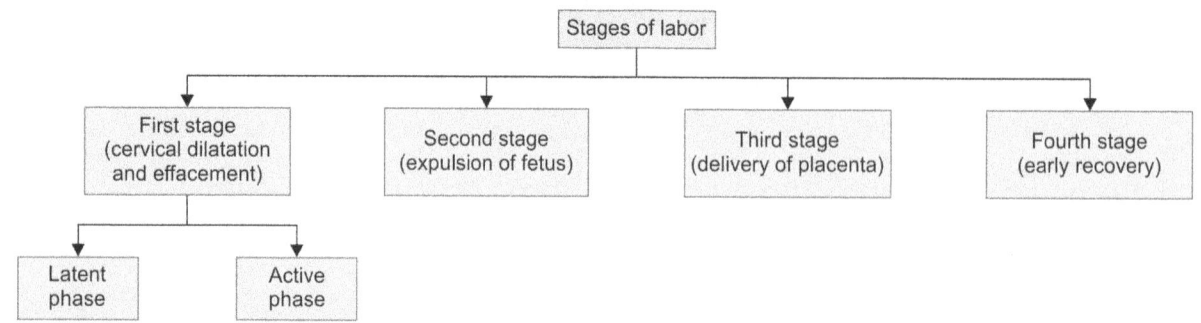

Algorithm 2: Stages of labor.

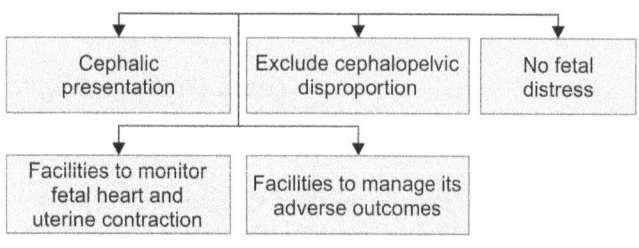

Algorithm 3: Criteria to be fulfilled before augmentation.

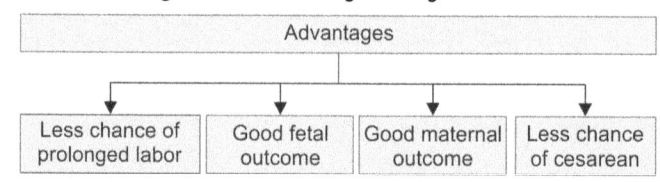

Algorithm 4: Advantages of augmentation.

- Routine assessments with digital vaginal examinations at 4-hour intervals
- Encouraging mobility and upright position
- Continuous companionship
- The use of oxytocin alone for treatment of delay in labor
- The use of amniotomy and oxytocin for treatment of *confirmed* delay in labor
- Respectful maternity care.

Not Recommended:
- The use of a package of care ("active management of labor") for prevention of delay in labor
- Administration of an enema
- The use of early amniotomy with early oxytocin augmentation
- The use of amniotomy alone
- Pain relief for preventing delay
- Restricting fluid and food intake for women at low risk
- The use of intravenous fluids to shorten labor
- Augmentation with intravenous oxytocin prior to confirmation of delay in labor
- High starting and increment dosage regimen of oxytocin
- Routine Perineal/pubic shaving prior to giving vaginal birth
- The use of oral misoprostol

- The use of internal tocodynamometry (compared with external tocodynamometry).

Although augmentation of labor may be beneficial in preventing prolonged labor, its inappropriate use may cause harm.[3]

FIRST STAGE OF LABOR (ALGORITHM 5)

The latent first stage is a period of time characterized by painful uterine contractions and variable changes of the cervix, including some degree of effacement and slower progression of dilatation up to 5 cm for first and subsequent labors.

The active first stage is a period of time characterized by regular painful uterine contractions a substantial degree of cervical effacement and more rapid cervical dilatation from 5 cm until full dilatation for first and subsequent labors.

The standard duration of the latent first stage has not been established and can vary from women to women. Duration of active phase does not exceed beyond 12 hours in first labors, beyond 10 hours in subsequent labors.

In active phase, rate of cervical dilatation is 1.2 cm/h in nulliparous women and 1.5 cm/h in multiparous women.

Labor may not accelerate until a cervical dilatation threshold of 5 cm is reached. Therefore, the use of medical

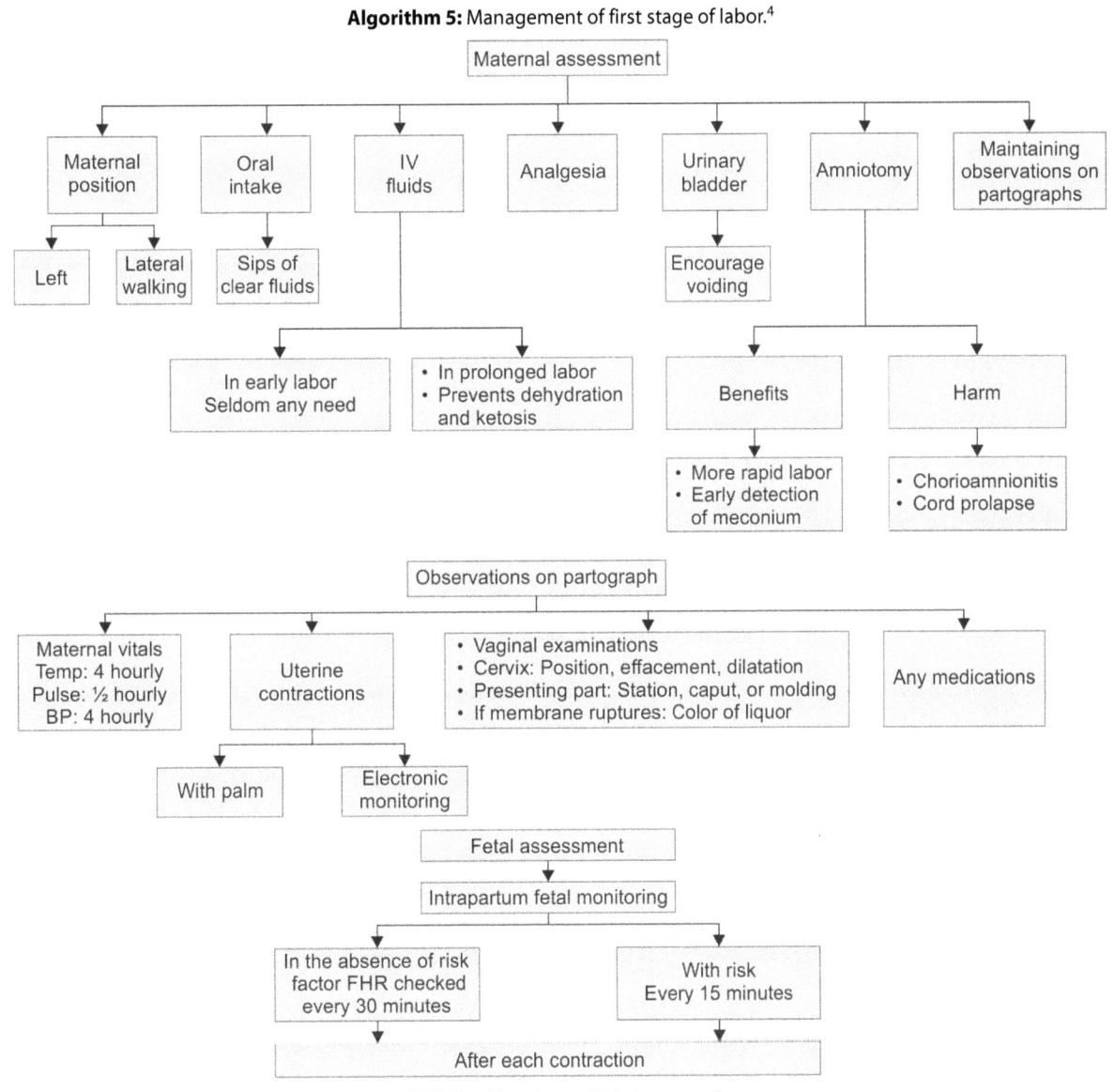

Algorithm 5: Management of first stage of labor.[4]

(FHR: fetal heart rate; IV: intravenous)

intervention to accelerate labor and birth such as oxytocin augmentation or cesarean section before this threshold is not recommended.[3]

MANAGEMENT OF SECOND STAGE OF LABOR (ALGORITHM 6)

Definition: It begins with full dilatation of cervix and ends with expulsion of fetus. Average duration of second stage 3 hours in first labors and 2 hours in subsequent labors.[3]

It is characterized by the onset of:
- Full cervical dilatation
- Appearance of bearing down efforts
- Urge to defecate
- Contractions become more prolonged
- Rupture of membrane.

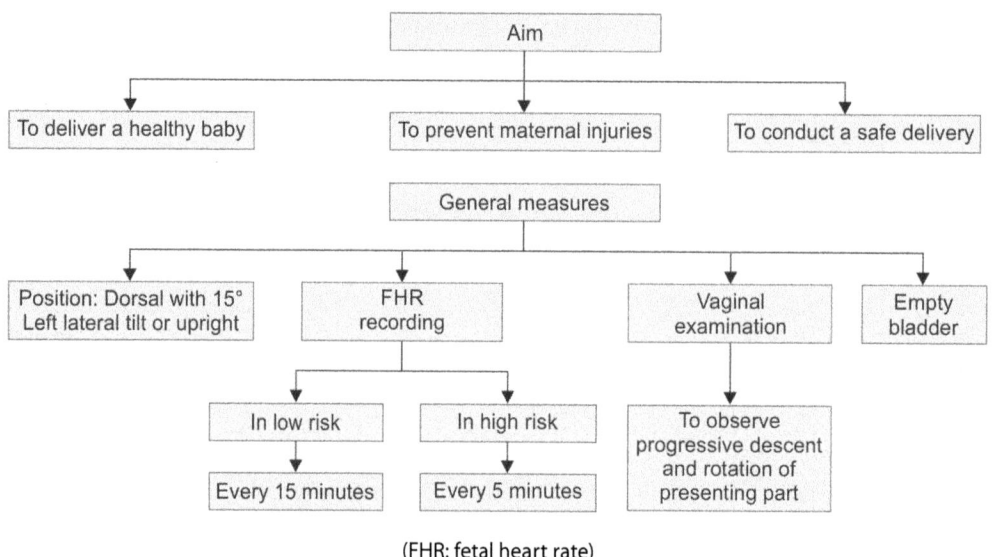

Algorithm 6: Management of second stage of labor.[5]

(FHR: fetal heart rate)

Algorithm 7: Management during delivery.[5]

(CPD: cephalopelvic disproportion; LSCS: lower segment cesarean section)

- There is no evidence that routine use of episiotomy causes significant reduction in laceration, severity of pain or pelvic organ prolapse compared with policy of restricted use.[3]
- Application of manual fundal pressure to facilitate child birth is not recommended.[3]

THIRD STAGE OF LABOR (ALGORITHM 8)

The part of labor from the birth of the baby until the placenta (afterbirth) and fetal membranes are delivered. The third stage of labor is also called the placental stage. The third stage of labor typically lasts between 10

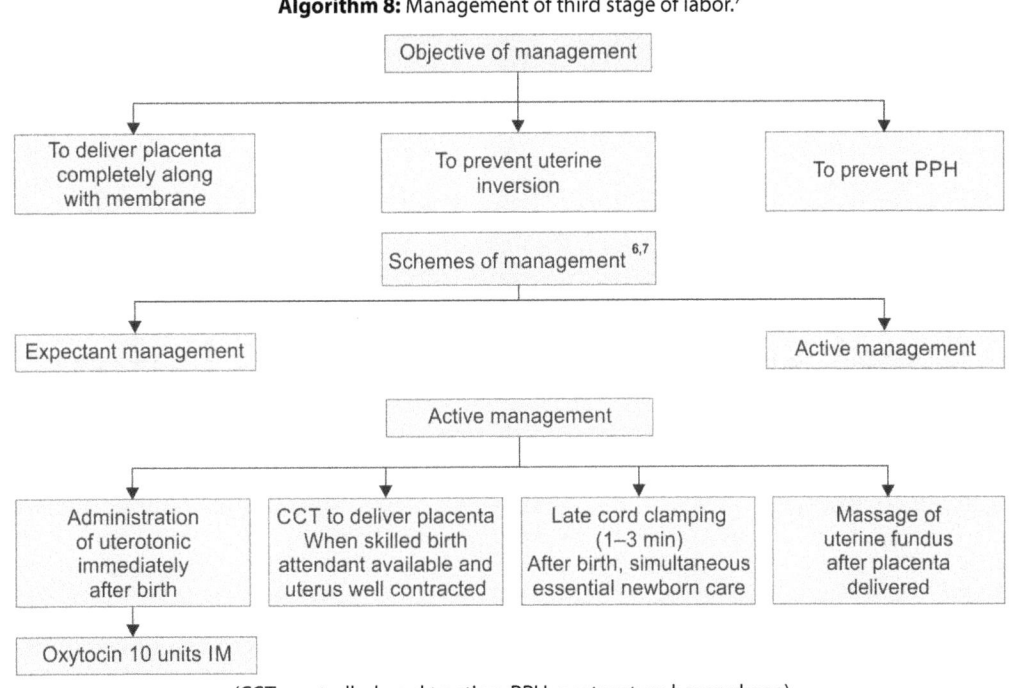

Algorithm 8: Management of third stage of labor.[7]

(CCT: controlled cord traction; PPH: postpartum hemorrhage)

and 30 minutes; if the placenta fails to separate within 30 minutes after childbirth, the third stage is considered to be prolonged.

Indications of early cord clamping:
- In cases of Rh incompatibility
- If baby is asphyxiated
- In babies of diabetic mother.

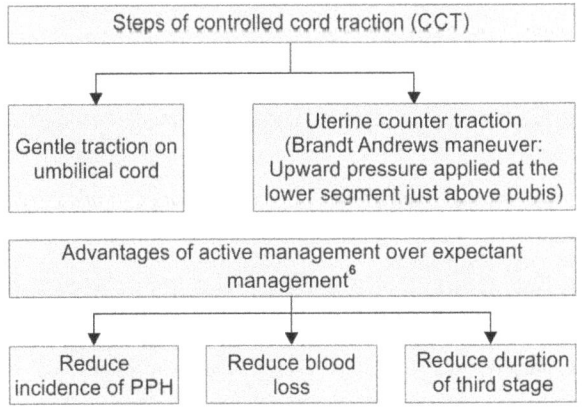

Algorithm 9: Steps of controlled cord traction (CCT).[7]

(PPH: postpartum hemorrhage)

FOURTH STAGE OF LABOR (ALGORITHM 10)

Stage of observation for at least 2 hours after the expulsion of afterbirths.

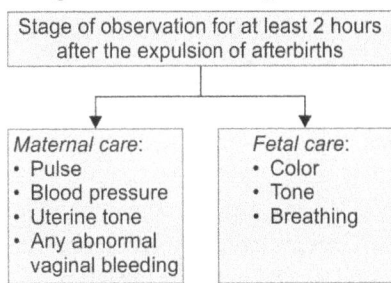

Algorithm 10: Fourth stage of labor.

REFERENCES

1. Joy S. Abnormal labor; 2011
2. National Institute for Health and Clinical Excellence. Available from: http://www.nice.org.uk/nicemedia/live/11037/36275/36275.pdf. 2007 Retrieved March 11 2015
3. WHO recommendation intrapartum care for a positive childbirth experience. Geneva; World Health Organisation; 2018.
4. Williams Obstetrics, 24th edition. Normal labour; 2014. pp. 447-51.
5. Management of second stage of labour. FIGO guidelines. Int J Gynecol Obstet; 2012. pp. 111-6
6. Begley CM, Gyte GM, Devane D, et al. Active versus expectant management for women in the third stage of labour. Cochrane Database Syst Review Rev. 2011; CD007412.
7. WHO recommendations on prevention and treatment of postpartum haemorrhage; 2012.

Chapter 32

Fetal Surveillance during Labor

Monika Gupta, Namrata Verma

INTRODUCTION

- The goal of fetal surveillance during labor is to detect fetal decompensation by assessing certain fetal heart characteristics that precede fetal brain injury.
- Intrapartum fetal monitoring helps us detect the changes in the fetal heart rate (FHR) that indicate a possibility of fetal hypoxia and metabolic acidosis so that timely action can be taken to prevent adverse outcomes.
- Intermittent auscultation, electronic fetal heart rate monitoring (EFM), fetal blood sampling for pH, blood lactate, ECG, pulse oximetry in resourceful settings are used for fetal surveillance during labor.

MODALITIES FOR INTRAPARTUM FETAL SURVEILLANCE

Intermittent Auscultation

- Intermittent auscultation (IA) is the recommended method for women without risk factors.
- Use either stethoscope or Doppler ultrasound.
- Carry out IA immediately after contraction for at least 1 minute.
- If any FHR abnormality is suspected, palpate the maternal pulse to differentiate between two heart rates.
- In active first stage, auscultate FHR every 15 minutes and every 5 minutes in second stage of labor [ACOG 2009, NICE 2014].[1,2]

Electronic Fetal Monitoring

- Electronic fetal monitoring involves the use of internal or external monitor to assess fetal well-being during labor and has formed the mainstay of fetal surveillance in high-risk pregnancies **(Table 1)**.
- Equipment required for the test is called a cardiotocograph (CTG), screening tool to detect fetal hypoxia during labor, which records FHR and uterine activity on a graph by means of internal and external transducers.
- *External monitoring:* It uses a Doppler ultrasound transducer to detect the movement of cardiac structures. The resulting signal requires signal

Table 1: Indications for electronic fetal monitoring.

Maternal	Fetal
Diabetes	Meconium-stained liquor
Intrauterine growth restriction (IUGR)	Abnormal Doppler velocimetry
Post-dated pregnancies	Oligohydramnios
Trial of labor after previous cesarean section	Chorioamnionitis
Epidural analgesia	Intrauterine infections
Antepartum hemorrhage	Preterm gestations
Hypertensive disorders	
Certain medical disorders	
Induced/augmented labor	

modulation and autocorrelation to provide adequate quality recordings. It can be used in antepartum and intrapartum fetal surveillance.
- *Internal fetal heart rate monitoring:* It uses a fetal electrode applied to scalp or breech, evaluates the time interval between successive heart beats by identifying R waves on the fetal ECG QRS complex, and therefore measures ventricular depolarization cycles. It is more accurate but requires rupture of membranes, so is used only for intrapartum monitoring.
- Electronic fetal monitoring is associated with overall increased rate of operative interventions in low-risk pregnancies. Although studies showed no reduction in perinatal mortality and cerebral palsy, but reduction in risk of neonatal seizures is evident.[3]
- Always consider the antenatal, intrapartum risk factors and current wellbeing of woman, fetus and progress of labor while interpreting CTG trace[4] **(Table 2)**.
- ACOG recommends evaluating CTG trace every 15 minutes during active first stage and every 5 minutes during second stage of labor **(Table 3)**. NICE recommends systematic assessment of condition of woman and fetus hourly or more frequently if there are concerns.

Three-tier system for classification of electronic FHR tracings and management has been described in **Table 4**.

Pattern	Definition

Baseline	• The mean FHR rounded to increments of 5 bpm during a 10 min segment, excluding:
	  – Periodic or episodic changes
	  – Periods of marked FHR variability
	  – Segments of baseline that differ by more than 25 bpm
	• Must be for minimum 2 min in any 10 min segment or the baseline for that time period is indeterminate. In this case, one may refer to the prior 10 min window for determination of baseline
	• Normal FHR baseline: 110–160 bpm; Tachycardia: >160 bpm; Bradycardia: <110 bpm

Baseline variability	• Fluctuations in the baseline FHR that are irregular in amplitude and frequency • Variability is visually quantified as the amplitude of peak-to-trough in bpm • Absent: Amplitude range detectable but 5 bpm or fewer • Moderate (normal): Amplitude range 6–25 bpm • Marked: Amplitude range greater than 25 bpm
Acceleration	• A visually apparent abrupt increase (onset to peak in less than 30 sec) in the FHR ≥32 weeks of gestation: an acceleration has a peak of ≥15 bpm above baseline, with a duration of ≥15 sec but <2 min from onset to return • <32 weeks, an acceleration has a peak of ≥10 bpm above baseline, with a duration ≥10 sec but <2 min from onset to return • Prolonged acceleration lasts ≥2 min but <10 min in duration • If an acceleration lasts ≥10 min, it is a baseline change
Early deceleration	• Visually apparent usually symmetrical gradual decrease and return of the FHR associated with a uterine contraction • A gradual FHR decrease is defined as from the onset to the FHR nadir of ≥30 sec • The decrease in FHR is calculated from the onset to the nadir of the deceleration • The nadir of the deceleration occurs at the same time as the peak of the contraction • In most cases, the onset, nadir, and recovery of the deceleration are coincident with the beginning, peak, and ending of the contraction, respectively
Late deceleration	• Visually apparent usually symmetrical gradual decrease and return of the FHR associated with a uterine contraction • A gradual FHR decrease is defined as from the onset to the FHR nadir of ≥30 sec or more • The decrease in FHR is calculated from the onset to the nadir of the deceleration • The deceleration is delayed in timing with the nadir of the deceleration occurring after the peak of the contraction • In most cases, the onset, nadir, and recovery of the deceleration occur after the beginning, peak, and ending of the contraction, respectively
Variable deceleration	• Visually apparent abrupt decrease in FHR • An abrupt FHR decrease is defined as from the onset of the deceleration to the beginning of the FHR nadir of <30 sec • The decrease in FHR is calculated from the onset to the nadir of the deceleration • The decrease in FHR is ≥15 bpm, lasting ≥15 sec, and <2 min in duration • When associated with uterine contraction, their onset, depth, and duration commonly vary with successive uterine contractions

Table 2: Interpretation of various CTG fetal heart rate patterns during labor.[4]

Contd...

Contd...

Pattern	Definition
Prolonged deceleration	• Visually apparent decrease in the FHR below the baseline • Decrease in FHR from the baseline that is ≥15 bpm, and <2 min in duration • If a deceleration last ≥10 min, it is a baseline change
Sinusoidal	• Visually apparent, smooth, sine waveline undulating pattern in FHR baseline with a cycle frequency of 3–5/min which persist for 20 min or more

Table 3: Potential causes of abnormal electronic FHR tracings and management.[5]

Pattern	Associated causes	Clinical actions
Bradycardia	*Maternal*: Hypotension, pyelonephritis, hypothermia, position, congenital heart block *Fetal*: Umbilical cord occlusion, hypoxia/acidosis, vagal stimulation due to head compression, cardiac conduction or structural defect	• Assess maternal pulse • Differentiate fetal from maternal heart rate • Vaginal examination (elevate presenting part if cord prolapse) • If cause is not correctable, consider intrapartum USG to evaluate dysrhythmia • If <100 bpm, obtain fetal scalp pH • Prepare for delivery
Tachycardia	*Maternal*: Fever, infection, dehydration, hyperthyroidism, anxiety, drugs, e.g. parasympathetic inhibiting (atropine) or sympathomimetic (terbutaline), anemia *Fetal*: Infection, prolonged fetal activity or stimulation, chronic hypoxemia or cardiac abnormalities, congenital anomalies, anemia	• Assess maternal temperature (manage if raised) • Assess medication or drugs • Reassess for duration of rupture of membranes, positive vaginal culture, especially *Group B Streptococcus* • If cause is not correctable, consider intrapartum USG to evaluate arrhythmia • If >160 bpm for >80 min, expedite delivery
Minimal/absent variability	Fetal sleep, prematurity, medications (analgesia/sedatives/corticosteroids/magnesium sulfate), hypoxic acidemia	• If <5 bpm for >80 minor sinusoidal • Attach fetal scalp electrode • Obtain fetal scalp pH if clinically appropriate • Prepare for delivery
Sinusoidal pattern	Fetal intracranial hemorrhage, fetal anemia, tissue hypoxia in brainstem, anti-D alloimmunization, twin-twin transfusion syndrome, vasa previa, maternal IV meperidine	• Attach fetal scalp electrode • Fetal transfusion if required • Obtain fetal scalp pH if clinically appropriate • Prepare for delivery
Variable decelerations	Vagal stimulation due to cord compression, fetal acidemia	• Observe in early first stage and observe for development of combined patterns • Very common in late first stage, occurs in more than half second stages, no action required as a normal response • If persistent variable deceleration • Amnioinfusion may ameliorate • Confirm fetal well being • Obtain fetal scalp pH if clinically appropriate • Prepare for delivery
Late decelerations	Fetal chemoreceptor/vagal result due to decreased PO_2, altered blood flow to the placenta (maternal hypotension), reduced maternal arterial oxygen saturation, placental changes altering maternal–fetal gas exchange (placental insufficiency, uterine hypertonus or tachysystole), fetal acidemia	• When occasional, ensure mother in left lateral, check maternal vital signs and continue observing • When repetitive: Obtain fetal scalp pH if clinically appropriate • Prepare for delivery
Prolonged decelerations	Fetal baroreceptor and chemoreceptor responses to profound changes in the fetal environment due to uterine hypertonus, unresolving umbilical cord compression, maternal hypotension, maternal seizure, and rapid fetal descent	• Vaginal examination to rule out cord prolapse • Prepare for delivery

Table 4: Three-tier system for classification of electronic FHR tracings and management.[6,7]

Category	Type of tracing	Management
I	• Baseline rate: 110–160 bpm • Baseline FHR variability: Moderate • Late or variable decelerations: Absent • Early decelerations: Present or absent • Accelerations: Present or absent	Manage as per protocol
II	*Baseline rate:* • Bradycardia not accompanied by absent baseline variability • Tachycardia *Baseline FHR variability:* • Minimal baseline variability • Absent baseline variability not accompanied by recurrent decelerations • Marked baseline variability *Accelerations:* • Absence of induced accelerations after fetal stimulation • Periodic or episodic decelerations • Recurrent variable decelerations with minimal or moderate baseline variability • Prolonged deceleration ≥2 min but <10 min • Recurrent late decelerations with moderate baseline variability • Variable decelerations with other characteristics, such as slow return to baseline, "overshoots", or "shoulders"	• Stop oxytocin drip • Left lateral position • Oxygen by mask • IV RL fast infusion • Amnioinfusion in variable decelerations

III	• Absent baseline FHR variability and any of the following
	   – Recurrent late decelerations
	   – Recurrent variable decelerations
	   – Bradycardia
	• Sinusoidal pattern
		Delivery

Current Recommendations

In both low- and high-risk pregnancies, IA or continuous EFM is considered an acceptable method of intrapartum surveillance. The recommended interval between checking the heart rate, however, is longer in the uncomplicated pregnancy **(Table 5)**.[8] When auscultation is used, it is recommended that it should be performed after a contraction and for 60 seconds. It also is recommended that a 1-to-1 nurse–patient ratio should be used if auscultation is employed.

Fetal Scalp Blood Sampling

- Invasive procedure
- Simple technique but requires facilities of blood gas analysis
- Estimation of pH and base excess helps in detecting acidosis and hence reduces the false positive rate of CTG
- If analysis is normal, repeat within 1 hour if indicated. If borderline, repeat in 30 minutes if indicated by CTG or earlier if additional nonreassuring or abnormal features are seen. If CTG remains unchanged and the analysis is stable after a second test, further samples may be deferred until additional nonreassuring or abnormal features are seen
- *Contraindications:* Fetal bleeding disorders and maternal to fetal transmittable infections

Table 5: Guidelines for methods of intrapartum fetal heart rate monitoring.[7]

Surveillance	Low-risk pregnancies	High-risk pregnancies
Acceptable methods		
Intermittent auscultation	Yes	Yes[a]
Continuous electronic monitoring (internal or external)	Yes	Yes[b]
Evaluation intervals		
First-stage labor (active)	30 min	15 min[a,b]
Second-stage labor	15 min	5 min[a,c]

[a] Preferably before, during, and after uterine contraction.
[b] Includes tracing evaluation and charting at least every 15 min.
[c] Tracing should be evaluated at least every 5 min.

- Failure rate is high as large sample of blood is required for the test (35–50 μL).[9]

ECG Waveform Analysis (ST Analyzer—STAN)

- ST analyzer combines standard CTG monitoring with concurrent assessment of the fetal ECG.
- ST analyzer software helps in identifying fetal hypoxia by detecting the changes in the ST segment of the fetal ECG, which reflects myocardial hypoxemia, which may also reflect cerebral oxygenation.
- It analyzes the average waveform of the fetal ECG signal over 30 consecutive heartbeats and compares this waveform with the average of each of the subsequent 30 complexes. It is thus able to determine the ST segment and T wave changes over time and alerts by signaling the occurrence of a "STAN event".
- ST analyzer monitoring with CTG in labor has shown a reduction in the operative delivery rates and metabolic acidosis than alone CTG in two randomized controlled trials (RCTs).[10]

Fetal Pulse Oximetry

- Continuously measures the intrapartum fetal oxygen saturation.
- A sensor is placed transvaginally through the cervix to rest against the fetal cheek or temple, requiring cervical dilatation (~ 2 cm or more) and ruptured amniotic membranes with a cephalic presentation.

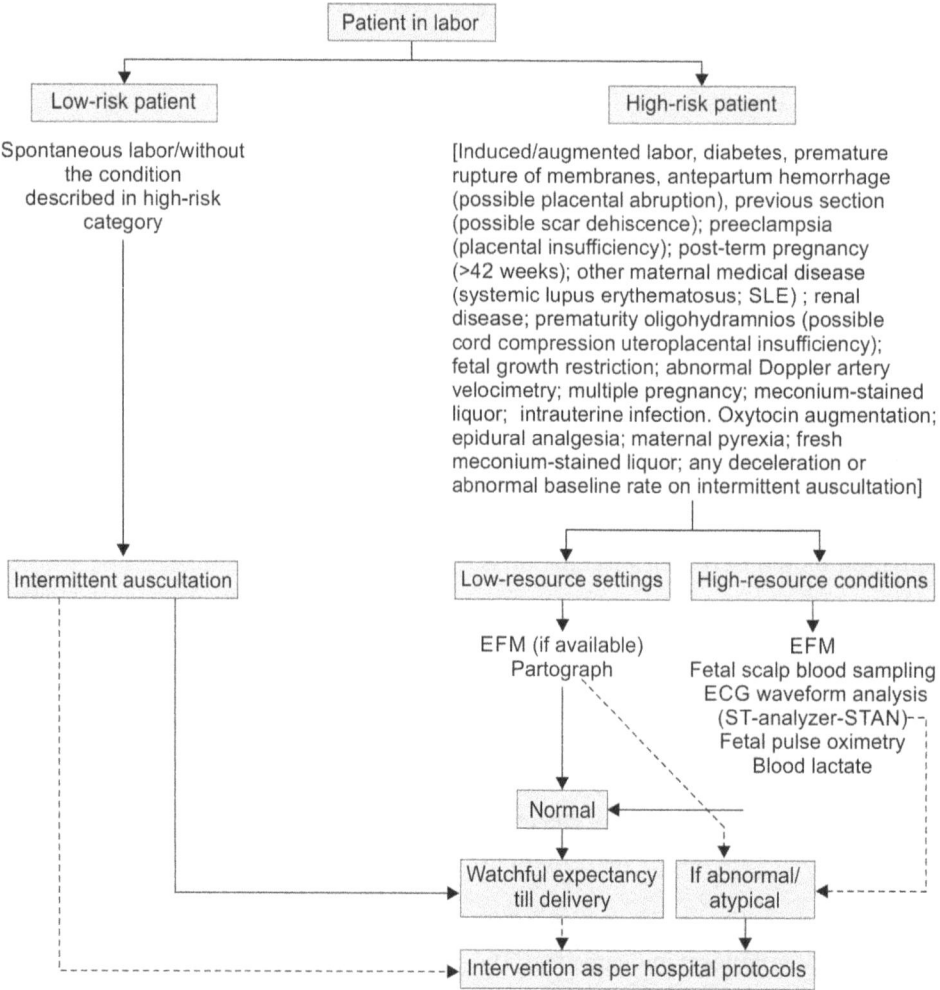

Algorithm for Intrapartum Fetal Surveillance

- SpO_2 >30% is associated with good fetal outcomes.
- It improves the specificity of the CTG and enables the direct and continuous assessment of fetal oxygenation.
- Not recommended for routine use.

Blood Lactate

- Directly measures lactate level and requires small amount of blood sample (5 µL).[9]
- Fetal scalp blood lactate levels correlate well with the umbilical arterial cord blood lactate level.
- Can distinguish between benign respiratory acidosis and potentially deleterious metabolic acidosis.
- Insufficient evidence to suggest any correlation between blood lactate levels and long-term neonatal outcome.

REFERENCES

1. Intrapartum fetal heart rate monitoring: nomenclature, interpretation, and general management principles. ACOG Practice Bulletin No. 106. American College of Obstetricians and Gynecologists. Obstet Gynecol. 2009;114(1):192-202.
2. NICE. (2014). Intrapartum care for healthy women and babies. NICE Clinical guideline. [Online]. Available from: nice.org.uk/guidance/cg190 [Last accessed October, 2019].
3. Alfirevic Z, Devane D, Gyte GML. Continuous cardiotocography (CTG) as a form of electronic fetal monitoring (EFM) for fetal assessment during labour. Cochrane Database Syst Rev. 2006;(3):CD006066.
4. Ayres-de-Campos D, Spong CY, Chandraharan E. FIGO consensus guidelines on intrapartum fetal monitoring: cardiotocography. Int J Gynecol Obstet. 2015;131(1):13-24.
5. Liston R, Sawchuck D, Yiung D; Society of Obstetrics and Gynaecologists of Canada; British Columbia Perinatal Health Programme. Fetal health surveillance: antepartum and intrapartum consensus guideline. J Obstet Gynecol Can. 2007;29(9):S3-56.
6. Macones GA, Hankins GD, Spong CY, et al. The 2008 National Institute of Child Health and Human Development workshop report on electronic fetal monitoring: update on definitions, interpretation, and research guidelines. Obstet Gynecol. 2008;112(3):661-6.
7. American College of Obstetricians and Gynecologists. (2010). Management of intrapartum fetal heart rate tracings. Practice Bulletin No. 116.
8. American Academy of Pediatrics and the American College of Obstetricians and Gynecologists. Guidelines for Perinatal Care, 8th edition. Elk Grove Village: AAP; 2017.
9. Nordstrom L, Chua S, Roy A et al. Quality assessment of two lactate test strip methods suitable for obstetric use. J Perinat Med. 1998;26(2):83-8.
10. Rosen KG, Amer-Wahlin I, Luzietti R, et al. Fetal ECG waveform analysis. Best Pract Res Clin Obstet Gynaecol. 2004;18(3):485-514.

Chapter 33

Pain Relief in Labor

Kartik Syal, Geetika Syal

WHY IS IT ESSENTIAL?

In a joint statement given in 1992, the American Anesthesiologists and Obstetrics and Gynecologists Society stated, "Labor pains are one of the most distressing pains a human being may have to bear; there is no other circumstance where it is considered acceptable for a person to experience such severe pain, amenable to safe intervention, while under a physician's care. Hence option of labor analgesia should be given to all pregnant females."[1]

This statement seals the fact that labor analgesia should be an essential part of obstetric care.

This advisory given long time back changed the outlook toward labor analgesia from being given to those who demanded offered to all laboring patients.

The severity of this pain has been described as "distressing," "horrible," or "excruciating" by most females during and after labor.[2]

Even when reported on objective pain scores like McGill pain questionnaires, labor pain is one of the most intense pain.[3]

Severe pain leads to *Sympathetic Stimulation*, which in its turn leads to rise in levels of *Catecholamines and Cortisol*. This rise in levels leads to decrease in both uterine contractions as well as placental perfusion which causes increase in fetal lactic acid levels along with *Maternal Acidosis*.

Also, severe pain causes *increased cardiac output and increased oxygen demand*; this in addition to maternal acidosis may lead to *significant fetal acidemia and fetal hypoxia*, especially in patients with heart or/and pulmonary diseases.

PHYSIOLOGY OF LABOR PAINS

In the first stage of labor:
- Myometrial ischemia due to uterine contractions causes release of pain transmitters like bradykinin, histamine, and serotonin.
- Also, there is stretching of mechanoreceptors in lower uterine segment and cervix.
- From these, the visceral pain impulses travel in A-d and C nerve fibers through paracervical ganglion and hypogastric plexus to cause pain in T_{10}-L_1 spinal cord segments.
- The pain is poorly localized over entire abdomen and may be transmitted to legs and gluteus.

In the second stage of labor:
- Pain is exaggerated extension of pain in first stage.
- It has principally somatic localized component.
- Distension of pelvic structures and perineum due to birthing fetus causes relative ischemia and even micro- and macroinjuries causing pain.
- Somatic pain is carried by branches of pudendal nerve in S_2-S_4 dermatomes.

INTERVENTIONS TO REDUCE LABOR PAINS

Different interventions to reduce labor pains and different ways to provide labor analgesia are described in **Figure 1** and **Table 1**, respectively.

Chapter 33
Pain Relief in Labor

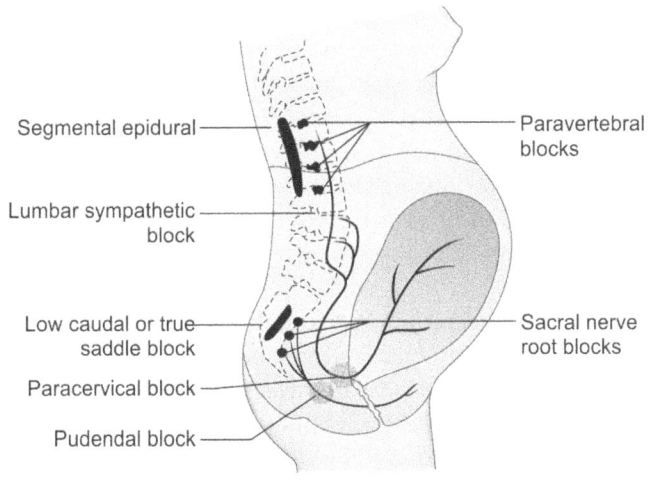

Fig. 1: Interventions to reduce labor pains.

Table 1: Different ways to provide labor analgesia.

Nonpharma-cological	Pharmacological		
	Inhalational	Systemic	Regional
• Birthing preparation • Hypnosis • Transcutaneous electrical nerve stimulation • Acupuncture • Electroanalgesia • Hydrotherapy • Aromatherapy	• Entonox • Sevoflurane • Desflurane • Trilene • Methoxyflurane	• Opioids • Sedatives • Ketamine • Tramadol	• Epidural • Subarachnoid block (spinal) • Combined spinal epidural • Lumbar sympathetic block • Paracervical block • Pudendal block

History of Labor Analgesia

- *1847:*
  - James Young Simpson administered the first obstetric general anesthetic using ether.
  - His action was widely criticized concerning maternal and fetal safety.
- *1853:*
  - Labor analgesia concept was popularized by John Snow who delivered Queen Victoria's eighth child under chloroform analgesia in 1853.
  - The history of labor analgesia progressed through the use of nitrous oxide (N_2O) by Klikovitch in Russia, use of morphine, hyoscine and later, pethidine.
- *1931:*
  - Use of present gold standard regional technique by Aburel in 1931.

The preferred technique of labor analgesia should be:
- Safe to mother and fetus
- Effective and controllable
- Predictable in its effects
- Should have a high technical success rate.
- Most importantly it should not weaken uterine contractions or maternal bearing down.

Programmed Labor

- Optimized labor protocol to ensure smooth progress of labor.
- Judicious use of labor inducers, appropriate obstetric-analgesic regimen, and partographic monitoring.
- Most suitable for low-risk primigravidae and can be carried out by the obstetrician in the active phase of labor.
- Low doses of different drug combinations are used to maximize analgesia and minimize side effects like respiratory depression and excess sedation.
- A simple regime described as follows:[4]
  - Injection diazepam 2 mg IV (total: 10 mg)
  - Injection tramadol 50 mg IM (total: 100 mg)
  - Injection pentazocine 6 mg IV (total: 30 mg)
  - Injection drotaverine 40 mg IV every 2 hours (maximum: three doses).
  - Injection ketamine 0.25–0.50 mg/kg IV (maximum: 1 mg/kg or 100 mg in 30 minutes) slow.

Programmed labor has been shown to produce good analgesia and amnesia, shorten the period of labor, decrease operative delivery, and blood loss as well as improve uterine flow.

Inhalational Analgesia

- Inhalational analgesia through face mask was the earliest form of obstetric analgesia.
- Subanesthetic concentrations of inhalational anesthetic agents, including N_2O.
- The advantages include that the mother remains awake with protective laryngeal reflexes, technique is self-administered (which makes it safe, as face mask

falls when patient goes to deepen plane), and progress of labor is unaltered.
- The earliest to be used were ether, chloroform, and cyclopropane, followed by trichloroethylene and methoxyflurane. Enflurane, isoflurane, sevoflurane, and desflurane are more recent additions; with Entonox (50% N_2O + 50% O_2) still the most widely used, but sevoflurane is believed to be the best agent.
- The disadvantage of using volatile agents is that sophisticated equipment is needed to administer these agents in a controlled way. Also, there is atmospheric pollution and chances of deepening of anesthetic depth and aspiration if face mask is held by someone other than patient herself.

Regional Analgesia

- Central neuraxial analgesia is the most versatile method of labor analgesia and is currently the gold standard technique for pain control in obstetrics.
- Local anesthetics administered in lower concentrations in combination with opioids provide effective, synergistic analgesia while reducing some of the unwanted side effects of local anesthetics, such as motor block.
- Regional analgesia is effective in preventing the increase in catecholamines associated with labor pain. Therefore, the sympathetic overactivity, which may lead to decrease in uterine blood flow and dysrhythmic contractions, is successfully blunted by regional analgesia
- Also, this pain relief allows parturient to be awake and be able to participate in labor and delivery.
- Regional anesthesia may be administered by the anesthetist using epidural, subarachnoid (spinal) block, combined spinal-epidural, or lumbar sympathetic block. Paracervical block, pudendal block, and local perineal infiltration are forms of labor analgesia practiced by obstetricians themselves.

Epidural Labor Analgesia

- The most important indication for labor analgesia remains maternal request for pain relief.
- Therapeutic indications like heart or/and pulmonary disease, pre-eclampsia: drastic hemodynamic changes during labor are avoided, thereby preserving both maternal and fetal well-being.
- Despite the supposed availability of many options, epidural analgesia remains the only effective technique to relieve severe pain as well as offer therapeutic benefits for high-risk parturients.
- Obstetric patients with previous cesarean section, anticipated difficult airway, multiple pregnancy, and obesity stand to benefit with an indwelling epidural catheter, in face of an emergency cesarean section.
- *Regimes:*
  - Intermittent bolus epidural analgesia (patient or anesthetist controlled epidural analgesia) with or without basal local anesthetic infusion
  - Continuous infusion epidural analgesia (at rate of 8–15 mL/hr)
  - Opioid alone or addition of opioid to local anesthetics
  - Opioid + local anesthetics most frequently used: Decrease latency, prolong duration, improve quality of analgesia, and allow lower doses of both drugs to be used.
- *Drugs:*
  - Bupivacaine in concentrations varying from 0.06% to 0.125% and ropivacaine 0.06–0.15%.
  - With or without opioids, which are fentanyl 50–100 μg in 10 mL saline (or 1–2 μg/mL) and sufentanil 10–25 μg in 10 mL saline.
- The use of lower concentrations or opioids alone as in combined spinal-epidural is what has come to be known as "*walking epidural.*"
- The proposed advantages of ambulation in labor include:[5]
  - The parturient's enjoyment of mobility
  - Autonomy and self-control in labor
  - Increased uterine activity and increased intensity of contractions
  - Decreased frequency of contractions
  - Decreased pain
  - Decreased duration of the first stage of labor
  - Decreased incidence of fetal heart rate (FHR) abnormalities
  - And decreased incidence of operative and/or assisted deliveries.

Labor Analgesia Using Subarachnoid (Spinal) Space

- Used in combination with epidural injection (combined spinal-epidural analgesia) due to its rapid reliable effect.

- Opioids like 25 µg fentanyl with low dose (2.5 mg) bupivacaine, in a concentration of 0.1%, can be used for practically immediate relief of pain and give time for epidural to act.
- Isolated spinal analgesia in the above doses can also be used, especially in patients coming for labor analgesia with almost full dilatation.

OTHER REGIONAL TECHNIQUES

Lumbar Sympathetic Block

Bilateral paravertebral lumbar sympathetic block at the level of L_2, though effective, is seldom used due to its limited duration and technical difficulty.

Paracervical Block

- Block is given by injecting local anesthetic agents into vaginal fornices lateral to the cervix.
- As it is simple to perform and can provide good analgesia in 40–80% of patients, it is still used by many obstetricians.
- The most deterrent complication is high incidence of fetal bradycardia after this block, due to uterine vasoconstriction and high fetal local anesthetic concentration.
- Hematoma, sacral neuropathy, and abscess being the other complications.

Pudendal Nerve Block

- Especially used for instrumental deliveries by obstetricians.
- It has been superseded by more reliable and safer spinal or epidural blocks.
- Bilateral nerve is blocked behind ischial spines adjacent to lateral vaginal walls by 10-15 mL of 1% lignocaine.
- Failure or partial block in 40–50% of cases and hematoma formation are complications associated with this block.

REFERENCES

1. American College of Obstetricians and Gynecologists (ACOG). Committee on Obstetrics: Maternal and Fetal Medicine. Pain Relief during Labor. ACOG Opinion Number 118. Washington, DC, USA: ACOG; 1992.
2. Brown ST, Campbell D, Kurtz A. Characteristics of labor pain at two stages of cervical dilation. Pain. 1989;38(3):289-95.
3. Melzack R, Taenzer P, Feldman P, et al. Labour is still painful after prepared childbirth training. Can Med Assoc J. 1981;125(4):357-63.
4. Daftary SN, Desai SV, Thanawala U, et al. Programmed labor-indigenous protocol to optimize labor outcome. South Asian Feder Obstet Gynecol. 2009;1(1):61-4.
5. Chamberlain G, Stewart M. Walking through labour. Br Med J (Clin Res Ed). 1987;295(6602):802.

Chapter 34

Meconium

Anshuja Singla, Charu Yadav

INTRODUCTION

Meconium is a greenish-black, sticky substance passed by the fetus during the first 48 hours after birth, though it begins to form in the fetal intestines by the 10th week of life. Meconium-stained amniotic fluid (MSAF) occurs in approximately 8–25% of all deliveries.

GRADES OF MECONIUM

Significant meconium is defined as a dark green or black amniotic fluid that is thick or tenacious or that has lumps of meconium.[1]

Nonsignificant/thin meconium is thin yellow-greenish tinged fluid containing nonparticulate meconium.[2]

Management Protocol in Case of Significant MSAF[2]

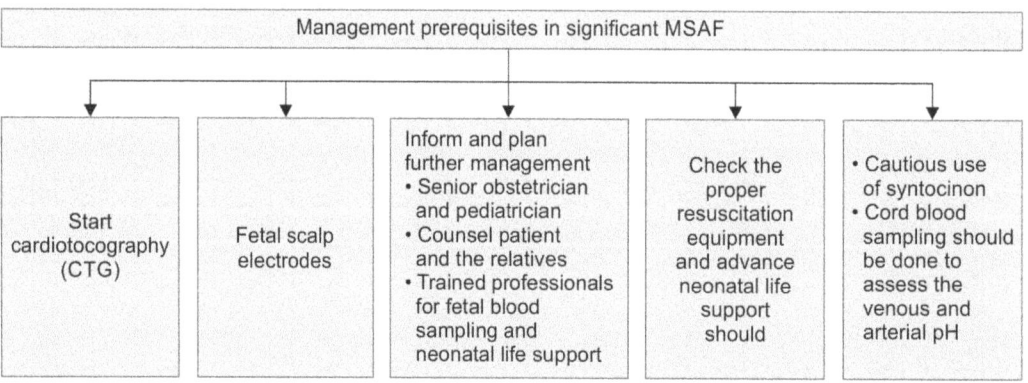

Meconium aspiration syndrome (MAS) is defined as respiratory distress in newborn infants born through MSAF.[3]

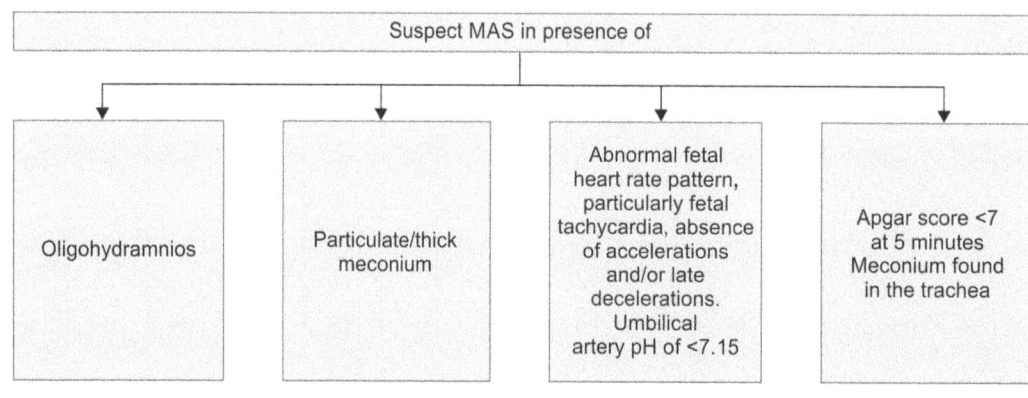

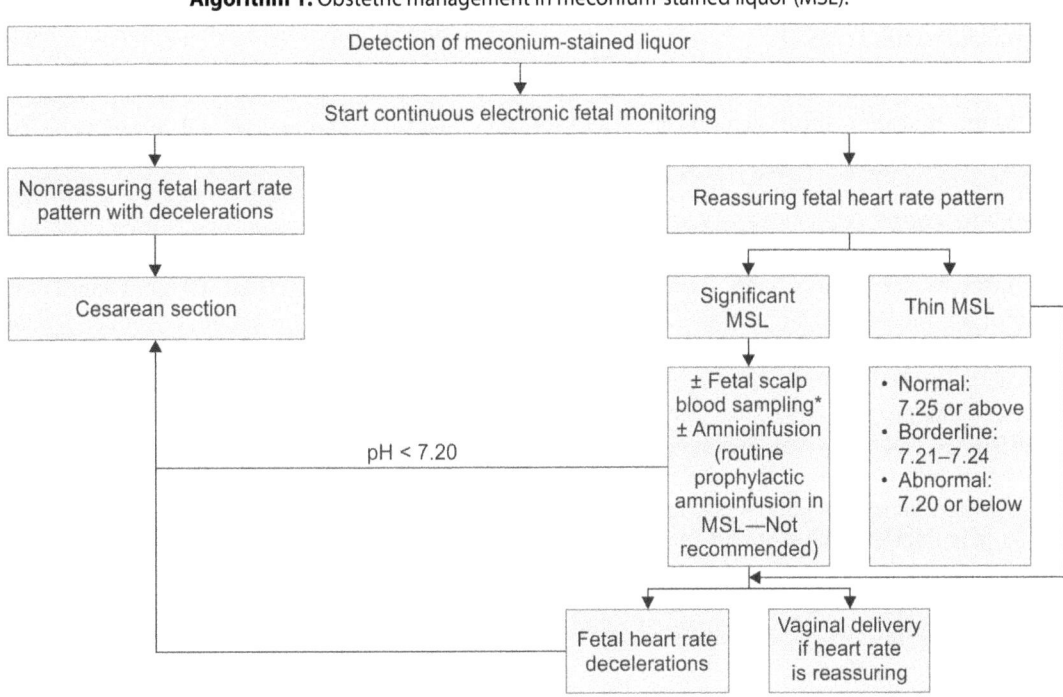

Algorithm 1: Obstetric management in meconium-stained liquor (MSL).

DELIVERY ROOM MANAGEMENT OF NEWBORN WITH MECONIUM-STAINED LIQUOR

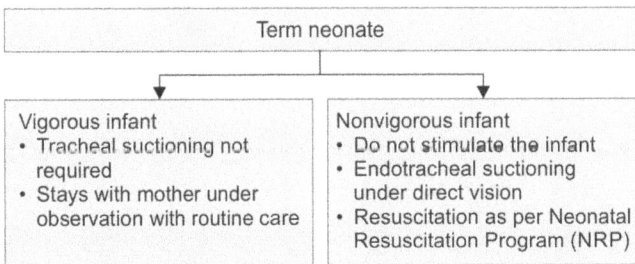

Algorithm 2: Neonatal care at birth.

STRATEGIES FOR PREVENTION OF MECONIUM ASPIRATION SYNDROME

- To detect fetal hypoxemia, continuous electronic fetal heart rate monitoring (EFM) should be done, thereby reducing the risk of adverse neonatal outcomes. Several studies have noted an increase in the frequency of FHR abnormalities in association with MSAF. In the presence of MSAF, fetal tachycardia, variable and late decelerations, and decreased long-term variability are risk factors for MAS.[4-8]

- Amnioinfusion has also been proposed as a method to reduce MAS by mechanical cushioning of the umbilical cord and dilution of meconium.[4] Amnioinfusion is associated with substantive improvements in perinatal outcome only in settings where facilities for perinatal surveillance are limited. It is not clear whether the benefits are due to dilution of meconium or relief of oligohydramnios. In settings with standard peripartum surveillance, amnioinfusion is either ineffective, or its effects are masked by other strategies to optimize neonatal outcome.[9]

Taking these results into account, it has been suggested that routine prophylactic amnioinfusion for labors complicated by meconium-stained amniotic fluid is not warranted.[10]

Dilemmas

Use of Prophylactic Antibiotics in the Prevention of Maternal or Neonatal Sepsis in Meconium-stained Amniotic Fluid

There is insufficient evidence to support the use of prophylactic antibiotics in women with MSAF because the rates of neonatal sepsis were not different in the two groups.[11]

Is there a Relation between the Duration of Labor and Fetal Outcomes in MSAF?

In a prospective study including 344 deliveries with MSAF, it was found that meconium aspiration (MA) was significantly related to longer length of labor.[12]

REFERENCES

1. National Institute for Health and Care Excellence. Intrapartum Care for Healthy Women and Babies. NICE Guideline (CG190). London, UK: National Institute for Health and Care Excellence; 2014.
2. Mid Essex Hospital Services NHS Trust. Management of Meconium Stained Liquor (Clinical Guidelines no. 04259); 2016.
3. Fanaroff AA. Meconium aspiration syndrome: historical aspects. J Perinatol. 2008;28(Suppl 3):S3-7.
4. Lin H, Wu S, Wu J, et al. Meconium aspiration syndrome: experiences in Taiwan. J Perinatol. 2008;28:S43-8.
5. Hernandez C, Little BB, Dax JS, et al. Prediction of the severity of meconium aspiration syndrome. Am J Obstet Gynecol. 1993;169:61-70.
6. Rossi EM, Philipson EH, Williams TG, et al. Meconium aspiration syndrome: intrapartum and neonatal attributes. Am J Obstet Gynecol. 1989;161:1106-10.
7. Starks GC. Correlation of meconium-stained amniotic fluid, early intrapartum pH, and Apgar scores as predictors of perinatal outcome. Obstet Gynecol. 1980;56:604-9.
8. Hageman JR. Meconium staining of the amniotic fluid: the need for reassessment of management by obstetricians and pediatricians. Curr Probl Pediatr. 1993;23:396-401.
9. Hofmeyr G, Xu H, Eke AC. Amnioinfusion for meconium-stained liquor in labor. Cochrane Database Syst Rev. 2014;(1):CD000014.
10. ACOG Committee Obstetric Practice. Amnioinfusion does not prevent meconium aspiration syndrome. ACOG Committee Opinion No. 346. Obstet Gynecol. 2006;108:1053-5.
11. Siriwachirachai T, Sangkomkamhang US, Lumbiganon P, et al. Antibiotics for meconium-stained amniotic fluid in labor for preventing maternal and neonatal infections. Cochrane Database Syst Rev. 2014;11:CD007772.
12. Alchalabi H, Abu-Heija AT, El-Sunna E, et al. Meconium-stained amniotic fluid in term pregnancies: a clinical view. J Obstet Gynaecol. 1999;19(3):262-4.

Chapter 35

Placental Adhesive Disorders

Taruna Sharma, Bindiya Gupta

INTRODUCTION

Placental adhesive disorders are a group of conditions with abnormal placental implantation and firm adherence, which are classified according to the depth of invasion. These disorders are associated with considerable maternal and fetal morbidity and mortality. The incidence of placental adhesive disorders is rising as the frequency of cesarean section has increased over the past few decades **(Table 1)**.[1] It occurs in 1:2500 deliveries and has increased tenfold in the past 50 years. Timely diagnosis during the antenatal period, on the contrary, allows for optimal planning of a multidisciplinary management approach and delivery at a tertiary care institution.

CLASSIFICATION (ALGORITHM 1)

- *Placenta accreta:* Chorionic villi adhered to the myometrium with no intermediate decidual layer.
- *Placenta increta:* Chorionic villi invade into the myometrium.
- *Placenta percreta:* Chorionic villi completely penetrate the myometrium reaching serosa and invading surrounding structures.

Placenta accreta is further classified on basis of the number of lobules involved:
- *Total placenta accreta:* Involve all lobes.
- *Partial placenta accreta:* Involve at least two but not all lobules.
- *Focal placenta accreta:* Involve only a single lobule.

Table 1: Risk of placenta accreta in women with previous cesarean section (CS).

No. of prior CS	Risk of placenta accreta (%)
0	3.3
1	11
2	40
3	61
4+	67

Algorithm 1: Classification of placental adhesive disorders.

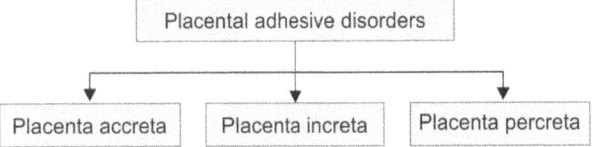

RISK FACTORS[2]

- Advanced maternal age (>35 years)
- Multiparity (>6 pregnancies)
- Prior cesarean delivery **(Table 1)**
- *Placenta previa:* Placenta previa is associated with 5–10% risk of accreta
- *Previous cesarean delivery with placenta previa:* Risk of placental adhesive disorders increase drastically
- Prior uterine surgery or curettage or intervention
- *Uterine pathology:* Adenomyosis, submucous fibroid, bicornuate uterus, Asherman syndrome

- Prior uterine artery embolization
- Endometrial ablation
- Manual removal of placenta
- Puerperal sepsis
- Postpartum endometritis
- In vitro fertilization (IVF) pregnancies
- Uterine irradiation
- Previous history of adherent placenta.

PATHOPHYSIOLOGY

The pathophysiology of placental adhesive disorders is discussed in **Algorithm 2**.

RADIOLOGICAL FINDINGS IN PLACENTAL ADHESIVE DISORDERS[3]

Grayscale Ultrasonography

- Obliteration of the clear space, defined as the obliteration of any part of the echolucent area located between the uterus and placenta.
- Interruption of the posterior bladder wall–uterine interface such that the usual continuous echolucent line appears instead of series of dashes.
- Visualization of placental lacunae (Swiss-cheese appearance).
- Thinning of myometrium overlying the placenta.

Color Doppler

- Vascular lakes with turbulent flow (peak systolic velocity >15 cm/sec).
- Diffuse or focal lacunar flow.
- Hypervascularity of serosa-bladder interface.
- Markedly dilated vessels over peripheral subplacental zone.

3D Power Doppler

- Hypervascularity
- Numerous coherent vessels involving the whole uterine serosa-bladder junction
- Inseparable cotyledonal and intervillous circulation, detour vessels, chaotic branching.

Magnetic Resonance Imaging

- Heterogeneous signal intensity within the placenta
- Uterine bulging
- Dark intraplacental bands on T2-weighted imaging.

MANAGEMENT[4-7]

Algorithms 3 to 6 discuss the management of placental adhesive disorders.

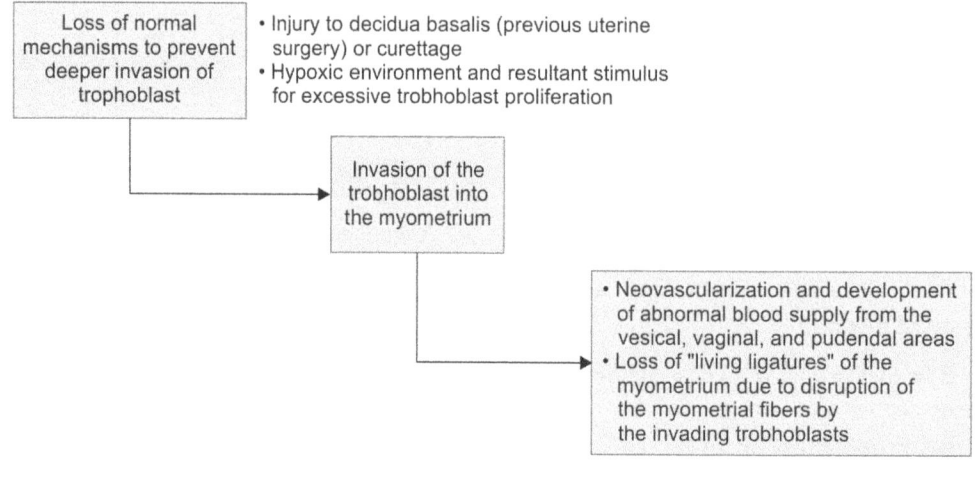

Algorithm 2: Pathogenesis of abnormal invasion of placenta.

Algorithm 3: Management in antenatal period.

- Give corticosteroid cover
- *Timing:* Electively scheduled cesarean delivery and hysterectomy at 34 weeks[5]

Preoperative checklist:[3]
- Referral to a tertiary center with experience in the management of placenta accreta preferably with facility for interventional radiology and intensive care unit.
- *Multidisciplinary team:* Senior obstetrician, neonatologist, and anesthetist. Surgical expertise from vascular surgeons, trauma surgeons, gynecological oncologists, and urologist may be required.
- A written informed consent of peripartum hysterectomy with consent for need for transfusion, intensive care unit (ICU) care, and ventilation should be taken. Consent regarding injury to pelvic structures should also be taken.
- All required blood products, including red blood cells, fresh frozen plasma, and platelets should be available. Facility for cell salvage techniques may be helpful.
- Arrange hemostatic agents like Factor VIIa, etc.
- The decision to use balloon occlusion or embolization catheters should also be determined in advance.
- Preoperative ultrasound for placental mapping to determine the upper edge of the placenta.

Counsel the woman and her family about suspected diagnosis, the need for operative delivery, massive hemorrhage, multiple blood transfusions, and possible hysterectomy.

Algorithm 4: Surgical management.

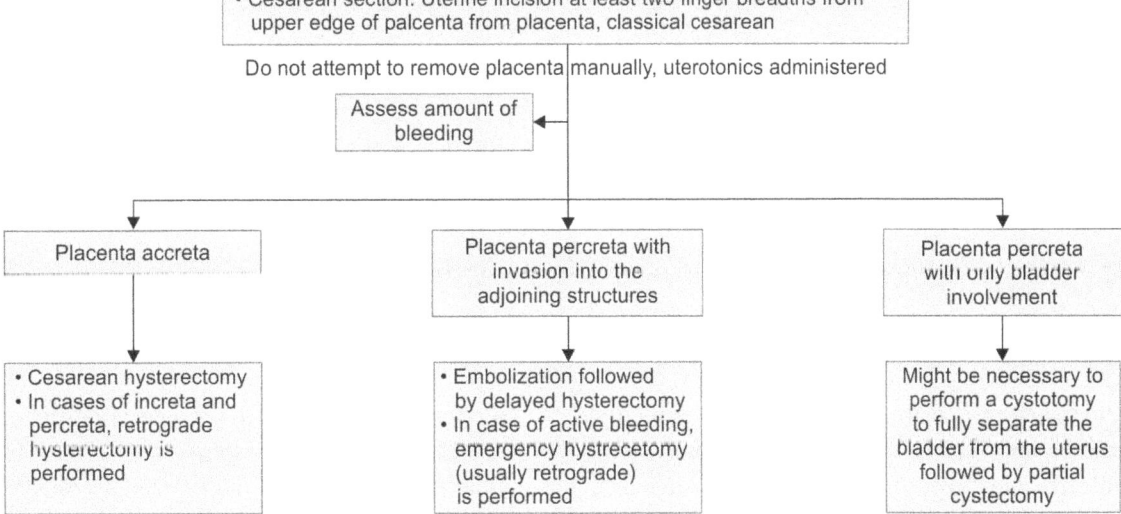

Measures to Prevent Urinary Tract Injuries

- Using preoperative cystoscopy to check for obvious bladder wall involvement.
- Placement of large bore ureteral stents to make for easier palpation.
- Filling the bladder with methylene blue prior to bladder mobilization.
- Postsurgery do a methylene blue dye test to check bladder integrity.

Measures to Reduce Blood Loss

- *Pelvic artery embolization:* Embolization catheters can be placed preoperatively under fluoroscopic guidance, balloon inflation done postdelivery in the internal iliac

Algorithm 5: Conservative management.[6]

Indications:
Only planned elective cases
- Preservation of fertility is of prime importance and/or upfront hysterectomy carries an unacceptably high risk of hemorrhage or injury to adjacent tissues

Prerequisites:
- No predisposing factor for sepsis
- Patient willing for close follow-up, highly motivated, and counseled
- Patient and relatives should be counseled of the complications including delayed hemorrhage, disseminated intravascular coagulopathy, endomyometritis, sepsis, need for delayed hysterectomy, recurrence (up to 30%), and adhesion formation (10–14%)

- **Hands off approach (Expectant management)**
  - Cut the cord at placental insertion and leave placenta in situ
  - Other adjunctive measures like uterotonics, compression sutures, balloon tamponade, internal iliac and/or uterine artery ligation reduce uterine perfusion, and embolization decrease postpartum hemorrhage, and expedite placental resorption.
  - Broad-spectrum antibiotics for 2 weeks
  - Weekly follow-up with βhCG and Doppler USG
  - Methotrexate not recommended
- **Placental-myometrial en bloc excision and repair***

If significant bleeding occurs on follow-up, do Doppler USG to
- *No vascularity*: Hysteroscopic resection of retained adherent placenta
- *If vascularity present*: Uterine artery embolization
- *If bleeding persists*: Delayed hysterectomy see vascularity of placenta

*Especially in cases with focal accreta with a margin of myometrium. Contraindicated in percreta, parametrial extension, and deep infiltration into the cervix.

Triple P procedure:[7]
This procedure involves three steps:
1. Preoperative placental localization to identify the superior border of the placenta and transverse cesarean scar is planned two fingerbreadths above the uppermost placental edge.
2. Preoperative placement of intra-arterial balloon catheters which are inflated after delivery or internal iliac artery ligation for proximal vascular control.
3. No attempt to remove the placenta with en bloc myometrial excision and uterine repair. During the excision, a 2 cm margin of myometrium is preserved above the bladder edge to allow hysterotomy closure.

Algorithm 6: Management of retained adherent placenta during vaginal delivery.[8]

The diagnosis is often made when plane of cleavage between placenta and uterine wall is not identified during manual removal

Focal placenta accreta
- Remove as much placental tissue as possible
- Achieve hemostasis with oxytocics and if required, uterine tamponade
- Uterine artery embolization if facilities available
- Do a follow-up ultrasound with Doppler
* An early decision of hysterectomy ± internal iliac artery ligation should be taken in case of excessive bleeding

Total placenta accreta
- **Bleeding persists**
  - Emergency hysterectomy
- **Not actively bleeding, stable vitals**
  - *Desirous of future fertility*: Conservative approach as detailed above
  - *Multiparous*: Hysterectomy can be offered after counseling

artery to secure proximal control of bleeding, if needed, hemostatic substances can then be administered via the catheters. To be used if bleeding ensues or in the case of patients with obstetric hemorrhage after delivery.
- Ligation of anterior division of internal iliac artery.

COMPLICATIONS

- Massive obstetrical hemorrhage with blood loss to the extent of 3,000–5,000 mL.[9]
- Surgical injury to bladder, bowel, ureters, or neurovascular structures.
- Requirement of blood and blood products—almost 90% patients may require blood transfusion.[10]
- Disseminated intravascular coagulation, acute transfusion reaction, adult respiratory syndrome, acute renal failure, and electrolyte imbalance.
- High maternal mortality (7–8%) in spite of planned approach to delivery, best surgical care, and availability of blood and blood products.[10]
- Most common indication for cesarean hysterectomy—38%.[11]

REFERENCES

1. Silver RM, Landon MB, Rouse DJ, et al. National Institute of Child Health and Human Development Maternal–Fetal Medicine Units Network. Maternal morbidity associated with multiple repeat cesarean deliveries. Obstet Gynecol. 2006;107:1226-32.
2. Fitzpatrick KE, Sellers S, Spark P, et al. Incidence and risk factors for placenta accreta/increta/percreta in the UK: a national case-control study. PLoS One. 2012;7(12):e52893.
3. RCOG. Placenta praevia, and vas praevia: diagnosis and management: Greentop guideline no. 27. [online] Available at: http://www.rcog.org.uk/files/rcog-corp/GTG27PlacentaPraeviaJanuary2011.pdf [Last accessed September, 2019].
4. Perez-Delboy A, Wright JD. Surgical management of placenta accreta: to leave or remove the placenta? BJOG. 2014;121:163-70.
5. Goh WA, Zalud I. Placenta accreta: diagnosis, management and the molecular biology of the morbidly adherent placenta. J Matern Fetal Neonatal Med. 2016;29(11):1795-800.
6. Fox KA, Shamshirsaz AA, Carusi D, et al. Conservative management of morbidly adherent placenta: expert review. Am J Obstet Gynecol. 2015;213(6):755-60.
7. Chandraharan E, Rao S, Belli AM, et al. The Triple-P procedure as a conservative surgical alternative to peripartum hysterectomy for placenta percreta. Int J Gynaecol Obstet. 2012;117(2):191-4.
8. Royal Cornwall Hospitals. Retained Placenta - Clinical Guideline For Diagnosis And Management. Treliske, UK: Royal Cornwall Hospitals, NHS; 2014.
9. Hudon L, Belfort MA, Broome DR. Diagnosis and management of placenta percreta: a review. Obstet Gynecol Surv. 1998;53:509-17.
10. O'Brien JM, Barton JR, Donaldson ES. The management of placenta percreta: conservative and operative strategies. Am J Obstet Gynecol. 1996;175:1632-8.
11. Shellhaas CS, Gilbert S, Landon MB, et al. The frequency and complication rates of hysterectomy accompanying cesarean delivery. Eunice Kennedy Shriver National Institutes of Health and Human Development Maternal-Fetal Medicine Units Network. Obstet Gynecol. 2009;114:224-9.

Section 4

Delivery

- **Episiotomy**
  Kalpana Negi, Aanya Sharma

- **Instrumental Vaginal Delivery**
  Reeti Mehra

- **Cesarean Section**
  Parul Kotdawala, Munjal Pandya

- **Breech**
  Kiran Guleria, Richa Sharma

- **Transverse Lie**
  Vaishali Korde Nayak, Parag Biniwale

- **Cord Prolapse**
  Taru Gupta, Mansi Dhingra, Snigdha Kumari

- **Shoulder Dystocia**
  Anupama Bahadur

- **Injuries of Birth Canal**
  Manju Puri, Shilpi Nain

- **Postpartum Hemorrhage**
  Sayeba Akhtar

- **Retained Placenta**
  Vandana Bhuriya

- **Maternal Collapse**
  Pratima Mittal, Jyotsna Suri

- **Uterine Inversion**
  Parneet Kaur

- **Sepsis and Septic Shock**
  Latika Chawla

Chapter 36

Episiotomy

Kalpana Negi, Aanya Sharma

DEFINITION

Episiotomy is a surgical incision given in the perineum and posterior vaginal wall in the second stage of labor to facilitate delivery. It is surgically planned second-degree tear and is one of the most common surgeries performed on woman.

AIM

- To enlarge the vaginal introitus and facilitate delivery
- To prevent soft tissue tearing which may involve anal sphincter and rectum
- To facilitate manipulation in malposition and malpresentations
- To prevent over-stretching of perineal muscles and fascia
- To prevent sudden compression and decompression of fetal head.

Episiotomy should be used in selective case. Routine use not recommended.

INDICATIONS

- Inelastic perineum causing arrest or delay in descent of presenting part
- Perineal tear anticipated, e.g. big baby, occipito-posterior, and face delivery
- Anticipating manipulation, e.g. breech delivery, shoulder dystocia, twin with second baby breech, or transverse
- Operative delivery, e.g. forceps delivery and ventouse delivery
- Previous perineal surgery, e.g. pelvic floor repair and pelvic reconstructive surgery.

ADVANTAGES

- Episiotomy is easy to repair and healing is better than lacerated wound
- Reduces trauma to the pelvic floor muscles—that reduces incidence of UV prolapse and perhaps urinary incontinence
- Minimizes intracranial injuries, especially in premature babies and after coming head of the breech
- Reduces duration of second stage.[1]

DISADVANTAGES

- Increases maternal blood loss
- Increases depth of posterior perineal injury[2]
- Postpartum pain is more as compared to natural tears[3]
- Risk of injury to anal sphincter in midline episiotomy
- Risk of laceration in subsequent vaginal delivery.[4]

TYPES

There are four main types of episiotomy (**Fig. 1**):
1. Median or midline
2. Mediolateral
3. Lateral
4. J-shaped.

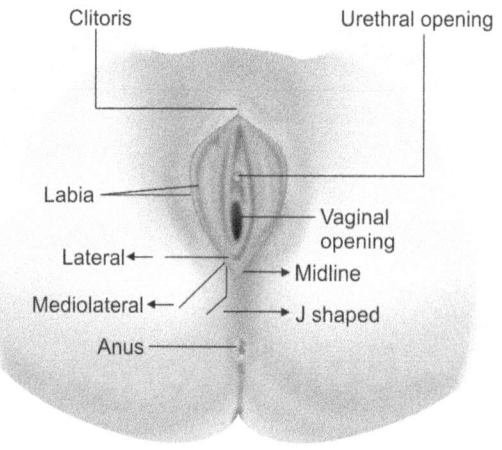

Fig. 1: Different types of episiotomy incisions.

	Midline	Mediolateral	Lateral	J-shaped
Merits	• Blood loss is less as muscles are not cut • Easy to repair • Healing is better • Wound gaping is rare • Postoperative pain and dyspareunia is least	• Involvement of anal sphincter and rectum rare • Episiotomy can be extended if required • Most commonly used method	Chances of injury to the sphincter and rectum not there	• Chances of injury to the anal sphincter and rectum less • Muscles cut are less
Demerits	Chances of injury to anal sphincter and rectum, especially in instrumental and manipulative deliveries where chances of extension is more[5]	• Blood loss is more than midline • Apposition of tissues not as good • Wound gaping is relatively more • Postoperative pain and dyspareunia is more	• Chances of injury to Bartholin's duct • Blood loss more • Tissue injury more • Not recommended	• Apposition of the tissues poor • Not done widely

Table 1: Merits and demerits of various types of episiotomy.

Midline: From the midpoint of the fourchette toward anus for about 2.5 cm.

Mediolateral: Starts from midpoint of fourchette, downward and outward, 45° to either right or left side for about 3–4 cm.

Lateral: Incision starts from about 1 cm away from center of the fourchette and extends laterally.

J-shaped: The incision starts from the center of fourchette toward anus for about 1 cm and then directed downward and outward in a J-shaped manner.

In current obstetrics, only midline and mediolateral procedures have someplace.

Relative merits and demerits of various types of episiotomy are listed in **Table 1**.

STEPS OF MEDIOLATERAL EPISIOTOMY

Equipment

- Sterile gown and gloves
- Sterile drapes
- Antiseptic solutions, e.g. povidone-iodine
- Gauze and swabs
- Episiotomy scissors, sponge holder, needle holder, tooth forceps, arteries
- 10 mL syringe, 1% lignocaine
- Suture material.

Preliminaries

- The patient should be preferably in dorsal or dorsolithotomy position.
- The perineum cleaned with swabs soaked in povidone-iodine and draped with sterile sheets.
- 10 mL of 1% lignocaine is infiltrated around the line of incision in a fan-shaped manner.

Procedure

- Index and middle finger of opposite hand are placed inside the vagina between the perineum and presenting part.
- The incision is made with episiotomy scissors with blunt side of the blade placed inside between fingers and posterior vaginal wall.
- The incision is made from midpoint of fourchette to either right or left as per surgeon's convenience, diagonally for about 2–3 cm or as per requirement.
- Incision should be given at the height of contraction.
- The scissors should be kept more laterally in a thin, stretched perineum so that when the tissues recoil after the delivery incision comes to about 45°.
- If delivery does not follow immediately, pressure should be applied at the site with a swab or gauze.
- Controlled delivery of the head should be done to avoid extension.

Timing of the Episiotomy

- The episiotomy should be given in second stage when presenting part is visible and is stretching the perineum.
- If done early, the blood loss may be more.
- Extent of incision to be given can be assessed accurately at this time.
- In case of forceps delivery, it should be done after application of the blades, i.e. after confirmation that forceps is properly placed and can be easily locked.

Structures Involved

- Posterior vaginal wall
- Superficial and deep transverse perineal muscles
- Bulbospongiosus and part of levator ani
- Fascia covering the muscles
- Transverse perineal branches of pudendal vessels and nerves
- Subcutaneous tissue
- Skin of the perineum.

REPAIR OF EPISIOTOMY

Purpose of Repair

- To control bleeding
- To assist healing
- To prevent infection.

Timing of Repair

- Repair is done soon after expulsion of placenta.
- If done earlier, disruption of wound may occur in case where manual removal of placenta or exploration of cervix and vagina is needed.
- If delayed, effect of local anesthesia may wear off and also chances of sepsis are more.

Suture Used

- Chromic catgut "0"
- Polyglactin 910 suture, e.g. Vicrylrapide "20"
- Polyglycolic acid, e.g. Dexone 11.

Prerequisite

- Adequate exposure
- Good light source from behind
- Adequate anesthesia
- Blood clots should be cleared from vagina
- Laceration should be looked for before the repair of episiotomy.

Principles of Repair

- Strict asepsis to be maintained
- Good anatomical reapproximation
- Hemostasis should be ensured
- All dead spaces should be closed
- Minimal sutures material and suture without tension.

Order of Repair

- Vaginal mucosa and submucosal tissue
- Perineal muscles
- Subcutaneous tissue and skin.

Method of Repair

There are wide variations in technique and the suture material used for repair of episiotomy:

- *Traditional interrupted technique:* This method is most commonly used. The repair is done in three stages. A continuous locking stitch starting from just above the apex and finishing at the level of fourchette with a loop knot. The perineal muscles are re-approximated by interrupted sutures. Finally, skin closed by interrupted mattress suture.
- *Two-staged method:* In this technique, vaginal mucosa and perineal muscles are closed as in traditional interrupted technique but skin is apposed, not sutured.
- *Continuous nonlocking technique:* Here the repair begins just above the apex of the tear, mucosa, and submucosal tissue closed with a single continuous nonlocking stitch. The muscles are then re-approximated using similar continuous nonlocking suture in one or two layers and repair completed with subcuticular stitch and secured with a knot in the vagina just above hymenal remnants. A single length of absorbable suture material is used with no knots other than first and the terminal knot. This method has an advantage in terms of less pain in the immediate postpartum period, less need for analgesia, and less use of suture material.[6]

POSTOPERATIVE CARE

Immediate Care

- Clean the area and check for bleeding.
- Remove all swabs or vaginal pack if used.
- Apply antiseptic ointment and keep a sterile pad.

Patient should be observed for 2 hours. She may be allowed to roll over or sit with thighs apposed. Patient may be allowed to move out of the bed as soon as she feels comfortable.

Postoperative Advice

- Patient should be advised to keep the area clean and dry. Wound should be cleaned with cotton swabs soaked in antiseptic solution after each time following urination and defecation. Antiseptic ointment should be applied.
- For pain relief, analgesics may be given. Sitz baths may be advised. Cold compressions or $MgSO_4$ compressions may also be used.

COMPLICATIONS

Immediate

- *Excessive blood loss:* Active bleeders should be secured with arteries, and if delay in delivery, incision should be pressed with sterile gauze.
- *Extension of incision through the sphincter and rectal mucosa:* Though it is more common with midline episiotomy, it may also occur with mediolateral episiotomy, e.g. when the episiotomy is inadequate, forceps delivery, shoulder dystocia, fetopelvic disproportion, fetal anomalies, and malpositions.

Early

- Vulval hematoma
- Infection
- Wound dehiscence
- Rectovaginal fistula
- Necrotizing fasciitis (rare).

Remote

- Dyspareunia
- Perineal tear in subsequent delivery
- Scar endometriosis.

CONCLUSION

- Episiotomy is useful in selective cases but should not be done routinely.[7]
- There is more chance of third and fourth-degree tear in midline episiotomy.[8]
- Mediolateral episiotomy is preferred especially in operative vaginal delivery.
- Continuous suture technique has many advantages over interrupted for repair of episiotomy.[6]

REFERENCES

1. Dutta DC, Konar H (Eds). Textbook of Obstetrics including Perinatology and Contraception, 8th edition. Kolkata: New Central Book Agency (P) Std.; 2016.
2. Wooley RJ. Benefits and risks of episiotomy: a review of the English-language literature since 1980-part II. Obstet Gynecol Surv. 1995;50(11):821-35.

3. Andrew V, Thakar R, Sultan AH, et al. Evaluation of postpartum perineal pain and dyspareunia: a prospective study. Eur J Obstet Gynecol Reprod Biol. 2008;137(2):152-6.
4. Alperin M, Krohn MA, Parvamen K. Episiotomy and increase in the risk of obstetric laceration in subsequent vaginal delivery. Obstet General. 2008;111(6):1274-8.
5. Yeomans ER, Hoffman BL, Gilstrap LC, Cunningham FG (Eds). Operative Obstetrics, 3rd edition. Chennai: McGraw Hill Education (India); 2018.
6. Kettle C, Dowsell T, Ismail KMK. Continuous and interrupted suturing techniques for repair of episiotomy or second degree tears. Cochrane Database Syst Rev. 2012;11:CD000947.
7. Jiang H, Qian X, Carroli G, et al. Selective versus routine use of episiotomy for vaginal birth. Cochrane Database Sys Rev. 2017;17:CD000081.
8. Helwig JT, Thorp JM Jr, Bowes WA Jr. Does midline episiotomy increase the risk of third and fourth degree lacerations in operative vaginal deliveries? Obstet Gynecol. 1993;82(2):276-9.

Chapter 37

Instrumental Vaginal Delivery

Reeti Mehra

INTRODUCTION

Operative vaginal delivery refers to a delivery in which the operator uses forceps or a vacuum device to assist the mother in delivering the fetus. The instrument is designed to be applied to the fetal head and then the operator uses traction to extract the fetus, typically during a contraction while the mother is pushing.

INCIDENCE

In the United States, 3.5% of all deliveries are accomplished via an operative vaginal approach. The overall rate of operative vaginal delivery has been diminishing, but the proportion of operative vaginal deliveries conducted by vacuum-assisted births has been increasing and is more than four times the rate of forceps-assisted births. In the United States, rate of forceps delivery decreased from 17.7% in 1980 to 4.5% in 2006 whereas vacuum delivery increased to 8.4%. This may be explicable by increase in fear of medicolegal cases and by lack of training.[1]

The reduced use of operative vaginal delivery (OVD) and increased use of cesarean delivery at many teaching institutions has reduced the resident competency in OVD. The important questions facing our specialty today are whether we want to passively witness OVD become "a lost art" while the cesarean delivery rate continues to climb.

INDICATIONS FOR OPERATIVE VAGINAL DELIVERY

Royal College of Obstetricians and Gynaecologists (RCOG) Practice Bulletin 2011 outlined the following indications for OVD (forceps or vacuum), recognizing that no indication is absolute; cesarean delivery is also an option in these clinical settings.

Maternal

- Inadequate expulsive efforts in second stage of labor
- Maternal exhaustion (distress) in second stage of labor
- Electively where expulsive efforts (Valsalva) are to be avoided: To shorten and reduce the effects of the second stage of labor on medical conditions (e.g. cardiac disease Class III or IV, hypertensive crises, myasthenia gravis, spinal cord injury patients at risk of autonomic dysreflexia, proliferative retinopathy, severe anemia in cardiac failure).

Fetal

- Nonreassuring fetal condition as evidenced by fetal bradycardia or tachycardia in second stage.
- Aftercoming head of the breech.
- Abruptio placentae or cord prolapse in second stage.

Others

Prolonged second stage of labor (nullipara >2 hr; multipara >1 hr, add 1 hr more if patient is in epidural analgesia).

OPERATIVE VAGINAL DELIVERY

Classification of Operative Vaginal Deliveries (Table 1)[2]

Table 1: Classification of operative vaginal delivery.[3]

Type of procedure	Criteria
Outlet	• Scalp is visible at the introitus without separating the labia • Fetal skull has reached the level of the pelvic floor • Sagittal suture is in the direct anteroposterior diameter or in the right or left occiput anterior or posterior position • Fetal head is at or on the perineum • Rotation is ≤45°
Low	• Leading point of the fetal skull (station) is station +2/+5 or more but has not as yet reached the pelvic floor • Rotation is ≤45° • Rotation is >45°
Mid-pelvic	The head is engaged in the pelvis but the presenting part is above +2 station
High	(Not included in this classification)

Prerequisites for Operative Vaginal Delivery

Prerequisites for Operative Vaginal Delivery (Forceps or Vacuum Application) (RANZOG 2009)[3,4]

Fetal and Maternal Criteria

- Fetal:
  - Fetal head engaged (head is <1/5 palpable per abdomen)
  - The cervix must be fully dilated
  - The membranes must be ruptured
  - Fetal head position and station is exactly known
  - Pelvis deemed adequate.
- Maternal:
  - Bladder must be emptied
  - Adequate maternal analgesia (regional block for mid-cavity or pudendal block)
  - Informed consent (verbal or written) with a prior clear explanation.

Others

- Experienced operator
- Aseptic techniques
- Back-up plan in case of failure
- Presence of a neonatologist
- Willingness to abandon the procedure when difficulties faced.

A mnemonic used to remember the prerequisites is:

FFFFORCE

F: Favorable presentation: cephalic, face with mento-anterior or aftercoming head of breech in forceps application
F: Favorable position: +2 or more
F: Favorable rotation: up to 45° rotation
F: Fully dilated cervix
O: No undue OBSTRUCTION, no undue cephalopelvic disproportion
R: Ruptured membranes
C: CONSENT taken and adequately CONTRACTING and relaxing uterus
E: EMPTY bladder and EPISIOTOMY.

Forceps

In present day practice, the commonly used forceps used are:

- Long curved forceps
- Short curved or outlet forceps, also called Wrigley's forceps
- Keilland forceps: only where technical expertise is available.

Long and short curved forceps: The long curved forceps measures 37 cm in length, distance between the tips is 2.5 cm and widest distance is 9.5 cm. The blades are fenestrated to provide a good grip on the fetal head and avoid slippage during extraction of the fetal head. The parts of the forceps are blades, shank, handle, and lock and are called right or left in relation to the maternal pelvis in which they lie. The long curved forceps may have a slot for the axis traction device. The blades have an upper pelvic curve and an inner fetal curve which grasps the fetal head. The lock is commonly the English lock which can be applied only when the left blade is applied first.

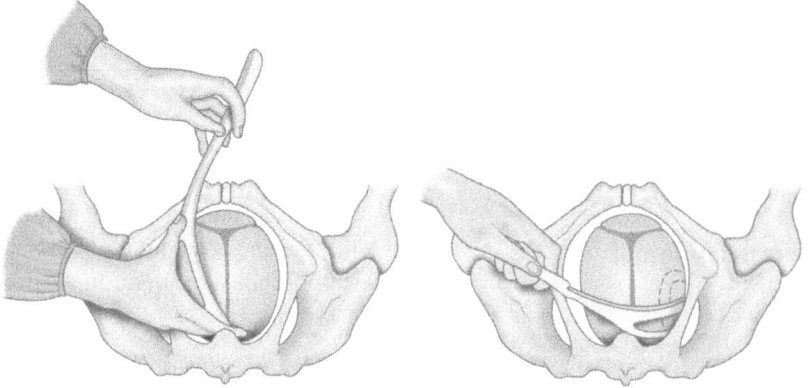

Fig. 1: Applying the left blade of the forceps.

The outlet forceps is also similar in every respect except for a shorter length of the shanks and is meant to be applied when the fetal head is on the perineum.

The Keilland forceps can be applied in relation to the position of the fetal head, i.e. in a cephalic manner. It can correct asynclitism. It is a diminishing art and is technically difficult to apply and can cause considerable maternal trauma, which is primarily why it has lost its popularity and in modern-day, most obstetricians are not familiar with its use.

Technique: Safe and effective use of forceps depends on good technique. Assemble the forceps before application. Ensure that the parts fit together and lock well. Lubricate the blades of the forceps. Wearing sterile gloves, insert two fingers of the right hand into the vagina on the side of the fetal head. Slide the left blade gently between the head and fingers to rest on the side of the head **(Fig. 1)**.

Repeat the same maneuver on the other side, using the left hand and the right blade of the forceps **(Fig. 2)**.

Depress the handles and lock the forceps. Difficulty in locking usually indicates that the application is incorrect. In this case, remove the blades and recheck the position of the head. Reapply only if rotation is confirmed.

After locking, apply steady traction inferiorly and posteriorly till the vertex reaches the pelvic floor, then directly posteriorly till the subocciput hinges under the symphysis pubis and then upward and forward to deliver the vertex and the face. Traction is given only with each contraction. After delivery of the head, remove the right blade first followed by the left one.[5]

Complications of forceps operation: The complication of the forceps operation is mostly related to the faulty technique and to the indication for which the forceps are applied rather than the instrument. The hazards are grouped into:

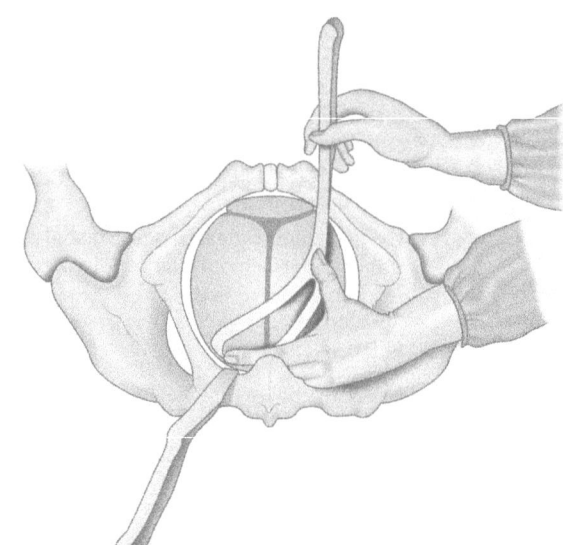

Fig. 2: Applying the right blade of the forceps.

Maternal:
- Immediate:
  - Injury: Vaginal laceration or sulcus tear, cervical tear, extension of episiotomy to involve the vaginal vault, complete perineal tear
  - Nerve injury:
    - Femoral (I.2, 3, 4)
    - Lumbosacral trunk (L4,5) with mid-forceps delivery.
  - Postpartum hemorrhage may be: (1) traumatic or (2) atonic, requiring blood transfusion or (3) both, may cause shock

- Anesthetic complications (following local or general anesthesia)
- Puerperal sepsis and maternal morbidity.
• *Remote:* Painful perineal scars, dyspareunia, low backache, genital prolapse, stress urinary incontinence, and anal sphincter dysfunction.

Fetal:
• Asphyxia, facial bruising, intracranial hemorrhage (rupture of the great vein of Galen). Cephalohematoma, facial palsy, skull fractures, cervical spine injury (rotational forceps).
• *Remote:* Cerebral or spastic palsy due to residual cerebral injury (rare).

Prophylactic forceps (Elective): This type of forceps operation was named after De Lee. It refers to forceps delivery only to shorten the second stage of labor when maternal and/or fetal complications are anticipated. The indications are: (1) eclampsia; (2) heart disease; (3) previous history of cesarean section; (4) postmaturity; (5) low-birth weight baby; and (6) to curtail the painful second stage.

It prevents possible fetal cerebral injury due to pressure on the perineum and spares the other from the strain of bearing down efforts. Prophylactic forceps should not be applied until the criteria of low forceps are fulfilled.

Trial forceps: It is a tentative attempt of forceps delivery in a case of suspected mid-pelvic contraction with a preamble declaration of abandoning it in favor of cesarean section if moderate traction fails to overcome the resistance. The procedure should be conducted in an operation theater keeping everything ready for cesarean section. The conduct of the fetal head, the delivery, is completed vaginally, if not, cesarean section is done immediately. Many unnecessary cesarean sections or difficult vaginal deliveries can thus be avoided.

Failed forceps: When a deliberate attempt in vaginal delivery with forceps has failed to expedite the process, it is called failed forceps. It is often due to poor clinical judgment and skill. Failure in the operative delivery may be due to improper application.

Causes: The common causes are: (1) incompletely dilated cervix; (2) unrotated occipitoposterior position; (3) cephalopelvic disproportion; (4) unrecognized malpresentation (brow) or hydrocephalus; (5) constriction ring; (6) clinically big baby (>4 kg); and (7) maternal body mass index (BMI) > 30.

The ACOG 2016 Practice Bulletin recommends that "judicious use of operative vaginal delivery for infants with suspected macrosomia is not contraindicated". The authors do point out that the adequacy of the pelvis and the progress of labor, especially the second stage, should be carefully considered in this setting and preparations made for possible shoulder dystocia.

Ventouse

Ventouse is an instrumental device designed to assist delivery by creating a vacuum between it and the fetal scalp.

Technique: A useful mnemonic, which was initially developed for forceps deliveries, has been adapted for vacuum extraction. This mnemonic is the first 10 letters of the English alphabet (given below). The vacuum should be applied with rigorous adherence to the prerequisites. Consent of the woman must be obtained and properly documented.

The proper function of the vacuum equipment should be determined before the cup is applied. The cup is applied by compressing it in an anteroposterior diameter and then introducing it into the posterior fourchette while protecting the maternal tissues and making space with the opposite hand at the flexion point which is 3 cm from the posterior fontanelle **(Figs. 3 and 4)**.

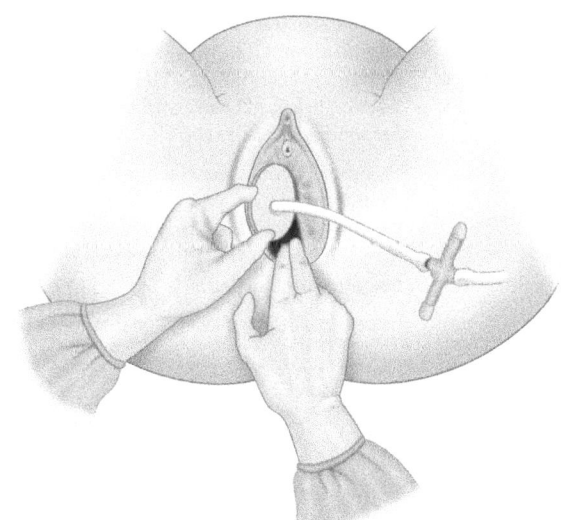

Fig. 3: Applying a vacuum cup. If using a 6 cm cup, to be over the flexion point, the leading edge should be 3 cm from the anterior fontanelle.

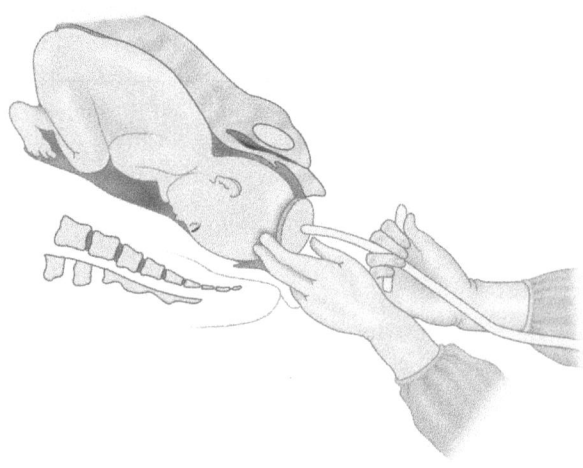

Fig. 4: Check that there is no maternal tissue included in the cup.

Vacuum Mnemonic

A	Anesthesia assistance	• Adequate pain relief • Neonatal support
B	Bladder	• Bladder empty
C	Cervix	• Fully dilated, membranes ruptured
D	Determine	• Position, station, and pelvic adequacy • Think possible shoulder dystocia
E	Equipment	• Inspect vacuum cup, pump, and tubing • Check pressure
F	Fontanelle	• Position the cup over the posterior fontanelle • Sweep finger around cup to clear maternal tissue
G	Gentle traction	• 0.2 kg/cm² initially and between contractions and increase pressure to 0.8 kg/cm² • Pull with contractions only: As contraction begins, prompt the woman for good expulsive effort • Traction in axis of birth canal and perpendicular to the cup
H	Halt	• No progress with three traction-aided contractions • Vacuum pops off three times • No significant progress after 20 minutes of operative vaginal delivery
I	Incision	Consider episiotomy if laceration imminent
J	Jaw	Remove vacuum when jaw is reachable or delivery assured

Contraindications of ventouse: (1) Any presentation other than vertex (face brow, breech); (2) preterm fetus (<34 weeks). Chance of scalp avulsion or subaponeurotic hemorrhage; (3) suspected fetal coagulation disorder; (4) suspected fetal macrosomia (>4 kg).

Contraindications for operative vaginal delivery (both for ventouse or forceps): (1) Unengaged fetal head; (2) obvious; (3) fetus having unacute bleeding diathesis (hemophilia).

Whenever operative delivery is considered, a healthcare provider skilled in newborn resuscitation should be present at the birth. This person's sole responsibility must be the care of the newborn selected.

When to Halt—beware:

- Three pulls over three contractions, no progress abandon procedure
- Three pop-offs: after one, reassess carefully before reapplying
- Reassess the patient if there is no progress in 20 minutes.

Vacuum versus Forceps Delivery

The relative benefits and risks for vacuum versus forceps delivery have been the subject of much study and debate.

A Cochrane systematic review of nine involving 1,368 women showed that soft vacuum cups compared with rigid cups were associated with a significant increase in the rate of failure (OR 1.6; 95% CI 1.2–2.3) but a significant reduction in puerperal scalp trauma (OR 0.4; 95% CI 0.3–0.6).[6]

One serious potential complication of vacuum extractions is subgaleal or subaponeurotic hemorrhage which can produce profound, irreversible, and fatal hypovolemic shock to the newborn; and can be fatal. Statistically, subgaleal hemorrhage occurs in approximately 1 in 1,000 normal spontaneous vaginal deliveries and in 46 in 1,000 vacuum extractions. Failure to recognize high pelvic station and/or cephalopelvic disproportion (CPD), and exceeding the recommended limits for the attempted vacuum extraction, are the two common errors that contribute to subgaleal hemorrhage.

Statistically, subgaleal hemorrhage occurs in approximately 1 in 1,000 normal spontaneous vaginal deliveries and in 46 in 1,000 vacuum extractions. Failure to recognize high pelvic station and/or CPD, and exceeding the recommended limits for the attempted vacuum extraction, are the two common healthcare provider errors associated with subgaleal hemorrhage.

The relative merits of vacuum extraction and forceps have been evaluated in a Cochrane systematic review of 10 randomized controlled trials, involving 2,923 women.[7] Vacuum extraction compared with forceps shows:

- A higher rate of failed delivery (OR 1.7; 95% CI 1.3–2.2), cephalohematoma (OR 2.4; 95% CI 1.7–3.4), and retinal hemorrhage is associated with use of vacuum (OR 2.0; 95% CI 1.3–3.0).
- A vacuum delivery is more likely to be associated with maternal worries about baby (OR 2.2; 95% CI 1.2–3.9).
- Significant maternal perineal and vaginal trauma is, however, more with forceps (OR 0.4; 95% CI 0.3–0.5).
- There is not much difference in delivery by cesarean section (OR 0.6; 95% CI 0.3–1.0), 5-minute Apgar scores (OR 1.7; 95% CI 1.0–2.8) or need for phototherapy (OR 1.1; 95% CI 0.7–1.8).

DOCUMENTATION

The indication, definition, and method of operative technique employed must be clearly and completely documented in all operative deliveries.[8,9] The position and station of the fetal head at the commencement of the intervention must be stated. A written note should be prepared for both the woman's and the baby's charts.

The need for the intervention must be:
- Convincing
- Compelling
- Documented.

Suggested format for a chart note that may also serve as a template to dictate a delivery summary:
- Date and time of birth
- Name of physician or other primary healthcare provider
- Indication for operative delivery
- Record of informed discussion with the woman of the risks, benefits, and options
- Position and station of the fetal head and method of assessment (i.e. vaginally and/or abdominally)
- Amount of molding and caput present
- Assessment of maternal pelvis
- Assessment of fetal heart rate and contractions
- Type of analgesia or anesthesia used, if any
- Use of episiotomy, description and timing, and details of repair
- Ease of application of vacuum or forceps
- Number of attempts and duration of traction for forceps and duration of application for vacuum (start and stop time noted), and force used
- Apgar score
- Results of cord blood analysis, if done
- Neonatal resuscitation activities, if needed
- Description of maternal and neonatal injuries, if any.

CARE AFTER OPERATIVE VAGINAL BIRTH

- Active third stage management
- Prepare for newborn resuscitation
- Umbilical arterial blood gas analysis, where laboratory facilities exist
- Examination for maternal trauma
- *Examination for neonatal trauma:*
  - Scalp trauma
  - Signs of cerebral irritation (poor sucking, listless)
  - Signs of scalp swelling, cephalohematoma, or subaponeurotic bleeds
  - The newborn should be examined carefully at the time of the initial newborn exam. Careful monitoring should be continued in the immediate neonatal period and, at minimum, a second full examination of the newborn should be completed prior to discharge. Any abnormal findings will require further investigation.
- Documentation of the indication, definition, and method of operative technique
- Review birth with the family

RECOMMENDATIONS OF ROYAL COLLEGE OF OBSTETRICIANS AND GYNAECOLOGISTS: GREEN-TOP GUIDELINE NO. 26[10]

All women should be encouraged to have continuous support during labor as this can reduce the need for OVD. Use of upright or lateral positions and avoiding epidural analgesia can reduce the need for OVD. Delayed pushing in primiparous women with an epidural can reduce the need for rotational and mid-cavity deliveries. These recommendations have Level A evidence.

A recent Cochrane review concluded that using a partogram[11] does not lead to a reduction in the incidence of operative births and use of oxytocin in second stage also does not reduce OVD.[12]

Primiparous women who received epidurals should be encouraged to bear down and push when they feel the urge and should be given an extra hour or so for the same, to reduce rotational or mid-cavity operative interventions.[13]

Verbal consent should be obtained before an operative vaginal delivery and same should be documented in the delivery notes. If circumstances allow, written consent may also be obtained. Written consent is mandatory for trial of operative vaginal delivery in theater.

An operative vaginal delivery should be performed by an operator who has the knowledge, experience, and skills necessary to assess and to use the instruments and manage complications that may arise. The operator should choose the instrument most appropriate to the clinical circumstances and their level of skill. Forceps and vacuum extraction are associated with different benefits and risks.

Operative vaginal births that have a higher risk of failure should be considered a trial and conducted in a place where immediate recourse to cesarean section can be undertaken. Higher rates of failure are associated with:
- Maternal body mass index over 30
- Estimated fetal weight over 4,000 g or clinically big baby
- Occipitoposterior position
- Mid-cavity delivery or when 1/5th of the head palpable per abdomen.

The use of episiotomy may reduce the incidence of anal sphincter injury and pelvic floor injury especially in nulliparous women and should be used liberally in instrumental vaginal deliveries.[14,15] However, routine use of episiotomy for all assisted vaginal deliveries is not recommended.[16]

Use of vacuum rotation followed by forceps extraction is referred to as sequential application of instruments. This is associated with increased maternal and fetal trauma. The operator must balance the risks versus benefits of a cesarean section or forceps following failed vacuum extraction. The neonatologist must be informed about the sequential use when this occurs to ensure appropriate management of the baby.

Prophylactic antibiotics are not routinely recommended. Strict asepsis should be ensured. Thromboprophylaxis should be provided to the mother if indicated.

There is a need for evidence-based guidelines, including standardized documentation of operative vaginal procedures. Training strategies for junior practitioners to acquire these skills and for experienced practitioners to maintain and disseminate their skills should be prioritized.

REFERENCES

1. Yeoman ER. Operative vaginal delivery. Obstet Gynecol. 2000;115(3):645-53.
2. American College of Obstetricians and Gynecologists. ACOG Practice Bulletin No. 17: Operative Vaginal Delivery. Washington, USA: ACOG; 2000.
3. Royal Australian and New Zealand College of Obstetricians and Gynaecologists (updated 2016). College Statement C-Obs 16: Instrumental vaginal delivery. Melbourne, Australia: RANZCOG. [online] Available from www.ranzcog.edu.au/publications/statements/C-obs16.pdf
4. Society of Obstetricians and Gynaecologists of Canada. Guidelines for operative vaginal birth. J Obstet Gynaecol Can. 2004;26(8):747-53.
5. WHO. (2003). Managing complications in pregnancy and childbirth: a guide for doctors and midwives. Geneva: World Health Organization. [online] Available from http://www.who.int/reproductive-health/impac/mcpc.pdf [Last accessed September, 2019].
6. Johanson RB, Menon V. Soft versus rigid vacuum extractor cups for assisted vaginal delivery. Cochrane Database Syst Rev. 2000;(4):CD000446.
7. Johanson RB, Menon V. Vacuum extraction versus forceps for assisted vaginal delivery. Cochrane Database Syst Rev. 2000;(2):CD000224.
8. Bachman J, Johanson R, Menon V. A vacuum operation needs to be documented in the same manner as any other operative procedure. Forceps delivery correspondence. J Am Acad Fam Pract. 1989;29:4.
9. Touqmatchi D, Boret T, Nicopoullous J. The quality of operative consenting against RCOG advice as standard. J Obstet Gynaecol. 2010;30(2):159-65.
10. Royal College of Obstetricians and Gynaecologists. Green Top Guidelines No. 26: Operative vaginal delivery. London: RCOG; 2011.
11. Lavender T, Hart A, Smyth RM. Effect of partogram use on outcomes for women in spontaneous labour at term. Cochrane Database Syst Rev. 2008;(4):CD005461.
12. Costley PL, East CE. Oxytocin augmentation of labour in women with epidural analgesia for reducing operative deliveries. Cochrane Database Syst Rev. 2012;5:CD009241.
13. Roberts CL, Torvaldsen S, Cameron CA, et al. Delayed versus early pushing in women with epidural analgesia: a systematic review and meta-analysis. BJOG. 2004;111(12):1333-40.
14. Deane RP. Operative vaginal delivery and pelvic floor complications. Best Pract Res Clin Obstet Gynaecol. 2019;56:81-92.
15. Boujenah J, Tigaizin A, Fermaut M, et al. Is episiotomy worthwhile to prevent obstetric anal sphincter injury during operative vaginal delivery in nulliparous women? Eur J Obstet Gynecol Reprod Biol. 2019;232:60-4.
16. Cargill YM, MacKinnon CJ. No. 148-Guidelines for Operative Vaginal Birth. J Obstet Gynaecol Can. 2018;40(2):e74-80.

Chapter 38

Cesarean Section

Parul Kotdawala, Munjal Pandya

DEFINITION

Cesarean section (CS) is a method by which the fetus is delivered through an incision over abdominal wall and uterus, after the age of viability.

The rate of CS is on rise all over the globe and the indications are changing over past few decades. The initial rise in the rates has reduced the maternal as well as neonatal morbidity and mortality. But there are claims that the rate can be decreased with cautious evaluation. Vigilant monitoring, rise in litigation, and patient preferences have contributed to the shift in the trend.

In the year 1985, at a consensus meeting organized by the WHO, International healthcare community concurred that ideal rate of cesarean sections should be between 5% and 15%.[1]

INDICATIONS

Indications can be categorized under four headings according to the urgency of terminating the pregnancy **(Algorithm 1)**. The emergency and urgent CS need to be performed within 30 minutes and 60–75 minutes, respectively after diagnosis of the conditions. CS can be scheduled or planned when there is no immediate threat to maternal as well as fetal well-being.[2]

Nonreassuring heart sound, severe cephalopelvic disproportion, and previous one or more CS are amongst the most common indications **(Algorithm 2)**.

INFORMED CONSENT

Once the CS is decided to be the preferred way of delivery, an informed consent should be taken. The patient and

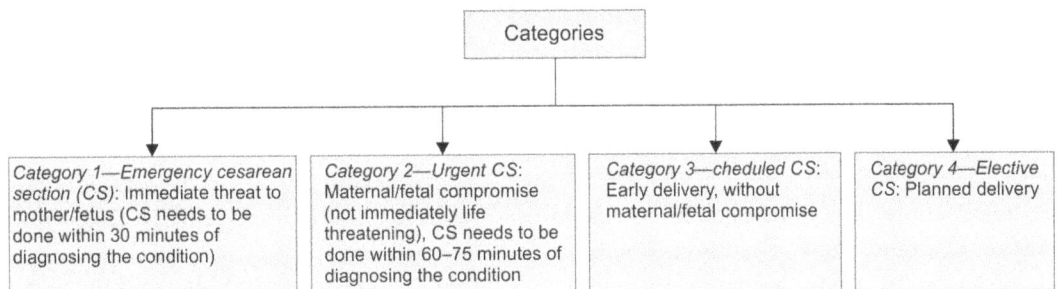

Algorithm 1: Categories of cesarean section.

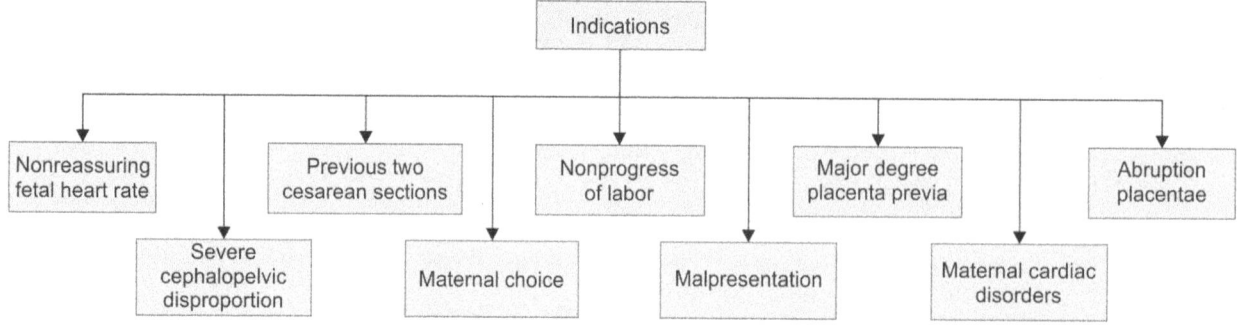

Algorithm 2: Indications of cesarean section.

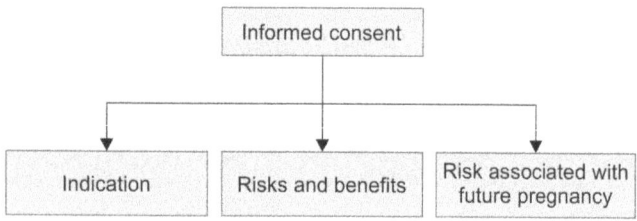

Algorithm 3: Informed consent.

relatives are explained about the indication and urgency for performing the surgery, the benefits as well as the potential risks associated.[3]

The caution regarding future pregnancy can be explained so as to make the patient aware **(Algorithm 3)**.

PREOPERATIVE PREPARATIONS

Routine blood investigations are done. Injection ceftriaxone (2 g) IV is given 1 hour before the surgery.[3]

Indwelling catheter is placed and fetal heart sounds are checked on table. X-matched packed cell volume should be available on standby in all CS and be available in OR for high-risk cases with the possibility of blood loss. Presence of neonatologist is preferred. Elastic stockings for lower limbs as a measure of thromboprophylaxis are preferred. For those who are high risk (obese, hypertensive, varicose veins), in consultation with physician, thrombolytic medications may be given **(Algorithm 4)**.

ANESTHESIA

Preanesthetic medications are administered so as to prevent chances of reflux and aspiration. Regional anesthesia is the preferred mode. Induction to delivery time is to be kept as short as possible to prevent neonatal morbidity of prolonged fetal exposure to general anesthesia **(Algorithm 5)**.

PROCEDURE

After inducing the patient, skin is prepared with antiseptic solutions. Shaving is avoided as the sharp cuts may lead to skin infection. When needed, clipping them short with scissors is preferred. A transverse incision is the norm now and the vertical incision is reserved for special situations only **(Algorithm 6)**.

Uterine incisions vary according to the condition. The most preferred one is lower segment transverse one, the edge of which may be extended upward if more space is required for delivery, on one side in form of J-shape or on both sides to make a "U." Old practice of inverted "T" by cutting up from the middle of the scar is tantamount to a classical scar and is deprecated. The classical vertical scar may not heal optimally, increasing the chances of rupture during subsequent pregnancy and delivery. In case of chorioamnionitis, extraperitoneal route can avoid spread of infection to the peritoneal cavity **(Algorithm 7)**.

Lower Uterine Segment Incision

- Visceral peritoneum is opened above the bladder fold.
- A sharp cut of 1" in the middle with knife, 1–2 cm above bladder fold is made in the lower uterine segment.
- The edges are extended by blunt extension of lower uterine segment incision, a preferred method over sharp cut with scissors as the former is associated with reduced blood loss and reduced chances of postpartum hemorrhage.
- Head is delivered after allowing liquor to be drained and delivered by guiding hand below the fetal head.

Algorithm 4: Preoperative preparation.

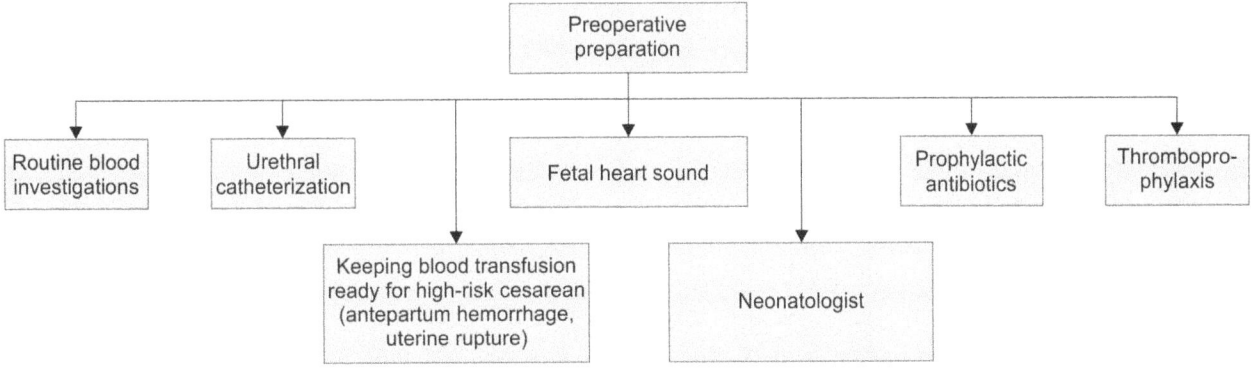

Algorithm 5: Anesthesia.

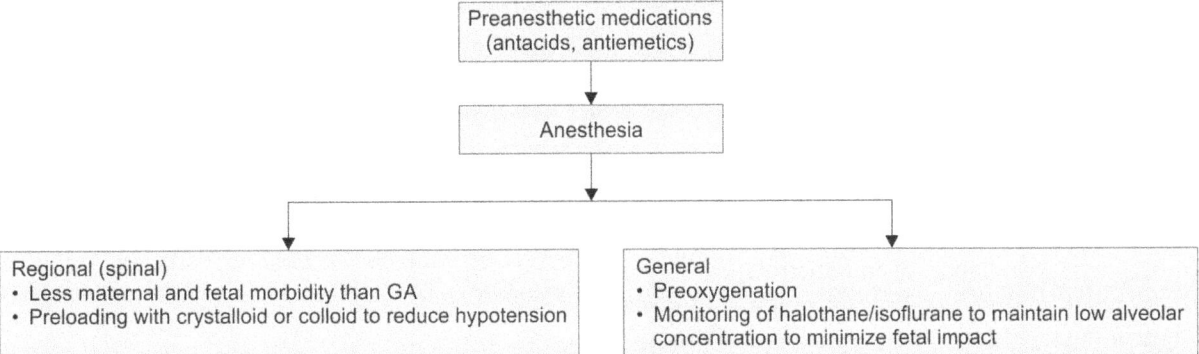

(GA: general anesthesia)

Algorithm 6: Procedure.

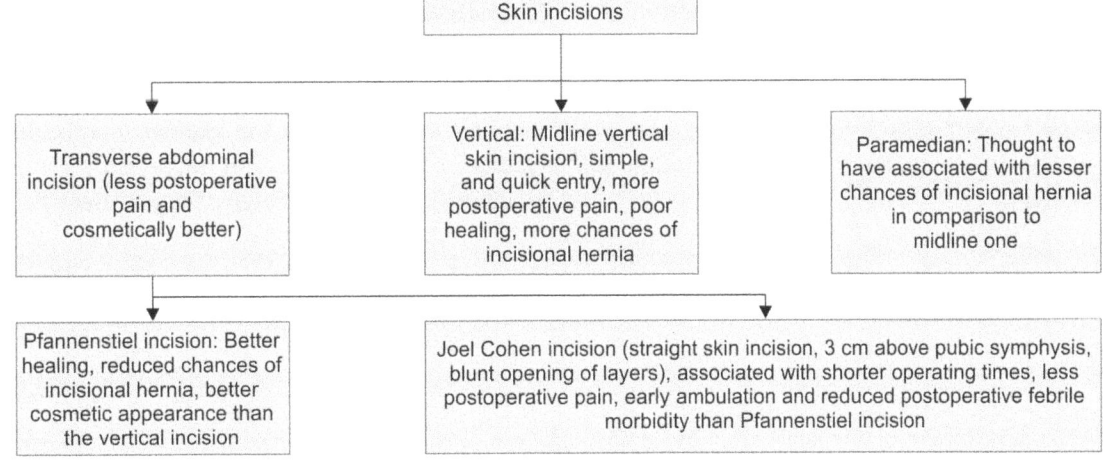

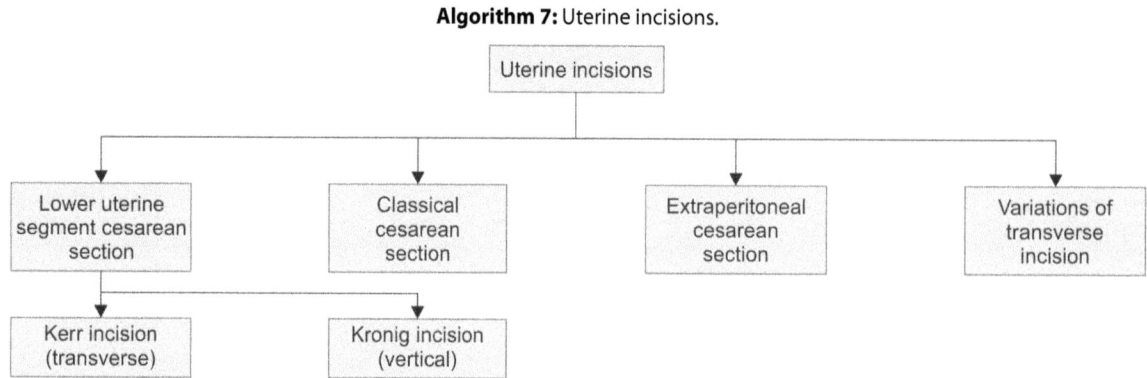

Algorithm 7: Uterine incisions.

- *Deeply engaged head:* Patwardhan, modified Patwardhan methods, elevate-rotate-reduce sequence (ERR), IV nitroglycerine. Pull from above is preferred over push from below (vagina), as the latter is associated with more maternal and neonatal morbidity.
- Vectis, Murless head extractor, head disengaging device, Snorkel are the devices tried successfully for deeply engaged head.
- *Floating head:* Forceps, vacuum, Kiwi Omni C cup.
- Uterotonics.
- Placenta removed by controlled cord traction (manual removal increases chances of endometritis).
- *Wound repair and closure:* Exteriorization of uterus is not recommended (more pain and does not improve operative outcomes), but there have been studies showing no superiority of exteriorization.
- *Single/double-layer uterine closure:* Still there are no enough conclusive evidences to support either of the methods.
- Nonclosure of visceral and parietal peritoneum (reduces operative time, postoperative analgesia, increases maternal satisfaction).

Classical Cesarean Section

- *Indications:* Huge fibroid in lower segment, placenta previa with vessels over lower segment occluding the lower segment.
- *Disadvantages:* Increased blood loss, less than optimal healing of the uterine closure, increased postoperative morbidity, and higher incidence of scar rupture in case of trial of labor in next pregnancy.

Extraperitoneal Cesarean Section

Parietal peritoneum over bladder dome exposed and incision kept over lower segment, in cases of chorioamnionitis.

Transverse incision variations: J-shaped and inverted T-shaped.

COMPLICATIONS

Surgery-related complications can be immediate and late. Mendelson syndrome can be a fatal complication related to anesthesia **(Algorithm 8)**.

POSTOPERATIVE CARE

Breastfeeding needs to be started as soon as the mother feels comfortable.[3] Patient is motivated to have early ambulation so as to get the bladder tone back, reducing chances of constipation and deep vein thrombosis, and facilitating involution of uterus **(Algorithm 9)**.

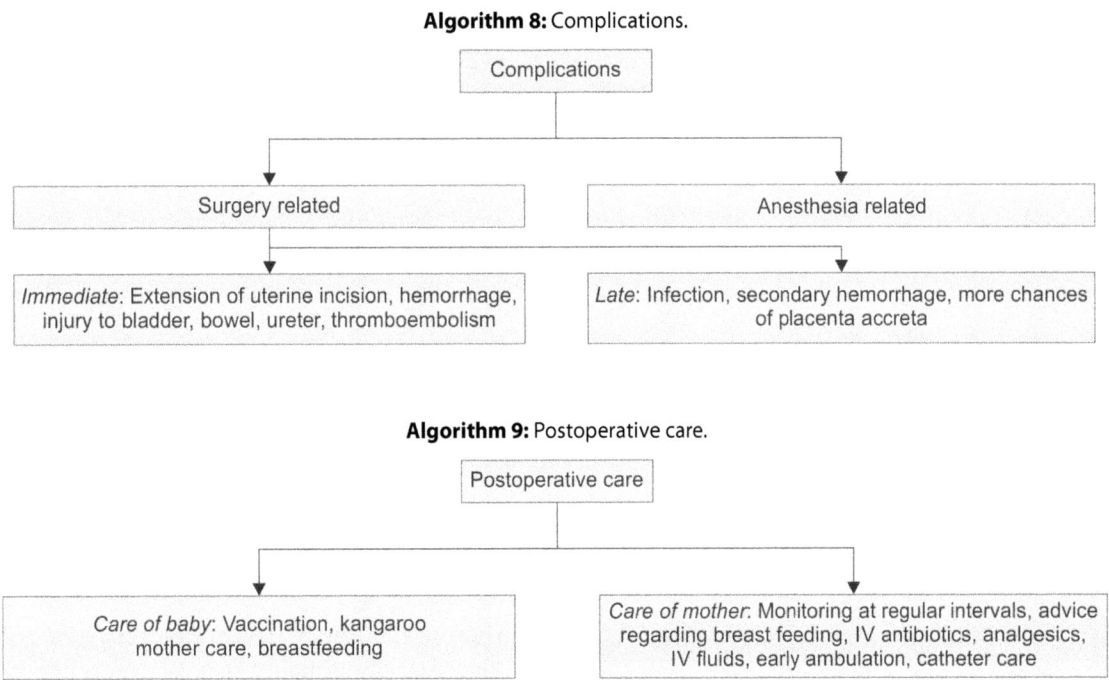

(IV: intravenous)

REFERENCES

1. World Health Organization. WHO Statement on Caesarean Section Rates. Human Reproductive Programme. Research for Impact. Geneva, Switzerland: World Health Organization; 2015.
2. Royal College of Obstetricians and Gynaecologists. Classification of Urgency of Cesarean Section – A Continuum of Risk (Good Practice No. 11). London, UK: Royal College of Obstetricians and Gynaecologists; 2010.
3. National Institute for Health and Care Excellence. (2017). Cesarean section overview. [online] Available from http://pathways.nice.org.uk/pathways/caesarean-section [Last accessed September, 2019].

Chapter 39

Breech

Kiran Guleria, Richa Sharma

INTRODUCTION

Breech presentation means that the baby is lying longitudinally with its buttocks and/or feet presenting first to the lower part of the maternal pelvis. It frequently occurs in early pregnancy, when the fetus is highly mobile within a relatively large volume of amniotic fluid.

The prevalence decreases with increasing gestational age, 20-25% of fetuses below 28 weeks present as breech, 7-16% at 32 weeks, and only 3-4% are breech at term.[1]

ETIOLOGY

Fifteen percent of breech may be due to fetal, maternal, or placental abnormalities.[1] It is hypothesized that a fetus with normal anatomy, activity, amniotic fluid volume, and placental location are likely, cephalic presentation near term because this position is best suited for the intrauterine space. In addition, a possible heritable component exists; parents who themselves were delivered as breech at term, are twice as likely to have firstborn offspring in breech presentation.

RISK FACTORS

Risk factors for breech presentation include:
- Advanced maternal age
- Multiparity (due to lax abdominal wall and more rounded intrauterine space)
- Contracted maternal pelvis
- Uterine abnormality (bicornuate or septate uterus)
- Placental abnormality (e.g. placenta previa, cornual placenta)
- Polyhydramnios or oligohydramnios
- Multiple gestations
- Short umbilical cord
- Preterm gestation
- Fetal anomaly (anencephaly, sacrococcygeal teratoma, neck masses)
- Fetal growth restriction
- Previous breech presentation.

Risk of recurrence—9% after first term breech pregnancy, 25% after two consecutive breech presentation at delivery, and almost 40% after three consecutive breech deliveries.[2]

CLINICAL FINDINGS

Signs and symptoms of breech presentation are best appreciated in the third trimester.
- *Symptoms:* Women often complain of subcostal discomfort due to the fetal head in the fundus and may perceive kicking in the lower abdomen when the breech is complete or incomplete.
- *Physical examination:* On per abdomen examination, breech presentation is characterized by the presence of a soft, irregular, and nonballotable (buttocks) structure in the lower uterine segment. On per vaginal examination, the soft buttocks, anal orifice, or feet may be identified when the cervix is dilated. A foot

is differentiated from a hand by the presence of the heel **(Algorithm 1)**.

- *Diagnosis:* Although clinical examination is diagnostic, but in certain situations (e.g. maternal obesity, leiomyoma, polyhydramnios, anterior placenta, or multiple gestations, etc.), ultrasound is more helpful.

In a resource-poor country like ours, the delivery route should be chosen based on specific healthcare infrastructure available, stage of labor, individual case (first time undiagnosed breech presentation in labor are common), availability of skilled birth attendant, and the limitations inherent in available evidence. A policy of planned cesarean delivery may not be desirable, affordable or feasible. In an individual situation, the maternal risks of cesarean, or the mother's desire to avoid cesarean delivery, may outweigh the short-term risks of vaginal birth to neonate. As both routes of delivery have similar long-term outcomes and cesarean delivery has implications for future pregnancies, planned vaginal delivery for breech may have a greater place in our country **(Algorithm 2)**.

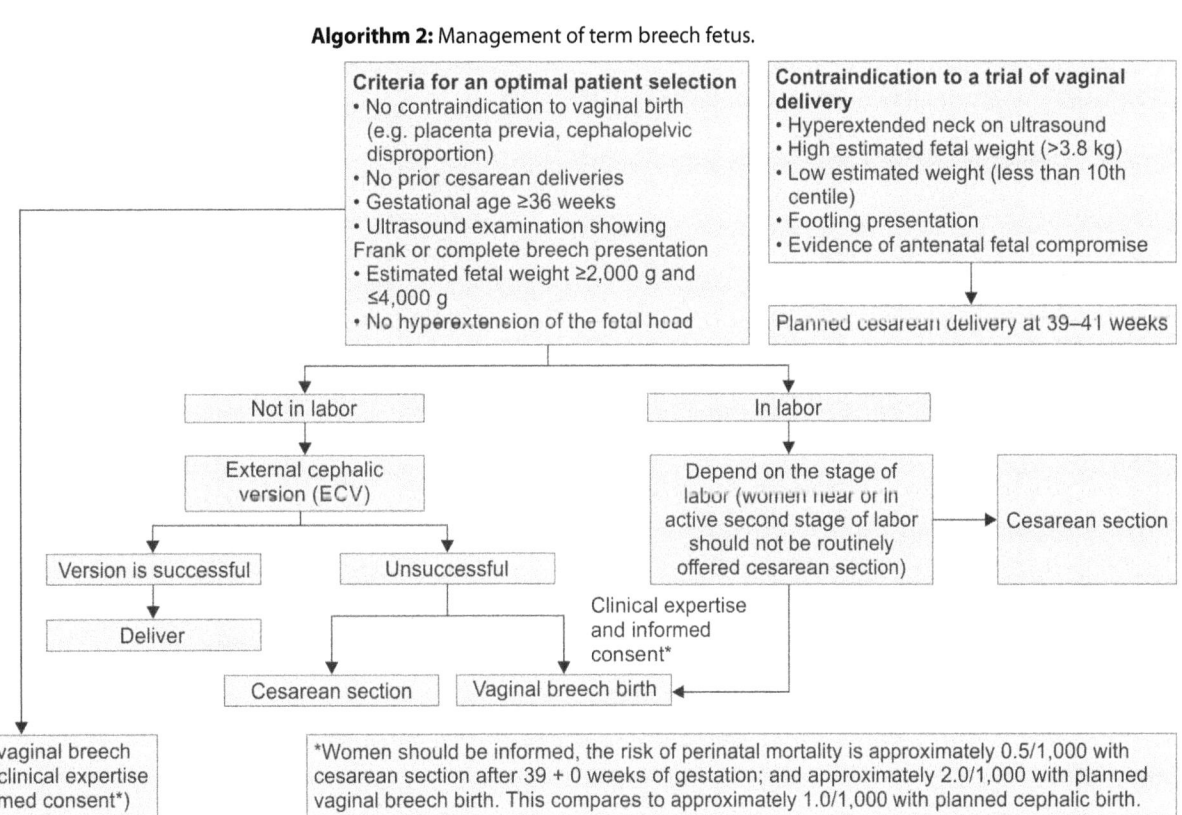

PRINCIPLES FOR THE MANAGEMENT OF VAGINAL BREECH BIRTH[3-5]

- Skilled supervision for vaginal breech birth in a hospital with facilities for immediate cesarean section.
- Assistance, without traction.
- Induction of labor is not usually recommended. Augmentation of slow progress with oxytocin should only be considered if the contraction frequency is less than 4 in 10 minutes in the presence of epidural analgesia.
- The first stage of labor should be managed according to the same principles as with a cephalic presentation.
- Continuous electronic fetal monitoring may lead to improved neonatal outcomes.
- Amniotomy is reserved for definite clinical indications.
- Selective rather than routine episiotomy.
- Descent is regarded as adequate if the breech reaches the level of the ischial spines when the cervix is 6 cm dilated and reaches the pelvic floor at full dilation.
- Passive second stage to allow the descent of the breech to the perineum prior to active pushing is recommended. If the breech is not visible within 2 hours of the passive second stage, cesarean section should be considered **(Algorithm 3)**.
- Semirecumbent or all four position for delivery.

Algorithm 3: Intrapartum management.

```
               "Hands-off" approach
                        │
         If (lack of tone, color, poor fetal
         condition, or delay of
         >5 minutes from delivery of the
         buttocks to the head,
         >3 minutes from the umbilicus
         to the head)
                        ▼
```

Assisted breech delivery
- Back to be kept anterior by gentle rotation without traction
- Once the scapula is visible, the arms can be hooked down by inserting a finger in the elbow and flexing the arms across the chest
- If nuchal, perform Lovset's maneuver for shoulder delivery
- Delivery of after coming head by Mauriceau-Smellie-Veit maneuver or with forceps
- Suprapubic pressure helps in flexion, if there is delay due to an extended neck
  Delivery using the Burns-Marshall technique is not advised due to risk of over extension of the fetal neck

Management of the Preterm Breech

Women should be informed that planned cesarean section is recommended for preterm breech presentation where delivery is planned due to maternal and/or fetal compromise. Routine cesarean section for breech presentation in spontaneous preterm labor is not recommended.[3] The mode of delivery should be individualized based on the stage of labor, type of breech presentation, fetal wellbeing, and availability of an operator skilled in vaginal breech delivery.

Management of the Twin Pregnancy with a Breech Presentation

Planned cesarean section for a twin pregnancy, where the presenting (first) twin is breech, is recommended. Routine emergency cesarean section for a breech first twin in spontaneous labor is not recommended.[3] The mode of delivery should be individualized based on cervical dilatation, station of the presenting part, type of breech presentation, fetal wellbeing, and availability of an operator skilled in vaginal breech delivery.

COMPLICATIONS

- *Maternal:* Perineal injuries, operative interventions, and increased cesarean section.
- *Perinatal:* Morbidity and mortality along with long-term neurologic sequelae are threefold higher in breech presentation than cephalic presentation particularly due to birth trauma (head and cervical spine) and asphyxia. Both intracranial and cervical spine trauma may result from head entrapment in either the uterine or abdominal incisions.

Head entrapment is a serious complication of breech delivery, where head of a term or preterm baby may be caught in a partially dilated cervix due to premature excessive maternal bearing down. It occurs in 0–8.5% of vaginal breech deliveries. This leads to acute asphyxia from compression of the umbilical cord and occipital bone damage **(Algorithms 4 and 5)**.[6]

Algorithm 4: Management of hydrocephalic fetus in breech presentation.

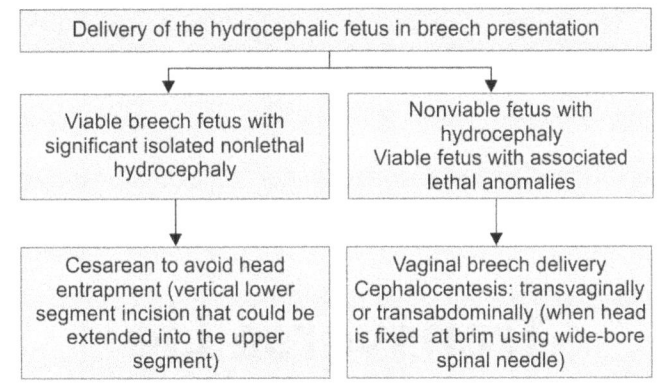

Algorithm 5: Head entrapment.

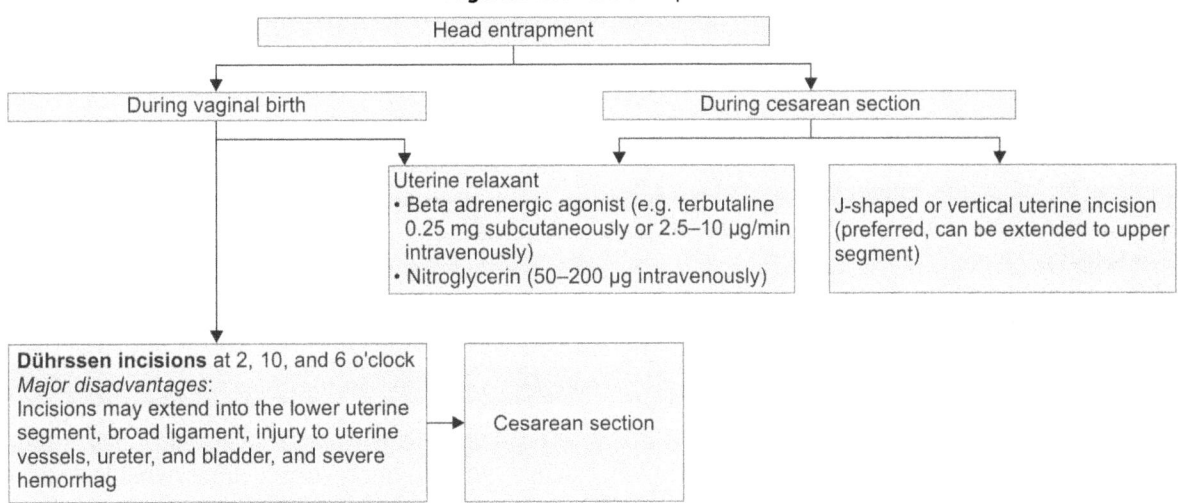

REFERENCES

1. Hickok DE, Gordon DC, Milberg JA, et al. The frequency of breech presentation by gestational age at birth: a large population-based study. Am J Obstet Gynecol. 1992;166:851-2.
2. Ford JB, Roberts CL, Nassar N, et al. Recurrence of breech presentation in consecutive pregnancies. BJOG. 2010;117:830-6.
3. Impey LWM, Murphy DJ, Griffiths M, et al. Management of breech presentation (Green-top Guideline No. 20b). BJOG. 2017;124(7):151-77.
4. Royal College of Obstetricians and Gynaecologists. External Cephalic Version and Reducing the Incidence of Term Breech Presentation. Green-top Guideline No. 20a. London: RCOG; 2017.
5. ACOG Committee on Obstetric Practice. ACOG Committee Opinion No. 340 reaffirmed. Mode of term singleton breech delivery. Obstet Gynecol. 2016;108:235-7.
6. Bin YS, Roberts CL, Ford JB, et al. Outcomes of breech birth by mode of delivery: a population linkage study. Aust N Z J Obstet Gynaecol. 2016;56:453-9.

Chapter 40

Transverse Lie

Vaishali Korde Nayak, Parag Biniwale

GENERAL CONSIDERATIONS

- *Transverse lie:* When the longitudinal axis of fetus lies perpendicular to maternal spine/longitudinal axis of uterus (**Fig. 1**).
  - *Dorsosuperior position (back-up):* Limbs are overlying the os, chances of cord prolapse.
  - *Dorsoinferior position (back-down):* Leading to shoulder presentation with or without cord prolapse. Denominator is scapula.

  The situation of head decides whether it is right or left position.
- *Oblique lie:* When longitudinal axis of the fetus is lying at an angle with the maternal spine or longitudinal axis of uterus:
  - The lower pole is empty and the head or the breech is in an iliac fossa.
  - Causes and management are similar to transverse lie.
- *Unstable lie:* When the fetal position/lie is repeatedly changing beyond 36 weeks gestation.

INCIDENCE OF TRANSVERSE LIE

At term, the incidence varies between 1:300[1,2] and 1:500[3] deliveries. Commonly seen in preterm babies[4] and at term in multiparas with lax abdomen.

A transverse lie may occur in association with the following conditions.

Maternal causes:[5]
- High parity
- Polyhydramnios
- *Uterine malformations:* Subseptate, arcuate uterus
- *Pelvic tumors:* Fibroids, ovarian cysts
- Placenta previa
- Contracted pelvis.

Fetal causes:[6]
- Multiple pregnancy
- *Fetal abnormality:* Hydrocephalous, fetal ascites
- Polyhydramnios
- Macrosomia
- Fetopelvic disproportion
- Intrauterine device (IUD).

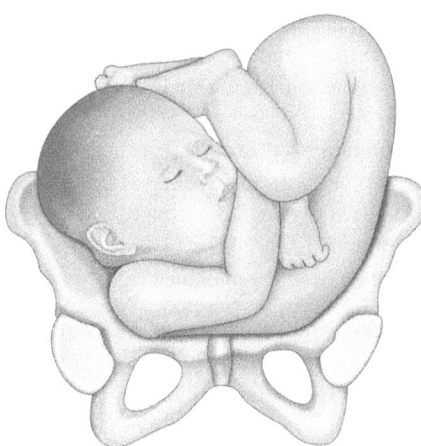

Fig. 1: Transverse lie.

This is a serious type of malposition where early detection and timely management will decrease the morbidities. If undetected/neglected, it can lead to serious complications like:
- Preterm rupture of membranes and cord prolapse → IUD
- Shoulder presentation and hand prolapse
- Impacted shoulder → obstructed labor → rupture uterus → maternal morbidity/mortality
- Fetal trauma → neonatal morbidity/mortality.

HISTORICAL ASPECT

Prior to cesarean section and development of good anesthesia, protracted labor leading to obstructed labor was inevitable. Maternal deaths were common due to uterine rupture, hemorrhage, shock, and infection. Shoulder presentation was the obstetrician's nightmare. A German midwife, Justine Siegemundin (1690), was the first one to describe a two-handed method of performing internal podalic version of the baby using a sling.[7] It was useful only if it was not an impacted uterus, otherwise destructive interventions were the only options to save the mother.[8]

CLINICAL EXAMINATION AND DIAGNOSIS OF TRANSVERSE LIE

Transverse lie is suspected when:
- Fundal height is less than weeks of gestation.
- Abdomen appears transversely stretched (squat uterus). Fundus near the umbilicus and wider than usual.
- By Leopold's maneuvers lower pole empty and fetal head/breech is palpable in either of the mother's flanks.[9]

Vaginal Examination

- The most important finding is the negative finding
- No head/breech palpable to the examining fingers
- High presenting part[10]
- Sausage-shaped bag of membranes
- Sometimes shoulder/hand/rib cage/back can be felt in combinations[10]
- Cord presentation/cord prolapse/hand prolapse.

Ultrasonography (USG) confirms the diagnosis and gives important information about liquor adequacy, any obvious cause leading to transverse position of the fetus and concealed cord presentation.

MECHANISM OF LABOR

Successful external version at term or spontaneous version to longitudinal lie in favorable situations has a good prognosis. But a persistent transverse lie cannot deliver spontaneously (except in preterm/macerated fetuses). If neglected, it leads to impacted shoulder, the head and breech stay above the inlet, and the neck gets stretched leading to obstructed labor. Cord prolapse, hand prolapse, and rupture uterus are the dreaded complications. So transverse lie is never to be left to nature at term.

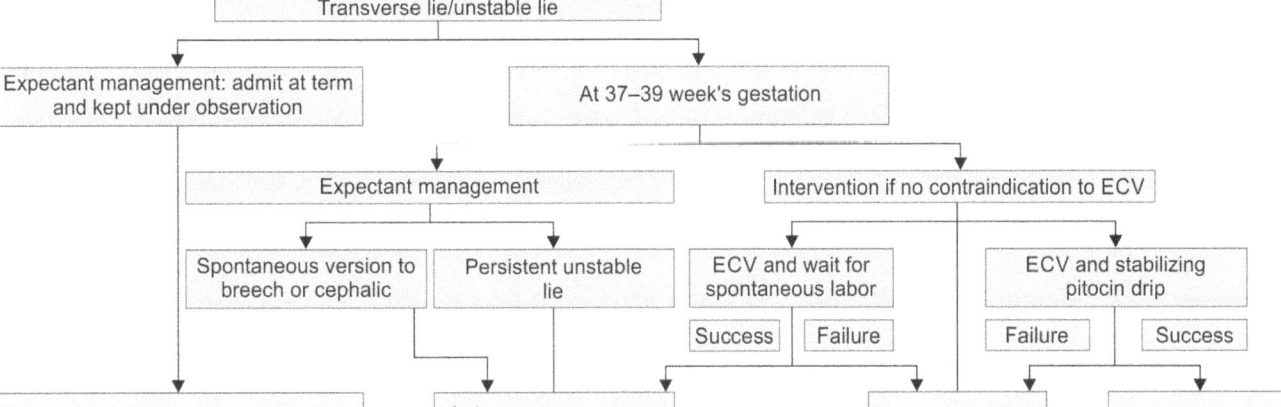

Algorithm 1: Management of transverse lie at term.

(ECV: external cephalic version)

MANAGEMENT OF TRANSVERSE LIE

It depends upon the clinical scenario at the time of presentation. While choosing the best option, we need to consider the following factors:
- Parity and previous mode of delivery
- Gestational age and estimated birth weight
- Placental localization
- Amount of liquor
- Whether labor has begun?
- Membranes are intact?

In case, the fetus is nonviable or dead macerated, vaginal delivery is possible with collapse of body/in doubled-up fashion, i.e. conduplicato corpore.

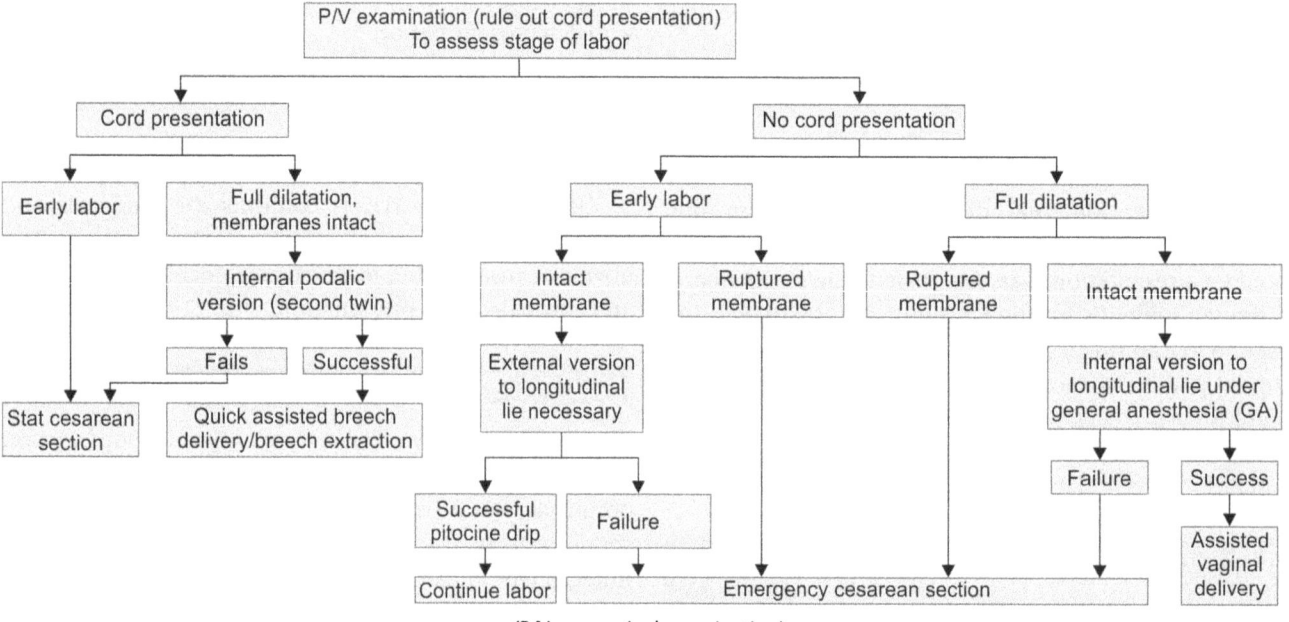

Algorithm 2: In labor with transverse lie.

(P/V: per vaginal examination)

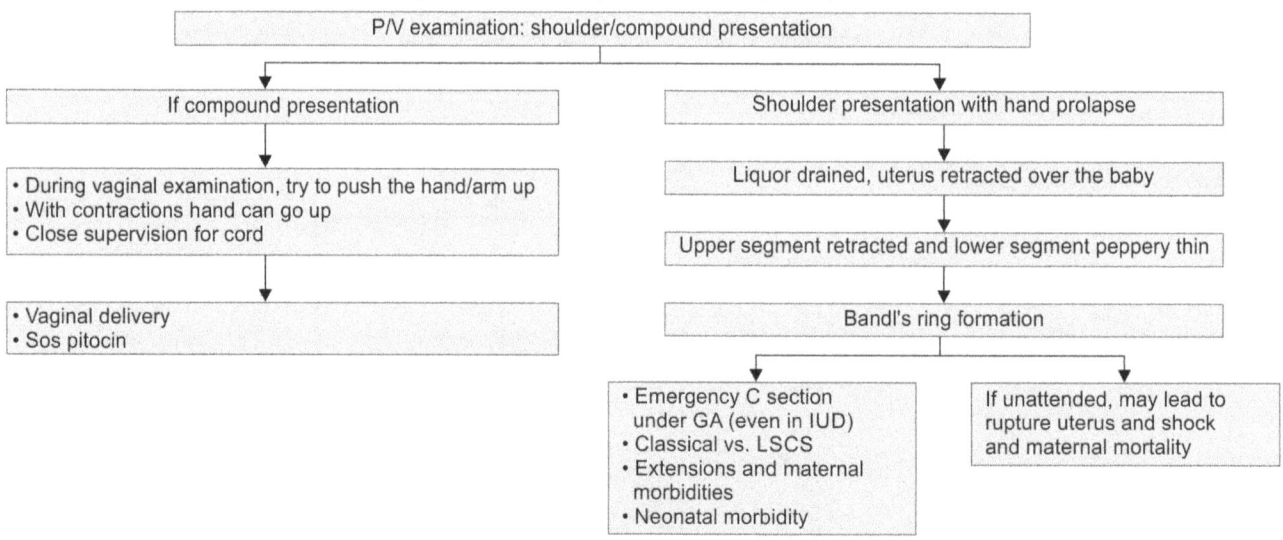

Algorithm 3: Management of shoulder presentation/compound presentation in labor.

(GA: general anesthesia; IUD: intrauterine device; LSCS: lower segment cesarean section; P/V: per vaginal examination)

COMPLICATIONS OF TRANSVERSE LIE

Maternal Complications

- Obstructed labor
- Difficult lower segment cesarean section (LSCS) with extensions
- Ruptured uterus
- Shock
- Postpartum hemorrhage (PPH)
- Septicemia
- Maternal death.

Fetal Complications

- Cord prolapse and fetal distress

Algorithm 4: Transverse lie. Summary of prenatal management.

- USG confirmation of lie
- Rule out possible causes for transverse lie
- Discuss pros and cons of ECV and about different modes of delivery

Expectant management
- Admit at 37 weeks for observation of lie and presentation
- Explain risk of cord prolapse in case of PROM
- Knee chest maneuver
- Chances of spontaneous version to cephalic/resolution to breech in 80% of cases before onset of labor/ROM[11-14]

Elective LSCS at term
- Scared uterus
- Any obstetrics contraindication for vaginal delivery
- Precious pregnancy
- Medical disorders like PIH, eclampsis, GDM, etc.

Intervention
- Admit at 37 weeks
- ECV after informed consent if no contraindications
- If successful, discharge after 24 hours and twice a week follow-up
- SOS stabilizing induction between 38 and 39 weeks
- If ECV fails, confirm fetal well being on CTG and discharge
- Second attempt of ECV after 1 week
- If fails, confirm fetal well-being, and elective LSCS at 38–39 weeks
- Any signs of fetal distress/labor → emergency LSCS
- If any contraindication of ECV or mechanical obstruction minimizing chances of vaginal delivery → elective LSCS at 38–39 weeks

ECV prerequisites[11-14]
- Facilities for immediate delivery
- LSCS available
- Explain risk of placental abruption
- Cord accidents, fetal distress, PROM
- Rh–prophylaxis
- Valid written informed consent
- Sos
- Terbutaline/ritodrin drip

(CTG: cardiotocography; ECV: external cephalic version; GDM: gestational diabetes mellitus; LSCS: lower segment cesarean section; PIH: pregnancy-induced hypertension; PROM: premature rupture of membrane; USG: ultrasonography)

Algorithm 5: Transverse lie. Summary of intrapartum management.

- Clinical examination to confirm the diagnosis
- To rule out cord presentation/cord prolapse
- To assess the stage of labor

Emergency LSCS
- Active labor with transverse/unstable lie
- PROM
- Cord presentation
- Cord prolapse
- Hand prolapse
- Shoulder presentation
- Impacted shoulder
- Obstructed labor
- Vaginal delivery not feasible due to mechanical obstruction

ECV
- Before labor/very early labor (uterus relaxing well), sos tocolysis.
- Membranes intact with good amount of liquor
- Baby average size
- No contraindication to vaginal delivery

IPV
Second baby of twins is the only indication of IPV in modern obstetrics

(ECV: external cephalic version; IPV: internal podalic version; LSCS: lower segment cesarean section; PROM: premature rupture of membrane)

- Fetal hypoxia
- Stillbirth
- Neonatal death
- Fetal trauma.

External or internal versions to be attempted by an experienced person after explaining the risks involved to the patient and ruling out the contraindications.

Cesarean delivery is the treatment of choice considering the safety of mother and child both. Some surgeons feel extraction of baby through the lower segment incision is difficult in certain situations and recommend vertical incision in lower segment, which if needed, can be extended upward. On the other hand, few series reports good success rates with lower segment transverse incision in delivering both dorsoinferior and dorsosuperior fetuses.[15,16]

REFERENCES

1. Gemer O, Segal S. Incidence and contribution of predisposing factors to transverse lie presentation. Int J Gynaecol Obstet. 1994;44:219-21.
2. Cruikshank DP, White CA. Obstetric malpresentations: twenty years' experience. Am J Obstet Gynecol. 1973;116:1097-104.
3. Okonofua FE. Management of neglected shoulder presentation. BJOG. 2009;116:1695-6.
4. Scheer K, Nubar J. Variation of fetal presentation with gestational age. Am J Obstet Gynecol. 1976;125:269-70.
5. Coates T. Malpositions of the occiput and malpresentations. In: Marshall J, Raynor M (Eds). Myles Textbook for Midwives, 16th edition. Edinburgh: Churchill Livingstone/Elsevier; 2014. pp. 435-54.
6. Mackenzie IZ. Unstable lie, malpresentations and malpositions. In: James D, Steer PJ, Weiner CP, et al. (Eds). High Risk Pregnancy Management Options, 4th edition. Nottingham: Elsevier Saunders; 2011. pp. 1123-37.
7. Speert H. Iconographia Gyniatrica, Philadelphia, US: F.A. Davis; 1973. p. 257.
8. Mann RM. Case of arm and shoulder presentation in which evisceration was performed. Assoc Med J. 1856;4(172):308.
9. Leopold, G, Spörlin L. Conduct of normal births through external examination alone (German). Arch Gynecol. 1984;45:337.
10. Nassar N, Roberts CL, Cameron CA, et al. Diagnostic accuracy of clinical examination for detection of non-cephalic presentation in late pregnancy: cross sectional analytic study. BMJ. 2006;333:578-80.
11. Tan JM, Macario A, Carvalho B, et al. Cost-effectiveness of external cephalic version for term breech presentation. BMC Pregnancy Childbirth. 2010;10:3.
12. Gifford DS, Keeler E, Kahn KL. Reductions in cost and cesarean rate by routine use of external cephalic version: a decision analysis. Obstet Gynecol. 1995;85:930-6.
13. Rosman AN, Guijt A, Vlemmix F, et al. Contraindications for external cephalic version in breech position at term: a systematic review. Acta Obstet Gynecol Scand. 2013;92:137-42.
14. Holmes WR, Hofmeyr GJ. Management of breech presentation in areas with high prevalence of HIV infection. Int J Gynaecol Obstet. 2004;87:272-6.
15. Shoham Z, Blickstein I, Zosmer A, et al. Transverse uterine incision for cesarean delivery of the transverse-lying fetus. Eur J Obstet Gynecol Reprod Biol. 1989;32:67-70.
16. Segal S, Gemer O, Sassoon E. Transverse lower segment uterine incision in cesarean sections for transverse lie. A retrospective survey. Arch Gynecol Obstet. 1994;255:171-2.

Cord Prolapse

Taru Gupta, Mansi Dhingra, Snigdha Kumari

INTRODUCTION

Umbilical cord prolapse is one of the most urgent emergencies in obstetrics. It is associated with increased neonatal morbidity and mortality. Birth asphyxia, prematurity, and congenital malformations account for the majority of adverse outcomes. It requires training of all staff involved in maternity care for proper management.

DEFINITION

Cord prolapse is defined as descent of the umbilical cord through the cervix in the presence of ruptured membranes.[1] Cord prolapse can either be:

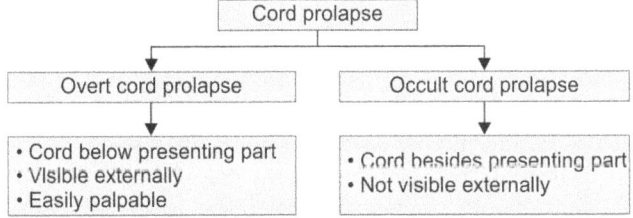

Cord presentation: Cord presentation is the presence of the umbilical cord between the fetal presenting part and the cervix, in the presence of intact membranes.

EPIDEMIOLOGY

The reported incidence of cord prolapse has fallen to about 0.2% or 1 in 500 of all deliveries in recent years. This is mainly as a result of changing obstetric management, including antenatal ultrasound diagnosis of funic presentation, greater use of continuous electronic fetal monitoring, and increasing rates of cesarean sections for malpresentation.[2] Perinatal mortality rate associated with cord prolapse has also come down to as low as 91 per 1,000.[2] Adverse fetal outcomes have mainly been attributed to asphyxia caused by direct cord compression and vasospasm. In hospital settings, however, prematurity and congenital malformation also play a major role.

RISK FACTORS

Risk factors associated with cord presentation can be general or procedure-related **(Algorithm 1)**.[3]

Umbilical cord prolapse mostly is seen in cases of poorly engaged or unengaged presenting part such as multiparous females, prematurity, contracted pelvis, polyhydramnios, breech presentation, transverse, and oblique lie. Among the breech fetuses, footling has the maximum risk of cord prolapse. The frequency of cord prolapse in vertex presentation is 0.24%; breech is 3.5%, and transverse is 9.6%.[4] Premature fetuses apart from filling in the pelvis inadequately are also more prone to malpresentation thus facilitating cord prolapse. Anomalous fetuses by the virtue of their irregular presenting parts and greater likelihood of malpresentation are more susceptible to cord prolapse. Minor degrees of placenta previa prevent fetal engagement. Also the cord insertion is near the cervix and more prone to prolapse. Iatrogenic obstetric interventions account for as high as 47% of the cases.[5] In most of the cases, two or more of the above factors coexist.

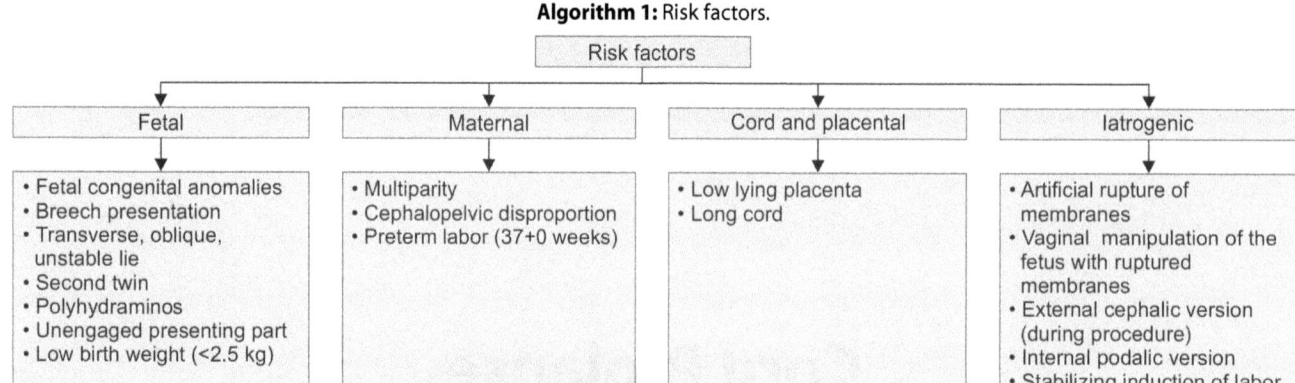

Algorithm 1: Risk factors.

AVOIDING CORD PROLAPSE

Fifty percent of cases of cord prolapse are a result of obstetric intervention:

- Artificial rupture of membranes (ARM) should be avoided if the presenting part is mobile. If ARM is clinically indicated, in the presence of risk factors for cord prolapse, this should be performed with arrangements in place for an immediate cesarean section.[3]
- Vaginal examinations and obstetric interventions carry the risk of upward displacement and cord prolapse, particularly with a high presenting part and ruptured membranes. Upward pressure should be kept to a minimum in such cases.[3]
- With transverse, oblique, or unstable lie, elective admission after 37 + 0 weeks gestation should be considered. Such women should be advised to present immediately if there are signs of labor or suspected rupture of membranes.[3]
- Women with noncephalic presentations and preterm prelabor rupture of membranes should be offered admission.[3]
- Rupture of membranes should be avoided if on vaginal examination, the cord is felt below the presenting part. When cord presentation is diagnosed in established labor, cesarean section is usually indicated.[3]
- Cord prolapse should be suspected when there is an abnormal fetal heart rate pattern, especially if such changes commence soon after membrane rupture, either spontaneous or artificial.[3]

DIAGNOSIS

- *Ultrasonography:* Cord presentation can be diagnosed by ultrasound especially by color Doppler in the antepartum period. However, routine ultrasound screening for the same is not recommended.[3] Selective ultrasound screening can be considered for women with breech presentation at term who is considering vaginal birth.[3]
- *Per speculum/per vaginum:* Cord presentation may be picked up in routine per vaginal examination during labor. In all cases where one or more of the aforementioned risk factors are present, a per vaginal examination should be done after rupturing of membranes to rule out cord prolapse. Persistent variable decelerations or persistent bradycardia especially after spontaneous or artificial rupture of membranes warrant a per vaginal examination to rule out cord prolapse.

A pulseless cord does not necessarily mean intrauterine demise. Fetal heart sound (FHS) auscultation and an ultrasound should be done to establish a diagnosis of intrauterine death (IUD).

MANAGEMENT (ALGORITHM 2)

After diagnosing cord prolapse, the first step is to call for help. The anesthetist and the neonatology team should be informed. The viability of the fetus (depending on the gestational age, presence of associated congenital anomalies) is assessed. Fetal heart sound is examined.

- *Fetal heart sound absent:* IUD is confirmed by ultrasonography (USG) (preferably bedside) after which spontaneous delivery is awaited.
- *Fetal heart sound present:* In such an event unless vaginal delivery is imminent, an abdominal delivery is indicated. While preparing the patient for cesarean, every effort should be made to elevate the presenting part in order to prevent cord compression by the

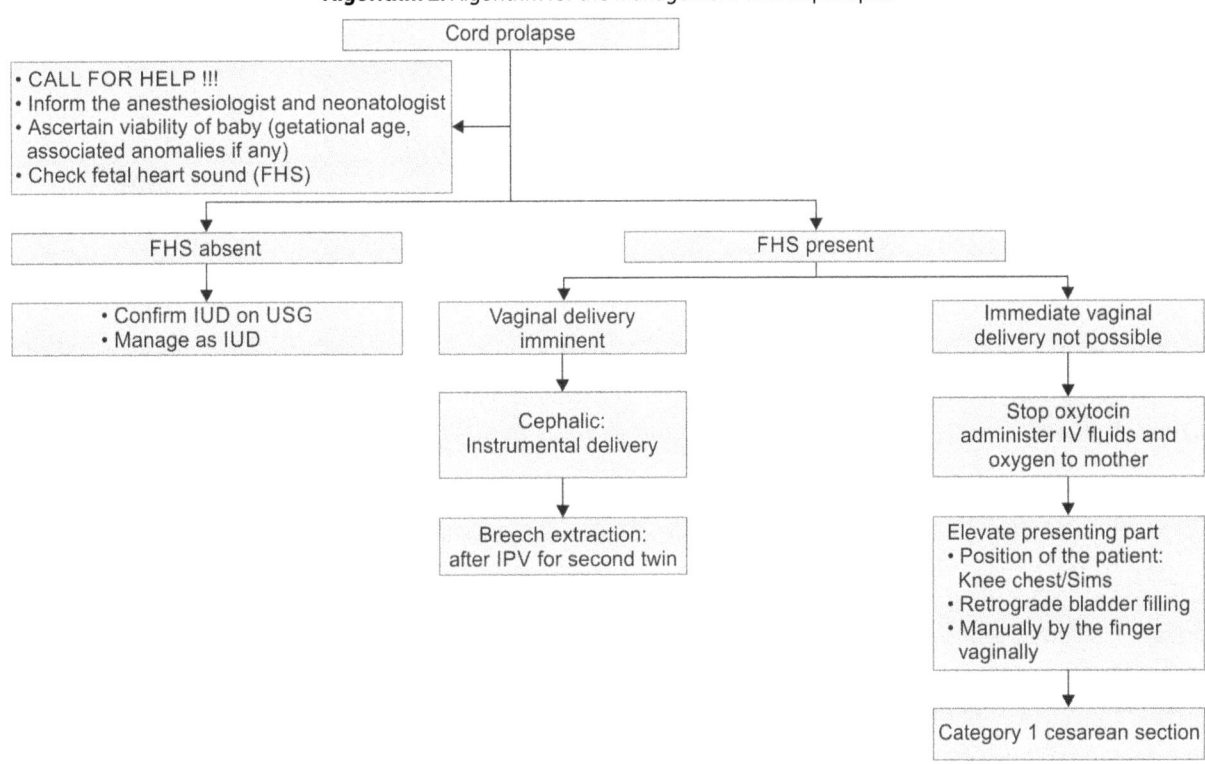

Algorithm 2: Algorithm for the management of cord prolapse.

(IPV: internal podalic version; IUD: intrauterine death; IV: intravenous; USG: ultrasonography)

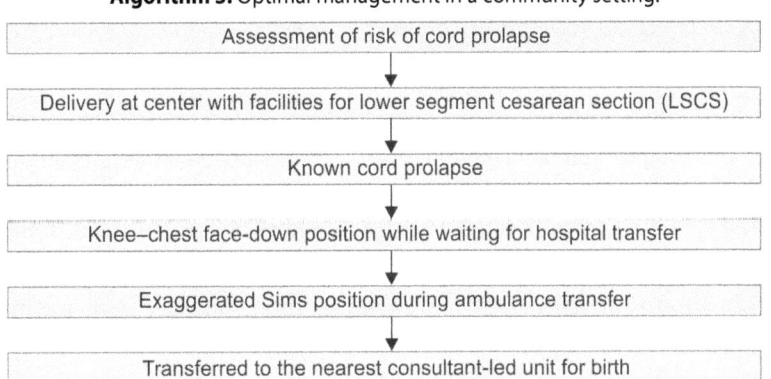

Algorithm 3: Optimal management in a community setting.

presenting part. This can be done by the following methods:
- Manually by the finger in the vagina.
- Retrograde filling of the bladder by 500–1,000 mL of saline and then clamping the catheter.[6]
- Putting the patient in knee—chest or exaggerated Sims' or Trendelenburg position.
- Role of tocolysis: Tocolysis may be used in order to reduce uterine contractions. The suggested tocolytic regimen is terbutaline 0.25 mg subcutaneously.[7]

An attempt to reposit the cord may incite vasospasm and further fetal hypoxia and hence is not advocated. Cord lying outside the vagina may be wrapped in warm moist mop till the patient is transferred to the operation theater in order to prevent vasospasm due to hypothermia.

A category 1 cesarean section should be performed with the aim of achieving birth within 30 minutes or less if the cord prolapse is associated with a suspicious or pathological fetal heart rate pattern but without compromising maternal safety.[3]

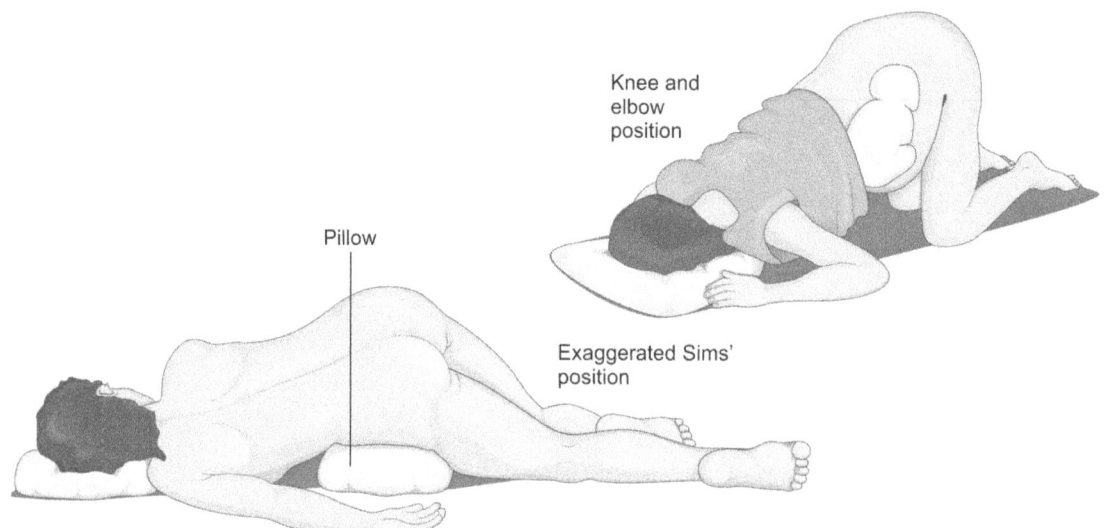

Fig. 1: Recommended positions to elevate the presenting part to minimize pressure on cord.

Anesthesia: The preferred type of anesthesia is general. Regional anesthesia may only be given when the fetal heart rate pattern is reassuring.

Breech extraction: Breech extraction is appropriate under some circumstances, e.g. after internal podalic version for a second twin.[3]

REFERENCES

1. Holbrook BD, Phelan ST. Umbilical cord prolapse. Obstetrics Gynecol Clin North Am. 2013;40(1):1-14.
2. Murphy DJ, MacKenzie IZ. The mortality and morbidity associated with umbilical cord prolapse. Br J Obstet Gynaecol. 1995;102:826-30.
3. Royal College of Obstetricians and Gynecologists: Umbilical Cord Prolapse. Guideline-2014. London, UK: Royal College of Obstetricians and Gynecologists.
4. Barclay M. Umbilical cord prolapse and other cord accidents. In: Sciarra JJ (Ed). Gynecology and Obstetrics. Philadelphia, PA: JB Lippincott; 1989. p. 1.
5. Usta IM, Mercer BM, Sibai BM. Current obstetrical practice and umbilical cord prolapse. Am J Perinatol. 1999;16(9): 479-84.
6. Vago T. Prolapse of the umbilical cord: a method of management. Am J Obstet Gynecol. 1970;107:967-9.
7. Ingemarsson I, Arulkumaran S, Ratnam SS. Single injection of terbutaline in term labor. I. Effect on fetal pH in cases with prolonged bradycardia. Am J Obstet Gynecol. 1985;153: 859-65.

Chapter 42

Shoulder Dystocia

Anupama Bahadur

INTRODUCTION

Shoulder dystocia is an obstetric emergency that occurs during a vaginal cephalic delivery. Additional obstetric maneuvers are required following failure of gentle downward traction on the fetal head to affect delivery of the shoulders.[1] It can also occur due to impaction of the posterior fetal shoulder on the sacral promontory. The other definition proposed is when there is a prolongation of head to body delivery time of more than 60 seconds but data is difficult to collect.[2,3] Anterior fetal shoulder gets wedged behind symphysis pubis and fails to deliver by applying downward traction and maternal efforts. It cannot be accurately predicted. Incidence of shoulder dystocia varies between 0.58 and 1.4%.[4,5] Maternal morbidity is a major concern especially postpartum hemorrhage (11%) due to uterine atony and vaginal lacerations and third- and fourth-degree perineal tears (3.8%).[6,7] There is significant perinatal morbidity especially brachial plexus injury complicating 2.3–16% of such deliveries with 10% resulting in permanent neurological dysfunction.[8]

RISK FACTORS ASSOCIATED WITH SHOULDER DYSTOCIA

- Previous history of shoulder dystocia
- Macrosomic baby weighing >4.5 kg
- Diabetes mellitus
- Body mass index (BMI) >30 kg/m^2
- Prolonged first/second stage of labor
- Parity >2
- Gestational age >42 weeks.

PROMPT RECOGNITION OF SIGNS OF SHOULDER DYSTOCIA

- Difficulty in delivery of face and chin
- "Turtle neck sign": Head remains tightly applied to vulva or even retracts
- Failure of restitution of fetal head
- Failure of shoulders to descend and deliver
- Immediately after recognition, call for help.

PREVENTIVE MANAGEMENT

- Anticipate shoulder dystocia if high-risk factors present
- Watch for labor abnormalities
- Avoid vacuum extraction
- Availability of senior obstetrician and experienced team
- Regular shoulder dystocia drill in labor room.

Remember HELPERR
- H: Call for help
- E: Evaluate episiotomy
- L: Legs (McRoberts' maneuver)
- P: Suprapubic maneuver
- E: Enter maneuvers (internal rotation)
- R: Remove the posterior arm
- R: Roll the patient (all four position).

MANAGEMENT OF SHOULDER DYSTOCIA

- Call for help, do not panic
- Note the time and document events
- Communicate with staff and patient

- Discourage patient to bear down as it exacerbates impaction of shoulders
- Avoid fundal pressure
- Avoid aggressive manipulations to prevent maternal and fetal injuries
- Consider episiotomy to make internal maneuvers easy.

McRoberts maneuver: Thighs to abdomen[9]
- "Knees to ear position"
- Hyperflexion and abduction of maternal hips
  - Cephalad rotation of pubic symphysis
  - Flattening of lumbar lordosis
  - Increases anteroposterior diameter

Suprapubic pressure and routine axial traction:
- In combination with McRoberts, reduces fetal bisacromial diameter
- Aim to bring the shoulders into oblique diameter
- Direct posteriorly and laterally—Rubin's method
- Deflect head toward floor
- Deliver anterior shoulder

Internal maneuvers or "all four" position and internal manipulation if McRoberts maneuver and suprapubic pressure fail.

Wood's corkscrew maneuver:[10]
- Fetal shoulders are rocked from side to side by applying force to maternal abdomen
- If unsuccessful pelvic hand reaches accessible fetal shoulder which is pushed toward anterior surface of chest
- Causes displacement of anterior shoulder from behind symphysis

Third-line maneuvers (salvage maneuvers) like Zavanelli, cleidotomy (deliberate fracture of clavicle), or symphysiotomy may be considered carefully to avoid maternal morbidity and mortality.

Zavanelli maneuver:
- Reversal of cardinal movements of labor
- Reverse restitution (rotation of head back to occipito-anterior)
- Flexion
- Manual replacement of vertex into uterus followed by Caesarean delivery

- Perform Gaskin maneuver
- Repeat the above steps as needed
- Each step should not take more than 30–60 seconds
- A total of 3–5 minutes for all maneuvers
- Baby to be examined by neonatologist for any injuries sustained.

COMPLICATIONS

Maternal Complications
- Prolonged second stage
- ↑ Operative deliveries
- ↑ Cesarean sections
- Postpartum hemorrhage
- Perineal trauma
- Uterine rupture.

Neonatal Complications
- Brachial plexus injury (recovery within 6–18 months)
- Fracture clavicle/humerus
- Arm weakness
- Hematoma
- Birth asphyxia
- Neonatal death.

CONCLUSION

Shoulder dystocia, a nightmare for obstetricians, is difficult to predict and prevent. Cesarean delivery cannot be recommended for all those women with an identifiable risk factor. All obstetricians must be prepared with a high level of awareness to manage this emergency by attending regular training. A team-oriented approach and appropriate documentation are necessary to manage shoulder dystocia.

REFERENCES

1. American College of Obstetricians and Gynecologists. ACOG Practice Bulletin No. 22. Fetal Macrosomia. ACOG: Washington, DC; 2000.
2. American College of Obstetricians and Gynecologists. ACOG practice bulletin no. 40. Shoulder dystocia. Obstet Gynecol. 2002;100:1045-50.
3. American College of Obstetricians and Gynecologists. Patient safety checklist no. 6: documenting shoulder dystocia. Obstet Gynecol. 2012;120(2):430-1.
4. Spong CY, Beall M, Rodrigues D, et al. An objective definition of shoulder dystocia: prolonged head-to-body delivery intervals and/or the use of ancillary obstetric maneuvers. Obstet Gynecol. 1995;86:433-6.
5. Gherman RB. Shoulder dystocia: an evidence-based evaluation of the obstetric nightmare. Clin Obstet Gynecol. 2002;45:345-62.
6. Gherman RB, Goodwin TM, Souter I, et al. The McRobert's maneuver for the alleviation of shoulder dystocia: how successful is it? Am J Obstet Gynecol. 1997;178:656-61.

7. Hoffman MK, Bailit JL, Branch W, et al. A comparison of obstetric maneuvers for the acute management of shoulder dystocia. Obstet Gynecol. 2011;117:1272-8.
8. Crofts JF, Attilakos G, Read M, et al. Shoulder dystocia training using a new birth training mannequin. BJOG. 2005;112:997-9.
9. Menticoglou SM. A modified technique to deliver the posterior arm in severe shoulder dystocia. Obstet Gynecol. 2006;108:755-7.
10. Rubin A. Management of shoulder dystocia. JAMA. 1964;189:835-7.

Chapter 43

Injuries of Birth Canal

Manju Puri, Shilpi Nain

INTRODUCTION

Birth canal is the passage through which the fetus is expelled during parturition. Both abnormal and mismanaged labor can lead to injuries of the birth canal. These injuries can pose concern because of the short- and long-term complications associated with it.

Birth canal can be divided into:

Lower genital tract	Upper genital tract
Perineum	Uterus
Vagina	
Cervix	

PERINEAL INJURIES

Applied Anatomy

The perineum comprises of two triangles: (1) the urogenital triangle, with the pubic symphysis being its apex, and (2) anal triangle with its apex at the coccyx. The urogenital triangle is covered by the perineal membrane, a connective tissue layer that is lying between the pubic rami and is penetrated by the vagina, urethra, and the rest of the external genitalia.

The anal triangle consists of the anal canal, the internal and external anal sphincters, the ischiorectal fossa, and the median raphe. The muscles of the external genitalia include the superficial and deep transverse perineal muscles, the ischiocavernosus muscles that cover the crura of the clitoris, and the bulbocavernosus muscles **(Fig. 1)**.

The anal wall is separated from the vaginal wall by perineal body which includes:
- External anal sphincter (EAS) and internal anal sphincter (IAS) muscles
- Superficial and deep transverse perineal muscles
- Bulbocavernosus muscle
- Levator ani muscle
- Perineal fascia and surrounding connective tissue
- Posterior vaginal wall
- Skin.

The apex of the perineal body is continuous with the rectovaginal septum.

The blood supply to the perineal structures is derived from the branches of the internal pudendal artery, which arises from the anterior division of the internal iliac artery. Main branches like inferior hemorrhoidal artery, superficial perineal artery, or transverse perineal artery are the source of hemorrhage from lacerations of the perineal body.

The veins of the perineum are valveless and have free anastomosis with the large intrapelvic venous plexuses and may be a cause of alarming hemorrhage or massive hematomas from obstetrical or surgical wounds of the vulva and vagina.

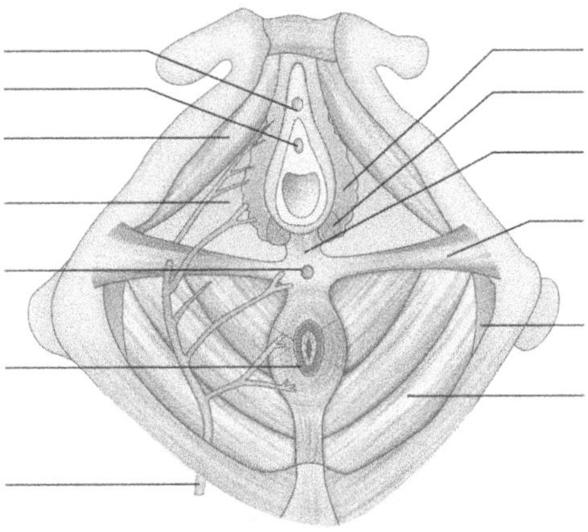

Fig. 1: Perineum.

Degrees of Perineal Tear[1]

A perineal tear may involve some or all of these structures and accordingly divided into various degrees **(Table 1, Figs. 2 to 5)**.

Table 1: Degrees of perineal tear.	
First degree	Vaginal mucosa and/or perineal skin
Second degree	Vaginal mucosa, perineal skin, superficial and or deep perineal muscles
Third degree	Vaginal mucosa, perineal skin, superficial and deep perineal muscles, EAS and IAS 3a: Less than 50% thickness of EAS is torn 3b: More than 50% tear of the EAS is torn 3c: Both EAS + IAS are torn
Fourth degree	Vaginal mucosa, perineal skin, perineal muscles, EAS, IAS, and anorectal mucosa
(EAS: external anal sphincter; IAS: internal anal sphincter)	

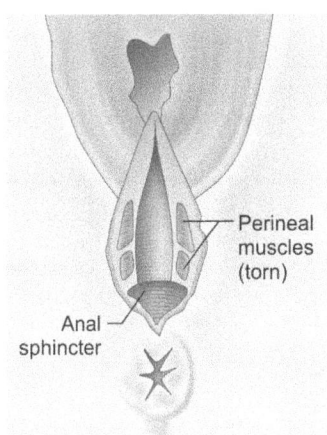

Fig. 3: Second-degree perineal tear.

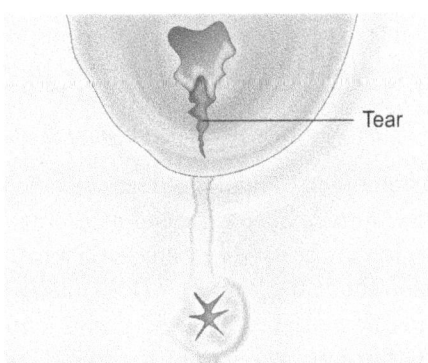

Fig. 2: First-degree perineal tear.

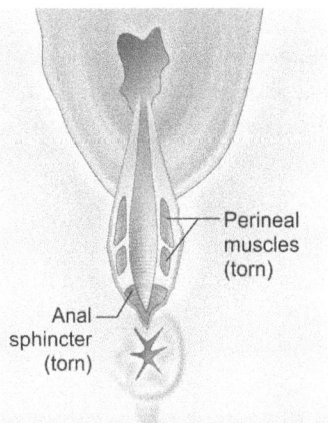

Fig. 4: Third-degree perineal tear.

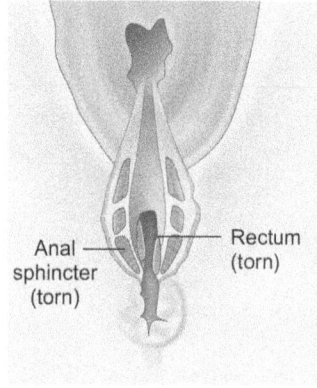

Fig. 5: Fourth-degree perineal tear.

Causes

The causes of perineal tears are listed in **Table 2**.

Table 2: Causes of perineal tear.		
Overstretched perineum	Rapid stretching	Rigid perineum
• Large baby • Face to pubis delivery • Narrow pubic arch • Shoulder dystocia • Instrumental delivery • Prolonged second stage of labor	• Precipitate labor • Aftercoming head of breech	• Elderly primigravida • Scarred perineum due to previous surgery like episiotomy or perineorraphy

Complications

Perineal injuries are a common cause of traumatic postpartum hemorrhage (PPH). After the repair, complications like puerperal infection, fecal urgency, fecal incontinence, chronic perineal pain, and dyspareunia may occur. Rarely rectovaginal fistula may be sequelae of an imperfectly repaired fourth-degree perineal tear.

Prevention

The various interventions suggested for prevention of perineal tears are:
- Perineal protection at crowning and delivery of shoulder.
- Application of warm perineal compresses during the second stage of labor.
- Timely episiotomy especially in instrumental deliveries.
- Mediolateral episiotomy should be preferred over median episiotomy.
- Slow delivery of fetal head in between contractions.

Management

Thorough exploration under adequate light is essential to know the extent of the injury and manage the same. In case of excessive bleeding, a vaginal pack should be inserted, and the woman should be taken to the operation theater for exploration and repair under regional or general anesthesia. An experienced surgeon should perform the exploration with good lighting and appropriate instruments.

Repair should be undertaken immediately, or as soon as appropriately trained person is available. If the time elapsed is more than 24 hours, a second-degree tear can be sutured after antibiotic coverage and wound is clean, however, in case of complete perineal tear, repair should be done after 3 months.

First-degree Tears

These tears are approximated by interrupted sutures with an absorbable material. These may be left as such if small and not bleeding.

Second-degree Tears

Under all aseptic precautions, repair the vaginal mucosa by continuous suture starting 1 cm beyond the apex of vaginal mucosa, subcutaneous tissue by interrupted sutures, and skin by interrupted sutures or continuous subcuticular stitch.

Perform a per-rectal examination after repair to ensure that no stitch is placed in the rectum. The suture material used is 1-0 or 2-0 absorbable.

Third- and Fourth-degree Tears (Complete Tears)

- The torn anorectal mucosa should be repaired using either continuous or interrupted technique. Fine 3-0 polyglactin may be used as it causes less irritation and discomfort than polydioxanone (PDS) sutures.
- Torn ends of external anal sphincter are identified, held with Allis forceps and repaired. If torn IAS is identified, it is advisable to repair this separately with interrupted

mattress sutures without any attempt to overlap the IAS.
- For repair of a full-thickness EAS tear, either an overlapping or an end-to-end method can be used with equivalent outcomes. For partial-thickness tears, an end-to-end technique should be used.
- Figure-of-eight sutures to prevent tissue ischemia.
- Surgical knots should be buried beneath the superficial perineal muscles to minimize the risk of knot and suture migration to the skin.
- Then stitch the rectal muscle and para-rectal fascia by interrupted suture.
- Either monofilament sutures such as 3-0 PDS or modern braided sutures such as 2-0 polyglactin can be used with equivalent outcomes.
- Stitch the vaginal mucosa in continuous and perineal muscles by interrupted sutures.
- Skin is approximated by interrupted sutures or continuous subcuticular stitch.

A gentle rectal examination should be performed after the repair to ensure that sutures have not been inadvertently inserted through the anorectal mucosa in case of third-degree tear repairs. If a suture is identified, it should be removed.

Care after Repair

- Broad-spectrum antibiotics for 5 days
- Low residual diet for 3–5 days
- Lactose 8 mL twice a day for 2 weeks to soften the stool
- Perineal care
- Avoid enema and rectal examination for 2 weeks
- Pelvic floor exercises.

Future Pregnancies

Obstetric anal sphincter injuries (OASIS) may occur in up to 11% of women giving birth vaginally. If there is any doubt about the degree of tear, it is advisable to classify it to a higher degree rather than a lower degree. Efforts should be made to repair the tears which are bleeding or distort anatomy.

About 60–80% of women are asymptomatic 12 months following repair of a third or fourth-degree perineal tear.

All women who sustained OASIS should be counseled about the mode of delivery in subsequent pregnancies and this should be clearly documented in the case sheet and discharge slip.

- *Previous third-degree tear repaired and asymptomatic*: Allow vaginal delivery. Episiotomy is given only if clinically indicated.
- *Previous third-degree tear repaired but symptomatic*: Advise elective cesarean section.

VAGINAL INJURIES

Applied Anatomy

The vagina is lined by stratified squamous epithelium thrown up into rugae providing distensibility without laceration. A dense, thin layer of elastic fibers is found immediately beneath the epithelium. Beneath this is a well-developed fibromuscular layer. The fibrous capsule external to this muscular coat is rich in elastic fibers and large venous plexuses.

The vagina receives its blood supply from the vaginal arteries and their anastomoses with branches of the uterine, inferior vesical, and internal pudendal arteries **(Fig. 6)**. The confluence of these anastomotic branches forms longitudinal azygous vaginal arteries in the midline of the anterior or posterior vaginal walls. Vaginal artery arises from internal iliac artery slightly cephalad and posterior to the origin of uterine and inferior vesical artery. Arterial hemorrhage may follow laceration or inadvertent surgical trauma to the vagina, especially in the vault of the vagina even after ligating the uterine arteries.[2]

The connective tissue lateral to the lower third of vagina is attached to fibers of the pubococcygeal muscle (fibers of Luschka) and to fibers fixing it to the perineal membrane.

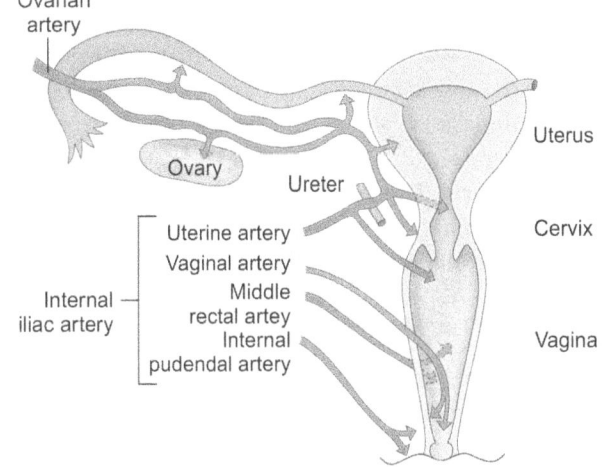

Fig. 6: Vascular supply to uterus, cervix, and vagina.

Causes

These injuries can be in the form of vaginal tears, lacerations, or vulvovaginal hematomas.

The causes of vaginal injuries are listed below:
- Instrumental delivery
- Along with cervical or perineal tears
- Prolonged labor with multiple per vaginum examinations
- Pre-existing vaginal infection, e.g. candidiasis

Complications

These injuries are associated with complications like hemorrhage, sepsis, vaginal stenosis, dyspareunia, vesicovaginal fistula, and rectovaginal fistula.

Prevention

- Treating vaginal infections like candidiasis in antenatal period.
- Avoiding multiple per vaginum examinations.
- Timely episiotomy especially in instrumental delivery.

Management

Vaginal Tears and Lacerations

- Thorough exploration under adequate light and relaxation under all aseptic precautions is essential for appropriate management.
    - *If the apex is reached:* First stitch is taken 1 cm above the apex to secure any retracted vessel.
    - *If the apex is not reached:* Patient should be taken to operation theater, explored under adequate anesthesia and repair in interrupted or continuous stitches with a 2-0 absorbable suture.
- Local packing is indicated in cases with multiple small lacerations and generalized oozing due to repeated handling.
- *Colporrhexis:* Laparotomy followed by repair along with internal iliac artery ligation or uterine artery embolization if indicated.

Vulvovaginal Hematomas

These can be infralevator or supralevator hematomas. Infralevator hematomas are more common. The differences between the two are as listed in **Table 3**.

Table 3: Difference between infralevator and supralevator hematomas.

	Infralevator	Supralevator
Causes	• Improper hemostasis during episiotomy repair • Rupture of paravaginal venous plexus	• Extension of cervical laceration • Along with uterine rupture (lower segment) • Rupture of veins in connective tissue at the base of broad ligament
Symptoms	• Persistent severe pain • Tenesmus • Urinary retention	Pain in lower abdomen or flanks
Signs	• Tender bluish-purple swelling • Rarely shock	• Swelling above the inguinal ligament pushing uterus to opposite side • Bogginess in fornices • Shock
Management	• <5 cm • Analgesics • Ice packing • >5 cm • RA/GA • Incision over most prominent part • Evacuation of clots • Secure bleeding points and or figure of eight sutures over oozing area to obliterate dead space and packing	• Ultrasonography (USG) confirmation • *Stable patient + nonexpanding hematoma:* Conservative management • *Hemodynamic instability:* Resuscitation + laparotomy with internal iliac ligation and hysterectomy or uterine artery embolization

(GA: general anesthesia; RA: regional anesthesia)

Periurethral/Periclitoral Lacerations

In case of slight bleeding, pressure for 1–2 minutes is enough. In case of significant bleeding, repair with a fine 2-0 or 3-0 absorbable suture after inserting urethral catheter if periurethral tear is done.

CERVICAL INJURIES

Applied Anatomy

The cervix projects into the anterior part of the vault of vagina.

Blood supply is from the internal iliac artery via its vaginal, uterine, internal pudendal, and middle rectal branches. A venous plexus drains via the vaginal vein into the internal iliac vein.

Left lateral cervical tear is more common. The tears can be unilateral or stellate (multiple on both lips). Rarely, there can be partial detachment or complete or annular detachment of the cervix.

Causes

The causes of cervical injuries can be enumerated in **Table 4**.

Table 4: Causes of cervical injuries.

Forceps delivery	Excess uterine contraction	Spontaneous detachment	Rigid cervix
• Breech delivery through an incompletely dilated cervix • Attempted manual dilatation	Precipitate labor	• Prolonged labor • Cervical dystocia	• Congenital • Scarring due to previous surgery (amputation, conisation)

Complications

Cervical tear is the most common cause of traumatic PPH. It can also lead to broad ligament hematoma, rupture of uterus due to extension into base of broad ligament, and ureteric injury consequent to the extension of the tear or during its repair.

Long-term sequelae include cervical incompetence, ectropion, or chronic cervicitis.

Prevention

Instrumental delivery should be performed by experienced clinician. No attempts to manually dilate the cervix should be made. Judicious use of oxytocics and partographic monitoring of labor to detect prolonged or precipitate labor may help in decreasing the incidence of cervical tears.

Management

Cervical tears should be repaired immediately after proper exploration **(Fig. 7)**:
- Insert speculum and retract the posterior vaginal wall.
- Explore the cervix in a clockwise manner to identify the tear. For this, we need two to three sponge holding forceps. Apply one at 12 o'clock position on cervix, another at 3 o'clock position, and inspect the cervix in between. Then apply another at 6 o'clock position, see between 3 o'clock and 6 o'clock positions and finally remove the one at 3 o'clock position and apply at 9 o'clock position and inspect the cervix between 6 o'clock and 9 o'clock position and then finally between 9 o'clock and 12 o'clock positions.
- Now grasp both margins of the tear and start repairing 1 cm above the apex of tear.
- Stitch the cervical tear by interrupted sutures taking the whole thickness of cervix with 1-0 chromic catgut on round body needle.
- Mattress suture may be taken to prevent rolling of the edges.
- In case the apex of tear is not visualized, clearly ask the assistant to push down the fundus of uterus gently to improve visualization or apply gentle traction on the sponge holders grasping the two margins of the tear or apply a suture as high as possible and then apply traction on that suture to take another above it and keep repeating till you reach beyond apex.
- If the cervical tear is extending to the lower segment or vault or the apex cannot be reached, it warrants laparotomy.

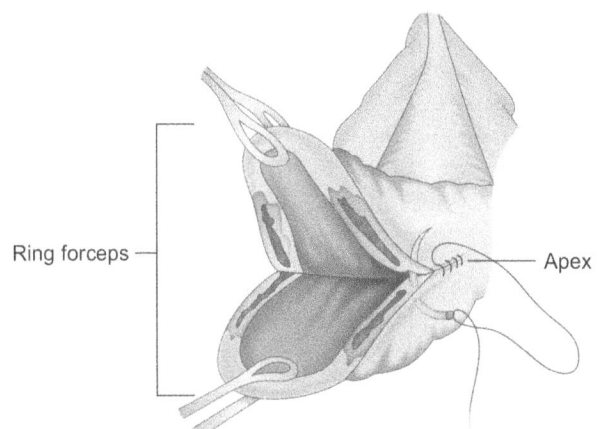

Fig. 7: Cervical tear exploration and repair.

UTERINE INJURIES

Uterine rupture is an acute obstetric emergency often resulting in fetal and/or maternal death. It commonly occurs in labor but can occur in late pregnancy.

Applied Anatomy

The uterus is made up of the fundus, body, and cervix. The body of the uterus narrows at isthmus which becomes the lower segment in pregnancy.

Relations

- *Anteriorly*: Uterovesical pouch of the peritoneum; the supravaginal cervix is related directly to bladder, separated only by connective tissue.
- *Posteriorly*: Pouch of Douglas, with coils of intestine within it.
- *Laterally*: The broad ligament and its contents; the ureter lies 12 mm lateral to the supravaginal cervix.

The ureter lies just above the level of the lateral fornix, below the uterine vessels as these pass across within the broad ligament. While performing a hysterectomy or ligation of uterine arteries, the ureter may be accidentally injured.

The uterine artery, a branch of internal iliac artery, runs in the base of the broad ligament and crosses above and at right angles to the ureter to reach the uterus at the level of the internal os. The artery then ascends in a tortuous manner alongside the uterus, supplying the corpus, and then anastomoses with the ovarian artery. The uterine artery also gives off a descending branch to the cervix and branches to the upper vagina.

Causes

Causes of uterine rupture are listed in **Table 5**.

Diagnosis

Diagnosis of uterine injuries is discussed in **Table 6**.

Complications

Complications associated with uterine rupture are PPH, surgical morbidity, sepsis, scar dehiscence in subsequent pregnancies, elective cesarean section in next pregnancy, and psychological morbidity consequent to hysterectomy.

Prevention

Uterine injuries can be prevented by optimizing labor protocols:
- Continuous maternal and fetal monitoring in labor.
- Careful monitoring of labor with partograph.

Table 5: Causes of uterine rupture.

Spontaneous	Scar rupture	Iatrogenic
- Previous D and C - Previous manual removal of placenta - Grand multipara - Congenital malformation of uterus - Previous resection of cornual ectopic pregnancy - Previous uterine perforation	- Previous classical cesarean section - Previous hysterotomy - Previous myomectomy - Previous lower segment cesarean section with extensions	- Injudicious use of oxytocin or prostaglandin - Internal podalic version or external cephalic version - Trauma - Destructive operations - Manual removal of placenta - Instrumental delivery - Obstructed labor cephalopelvic dispropotion, malpresentation

Table 6: Diagnosis of uterine injuries.

Scar dehiscence (**Fig. 8**)	Scar/uterine rupture (**Figs. 9 and 10**)
- Unexplained maternal tachycardia - Scar tenderness - Fetal distress - Prolonged deceleration on CTG - Difficulty in urination	- Hypovolemic shock - Sudden cessation of uterine contractions - Vaginal bleeding - Hematuria - Loss of uterine contour - Palpation of fetal parts superficially - Absent fetal heart - Loss of station of presenting part on per vaginum examination

(CTG: cardiotocography)

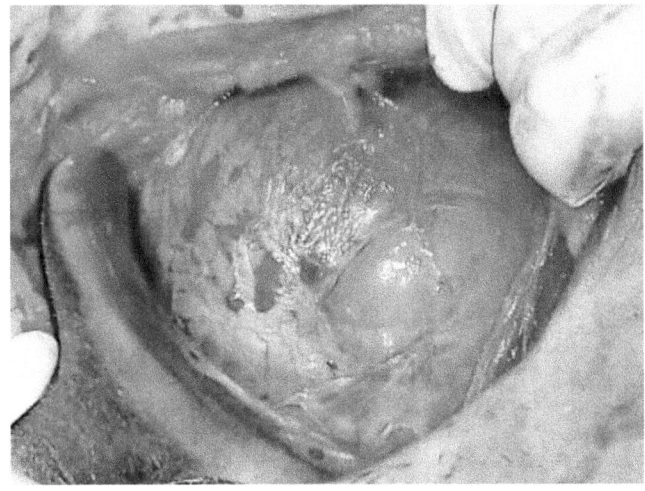

Fig. 8: Uterine scar dehiscence.

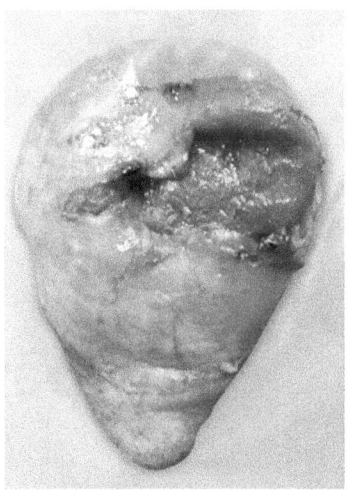

Fig. 10: Posterior wall rupture uterus.

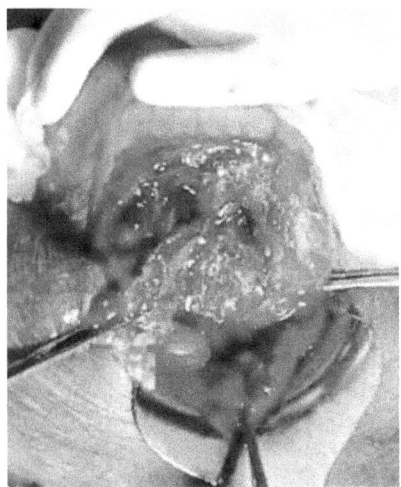

Fig. 9: Uterine scar rupture.

- Judicious use of oxytocics and instrumental delivery.
- Continuous maternal and fetal monitoring in labor.
- Judicious use of oxytocics and instrumental delivery.
- Reduce the rates of primary cesarean section.
- Proper suturing and adequate hemostasis during primary cesarean section.
- Mandatory hospital delivery of patients with previously scarred uterus.
- Appropriate case selection for trial of labor in patients with previous cesarean section.
- Timely referral of at-risk cases like obstructed labor contracted pelvis or malpresentation.

Management

After informed and written consent and arranging blood and blood products, patient is taken to operation theater for laparotomy. Surgical repair of uterus or hysterectomy should be done depending upon the size and extent of uterine rupture, maternal condition, and desire for future childbearing.

Future Pregnancies

Patient and relatives should be explained about the increased risk of rupture with subsequent pregnancies, need for elective cesarean in subsequent pregnancies. Effective contraception should be offered.

- Women with history of rupture uterus should have a planned elective cesarean section (37–38 weeks' gestation) in their next pregnancy.
- If there are extensive tears involving the upper segment, future pregnancy may not be safe.

REFERENCES

1. Royal College of Obstetricians and Gynaecologists. (2015). Third- and Fourth-degree Perineal Tears, Management (Green-top Guideline No. 29). [online] Available from https://www.rcog.org.uk/en/guidelines-research-services/guidelines/gtg29/ [Last accessed September, 2019].
2. Ellis H. Clinical Anatomy A Revision and Applied Anatomy for Clinical Students, 11th edition. Hoboken, NJ: Wiley-Blackwell; 2002.

Chapter 44

Postpartum Hemorrhage

Sayeba Akhter

INTRODUCTION

Postpartum hemorrhage (PPH) is the major cause of maternal death and accounts for about one-quarter of it globally, especially in low-income countries.

DEFINITION

Postpartum hemorrhage may be defined as bleeding more than 500 mL in vaginal delivery and more than 1,000 mL in cesarean section. For clinical purpose, any amount of bleeding that leads to hemodynamic instability may be considered as PPH.

CLASSIFICATION

Postpartum hemorrhage occurring within 24 hours of delivery is called primary PPH and that occurring after 24 hours up to 12 weeks postpartum is known as secondary PPH. Depending on the amount, it can again be divided as minor and major, moderate, and severe. The classification is shown below in **Algorithm 1**.

Algorithm 1: Classification of postpartum hemorrhage.

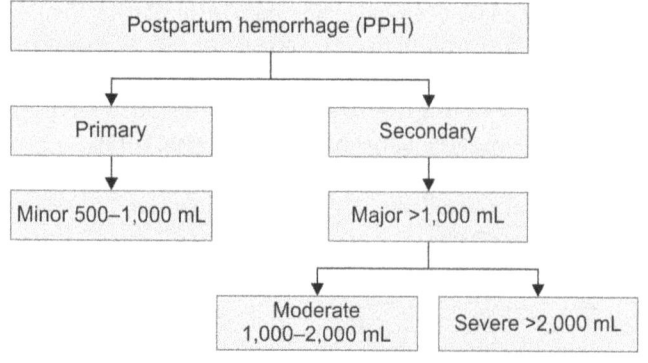

CAUSES

Causes of PPH are commonly described as 4 "T"s namely Tone, Trauma, Tissue, and Thrombin. Among all the causes, atonic PPH is the most common. The causes of PPH are many. Some common and important causes are shown in **Algorithm 2**.

PREVENTION

Postpartum hemorrhage is a potentially life-threatening condition and a leading cause of maternal mortality. So prevention has immense importance. Antepartum prevention by identification of risk factors and active management of third stage of the labor are the key points of prevention. Steps of prevention are shown in **Algorithm 3**.

Use of prophylactic uterotonics and antifibrinolytic agent:[1-5]
- *Inj. oxytocin:* 10 IU IM/IV, first-line drug.
- *Inj. carbetocin:* 100 μg IM/IV, long-acting, heat-stable, and has fewer side effects.[4,6]
- *Tab. misoprostol:* 600 μg orally, preferred in low-resource settings where inj. oxytocin is not available/difficult to administer.
- *Inj. ergometrine/methylergometrine*: 200 μg IM/IV. Contraindicated in hypertensive disorder and heart disease.
- *Inj. oxytocin + ergometrine*: Fixed dose combination (5 IU/500 μg).
- Inj. oxytocin + Inj. Tranexamic acid (in C/S).[5]

Algorithm 2: Causes of postpartum hemorrhage (PPH).

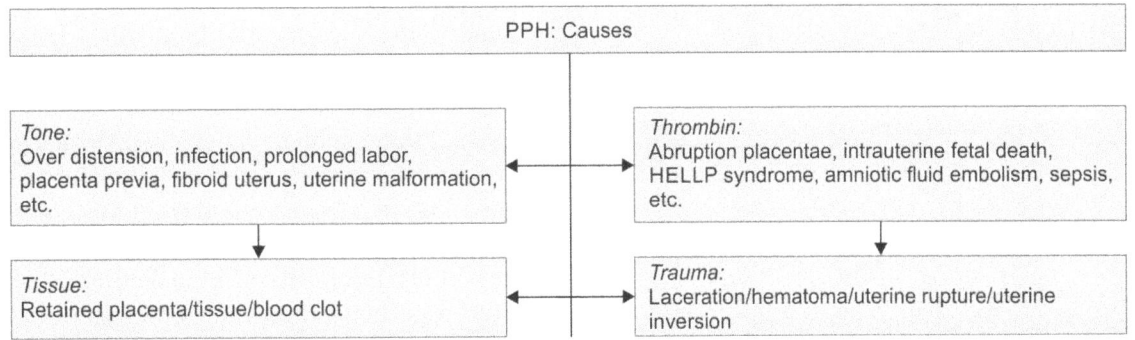

Algorithm 3: Steps of postpartum hemorrhage (PPH) prevention.

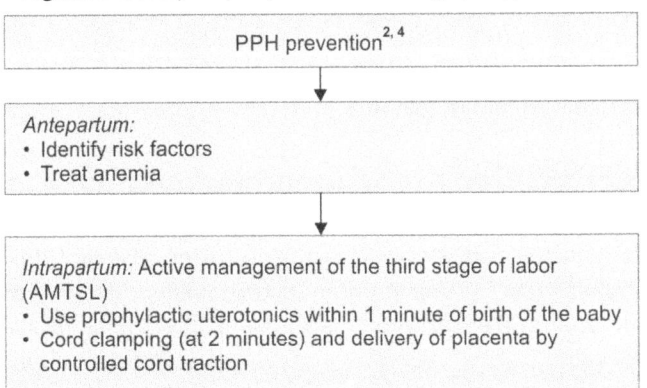

MANAGEMENT OF PRIMARY POSTPARTUM HEMORRHAGE

Management of PPH comprises of general and specific management.

General Management

- Start resuscitation immediately
- Call for help
- *Assess*: Airway, breathing, and circulation (ABC)
- Give supplementary oxygen at the rate of 10–12 L/min by face mask
- *Assess*: Shock Index (heart rate/systolic BP) to determine hemodynamic compromise[2]
- Keep the patient warm
- Give fundal massage
- Secure 2 IV channel with wide bore (14 G) cannulae
- Start IV fluid replacement with warm crystalloid solution
- Draw blood sample and send for baseline investigations—complete blood count (CBC), blood grouping and Rh typing, cross-matching, coagulation profile including fibrinogen, liver function test (LFT), and renal function test (RFT)
- Catheterize urinary bladder and check urine output
- Continuous monitoring of pulse, blood pressure, respiration, and oxygen saturation
- Start blood transfusion once available and if needed
- Inform the patient and family about the condition of the patient and steps need to be taken
- Involve multidisciplinary team with experienced doctors and staffs for management of major PPH.

Specific Management

Identification of cause is very important for starting cause-specific management. Simple palpation of uterus and checking placenta for integrity can give a clue to the underlying cause. Contracted uterus with bleeding suggests traumatic cause; whereas flabby uterus with bleeding indicates atony. Specific management according to causes is described below:

Atonic Postpartum Hemorrhage

Refer to **Algorithm 4**.

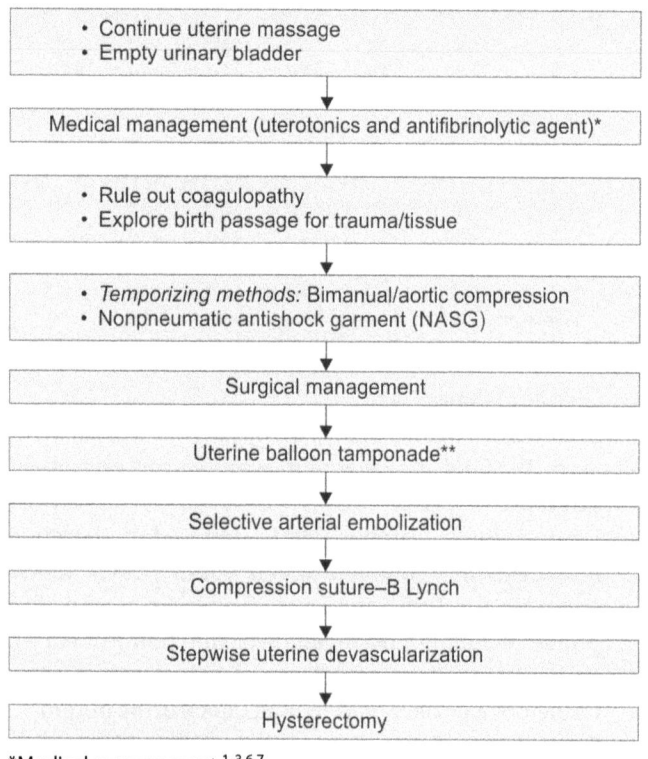

Algorithm 4: Management in atonic postpartum hemorrhage.[2,3,8]

Medical management:[1-3,6,7]

Use of uterotonic drugs:
First line: Inj. oxytocin 5 IU IV or 10 IU IM followed by 20–40 IU in IV infusion.
Other drugs:
- Inj. carbetocin 100 µg IV or IM
- Tab. misoprostol 800 µg sublingual
- Inj. ergometrine 0.2 mg IM, can be repeated hourly up to 5 doses (max—1 mg/24 hours)
- Inj. ergometrine + Inj. oxytocin (500 µg/5 IU)
- Inj. carboprost 0.25 mg IM (max—2 mg)
- Antifibrinolytic agent:
- *Inj. tranexamic acid:* 1 g IV within 3 hours of birth, can be repeated after 30 minutes.[9]

Uterine balloon tamponade*[8]:* Sayeba's UBT/Bakri/ Sengstaken–Blakemore/Rusch balloon can be used according to availability **(Fig. 1).

Traumatic Postpartum Hemorrhage (Algorithm 5)

Trauma can occur in the form of tear/laceration/hematoma involving perineum, vagina, cervix, or even high-up involving uterus or broad ligament/uterine inversion. Examination under analgesia with a good light source may be enough to detect lower genital tract trauma but broad ligament hematoma may need ultrasonographic evaluation. Inj. tranexamic acid within 3 hours of delivery improves PPH. Tear needs to be repaired. Small hematoma can have expectant management but large and expanding hematoma needs evacuation. Inversion of uterus needs immediate reposition to prevent neurogenic shock. In case of failure of immediate reposition, manual/hydrostatic/surgical reposition under general anesthesia (GA) is done. Laparotomy is needed for suspected uterine rupture/broad ligament hematoma.

Coagulopathy

Dilutional coagulopathy occurs in massive blood transfusion without adequate fresh frozen plasma (FFP) replacement. Consumption coagulopathy occurs in situations like abruptio placentae, HELLP (Hemolysis, Elevated Liver enzymes and Low Platelet count syndrome), intrauterine fetal death (IUFD), amniotic fluid embolism, etc. Vigilance and frequent monitoring of coagulation profile (PT, aPTT, fibrinogen, platelet count) are necessary. It can be prevented by early transfusion of FFP in suspected conditions. Treatment is done by transfusion of deficient coagulation factors **(Algorithm 6)**.

Retained Placenta/Retained Tissue

Placenta may not be delivered even after 30 minutes of delivery (retained placenta) or partially delivered (retained tissue). If patient is hemodynamically stable, spontaneous expulsion can be awaited up to another

Chapter 44
Postpartum Hemorrhage

1. Instruments and logistics needed for condom catheter tamponade by Sayeba's method should be ready	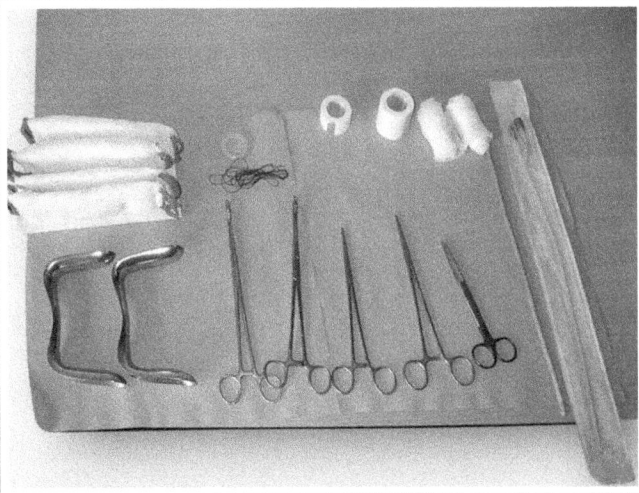
2. The condom is tied over the rubber catheter by thread	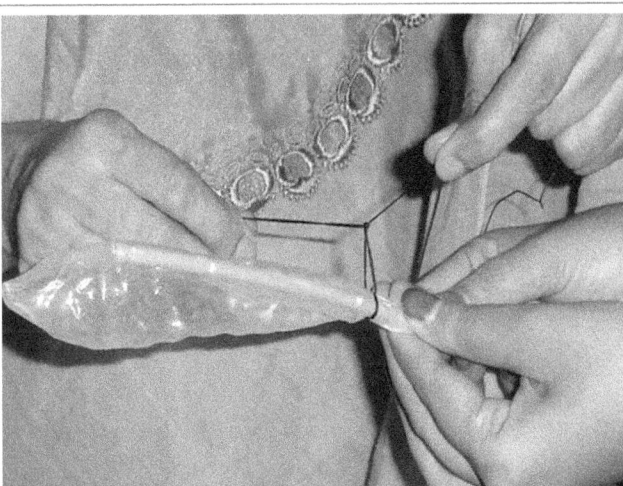
3. Lip of cervix held by sponge holding forceps	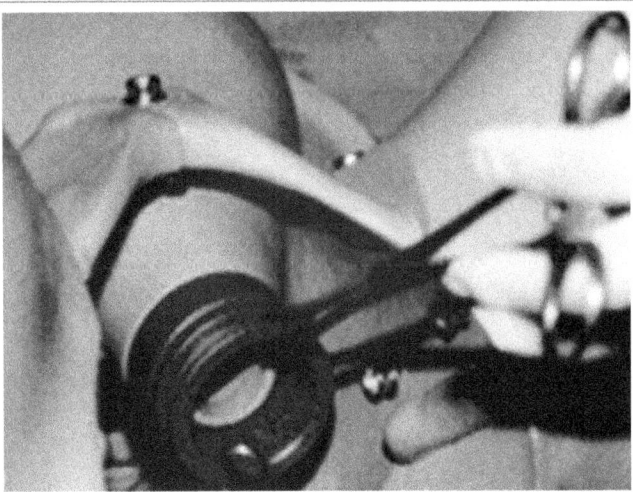

Contd...

Contd...

4. The fitted condom is inserted within the uterine cavity	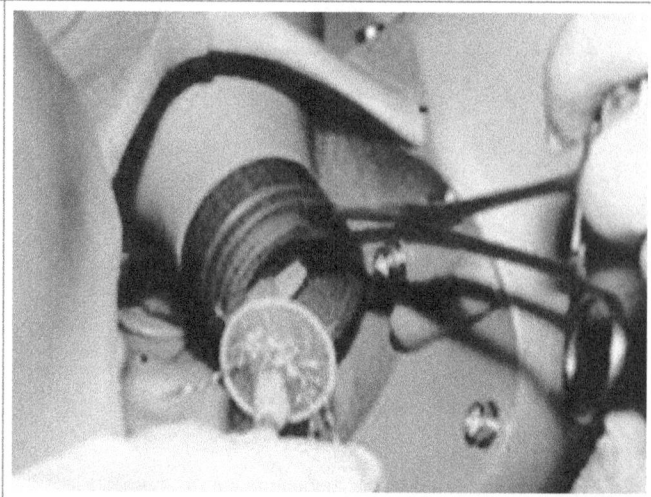
5. The vaginal pack is inserted to prevent slippage of condom from the uterine cavity	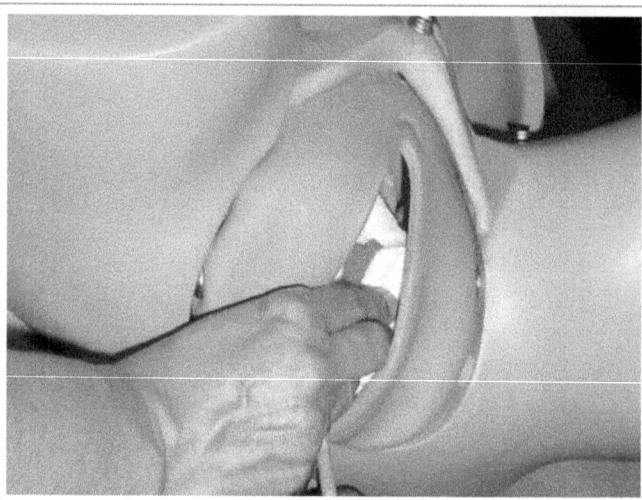
6. The distal end of rubber catheter is connected with saline set	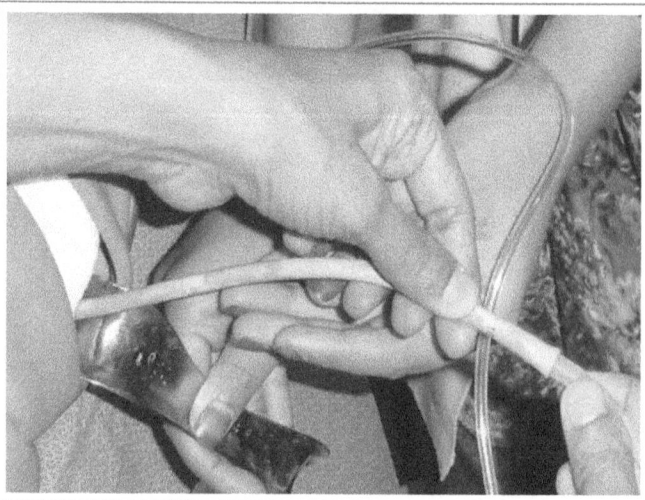

Contd...

Contd...

7. The regulator is opened up fully to inflate condom within uterine cavity by 250–500 mL of saline. 1,500 mL (severe atony)

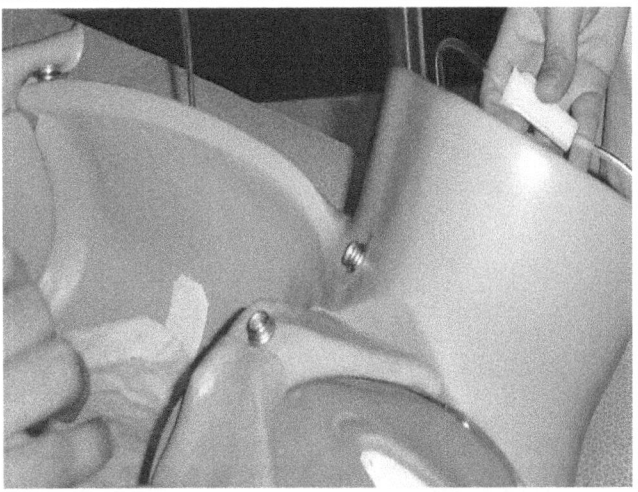

8. If saline bag is compressed and resistance felt that indicates tamponade has been produced. As an alternative to saline set, a 100 cc Tommy syringe may be used for rapid inflation of condom by saline

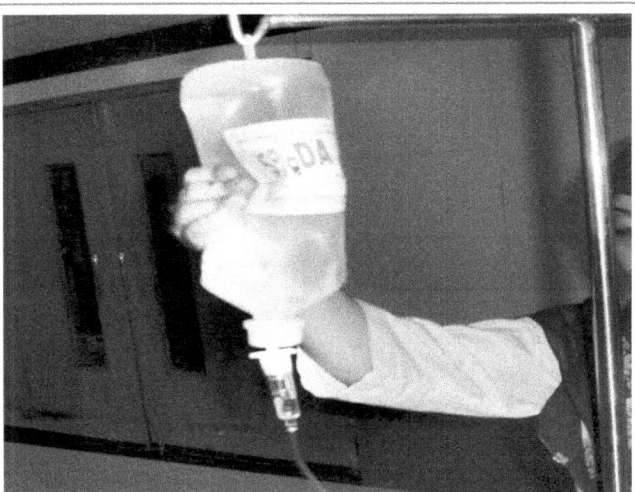

9. Inflated condom causes distension of the uterus and thereby compresses sinuses

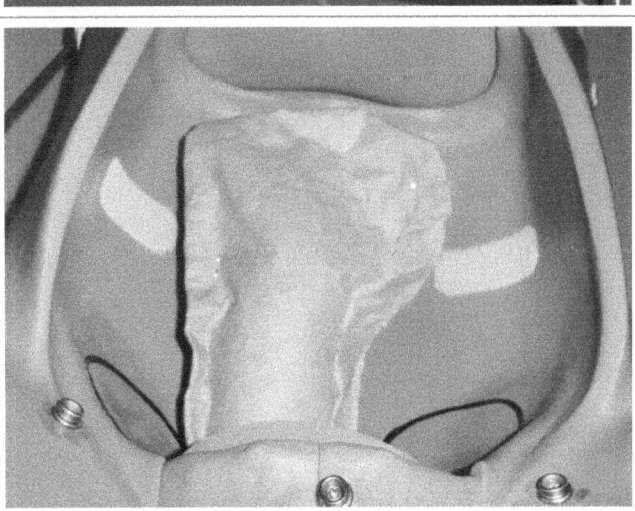

Contd...

Contd...

10. The catheter is detached, folded, tied, and is strapped on the thigh	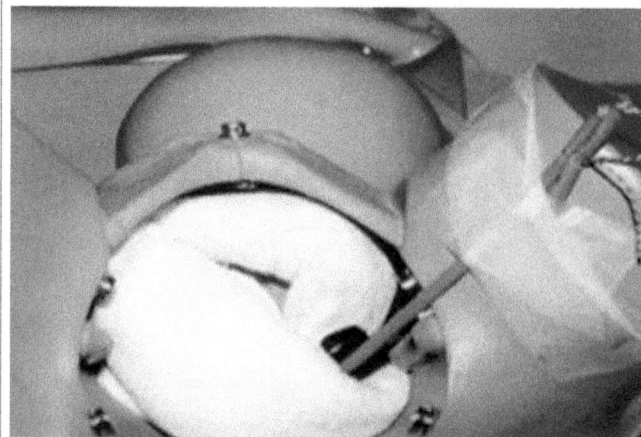
11. After 24 hours, If no more bleeding, the suture is cut and balloon is deflated gradually and removed.	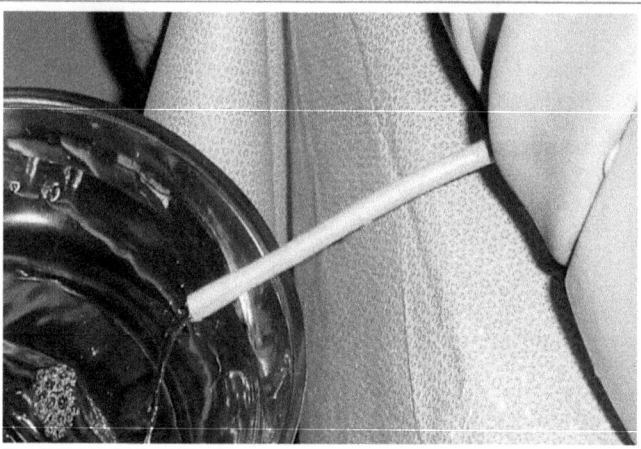
12. Continue monitoring vital signs, per vaginal bleeding, and use antibiotic.	

Fig. 1: Steps of condom catheter tamponade by Sayeba's method.[7]

Algorithm 5: Management in traumatic postpartum hemorrhage.

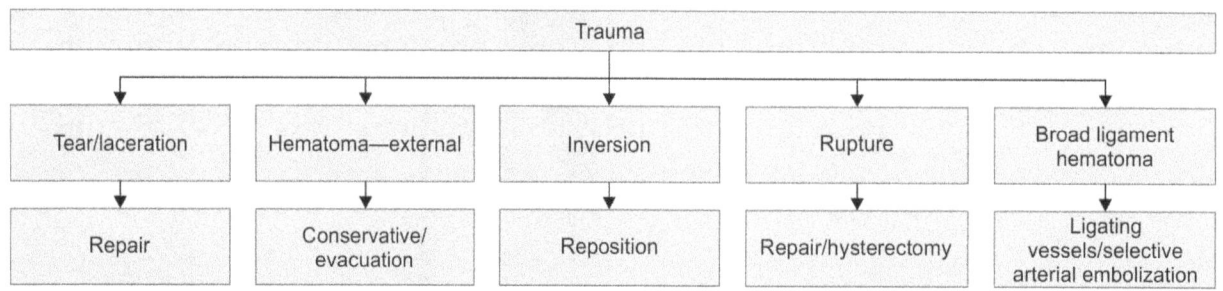

Algorithm 6: Management in coagulopathy.

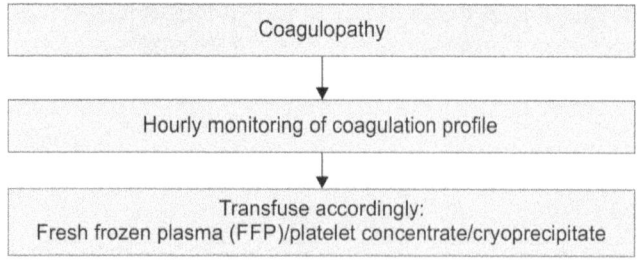

30 minutes with administration of inj. oxytocin 10 U IM or IV. Then manual removal is to be done under GA with antibiotic coverage. If patient is unstable then resuscitation followed by immediate manual removal is needed. In case of retained tissue, manual exploration followed by evacuation and curettage with antibiotic coverage is the treatment of choice. Uterotonics are needed to be continued **(Algorithm 7)**.

Algorithm 7: Management in retained placenta/retained tissue.

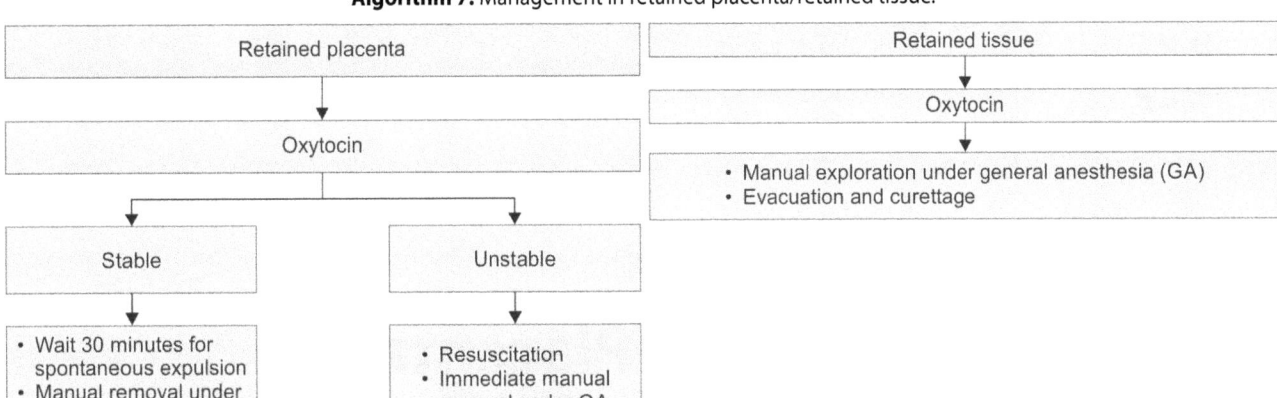

MANAGEMENT OF SECONDARY POSTPARTUM HEMORRHAGE

The predominant causes of secondary PPH are retained tissue and infection. However, the possibility of gestational trophoblastic disease must be kept in mind. Patient may present with fever, foul-smelling discharge, tender abdomen with subinvoluted uterus and open os. Some necessary investigations needed to be sent immediately are: high vaginal, endocervical, and rectal swab for C/S, urine C/S, blood C/S, CBC and C-reactive protein (CRP), serum beta-human chorionic gonadotropin (β-hCG), and coagulation profile. USG must be done to exclude retained product of conception. Immediate starting of uterotonics and antibiotics (ampicillin + metronidazole + gentamicin/clindamycin + gentamicin) are recommended. Surgical evacuation should be done immediately in patients with heavy bleeding and followed by UBT/devascularization/hysterectomy as appropriate. In stable patients, surgical procedures can be delayed for 24 hours of antibiotic therapy **(Algorithm 8)**.

Algorithm 8: Management of secondary postpartum hemorrhage (PPH).

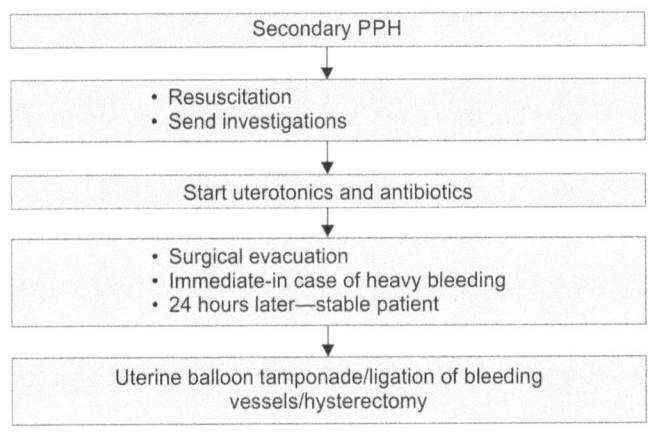

REFERENCES

1. FIGO Safe Motherhood and Newborn Health (SMNH) Committee. Prevention and treatment of postpartum hemorrhage in low resource settings. Int J Gynaecol Obstet. 2012;117:108-18.
2. Mavrides E, Allard S, Chandraharan E, et al. Prevention and management of postpartum haemorrhage. BJOG. 2016;124:e106-49.
3. WHO. WHO Recommendations for the Prevention and Treatment of Postpartum Hemorrhage. Geneva: WHO Press; 2012.
4. WHO recommendations: uterotonics for the prevention of postpartum haemorrhage. Geneve: World Health Organization; 2018. Licence: CC BY-NC-SA 3.0 IGO.
5. Su LL, Chong YS, Samuel M. Carbetocin for preventing postpartum hemorrhage. Cochrane Database Syst Rev. 2012;(2):CD005457.
6. Widmer M, Piaggio G, Nguyen TMH, Osoti A, Owa O, Misra S, et al for the WHO CHAMPION Trial Group. Heat Stable Carbetocin versus Oxytocin to Prevent Hemorrhage after Vaginal Birth. N Engl J Med. 2018;379:743-52. DOI: 10.1056/NEJMoa1805489.
7. WOMAN Trial Collaborators. Effect of early tranexamic acid administration on mortality, hysterectomy, and other morbidities in women with post-partum hemorrhage (WOMAN): an international, randomized, double-blind, placebo-controlled trial. Lancet. 2017;389(10084):2105-16.
8. Akhter S, Begum MR, Kabir Z, Rashid M, Laila TR, Zabeen F. Use of a condom to control massive postpartum hemorrhage. Med Gen Med. 2003;5(3):38.
9. WHO recommendation on tranexamic acid for the treatment of postpartum haemorrhage. Geneva: World Health Organization; 2017. Licence: CC BY-NC-SA 3.0 IGO.

Retained Placenta

Vandana Bhuriya

INTRODUCTION

The third stage of labor is the period after delivery of baby up to delivery of placenta. This stage comprises of:

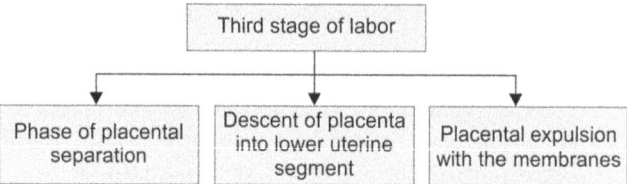

MECHANISM OF PLACENTAL SEPARATION (ALGORITHM 1)

Duration of third stage of labor is usually between 5 and 15 minutes. Third stage is diagnosed to be delayed if it takes longer than 30 minutes to deliver the placenta with active management of labor OR 60 minutes if allowed to deliver the placenta physiologically with maternal effort (NICE intrapartum guidelines).[1]

In developing countries, it affects about 0.1% of deliveries but has up to 10% case fatality rate. In developed countries, it is more common (about 3% of vaginal deliveries) but very rarely associated with mortality due to easy availability of medical care.[2]

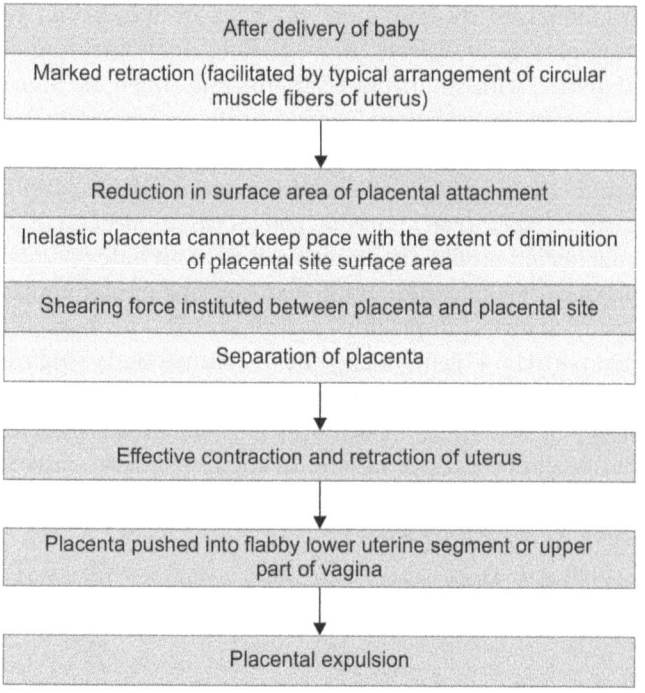

Algorithm 1: Mechanism of placental separation.

TYPES OF RETAINED PLACENTA

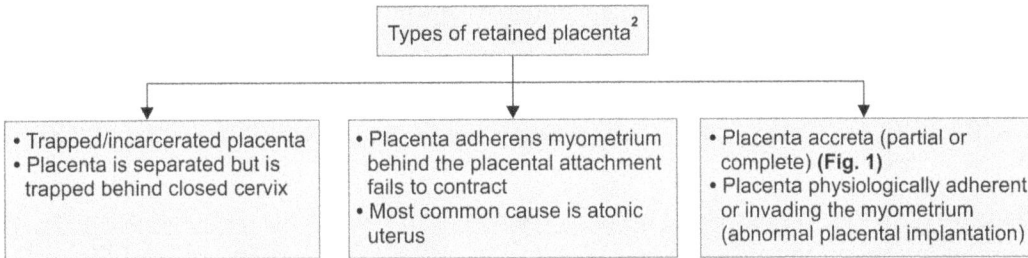

RISK FACTORS

- Preterm delivery
- Previous history of abortion
- Previous history of retained placenta
- Previous cesarean section or any other surgery on uterus (myomectomy)
- Induced labor
- Uterine malformations (bicornuate uterus)
- Leiomyoma uterus.

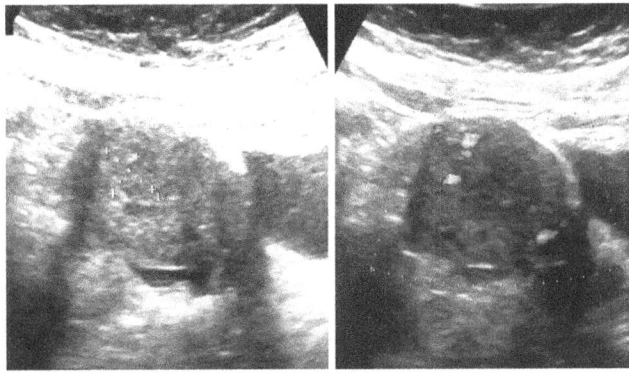

Fig. 1: Echogenic mass within the endometrial cavity with few hyperechoic foci giving stippled appearance and with areas of increased vascularity within it suggestive of retained placenta.

MANAGEMENT OF RETAINED PLACENTA (ALGORITHM 2)

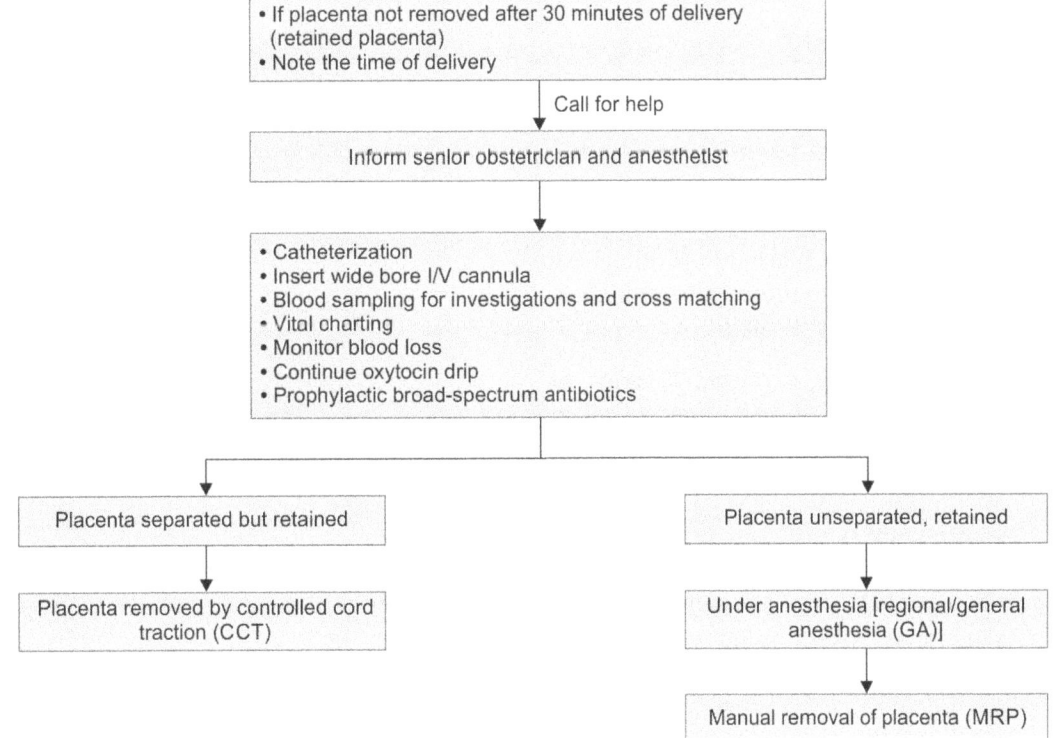

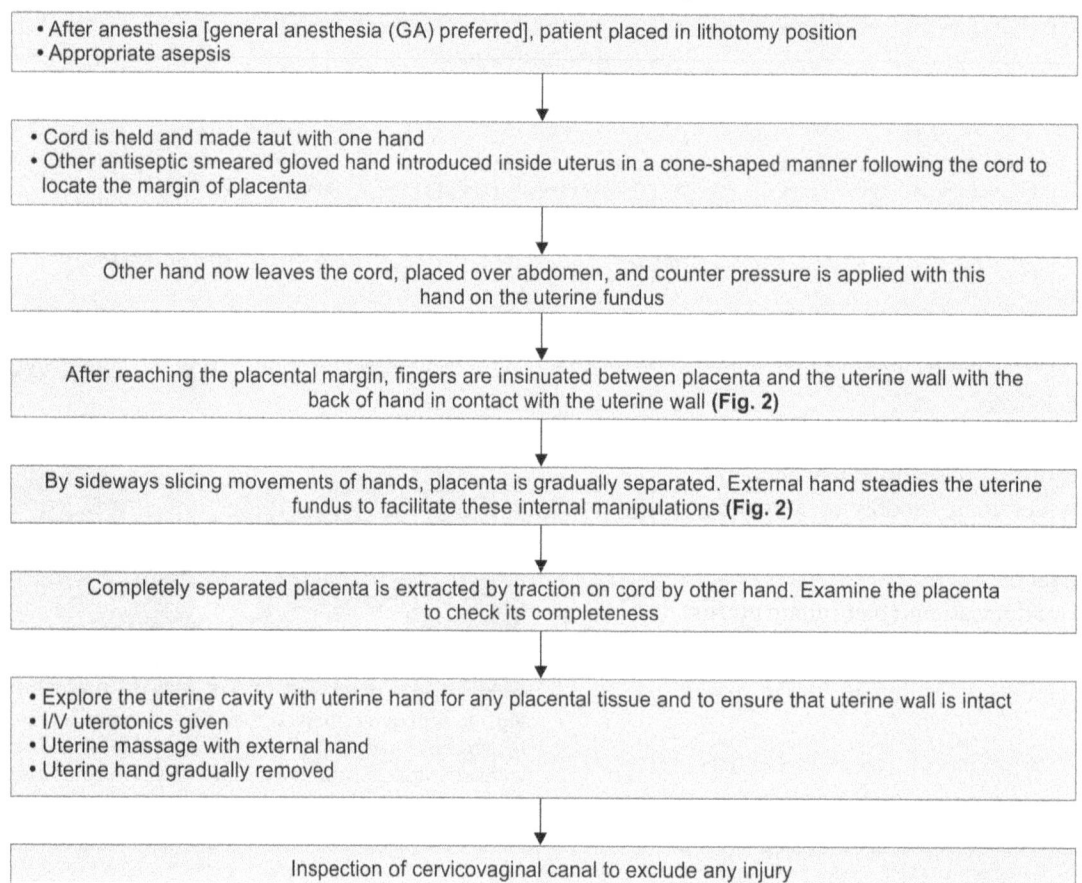

Algorithm 3: Procedure of manual removal of placenta (MRP).

Procedure of Manual Removal of Placenta (Algorithm 3)

Medical Management

Some attempts have been made to increase the uterine contractility so that retained placenta is expelled without the need of manual removal of placenta (MRP). These methods may be attempted before resorting to anesthesia or in areas where anesthesia is not available.

Intraumbilical vein injection of oxytocin: 20 units of oxytocin are mixed in 20 mL saline and injected up to umbilical vein have been studied. Not recommended by a Cochrane review[3] and NICE.[1]

Sulprostone: A potent stimulator of uterine smooth muscle contractions with high abortifacient activity. It has been shown to reduce the need of MRP by 49% in one study.[4]

Multicentric randomized trials are required for proving the beneficial effect of these agents for retained placenta.

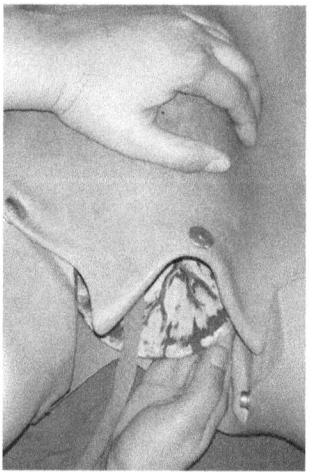

Fig. 2: Manual removal of placenta.

COMPLICATIONS OF RETAINED PLACENTA

- Infection
- Hemorrhage

- Shock
- Subinvolution
- Hysterectomy.

REFERENCES

1. NICE. Intrapartum Care: Care of Healthy Women and their Babies during Childbirth. NICE Clinical Guideline. London, UK: NICE; 2014.
2. Weeks AD. The retained placenta. Best Pract Res Clin Obstet Gynaecol. 2008;22:1103-17.
3. Nardin JM, Weeks A, Carroli G. Umbilical vein injection for management of retained placenta. Cochrane Database Syst Rev. 2011;(5)13:CD001337.
4. van Beekhuizen HJ, de Groot AN, De Boo T, et al. Sulprostone reduces the need for the manual removal of placenta in patients with retained placenta: a randomized controlled trial. Am J Obstet Gynecol. 2006;194(2):446-50.

Chapter 46

Maternal Collapse

Pratima Mittal, Jyotsna Suri

DEFINITION

Maternal collapse is an acute event involving the cardiorespiratory system and/or brain, resulting in reduced/absent conscious levels and potentially death at any stage of pregnancy and up to 6 weeks postpartum.[1]

HOW TO RESPOND TOWARD A WOMAN WITH MATERNAL COLLAPSE?

The initial approach aims to resuscitate the collapsed woman **(Algorithm 1)**. Shout and tap shoulders of woman from front to check for response.[2]

If woman is not responsive then:
- Do not waste time in starting resuscitation. Even if there is nobody around, start resuscitation immediately and shout for help.[2,3]
- Turn the woman on her back and quickly open airway with head tilt and chin lift, at the same time, look, listen, and feel for breathing.[2]

If there are no sounds or movements of breathing or carotid pulse (do not waste precious time on looking for carotid—maximum time 10 seconds—checking for breathing and carotid pulse can be simultaneous), proceed to high-quality chest compressions.[2,3]

Algorithm 1: Initial approach toward woman with maternal collapse.

Definition: An acute event involving the cardiorespiratory system and/or brain, resulting in reduced/absent conscious levels and potentially death at any stage of pregnancy and up to 6 weeks postpartum.

Maternal collapse → Responsive? → Shout for help

Yes:
- Put in left lateral position
- Assess maternal condition
- Perform obstetric evaluation
- Assess fatal well being
- Call for obstetric review

No:
- Tilt the women head, keep it tilted and lift chin and open airway
- Inspect the mouth and remove the foreign body, if present and easily visible
- Check airway by looking for chest movements, listening for breath sounds and feeling for the breath movements
- ***Simultaneously feel carotids for no more than 10 seconds***

Agonal breaths are irregular, slow, and deep breaths, frequently accompanied by a characteristic snoring sound. They originate from the brain stem, which remains functioning for some minutes even when deprived of oxygen. The presence of agonal breathing can be interpreted incorrectly as evidence of circulation and that cardiopulmonary resuscitation (CPR) is not needed. Agonal breathing may be present in up to 40% of victims in the first minutes after cardiac arrest and, if correctly identified as a sign of cardiac arrest, is associated with higher survival rates.[2]

Note: The focus is more on response of woman and breathing rather than pulse as a trigger to start chest compressions.

FEATURES OF GOOD QUALITY COMPRESSIONS (ALGORITHM 2)

- Rate of CPR should be 100–120/min.[3]
- The ratio of compressions to ventilation is 30:2.[3]
- Compression should be given at the lower half of the sternum between the nipples with heel of one hand and the other hand on top with fingers interlocked.[3]
- Push chest hard and fast. It should be compressed at least by 5–6 cm.[3]
- Allow complete recoil of the chest wall.[3]
- Do not bend your elbows when doing chest compressions; doing so will deliver weak, ineffective chest compression.[3]
- The time interval between each compression and relaxation should be approximately the same.[3]
- Minimize any interruptions to chest compression (hands-off time).[3]
- If available, use a prompt and/or feedback device to help ensure high-quality chest compressions.[4]
- Do not rely on palpating carotid or femoral pulses to assess the effectiveness of chest compressions.[5]
- Resume compressions without any delay; place your hands back on the center of the patient's chest (lower part of sternum).[3]
- Ideally, the person doing compression should be changed every 2 minutes if there are enough team members so that fatigue does not compromise the quality of compression. This change should be done with minimal interruption to compressions and should be done during planned pauses in chest compression such as during rhythm assessment.
- Use a bag and mask to start ventilation and supplemental oxygen should be added as soon as possible. A tight seal should be formed over the nose and with one hand such that a "C" is formed **(Fig. 1)**. The other hand should be used to inflate the bag. The inspiratory time should be around 1 second. Give enough volume to produce a visible rise of the chest wall. Avoid rapid or forceful breaths.[2,3]
- The compression/ventilation ratio should be no more than 30:2. Once advanced airway is in place, the breaths should be given at a rate of 10/min and compressions at 100–120/min.[3]
- As soon as a defibrillator is available, the self-adhesive pads should be applied to the chest. Do not interrupt compressions during this process. The heart rhythm

Algorithm 2: Cardiopulmonary resuscitation (CPR) in pregnant women.

During CPR:
- Rate of CPR should be 100–120/min
- Compression should be given at the lower border of the sternum between the nipples with heel of one hand and the other hand on top with fingers interlocke
- If pregnant uterus more than 20 weeks LUD to be done
- Depth 5–6 cm: Push hard and fast
- Allow complete recoil of the chest wall
- Attempt/verify IV access, airway and oxygen
- Give Inj. Epinephrine in a dose of 1 mg every 3–5 minutes if non-shockable rhythm

- Tilt the women head, keep it tilted and lifted chin and open airway
- Inspect the mouth and remove the foreign body, if present and easily visible
- Check airway by looking for chest movements, listening for breath sounds and feeling for the breath movements.
- *Simultaneously feel carotids for no more than 10 seconds*

↓ Palpable but no breathing
- Ventilate with bag and mask or mouth every 5–6 seconds
- Ensure chest rises visibly
- Check carotid pulse every 2 minutes

↓ Not palpable/not clearly defined with no breathing/agonal breathing
- CPR 30:2 until defibrillator/monitor attached
- If no response after 4 minutes, of CPR/ proceed with perimortem cesarean section

(IV: intravenous; LUD: left uterine displacement)

will be assessed with the electrodes during a brief pause (less than 5 seconds) in compressions.[2]
- If the rhythm is ventricular fibrillation/pulseless ventricular tachycardia (VF/pVT), start defibrillation. All other team members are informed to stand clear of the patient, the fetal monitors and oxygen are placed away, and shock is delivered.[2,3] The energy used is the same as for nonpregnant patients.
- Restart chest compressions immediately. Do not delay restarting chest compressions to check the cardiac rhythm.[2,3]
- If rhythm is nonshockable asystole or pulseless electrical activity, do not defibrillate but continue CPR.[2,3]
- Using a manual defibrillator, it is possible to reduce the pause between stopping and restarting of chest compressions to less than 5 seconds.[3]
- If staff cannot use a manual defibrillator, use an automated external defibrillator (AED). Switch it on and just follow the instructions.
- If there is no access, IV access should be established once resuscitation is underway so as to deliver the drugs. Injection adrenaline 1 mg IV, every 3–5 minutes, if nonshockable rhythm. In case of refractory ventricular fibrillation, Inj. amiodarone 300 mg IV.

HOW IS RESUSCITATION DIFFERENT IN PREGNANT WOMEN?

Chest compressions are performed in the same way as in a nonpregnant person *except* that if the pregnant uterus is above the umbilicus, it should be tilted toward the left side with one hand or both hands by the assisting personnel. This is to relieve the aortocaval compression effect of the uterus so as to increase the cardiac output and make the compressions more effective **(Fig. 2)**. The 15° tilt of the patient which was practiced earlier is not recommended anymore as it hampers effective compressions.[3]

Remember...
Leftward Displacement of Uterus During CPR Either with Single Hand or with Both Hands

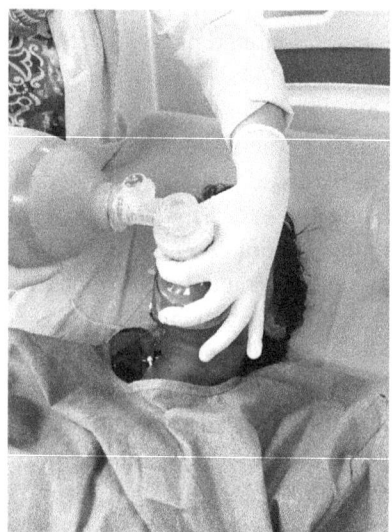

Fig. 1: Technique for giving bag and mask ventilation.

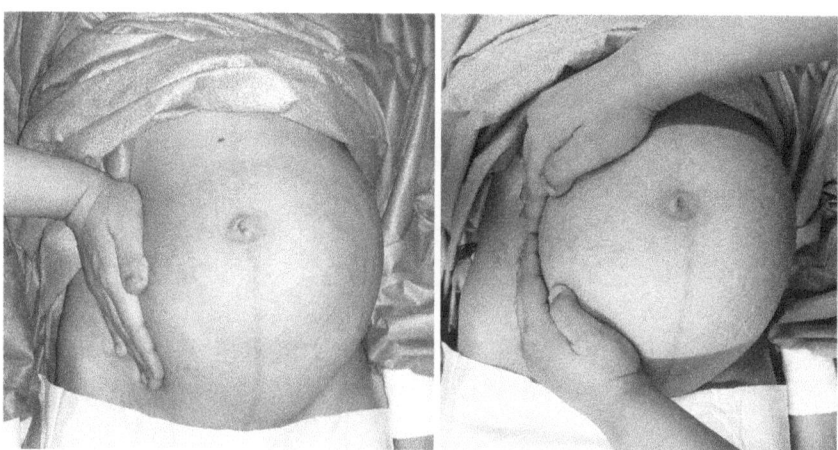

Fig. 2: One-handed and two-handed methods to achieve left uterine displacement.

EVALUATION OF THE CAUSE OF MATERNAL COLLAPSE

Evaluate the causes of maternal collapse after initial resuscitation. The causes of cardiac arrest in pregnancy can be remembered by mnemonic "BEAU CHOPS."
- **B**leeding
- **E**mbolism:
  - Pulmonary
  - Amniotic fluid
- **A**nesthetic complication
- **U**terine atony
- **C**ardiac disease
- **H**ypertension:
  - Preeclampsia
  - Eclampsia
- **O**ther:
  - Mg toxicity
  - Other differential diagnosis of standard ACLS, i.e. 5 Ts and 5 H
- **P**lacenta abruption/previa
- **S**epsis

Immediately after resuscitation steps should be taken to identify and treat the underlying cause.

ROLE OF PERIMORTEM CESAREAN DELIVERY SECTION

If CPR is not effective, consider resuscitative hysterotomy [also called perimortem cesarean delivery (PMCD)]:
- Perimortem cesarean delivery should be considered at 4 minutes after onset of maternal cardiac arrest or resuscitative efforts (for the unwitnessed arrest) if there is no maternal return of spontaneous circulation (ROSC)—AHA 2015 Guidelines.
- In patients who are >20 weeks of pregnancy. Before 20 weeks of gestation, there is no proven benefit from the delivery of the fetus and placenta. Perimortem cesarean section should be considered a resuscitative procedure to be performed primarily in the interests of maternal, not fetal, survival.

The time frame can be extended to 6–14 minutes with good results as reported recently:[4]
- A study by Rose et al. reinforced the concept that arrangements for delivery should be made at the same time with initiation of maternal resuscitative efforts if the uterus is palpable at or above the umbilicus. The authors also added that if maternal condition is not rapidly reversible, hysterotomy with delivery should be performed regardless of fetal viability or elapsed time since arrest.[5]

- The resuscitation is more effective as the aortocaval compression is relieved, the maternal oxygen requirement reduces, and lung mechanics improve.[6,7]
- Perimortem cesarean section should not be delayed by moving the woman—it should be performed where resuscitation is taking place and there is no need to administer anesthesia.
- A perimortem cesarean section tray should be available on the resuscitation trolley in all areas where maternal collapse may occur, including the accident and emergency department.
- The principle of successful CS delivery is rapid incision, rapid delivery, and rapid closure. It is best obtained with large vertical abdominal incisions, classical lower segment cesarian section (LSCS), and closure with large running sutures in a single layer.[6,7]
- Cesarean section will be relatively bloodless since there is no circulation and cardiac output. Chest compressions and ventilation should be continued. If mother is resuscitated then she can be shifted to OT for proper closure of uterus and abdomen; and subsequently to ICU.
- Best survival rate for infants >28 weeks occurs when delivery of infant occurs in <5 minutes after the mother's heart stops beating.

REFERENCES

1. Royal College of Obstetricians and Gynaecologists. (2011). Maternal Collapse in Pregnancy and the Puerperium (Green-top Guideline No. 56). [Online] Available from: https://www.rcog.org.uk/globalassets/documents/guidelines/gtg_56.pdf [Last accessed September, 2019].
2. Resuscitation Council UK. Adult basic life support and automated external defibrillation. London, UK: Resuscitation Council UK; 2015.
3. American Heart Association. American Heart Association Guidelines for CPR & ECC, 2015. Dallas, USA: American Heart Association; 2015.
4. Baghirzada L, Mrinalini B. Maternal cardiac arrest in a tertiary care centre during 1989-2011: a case series. Can J Anesth. 2013;60:1077-84.
5. Rose CH, Faksh A, Traynor KD, et al. Challenging the 4- to 5-minute rule: from perimortem cesarean to resuscitative hysterotomy. Am J Obstet Gynecol. 2015;213(5):653-6, 653.e1.
6. Katz V, Balderston K, DeFreest M. Perimortem cesarean delivery: were our assumptions correct? Am J Obstet Gynecol. 2005;192(6):1916-20; discussion 1920-1.
7. Smith S. Mother and baby survive near-death experiences. [online] CNN website. Available at: http://www.cnn.com/2010/HEALTH/01/05/mother.baby.revived/index.html [Last accessed September, 2019].

Chapter 47

Uterine Inversion

Parneet Kaur

INTRODUCTION

It is one of the rare but life-threatening complications of third stage of labor with high maternal morbidity and mortality if not recognized and rectified in time.

DEFINITION

It is the turning inside out of the uterus.

INCIDENCE

In India, the incidence reported is 1:2,000–1:50,000 deliveries.[1]

CLASSIFICATION OF INVERSION (ALGORITHM 1)

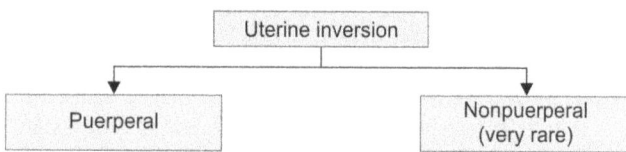

Algorithm 1: Classification of inversion.

- In puerperal inversion, part of the uterus indents toward the dilated cervix and eventually passes through it. For the initial indentation, relaxation of the uterus is required followed by resumption of contractions in such a way that inversion ensues.
- Nonpuerperal inversion is very rare and occurs in nonpregnant patients when it is usually associated with prolapsing uterine fibroids or other benign pathologies. The nonpuerperal uterine inversion is beyond the scope of this book.

TYPES OF INVERSION (ALGORITHM 2)

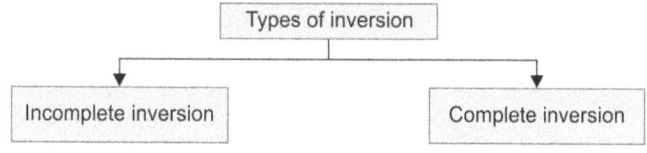

Algorithm 2: Types of inversion.

- In incomplete inversion, the fundus turns inside out but it has still not come out through the cervix.
- In complete inversion, the fundus passes through the cervix and may be lying inside the vagina or outside introitus.

The obstetric inversion is mostly complete but it may be incomplete at times.

DEGREES OF INVERSION (ALGORITHM 3)[1]

The placenta may or may not have been separated from the uterine wall before the inversion occurred.

Chapter 47: Uterine Inversion

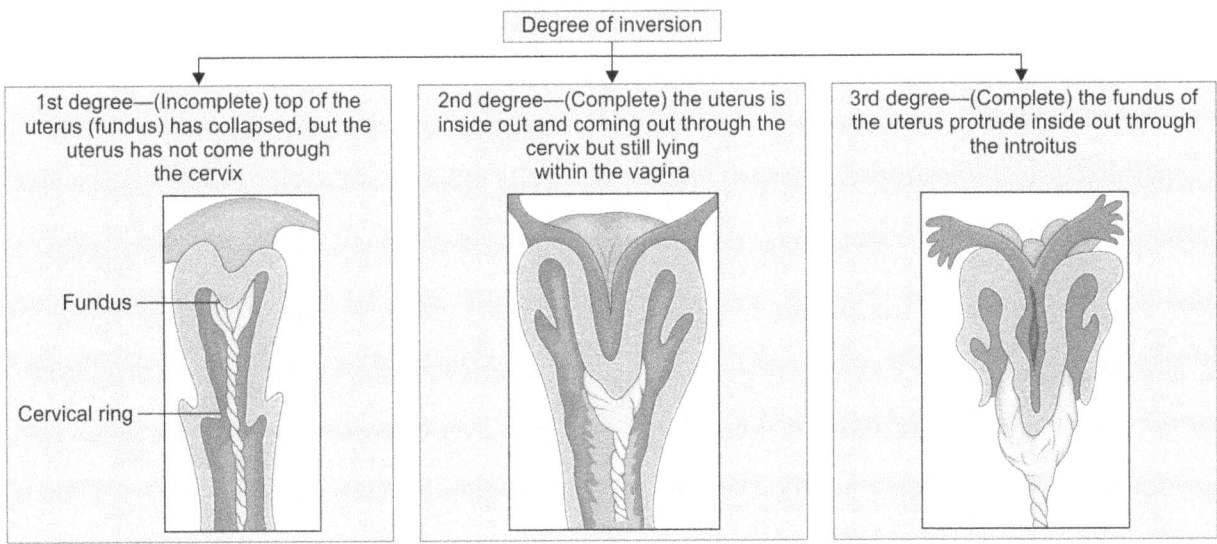

Algorithm 3: Degrees of inversion.

TIMING OF INVERSION (ALGORITHM 4)[2]

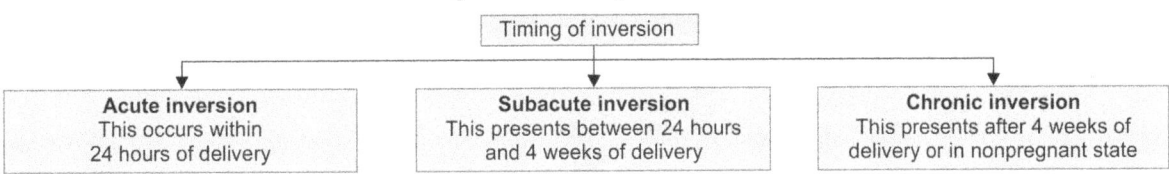

Algorithm 4: Timing of inversion.

ETIOLOGY (ALGORITHM 5)

- For inversion to occur, uterus must be relaxed.
- Many predisposing factors are incriminated as a cause for uterine inversion.
- Still, in up to 50% of cases, no precipitating factor is identified.

DIAGNOSIS

Prompt diagnosis is crucial and life-saving for the patient:
- If a mass appears in the vagina/outside introitus, the diagnosis is obvious. Placenta may or may not be attached.
- Always have suspicion of inversion when:
  - When the degree of shock is inconsistent with visible blood loss.
  - Postpartum hemorrhage (PPH) is associated with severe and sustained lower abdominal pain.
  - There is a feeling of "dimple" in the uterine fundus on per abdomen examination or fundus is not palpable.
  - On P/V examination, mass is felt in the vagina and this confirms the diagnosis (**Fig. 1**).
- Very rarely when diagnosis is not clear by physical examination and patient is hemodynamically stable, an ultrasound can confirm the diagnosis.[3]

Shock in cases of inversion uterus is always out of proportion to visible blood loss (**Algorithm 6**).

Algorithm 5: Etiology of uterine inversion.

```
                    Etiology
                       │
        ┌──────────────┴──────────────┐
        ▼                             ▼
```

Mismanaged third stage of labor
It is the most common (80%) cause of acute inversion of uterus:
- Pulling on the umbilical cord in the absence of a uterine contraction in an effort to deliver the placenta before placental separation has occurred
- Fundal pressure when uterus is relaxed.

Other causative factors:
- Sudden increase in intra-abdominal pressure due to coughing/sneezing after delivery of infant when the uterus has still not contracted
- Fundal attachment of placenta
- Morbidly adherent placenta
- Short cord
- Precipitate delivery
- Previous uterine inversion
- Inversion may occur, following manual removal of placenta (MROP) under general anesthesia (GA) if the manipulating hand is removed too soon, even before the uterine tone has returned
- A spontaneous inversion without any cause is also seen during lower segment cesarean section (LSCS) under anesthesia
- Magnesium sulfate has been recently incriminated as a cause for inversion[3]
- Connective tissue disorders (Marfan's syndrome, Ehler-Danlos syndrome) are very rare causes

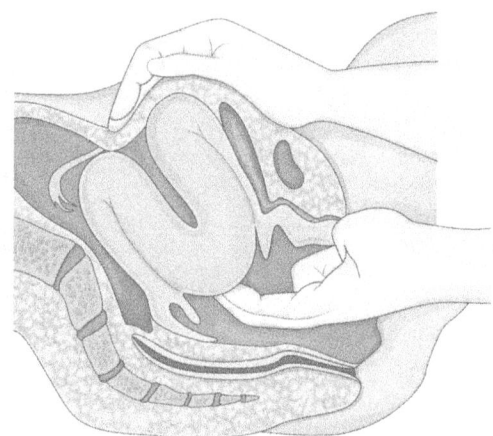

Fig. 1: Incomplete uterine prolapse can be diagnosed by bimanual examination.

Algorithm 6: Causes of shock in uterine inversion.

```
              Causes of shock in uterine inversion
    ┌──────────────┬──────────────┬──────────────┐
    ▼              ▼              ▼              ▼
```

| The prolapsed uterus stretching the cervix causes vagal stimulation thus the woman has signs of cardiovascular collapse and shock | Due to tension on the nerves because of stretching of infundibulopelvic ligaments | There is pressure on the ovaries as they are dragged with the fundus through the cervical ring | Peritoneal irritation |

CLINICAL FEATURES (ALGORITHM 7)

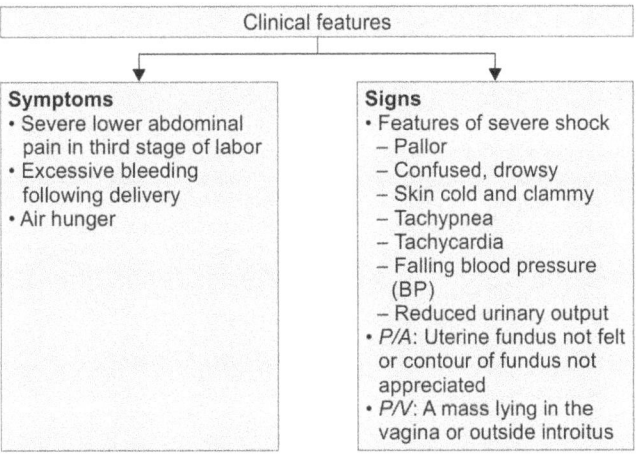

Algorithm 7: Clinical features.

DIFFERENTIAL DIAGNOSIS (ALGORITHM 8)

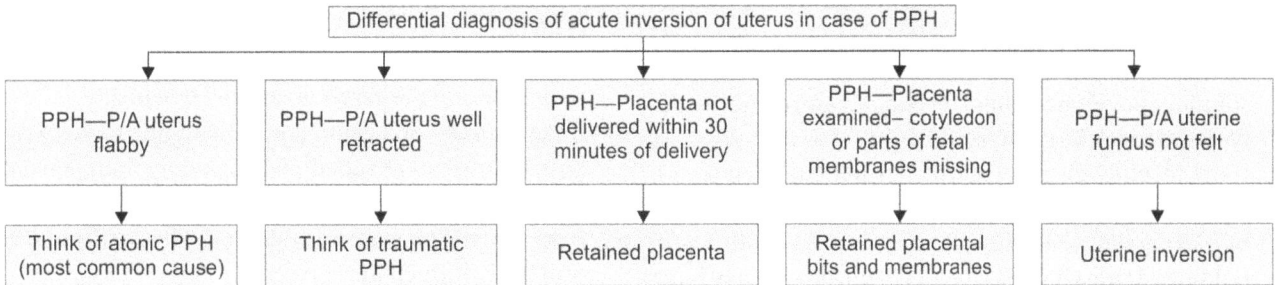

Algorithm 8: Differential diagnosis of uterine inversion in case of postpartum hemorrhage (PPH).

MANAGEMENT (ALGORITHM 9)

- The definitive management is immediate *manual replacement of uterus*.
- Thus, the best person to treat is the attendant present at the time of its occurrence.
- If the placenta is still attached, do not try to remove it (because of danger of massive hemorrhage). If the placenta is partially attached to the fundus, only then it should be removed.[4]
- Do not give uterotonics (oxytocin).[4]
- If not replaced immediately, usually within minutes the uterus and cervix contract and then due to increasing congestion and edema, replacement without anesthesia becomes impossible.

Once PPH has been identified, management involves four components, all of which must be undertaken simultaneously.[5]

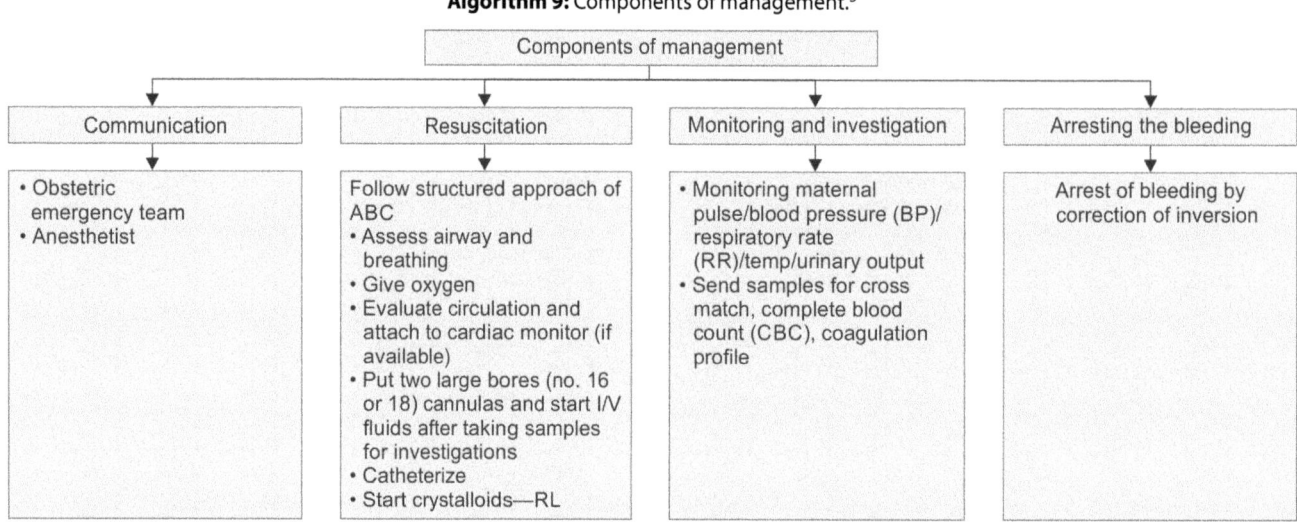

Algorithm 9: Components of management.[5]

Manual Replacement of Uterus

First-line management endorsed by all governing bodies (WHO, ACOG, RCOG):[5-7]

- The inverted uterus should be cleaned with antiseptic solution (povidone iodine) thoroughly and compressed with warm sterile sponge.
- If the recently inverted uterus has not contracted and retracted, then the uterus may be replaced immediately by placing the palm of the hand against the fundus as if holding a tennis ball and fingers in the direction of long axis of vagina.
- Keeping fingers at cervicouterine junction and resting fundus in palm, lift the uterus above the level of umbilicus by exerting upward pressure circumferentially. This maneuver was first described by AB Johnson in 1949 thus is known as Johnson maneuver **(Fig. 2)**.[8]
- Always push the part that has inverted last of all, i.e. the part closest to the cervix is reposed first of all.
- If the manual replacement is difficult due to increased bulk because of attached placenta, only then placenta may be removed and replacement tried again.
- Basically, the purpose and effort are to push the uterine wall back through the cervix.
- Put the other hand over the abdomen for counter support.
- The sooner inversion is replaced, more the chances of success.

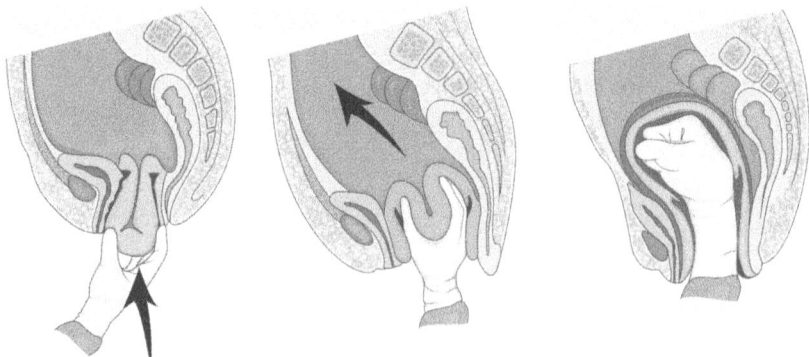

Fig. 2: Manual replacement of inverted uterus.

- If not successful then immediate manual replacement under tocolytic cover can be tried, e.g. Inj. terbutaline 250 μg subcutaneously or intravenously diluted in 5 mL of saline slowly over 5 minutes (other tocolytic that can be used are magnesium sulfate and nitroglycerine).[1,7]
- Terbutaline is preferred drug because of its rapid onset of action, short half-life, easy availability in labor room, ease of use, and more familiarity by the obstetricians.[8]
- Tocolysis should be stopped as soon as inversion is corrected.
- After a successful replacement, keep the hand in the uterus and give rapid oxytocin infusion (20 units in 500 mL of Ringer lactate solution) to contract the uterus.
- Feel that the uterus is contracted.
- Now proceed with manual removal of placenta (MROP) if placenta still attached.
- Slowly withdraw the hand from the uterus after ensuring that it is well contracted.
- Now maintain bimanual compression till uterus is firmly contracted.
- It is very satisfying to do P/S examination and see restored cervical lips.
- Continue monitoring the uterus for evidence of subsequent inversion.
- Prophylactic antibiotics are given as per the institute protocol.
- Give blood and blood products as per the estimated blood loss.
- If still unsuccessful then manual replacement is to be attempted under general anesthesia (GA).[6]
- Now the patient needs to be shifted to OT from labor room.
- If needs referral, repose the prolapsed uterus into vagina and refer after informing the referral center telephonically. If prolapsed part cannot be reposed then cover the prolapsed uterus with a sponge soaked in antiseptic solution.
- Manual replacement is again tried under general anesthesia as the cervical ring will be relaxed and replacement will be possible.

Hydrostatic Pressure Method

This is recommended by WHO as second line of management if manual replacement fails:[6]
- It was first popularized by O'Sullivan thus also known as O Sullivan's hydrostatic reduction method.
- Before attempting this procedure, lacerations of vagina and rupture uterus should be excluded first and if found they should be sutured.

Principle

The vagina is filled with a large amount of fluid which distends the vaginal fornices and helps in opening the cervical ring, thus allowing replacement of inverted fundus.

Method

- Reduce the uterus into vagina
- Place the woman in deep Trendelenburg position (lower her head below the level of perineum)
- We need:
  - Douche system with a large nozzle
  - Long tubing (2 m)
  - Warm irrigation fluid (3-5 L) is required (sterile water or normal saline)
- Place the nozzle of the douche in the posterior fornix **(Fig. 3)**
- Identification of posterior fornix is easy in cases of incomplete inversion when the uterus is still in vagina. In other cases, posterior fornix can be recognized by the upper limit of rugose vagina where it becomes smooth vagina.
- Occlude the vaginal introitus with forearm[4] or silicon suction cup **(Figs. 4 to 6)**[8-10]

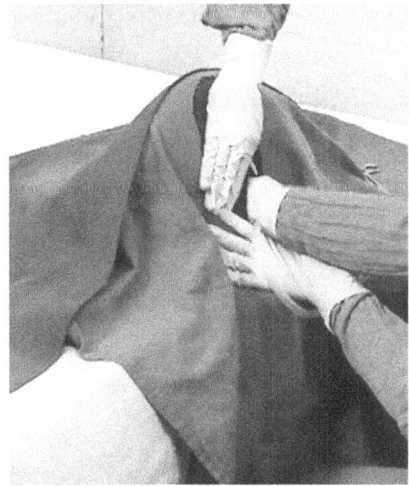

Fig. 3: Whole of hand along with tubing in posterior vaginal fornix. The assistant helps in sealing the introitus.

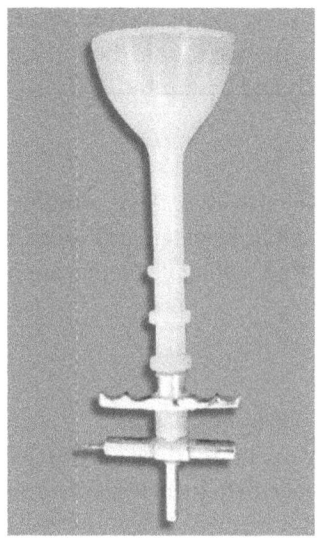

Fig. 4: Silicon ventouse cup which can be used to seal the introitus.

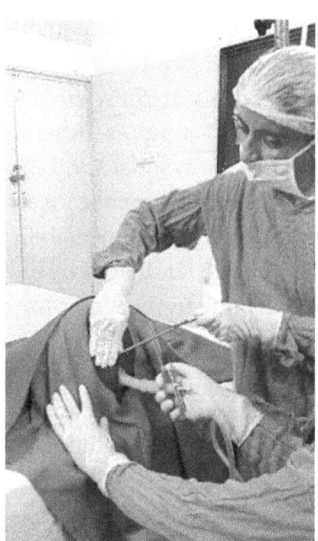

Fig. 6: The cup has to be kept in lower vagina at the inner aspect of introitus for proper sealing along with assistant helping with hand or applying Allis forceps.

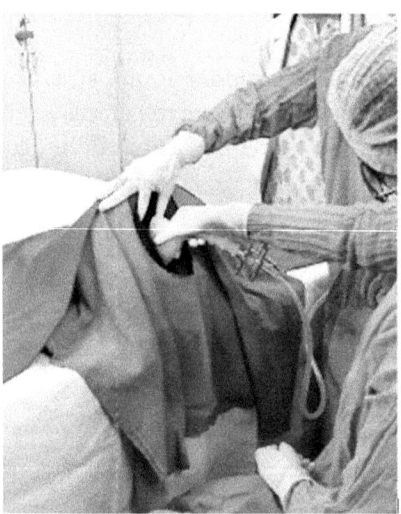

Fig. 5: The silicon ventouse cup being introduced in vagina after folding.

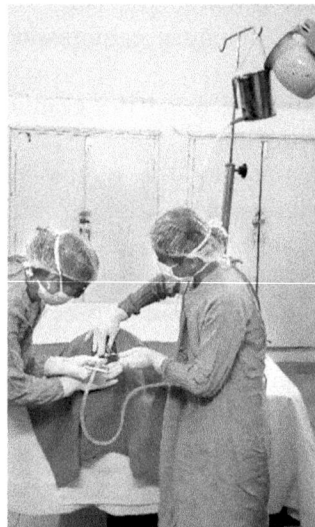

Fig. 7: An enema can which is available in all labor rooms can be utilized to instill irrigation fluid. An assistant keeps on pouring warm saline continuously.

- Douche with full pressure (**Figs. 7 and 8**)
- Raise the water reservoir to at least 2 m
- We can manually compress saline bottles to increase pressure
- The water pressure inflates the uterus and props it back into position
- Give oxytocin infusion and feel for the contour of retracted uterine fundus per abdomen before finishing the procedure

- This precautionary step ensures successful completion of procedure and will prevent recurrence and PPH
- MROP is done after uterus contracts if the placenta is still attached
- If rarely the inversion recurs then we can do balloon tamponade after correcting inversion and remove the balloon after 10–12 hours.[7]
- Patient is observed carefully in the labor ward for 24 hours and oxytocin drip is continued.

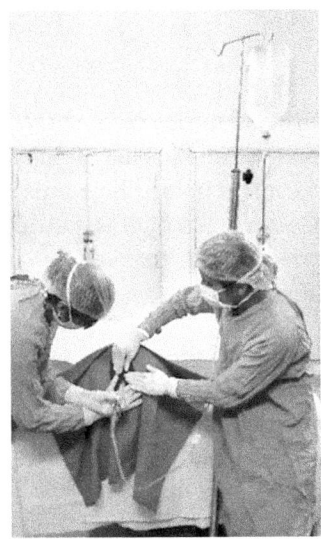

Fig. 8: A 3 L of normal saline bottle along with TUR set (trans urethral resection set) can be used to make water head. Even two bottles of normal saline can be used as TUR set has two inlets.

- Blood is replaced as per the estimated loss.
- Other uterotonic agents can be used as per need.

Surgical Methods

- Nonsurgical methods usually are successful but if unsuccessful then we need to consider surgical methods.
- The surgical methods at laparotomy are recommended as third-line management by WHO and ACOG after manual correction fails.[6,7]

Laparotomy

Huntington's Method

- The abdomen is opened in layers by subumbilical vertical skin incision under anesthesia.
- First, dilate the constricting cervical ring digitally.
- Then two Allis tissue forceps (or Babcock's) are placed inside the inverted fundus, approximately 2 cm below the ring to grasp the round ligaments.
- Using forceps on both sides, gentle continuous upward traction is applied to the fundus while an assistant attempts manual correction vaginally.
- New clamps are placed 2 cm below previous clamps and traction applied further till inversion is corrected.
- Alternatively, a silicon ventouse cup can be inserted into inverted fundus, vacuum created, and gentle traction is applied to correct inversion. Tissue trauma is much less with this technique and constriction ring is easy to negotiate.[8,11]

Haultains Method

- It is required rarely when at times constriction ring is too tight that Huntington's technique merely causes tearing of myometrium.
- In this technique, constricting cervical ring is divided posteriorly to protect the bladder lying in front.
- Repeat digital dilatation is done followed by application of Allis/Babcock's forceps for traction as in Huntington's method.
- After correction, the uterus is stitched posteriorly.

At times uterus again inverts immediately after correction, in such cases compression sutures may be applied.[12]

Vaginal Methods[2]

These methods are mentioned in the literature but as such not recommended by any major governing bodies:
- The following surgical procedures are done vaginally:
  - *Spinelli:* Anterior median colpohysterotomy is done for removal of cervical ring.
  - *Kustner:* Posterior median colpohysterotomy is done to cut the cervical ring and replace uterus followed by suturing of hysterotomy incision.
- The abdominal route is usually preferred over the vaginal route as hemorrhage is controlled more efficiently and incision over uterus is comparatively small.
- Postoperative care is to be done in the form of continuous oxytocin infusion, antibiotics, analgesics, and replacement of blood as per estimated loss.
- *Subacute inversion:* Here, hydrostatic reduction may be tried under antibiotic cover but mostly laparotomy and surgical procedures are needed.

Algorithm 10: Management of uterine inversion.

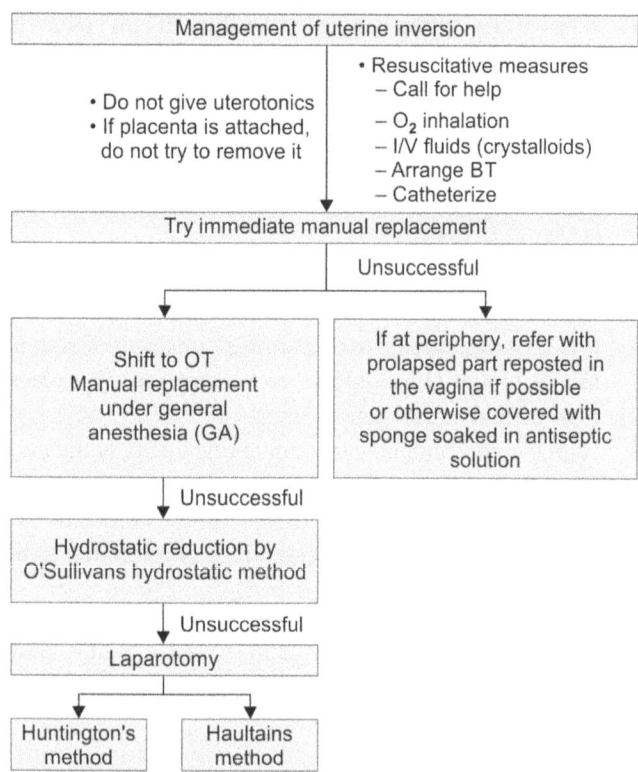

(After successful uterine replacement, give oxytocin infusion for 12–24 hours, antibiotics and blood transfusion as per estimated loss)

COMPLICATIONS (ALGORITHM 11)

Algorithm 11: Complications of uterine inversion.

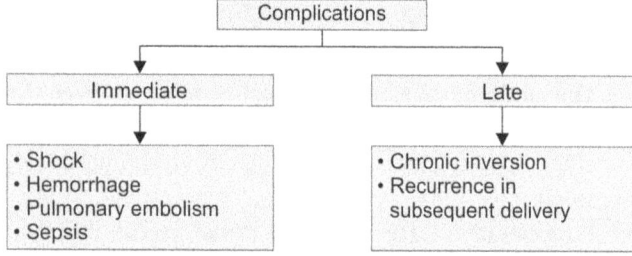

- Chronic puerperal uterine inversion may become apparent weeks after delivery. Here, correction is mostly done by surgical methods after the infection is controlled. Sometimes, hysterectomy may be necessary in these cases.
- Due to the risk of recurrence in subsequent delivery, the patient should be booked for hospital delivery in next pregnancy.

INVERSION UTERUS DURING CESAREAN SECTION[12,13]

- Inversion can occur during cesarean section, especially if manual removal of placenta is done routinely after delivery of the infant before the uterus has contracted.
- The incidence is twice as high as that of vaginal delivery but these cases are not that risky as the inversion is immediately corrected under the existing anesthesia.

ADVICE ON DISCHARGE

- Give iron and calcium supplements for 6 months.
- Appropriate contraceptive methods should be advised as per the need.
- She should be counseled and informed to avoid attempting the next pregnancy for minimum of 2 years.
- She should always go for institutional delivery in next pregnancy as inversion is known to recur.

PROGNOSIS

- If met in unfavorable surroundings, the prognosis is extremely gloomy.
- Death may occur suddenly due to hemorrhage, shock, and pulmonary embolism.
- Before modern management, very high mortality rates were reported but presently the mortality reported is much less (2.5%).[13,14]
- Even if the patient survives, infection, sloughing of the uterus and chronic inversion with ill-health may occur.

PREVENTION (ALGORITHM 12)

Algorithm 12: Prevention.[4]

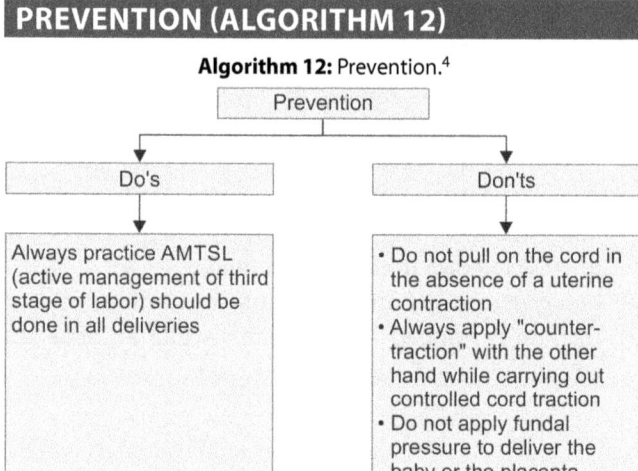

CONCLUSION

Uterine inversion is an obstetric emergency. It requires quick diagnosis and prompt action for correction with simultaneous resuscitative measures. As the incidence is low so drills for labor room staff are essential so that they are prepared for this untoward emergency. The prognosis for the patient is best if the replacement is done as early as possible.

REFERENCES

1. Baskett TF, Calder AA, Arulkumaran S. Munro Kerr's Operative Obstetrics, 11th (Centenary) edition. Philadelphia, USA: Elsevier; 2010.
2. Ziki E, Madombi S, Chidakwa C, et al. Reduction of subacute uterine inversion by Haultain's method: a case report. S Afr J Obstet Gynaecol. 2017;23(3):78-9.
3. Leal RFM, Luz RM, de Almeida JP, et al. Total and acute uterine inversion after delivery: a case report. J Med Case Rep. 2014;8:347.
4. Lalonde A, International Federation of Gynecology and Obstetrics. Prevention and treatment of postpartum hemorrhage in low-resource settings. Int J Gynecol Obstet. 2012;117:108-18.
5. Royal College of Obstetricians and Gynaecologists. Prevention and Management of Postpartum Haemorrhage. Green-top Guideline No. 52 BJOG. 2017;124(5):e106-49.
6. World Health Organization. Correcting Uterine Inversion. Managing Complications in Pregnancy and Childbirth: A Guide for Midwives and Doctors, 2nd edition. Geneva: World Health Organization; 2017. pp. 109-12.
7. Committee on Practice Bulletins-Obstetrics. Postpartum hemorrhage. ACOG Practice Bulletin 183. Obstet Gynecol. 2017;130(4):e168-86.
8. Bhalla R, Wuntakal R, Odejinmi F, et al. Acute inversion of the uterus. Obstet Gynaecol. 2009;11:13-8.
9. Gupta P, Sahu RL, Huria A. Acute uterine inversion: a simple modification of hydrostatic method of treatment. Ann Med Health Sci Res. 2014;4(2):264-7.
10. Ogueh O, Ayida G. Acute uterine inversion: a new technique of hydrostatic replacement. Br J Obstet Gynaecol. 1997;104:951-2.
11. Antonelli E, Irion O, Tolck P. Subacute uterine inversion: description of a novel replacement technique using the obstetric ventouse. BJOG. 2006;113:846-7.
12. Cunningham FG, Leveno KJ, Bloom SL, et al. (Eds). Williams Obstetrics, 24th edition. United States of America: The McGraw-Hill Education; 2014.
13. Baskett TF. Acute uterine inversion: a review of 40 cases. J Obstet Gynaecol Can. 2002;24:953-6.
14. Kittur S. A study of maternal mortality at the teaching hospital, Hubli, Karnataka. Int J Reprod Contracept Obstet Gynecol. 2013;2:74-9.

Chapter 48

Sepsis and Septic Shock

Latika Chawla

INTRODUCTION

Sepsis is one of the leading causes of maternal mortality worldwide accounting to around 15% of maternal deaths.[1] Major killer in the Indian population is still postpartum hemorrhage, preeclampsia, and eclampsia, however, sepsis still accounts for around 11% of maternal deaths in India. Sepsis is an intense response generated by the body in acknowledgment of presence of infection, which in turn damages its own tissues and organs. It is a medical emergency and has high mortality rates if not appropriately and timely dealt with.

Definitions as per the "The Third International Consensus Definition for Sepsis and Septic Shock (2016)[2]
- *Sepsis*: A life-threatening organ dysfunction caused by a dysregulated host response to infection
- Organ dysfunction is to be identified using SOFA score
- Patients with suspected infection can be quickly identified by using a rapid bedside test, the qSOFA score
- *Septic shock:* Subset of sepsis in which underlying circulatory and cellular/metabolic abnormalities are profound enough to substantially increase mortality. Clinically, sepsis with persisting hypotension that requires vasopressors to maintain mean arterial pressure (MAP) ≥65 mm Hg and with serum lactate level >2 mmol/L (18 mg/dL) despite adequate volume resuscitation is septic shock.

According to the Third International Consensus Definition for Sepsis and Septic Shock (2016),[2] sepsis is now defined as "a life-threatening organ dysfunction caused by a dysregulated host response to infection."

Patients with suspected infection can be quickly identified, without the need for laboratory tests by using a newly developed tool, the qSOFA score. Presence of any two of the following three clinical criteria (respiratory rate of 22 breaths/min or greater, altered mentation, or systolic blood pressure of 100 mm Hg or less) allows rapid identification of such patients with poorer outcomes.[3]

Organ dysfunction can be identified by an increase in the sequential (sepsis-related) organ failure assessment (SOFA) score by ≥2.[3] The SOFA score can be calculated as in **Table 1**.[3] Baseline SOFA score for a person without infection is taken as zero. A score of ≥2 reflects organ dysfunction and is suggestive of an overall mortality rate of >10%.[3]

The consensus has defined septic shock as a "subset of sepsis in which underlying circulatory and cellular/metabolic abnormalities are profound enough to substantially increase mortality."[2] Clinically, a patient with sepsis with persisting hypotension that requires vasopressors to maintain mean arterial pressure (MAP) ≥65 mm Hg and with serum lactate level >2 mmol/L (18 mg/dL) despite adequate volume resuscitation is said to be in septic shock. Mortality rates with septic shock reach up to 40% and are even higher in pregnant women reaching up to 60%.[4]

The terms "severe sepsis" and "systemic inflammatory response syndrome (SIRS)" have been abandoned. The SOFA score is not applicable to the pregnant population.

Table 1: Sequential (sepsis related) organ failure assessment (SOFA) score.[a]

	Score				
System	0	1	2	3	4
Respiration PaO$_2$/FiO$_2$, mm Hg (kPa)	≥400 (53.3)	<400 (53.3)	<300 (40)	<200 (26.7) with respiratory support	<100 (13.3) with respiratory support
Coagulation Platelets, × 10^3/μL	≥150	<150	<100	<50	<20
Liver Bilirubin (mg/dL)	<1.2	1.2–1.9	2.0–5.9	6.0–11.9	>12.0
Cardiovascular	MAP ≥ 70 mm Hg	<70 mm Hg	Dopamine <5 or dobutamine (any dose)[b]	Dopamine 5.1–15 or epinephrine <0.1 or norepinephrine <0.1[b]	Dopamine >15 or epinephrine >0.1 or norepinephrine >0.1[b]
Central nervous system Glasgow Coma Scale[c]	15	13–14	10–12	6–9	<6
Renal Creatine (mg/dL) Urine Output mL/d	<1.2	1.2–1.9	2.0–3.4	3.5–4.9 <500	>5 <200

[a]Adapted from Vincent JL et al, 1998[3]
[b]Catecholamine doses are given as μg/kg/min for atleast 1 hour
[c]Glasgow Coma Scale Scores range from 3–15: Higher score indicates better neurological function
(FiO$_2$: fraction of inspired oxygen; MAP: mean arterial pressure; PaO$_2$: partial pressure of oxygen)

However, till date, there are no universally validated scores/guidelines that can be accepted for diagnosing/monitoring sepsis in pregnant women.

The overall incidence of sepsis is on the rise due to the increase in life span, presence of multiple co-morbidities in the older population, and use of immune-suppressants.

RISK FACTORS

Risk factors for the development of sepsis in the pregnant population have been identified in **Box 1**.[5]

Box 1 Risk factors.

- African American ethnicity
- Anemia
- Obesity
- Impaired glucose tolerance/diabetes
- Immunosuppressant medication
- Vaginal discharge
- History of group B streptococcal infection
- Amniocentesis/invasive procedures
- Cervical cerclage
- Prolonged spontaneous rupture of membranes
- Group A streptococcal infection in close contacts/family members

Causes of sepsis vary in the antepartum and postpartum period[6,7] and are enlisted below in **Algorithm 1**.

Algortithm 1: Sepsis in pregnancy.

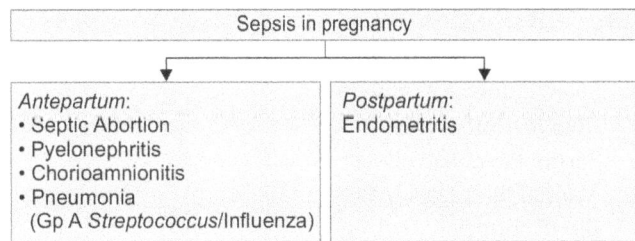

The most commonly implicated bacteria in sepsis leading to maternal mortality include *Escherichia coli* and Group A beta-hemolytic *Streptococcus*. Endometritis and chorioamnionitis are usually as a result of mixed bacterial flora.[4]

RECOGNITION OF SEPSIS

A patient with sepsis commonly presents with fever, tachycardia, tachypnea, and raised white blood cell (WBC) counts. Additionally, signs and symptoms due to the primary organ involvement may be there (e.g. cough, default in breathing, chest pain or flank pain, painful micturition, frequency of micturition, etc.). With worsening of the condition, signs of shock manifest (arterial hypotension with MAP less than 65 mm Hg). Tissue hypoperfusion may lead to organ dysfunction which may manifest as decreased urine output, anuria, and altered mental status.

A high index of suspicion is needed to diagnose sepsis in the pregnant population. If sepsis is clinically suspected, prompt action is needed to decrease maternal and fetal morbidity and mortality. As discussed before, no validated scores are available to diagnose/monitor sepsis in the pregnant women, however, the Royal College of Obstetricians and Gynaecologists (RCOG) has adopted the modified early obstetric warning score (MEOWS) to facilitate early detection of worsening of physical condition of a woman in labor.[5]

MANAGEMENT

Early involvement of a critical care specialist/intensivist/physician should be considered. Patient should be cared for in an intensive care unit (ICU) setup. If such facilities are not available, referral to a higher center should be considered but only after stabilization of the patient.

INVESTIGATIONS

Following investigations need to be done for a patient with suspected sepsis/sepsis:
- Complete blood count
- Liver/kidney function test
- Coagulation profile
- Serum lactate levels
- Arterial blood gas (ABG)
- Blood culture
- Other cultures as necessary
- Blood glucose levels.

The "Sepsis Six Bundle" is an initiative developed by the UK Sepsis Trust that should be carried out in entirety within 1 hour of recognition of sepsis.[8] The bundle includes the following six points:
1. Administer oxygen to maintain SpO_2 at >94%
2. Take blood cultures and consider infective source
3. Administer intravenous antibiotics
4. Consider intravenous fluid resuscitation
5. Check serial lactates
6. Commence hourly urine output measurement.

Oxygen should be administered to maintain SpO_2 to more than 94%. Blood cultures should always be obtained before administering intravenous antibiotics. Taking two blood cultures increases the probability of detecting the organism involved in the infective process. A broad-spectrum antibiotic should be administered intravenously according to the primary source of infection/local hospital protocol. Combination of antibiotics should be used in the presence of septic shock. Early administration of antibiotics is the single most important component of the Sepsis Six Bundle which helps in decreasing morbidity/mortality. Intravenous fluid resuscitation should include administration of fluids at the rate of 30 mL/kg in the first 3 hours and subsequently to maintain an output of more than 0.5 mL/kg/hr. Crystalloids are the fluids of choice. Central venous pressure (CVP) line insertion should be considered. Blood should be administered if hemoglobin levels are less than 7 g% or if there is ongoing hemorrhage.

Platelets should be administered only if counts are less than $10,000/mm^3$ or if less than $20,000/mm^3$ with bleeding. Serial monitoring of serum lactate levels should be done. Also despite adequate fluid resuscitation, if vasopressors are needed to maintain MAP >65 mm Hg and serum lactate level of >2 mmol/L (18 mg/dL), septic shock is diagnosed. Serum lactate level is an important predictor of outcome in patients with sepsis and mortality rates are directly proportional to the lactate levels. Vasopressor of choice in a patient with sepsis (including pregnant women) is norepinephrine.[5] Glucocorticoids (hydrocortisone) can be considered if hypotension persists despite adequate fluid resuscitation and vasopressor therapy. Consideration should also be given to thromboprophylaxis.

The importance of close monitoring of the vitals, SpO_2, hourly input, and urine output cannot be overemphasized.

After stabilization of the patient, removal of the primary source of infection can be considered if possible (e.g. removal of infected retained products of conception).

TERMINATION OF PREGNANCY

Termination of pregnancy should be considered (after discussion with a senior obstetrician and neonatologist) if pregnancy-related cause for sepsis is suspected (e.g. chorioamnionitis) or if delivery would benefit the mother or baby or both.[5] Antenatal corticosteroids should be used with caution in a woman with sepsis. Fetal surveillance in the intrapartum period should be done with continuous **cardiotocography** (CTG).

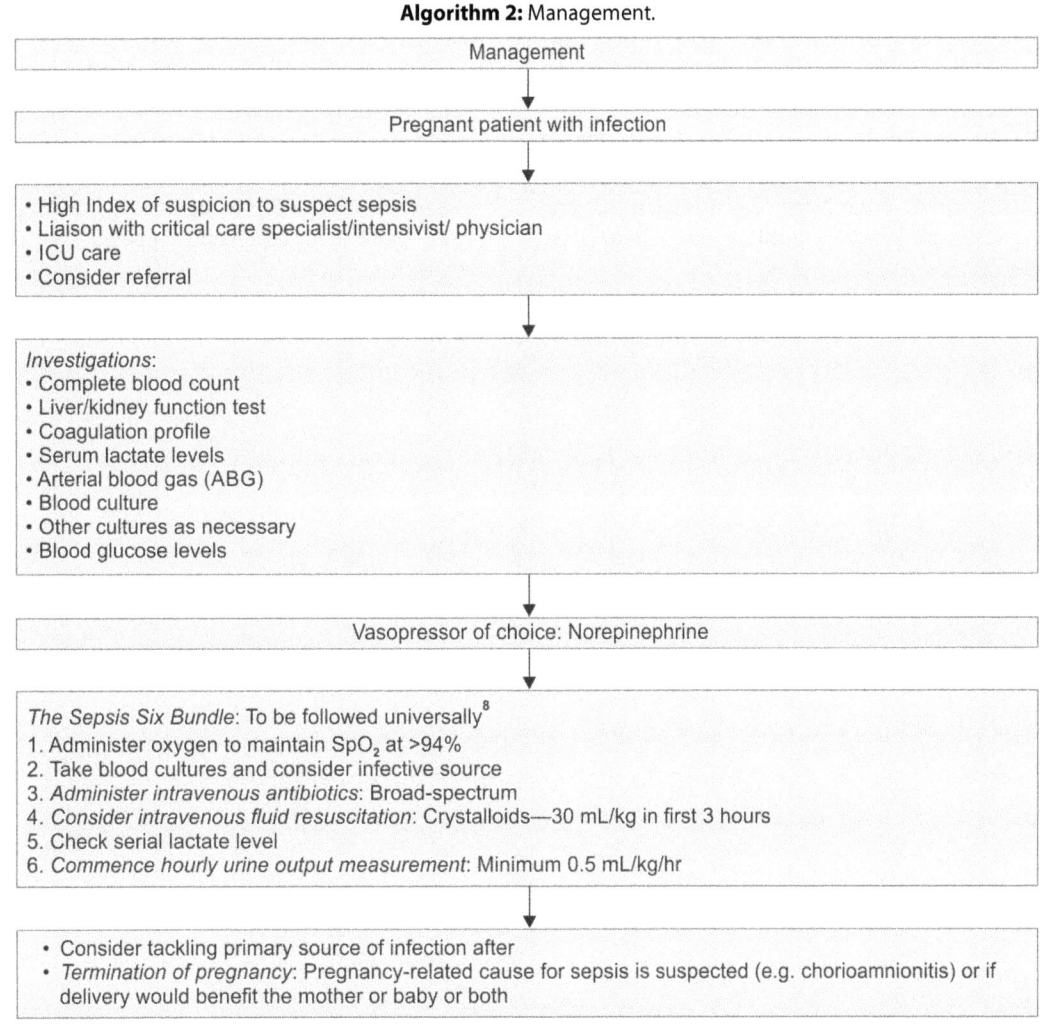

Algorithm 2: Management.

(ICU: intensive care unit; SpO$_2$: peripheral capillary oxygen saturation)

CONCLUSION

Sepsis and septic shock is considered to be a medical emergency with high rates of morbidity and mortality, which may be even higher in pregnant women. At the moment, there are no guidelines that are specific to the pregnant females for the diagnosis and management of sepsis. Hence the general principle for management of sepsis in pregnant female should be derived from the clinically available guidelines. Management of a pregnant patient with sepsis/septic shock is best carried out in an ICU setting in liaison with critical care specialists. However, the role of the obstetrician and medical staff in early diagnosis and resuscitation should not be underestimated. The former thus needs to be well educated in early recognition and stabilization of patients with sepsis/septic shock.

REFERENCES

1. Padilla C, Palanisamy A. Managing maternal sepsis: early warning criteria to ECMO. Clin Obstet Gynecol. 2017;60(2):418-24.
2. Singer M, Deutschman CS, Seymour CW, et al. The third international consensus definitions for sepsis and septic shock (Sepsis-3). JAMA. 2016;315:801.
3. Vincent JL, de Mendonça A, Cantraine F, et al. Working Group on "Sepsis-Related Problems" of the European Society of Intensive Care Medicine. Use of the SOFA score to assess the incidence of organ dysfunction/failure in intensive care units: results of a multicenter, prospective study. Working Group on "Sepsis-Related Problems" of the European Society of Intensive Care Medicine. Crit Care Med. 1998;26(11):1793-800.

4. Lewis G (Ed). Saving Mothers' Lives: Reviewing Maternal Deaths to Make motherhood safer—2003-2005. The Seventh Report on Confidential enquiries into Maternal Deaths in the United Kingdom. London: RCOG Press; 2007.
5. Royal College of Obstetricians and Gynaecologists. (2012) Bacterial Sepsis in Pregnancy. Green-top Guideline No 64a. [online] Available from: https://www.rcog.org.uk/en/guidelines-research-services/guidelines/gtg64a/ [Last accessed September, 2019].
6. Barton JR, Sibai BM. Severe sepsis and septic shock in pregnancy. Obstet Gynecol. 2012;120:689.
7. Sheffield JS, Cunningham FG. Community-acquired pneumonia in pregnancy. Obstet Gynecol. 2009;114:915.
8. Dellinger RP, Levy MM, Carlet JM, et al. Surviving sepsis campaign: International guidelines for management of severe sepsis and septic shock. Crit Care Med. 2008;36:296-327 [Published correction appears in Crit Care Med. 2008;36:1394-6].

Section 5

Postpartum Period

- **Puerperal Pyrexia**
  Shail Kaur

- **Secondary Postpartum Hemorrhage**
  Saswati Sanyal Choudhury

Chapter 49

Puerperal Pyrexia

Shail Kaur

INTRODUCTION

Infections in the peripartum period are one of the leading causes of maternal morbidity and mortality, accounting for one-tenth of maternal deaths worldwide.[1] Severe infections associated with sepsis have mortality rates of 20–40% which rise to 60% if multiorgan failure sets in. These patients are eventually at risk for pelvic inflammatory disease (PID), tubal blockage, infertility, and chronic pelvic pain.

DEFINITION

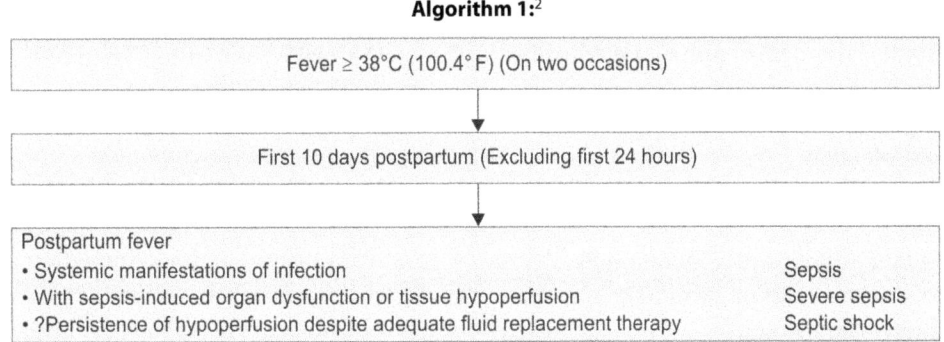

Algorithm 1:[2]

Fever ≥ 38°C (100.4°F) (On two occasions)
↓
First 10 days postpartum (Excluding first 24 hours)
↓
Postpartum fever
- Systemic manifestations of infection — Sepsis
- With sepsis-induced organ dysfunction or tissue hypoperfusion — Severe sepsis
- ?Persistence of hypoperfusion despite adequate fluid replacement therapy — Septic shock

Section 5
Postpartum Period

STEP 1

Evaluate

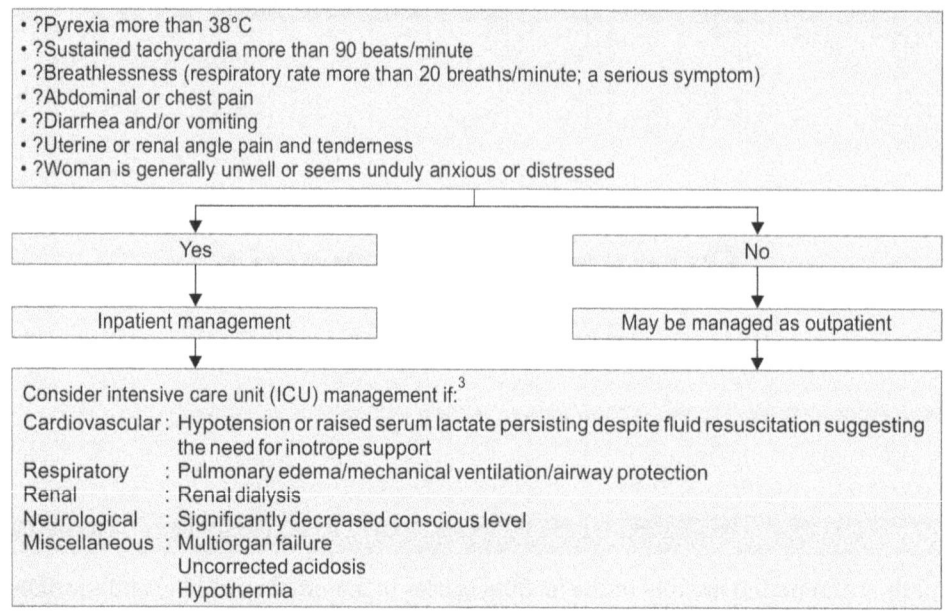

STEP 2

Review Risk Factors

- Obesity
- Impaired glucose tolerance/diabetes
- Impaired immunity/immunosuppressant medication
- Anemia
- Vaginal discharge
- History of pelvic infection
- Amniocentesis and other invasive procedures
- Cervical cerclage
- Prolonged spontaneous rupture of membranes
- Vaginal trauma, cesarean section, wound hematoma
- Retained products of conception
- Group A *Streptococcus* infection in close contacts/family members

STEP 3

Evaluation and treatment of these patients should be prompt and targeted.

The most common cause is *endometritis*[4] (2% following vaginal delivery and 10–15% following cesarean section).

- Streptococcal infection [especially Group A *Streptococcus* (GAS)] present very early, maybe within 12 hours postpartum.
- Recently delivered women who present with bleeding or abdominal pain should be promptly evaluated for infections.
- The major pathogens causing sepsis in the puerperium are:[3]
  - GAS, also known as *Streptococcus pyogenes*
  - *Escherichia coli*
  - *Staphylococcus aureus*
  - *Streptococcus pneumoniae*
  - Methicillin-resistant *S. aureus* (MRSA), *Clostridium septicum*, and *Morganella morganii*
- Detailed history and a systematic head-to-toe evaluation are critical to establishing a correct diagnosis which is imperative to direct the investigations required and to treat correctly and promptly. Possible source of infection from outside the genital tract should be carefully looked for.

History

- History of recent exposure to any infections should be inquired into
- A history of recent sore throat or streptococcal infection in family members
- Intravenous drug misuse
- Recent fever with chills and rigors, suggest bacteremia

- Diarrhea and vomiting may be attributable to food-borne pathogens
- Ask for history of antimicrobial therapy for any illness recently
- History of exposure to farm animals or ingestion of unpasteurized or uncoiled milk (*Salmonella, Campylobacter, Listeria, Chlamydophila psittaci, Coxiella burnetii*)

Symptoms to be Evaluated

- Fever and rigors (persistent spiking temperature suggests abscess). Beware that normal temperature may be attributable to antipyretics or nonsteroidal anti-inflammatory drugs (NSAIDs).
- Diarrhea or vomiting may indicate exotoxin production (early toxic shock)
- Breast engorgement/redness
- Rash (generalized maculopapular rash)
- Abdominal/pelvic pain and tenderness
- Wound infection—spreading cellulitis or discharge
- Offensive vaginal discharge (smelly—suggestive of anaerobes; serosanguineous—suggestive of streptococcal infection)
- Productive cough
- Urinary symptoms
- Delay in uterine involution, heavy lochia
- General—nonspecific signs such as lethargy, reduced appetite.

Sources from Outside the Genital Tract

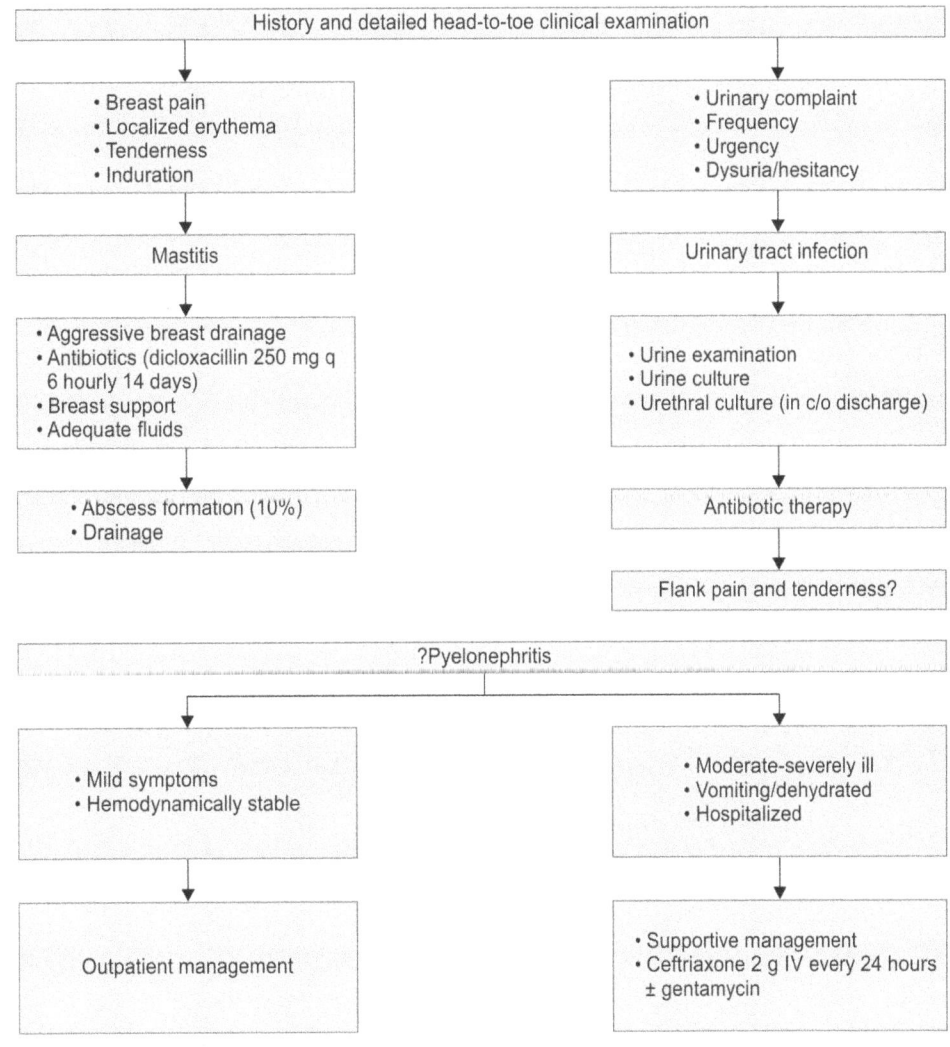

PNEUMONIA

Pneumonia[5] is one of the most common nonobstetric infections to cause maternal mortality in the peripartum period. Recent changes in treatment have helped bring the mortality rates to 0–4% from earlier rates of 24%.

In most cases, etiologic pathogen is not isolated, however, *Streptococcus pneumoniae* and *Haemophilus influenzae* remain the most common isolates. Unusual pathogens are sometimes responsible for pneumonia probably due to alterations in the maternal immune status that characterize pregnancy.

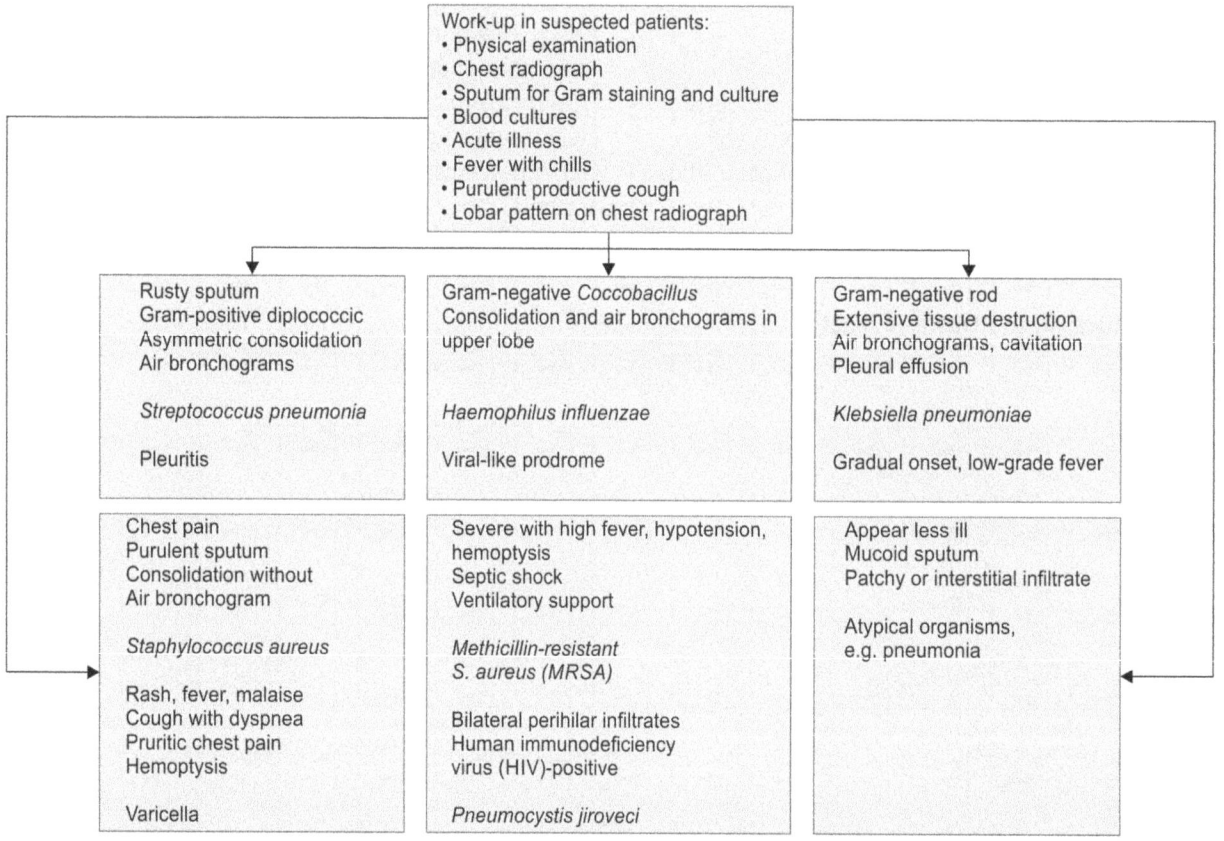

SKIN AND SOFT TISSUE INFECTIONS

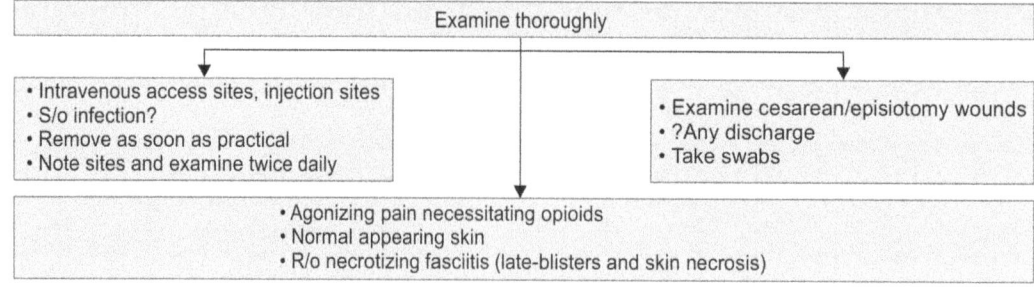

GASTROENTERITIS

- Normal pathogens usually do not present with systemic manifestations.
- *Clostridioides difficile* is increasing in incidence among obstetric population.
- Toxic shock syndrome may sometimes manifest with nausea and vomiting.

PHARYNGITIS

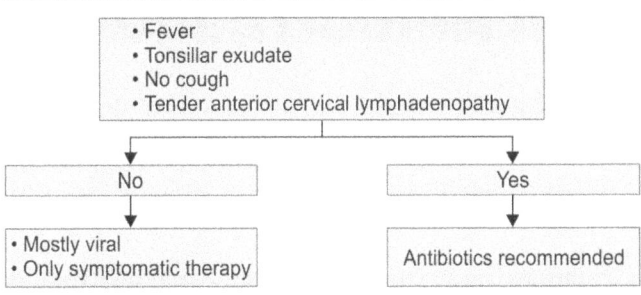

INFECTION RELATED TO REGIONAL ANESTHESIA

- Spinal abscess
- Investigate and treat promptly

MANAGEMENT

- Routine blood tests should include full blood count, urea, electrolytes, and C-reactive protein (CRP).
- Swabs and imaging should be advised as guided by history and examination.
- Antibiotic therapy should be initiated as soon as feasible and one need not wait for sensitivity reports.
- The choice of antibiotics may be guided by possible type and source of infection as assessed on clinical examination.

Without Sepsis

Considerations to be kept in mind when deciding antibiotics:
- *Co-amoxiclav:* Does not cover MRSA, *Pseudomonas* or ESBL-producing organisms
- *Metronidazole:* Only covers anaerobes
- *Clindamycin:* Covers most streptococci and staphylococci, including many MRSA, and switches off exotoxin production with significantly decreased mortality. Not renally excreted or nephrotoxic
- *Piperacillin/tazobactam:* Covers most organisms except MRSA and are renal sparing (in and carbapenems contrast to aminoglycosides) but does not cover ESBL producers
- *Gentamicin (as a single dose of 3–5 mg/kg):* Poses no problem in normal renal function but if doses are to be given regularly serum levels must be monitored

Patients with Sepsis

Obtain blood cultures prior to antibiotic administration:
- Broad-spectrum antibiotic within 1 hour of recognition of severe sepsis (a combination of either piperacillin/tazobactam or a carbapenem plus clindamycin).
- Vancomycin or teicoplanin may be added if there is suspicion of MRSA.

Measure Serum Lactate

In the event of hypotension and/or serum lactate greater than 4 mmol/L:
- Deliver an initial minimum of 20 mL/kg of crystalloid or an equivalent.
- Apply vasopressors for hypotension not responding to initial fluid resuscitation to maintain mean arterial pressure above 65 mm Hg.

In the event of persistent hypotension despite fluid resuscitation (septic shock) and/or serum lactate greater than 4 mmol/L:
- Achieve a central venous pressure of ≥8 mm Hg.
- Achieve a central venous oxygen saturation ≥70% or mixed venous oxygen saturation ≥65%.

REFERENCES

1. Isley MM, Katz VL. 'Postpartum care and long term health considerations'. Obstetrics: Normal and Problem Pregnancies. Elsevier, 2017. pp. 499-516.
2. WHO recommendations for prevention and treatment of maternal peripartum infections, WHO 2015. Available from: https://apps.who.int/iris/bitstream/handle/10665/186171/9789241549363_eng.pdf [Last accessed on January, 2020]
3. RCOG Green-top Guideline No. 64b. Available from: https://www.rcog.org.uk/globalassets/documents/guidelines/gtg_64b.pdf [Last accessed on January, 2020]
4. Dalton E, Castillo E. Post-partum infections: A review for the non-OBGYN. Obstet Med. 2014;7(3):98-102.
5. Kansara TN, Shah TM, Lalcheta FR. A study of maternal mortality due to non-obstetric causes. Int J Reprod Contracept Obstet Gynecol. 2019;8(5):2027-33.

Chapter 50

Secondary Postpartum Hemorrhage

Saswati Sanyal Choudhury

INTRODUCTION

Postpartum hemorrhage (PPH) is the most important cause of maternal mortality, especially in low-resource setting countries. PPH is defined as blood loss more than 500 mL after birth of the baby till 12 weeks quantitatively. Secondary or late PPH is defined as bleeding after 24 hours to 12 weeks after delivery.[1] Clinical definition of PPH is blood loss irrespective of its amount postdelivery up to the end of puerperium as a consequence of which the patient becomes hemodynamically unstable as is evidenced by tachycardia and hypotension. American College of Obstetricians and Gynecologists (ACOG) also defined it as a drop of hematocrit of 10% or hemorrhage requiring immediate transfusion. Unlike primary PPH, secondary or late PPH does not have a clear definition for quantity of blood loss and can vary from increased lochia to massive hemorrhage. It usually manifests between 8th day and 14th day. The incidence in the developed world is reported to be 0.47–1.44%.[2,3]

ETIOLOGY OF LATE POSTPARTUM HEMORRHAGE

- Retention of placental bits—placenta accreta.
- Subinvolution of uterus due to placental site infection **(Algorithm 1)**.
- Lower genital tract trauma which usually presents within first few days of delivery. Use of forceps and ventouse causing trauma, infected episiotomy wound, and hematomas.
- Retained product undergoes necrosis with fibrin deposition and may eventually form placental polyp.
- Cesarean wound dehiscence due to infection usually occurs within between 10 and 14 days due to separation of slough.
- *Coagulopathies*: Von Willebrand disease or other inherited coagulopathies.
- Infected fibroid or intramural fibroid transforming to submucous due to uterine contraction.
- Uterine inversion chronic type.
- Arteriovenous malformation resulting from venous sinuses becoming incorporated in the scar within myometrium after necrosis of chorionic tissue.
- Choriocarcinoma.
- Cervical cancer.

Algorithm 1: Causes of subinvolution.

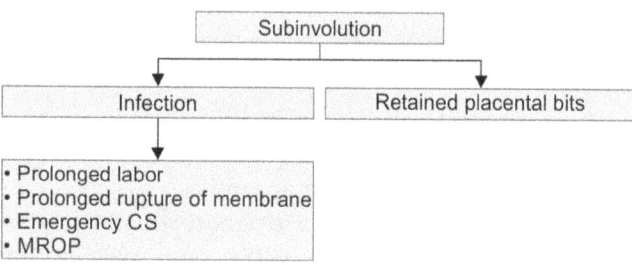

(CS: cesarean section; MROP: manual removal of placenta)

CLINICAL PRESENTATION

Hemorrhage may be mild, moderate, or severe. General physical examination will show pallor, hypotension, and tachycardia depending on the amount of hemorrhage. Fever may be present if sepsis is present along with abdominal tenderness bleeding. Vaginal examination shows patulous cervical os, subinvolution of uterus, and foul smell along with infected wound in vulva and vagina if any.

Investigations for secondary PPH are listed in **Algorithm 2**.

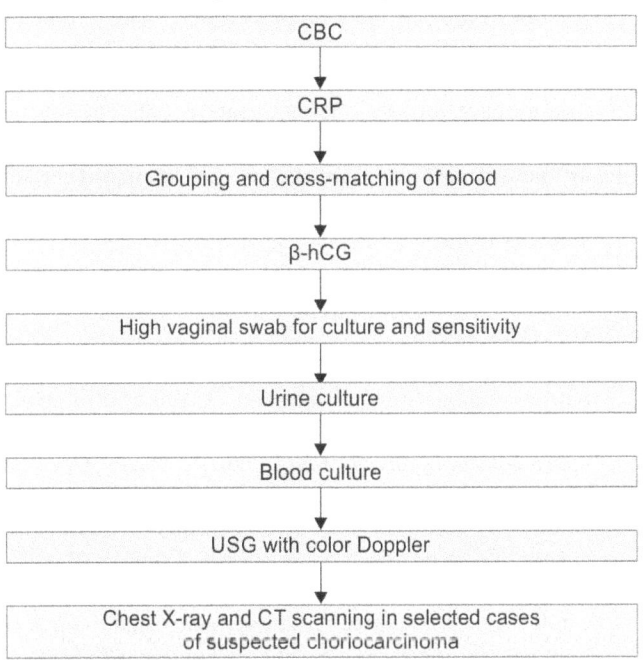

Algorithm 2: Investigations.

(β-hCG: beta-human chorionic gonadotropin; CBC: complete blood count; CRP: C-reactive protein; CT: computed tomography; USG: ultrasonography)

Box 1	A proposed standardized system for reporting postpartum ultrasound scan.[4]

- Normal endometrial cavity
- Endometrial cavity containing fluid only
- Endometrial cavity enlarged [anteroposterior (AP) depth >1 cm]. Maximum AP dimensions noted
- Endometrial cavity containing echogenic foci. Dimensions of large foci noted. Doppler evaluation of blood flow in foci

Source: Adapted from Neill et al. 2002

MANAGEMENT OF SECONDARY POSTPARTUM HEMORRHAGE

There is no evidence from randomized controlled trials (RCTs) to show effects of treatment for secondary PPH[5] and the aims of the management are resuscitation followed by establishment of the cause and then dealing the situation according to the cause **(Algorithm 3)**.

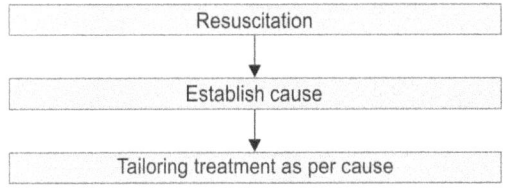

Algorithm 3: Aims of management.

Management of shock includes fluid and blood transfusion after assessing the amount of blood loss. Treatment with oxytocics like oxytocin, ergometrine, and prostaglandins is needed to deal with atonicity of uterus due to retained product or infection. Administration of antibiotics remains the mainstay of management for all secondary PPH as infection plays a major role in its occurrence. Choice of antibiotics includes broad-spectrum ones. Antibiotics recommended choice is amoxycillin and clavulanic acid, combined with metronidazole and gentamicin.[3,6] If ultrasonography (USG) shows retained product of conception, exploration is done after giving antibiotics and if no product is found, only conservative management with antibiotics is sufficient in majority of the cases unless there are other underlying pathology. Exploration of uterus is done by senior obstetricians as chance of injury is high especially in complicated cases like morbidly adherent placenta and postcesarean cases. Sharp curettage is avoided to prevent synechia. Other surgical procedures like repair of cesarean section (CS) wound dehiscence or other infected wound are done in indicated cases. Surgical procedures used to treat atonic PPH like brace sutures, tamponade, pelvic artery ligation, and if nothing works, hysterectomy may be considered in uncontrolled bleeding. Uterine artery embolization, if available, is a good alternative to save uterus where the facility is available. Other medical treatments like use of tranexamic acid, recombinant factor VIIa, and local vasopressin used in primary PPH may be considered although there are no reports of their use in secondary PPH.[6] Coagulation profile is sent to rule out coagulopathies in suspected cases and managed accordingly. Fibroids and chronic inversion are managed surgically **(Algorithm 4)**.

Most of the secondary hemorrhage reveal within 7–10 days after delivery. Retention of products and infection plays the major role in the causation but there is diverse etiology for which management is also variable and one must have the suspicion of unusual possibilities like choriocarcinoma, cancer cervix, and others so that management is done for the specific cause to have the best outcome.[7]

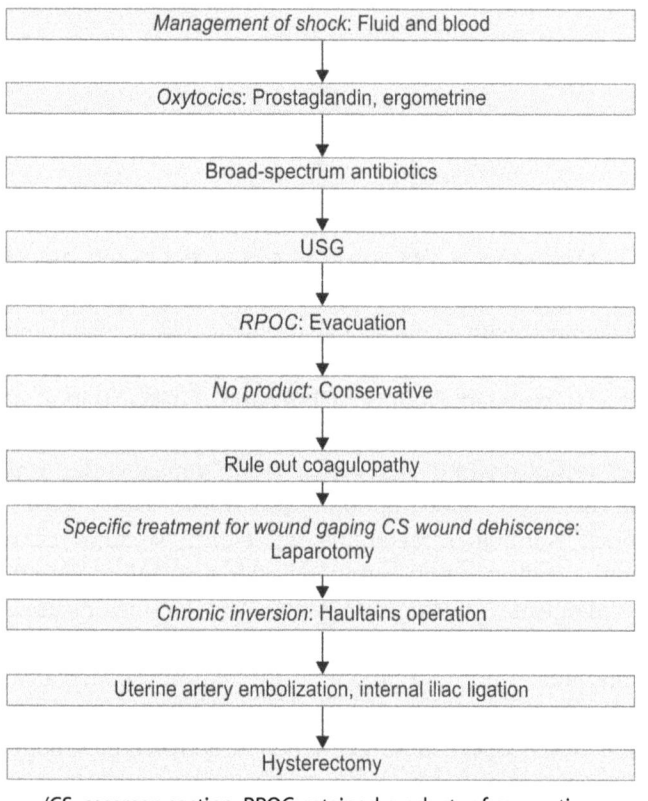

Algorithm 4: Management of secondary postpartum hemorrhage.

(CS: cesarean section; RPOC: retained products of conception; USG: ultrasonography)

REFERENCES

1. Thompson W, Harper MA. Post partum haemorrhage and abnormalities of the third stage of labour. In: Chamberlain G, Steer P (Eds). Turnbull's Obstetrics, 3rd edition. Edinburg: Churchill Livingstone; 2001. pp. 619-33.
2. Hoveyda F, Mackenzie IZ. Secondary post partum haemorrhage: incidence, morbidity and current management. Br J Obstet Gynaecol. 2001;108:927-30.
3. King PA, Duthie SJ, Dong ZG, et al. Secondary post partum haemorrhage. Aust NZ J Obstet Gynaecol. 1989;29:394-8.
4. Neill AC, Nxon RM, Thornton S. A comparison of clinical assessment with ultrasound in the management of secondary post partum haemorrhage. Eur J Obstet Gynacol. 2002;104:113-5.
5. Alexander J, Thomas P, Sanghera J. Treatments for secondary post partum haemorrhage. Cochrane Database Syst Rev. 2002;(1):CD002867.
6. Fernandez H, Claquin C, Guibert M, et al. Suspected post partum endometritis: a controlled clinical trial of single agent antibiotic therapy with Amox-CA vs ampicillin-metronidazole+aminoglycoside. Eur J Obstet Gynecol. 1990;36:69-74.
7. Groom KM, Jacobson TZ. The management of secondary postpartum hemorrhage. In: B-Lynch C, Lalonde AB (Eds). A Text Book of Postpartum Hemorrhage. A Comprehensive Guide to Evaluation, Management and Surgical Intervention, Special FOGSI edition. London, UK: Sapiens Publishing; 2006. pp. 316-23.

Section 6

Neonate

- **Care of Healthy Newborn**
  Piyush Gautam, Nivedita Sharma

- **Care of Preterm Newborns**
  Pancham Chauhan

- **Neonatal Resuscitation**
  Parveen Bhardwaj

- **Neonatal Jaundice**
  Ram Krishan Kaushal

Chapter 51

Care of Healthy Newborn

Piyush Gautam, Nivedita Sharma

INTRODUCTION

Most maternal and infant deaths occur in the first month after birth; almost half of neonatal deaths occur within the first 24 hours, and 66% occur during the first week.[1] Thus, the first days and weeks of life are critical for the future health of a child and care given during this time is critical in preventing complications and ensuring intact survival and wellbeing of a newborn infant.

NORMAL NEWBORN

A normal newborn:
- Weighs more than 2,500 g
- Breathes normally and regularly
- Has warm trunk and soles (temperature 36.5–37.4°C)
- Is pink in color
- Has spontaneous body movements and actively sucks on breast.[2]

Newborn care essentially starts with preparation in the delivery room. This includes providing warmth, place to do resuscitation, and equipment and supplies.

These are summarized below:
- A draught-free, warm room with temperature >25°C
- A clean, dry, and warm delivery surface
- A radiant warmer
- Two clean, warm towels
- A folded piece of cloth (1/2–1" thick)
- A newborn size self-inflating Ambu bag
- *Infant masks in two sizes*: size "1" for normal-weight baby and "0" for small baby
- Suction device
- Oxygen
- Clock (with seconds hand).

A newborn care corner is shown in **Figure 1**.

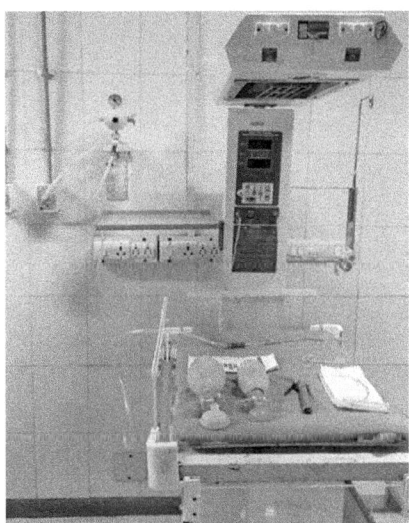

Fig. 1: Newborn care corner.

As 10% newborns require some assistance at birth, each delivery must be attended by a person skilled in basic neonatal resuscitation. The following algorithm depicts the steps to be followed while resuscitating a newborn **(Algorithm 1)**.

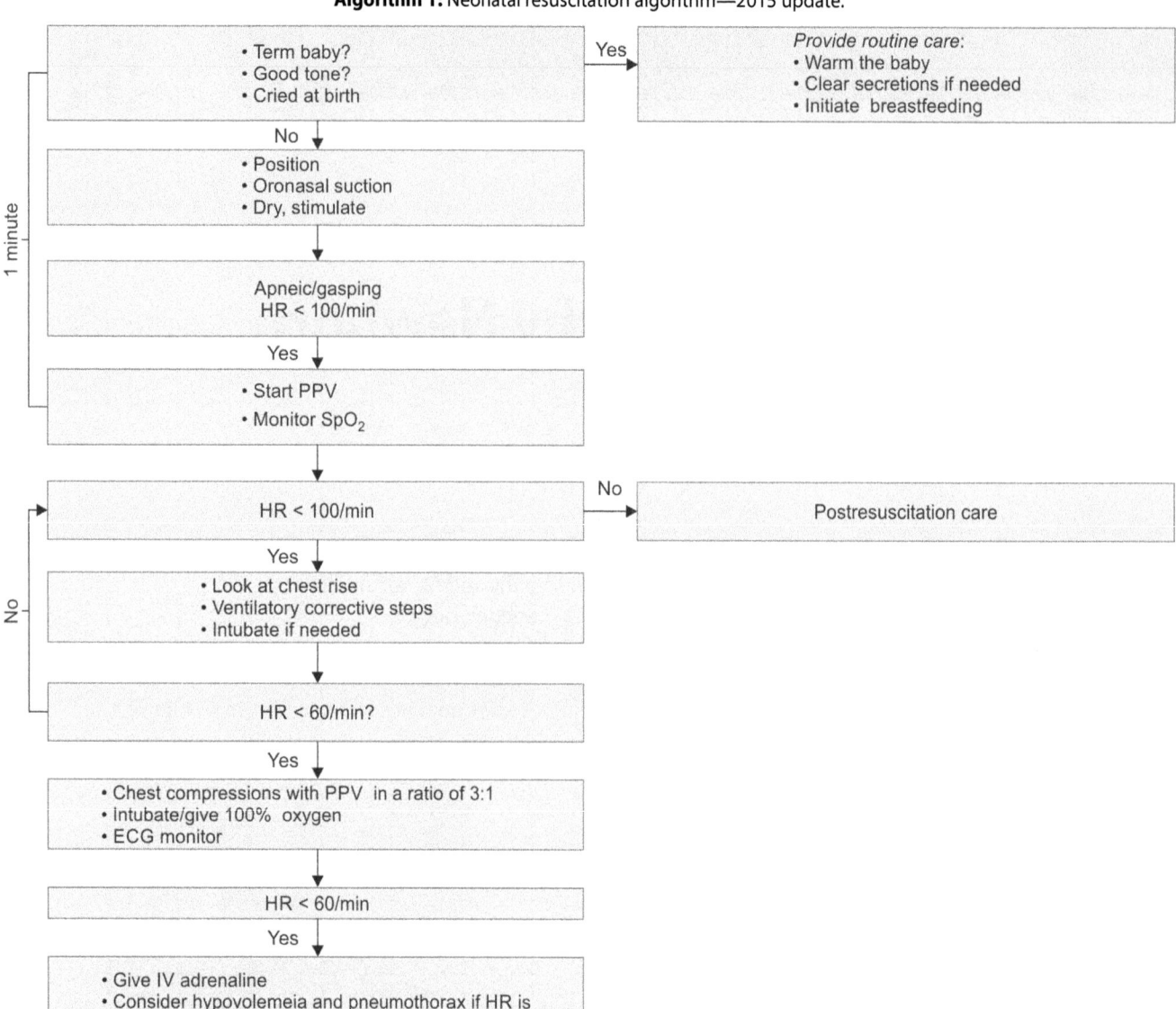

Algorithm 1: Neonatal resuscitation algorithm—2015 update.

(ECG: electrocardiogram; HR: heart rate; IV: intravenous; PPV: positive pressure ventilation; SpO$_2$: saturation of peripheral oxygen)

A stepwise approach to be followed while delivering a newborn is discussed below:[2]

- *Call out the time of birth:* Call out the time of birth loudly, as in addition to recording the time, it alerts other personnel in case any help is required.
- Receive the baby onto a warm, clean, and dry towel and kept on the mother's chest or in a clean, warm place close to the mother.
- *Clamp and cut the umbilical cord:* The umbilical cord should be clamped after 1–3 minutes using a sterile, disposable clamp or a sterile tie and cut using a sterile blade about 2 cm (1 inch) away from the skin.
- *Immediately dry the baby and wipe the eyes:*
  - Use a warm towel, remove the wet towels, and wrap the baby loosely in a clean, dry, and warm towel.

This will prevent hypothermia. Make sure not to wipe off the vernix.
- Drying also provides sufficient stimulation for breathing to start in a mildly depressed newborn.
- Wipe both eyes with a sterile gauze. Clean the eyes using sterile gauze. Use separate gauze for each eye, wiping from the medial to the lateral side.
- *Keep the baby and the mother warm:* Leave the baby between the mother's breasts to start skin-to-skin care. This will ensure euthermia, as well as promote early breastfeeding. Both mother and baby are covered with a warm cloth. The baby's head should be covered with a cap since head is the major contributor to the surface area of the body.
- Place an identity label on the baby. This helps in easy identification of the baby, avoiding any confusion. The label should be placed on the wrist or ankle.
- Encourage the initiation of breastfeeding. Breastfeeding should be initiated within 1 hour of birth in all babies.

A newborn who has cried and is stable is provided "routine care" that includes:
- Provide warmth
- Suction mouth and nose (if necessary)
- Cut the cord in 1–3 minutes
- Keep baby with mother
- Initiate breastfeeding.

TEMPERATURE CONTROL: ENSURING WARMTH, THE "WARM CHAIN"

Warmth is one of the basic needs of a newborn baby, being critical to the baby's survival and wellbeing. A newborn is more prone to develop hypothermia because of a large surface area per unit of body weight. In addition, low-birth weight babies have decreased thermal insulation due to less subcutaneous fat and decreased heat production due to less brown fat.

Assessment of Baby's Temperature by Touch

Baby's temperature can be assessed with reasonable precision by touching the abdomen, hands, and feet with the dorsum of the hand. In newborns, abdominal temperature represents core temperature. When feet are cold and abdomen is warm, it indicates that the baby is in cold stress. In hypothermia, both feet and abdomen are cold to touch. The assessment, clinical features, and management of hypothermia are summarized in **Table 1**.

Table 1: Assessment of body temperature and management of hypothermia.

Temperature	Clinical assessment	Condition	Intervention
36.5–37.5°C	• Warm trunk • Warm extremities	Normal	Continue routine care
36–36.4°C	• Warm trunk • Cold extremities	Cold stress	Skin-to-skin contact: • Cover adequately • Ensure room is warm • Provide warmth • Encourage breastfeeding
32–35.9°C	• Cold trunk • Cold extremities	Hypothermia	Active rewarming under radiant warmer

Warm Chain

The "warm chain" is a set of interlinked procedures carried out at birth and later which will minimize the likelihood of hypothermia in all newborns.

Following measures must be adopted to prevent heat loss in the labor room:[2]
- Warm delivery room (25°C)
- Newborn care corner temperature to be maintained at 30°C
- Drying the baby immediately
- Skin-to-skin contact between mother and baby
- Wrapping and covering the baby (**Fig. 2**).

The correct method for wrapping and covering the baby is shown in **Figure 2**.

 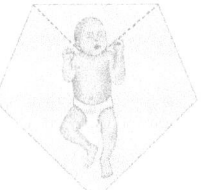 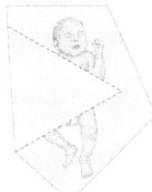
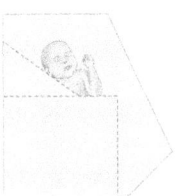 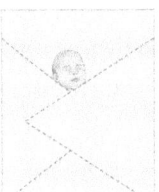

Fig. 2: Wrapping and covering the baby.

PREVENTION OF INFECTIONS: THE "CLEAN CHAIN"

Sepsis is the most important cause of neonatal death in hospital. Prevention of infections is more cost-effective than treating them.

Similar to the warm chain, the "clean chain," if practiced from the time of delivery till discharge, will prevent infections.

The components of a clean chain are:
- *Clean delivery* (*WHO six cleans*):
  - Clean attendant's hands
  - Clean delivery surface
  - Clean cord-cutting instrument (scissor, blade)
  - Clean string/clamp to tie the cord
  - Clean cloth to wrap the baby
  - Clean cloth to cover the mother
- *After delivery:*
  - All caregivers should wash hands before handling the baby
  - Feed only breast milk
  - Keep the cord clean and dry; do not apply anything
  - Use a clean cloth as a diaper/napkin
  - Wash your hands after changing diaper/napkin.

FEEDING

It is essential to help mothers of healthy newborn babies to establish breastfeeding as soon as possible after delivery. Exclusive breastfeeding should be continued till 6 months of age.

Advantages of Breastfeeding

Exclusive breastfeeding helps establish a bond between the mother and baby, and in addition to its nutritive value, decreases the risk of:[1]
- Diarrhea
- Pneumonia
- Otitis media
- Death in the first year of life.

Preparing the Infant and the Mother for Breastfeeding

Ensure that the infant is clinically stable and alert. The mother can feed in sitting or lying down position, according to her comfort. The mother must be encouraged to breastfeed as soon as possible and her fears about breastfeeding, if any, must be allayed. One should look for the following signs of correct attachment to the breast:
- Baby's mouth is wide open
- Lower lip is turned outward
- Chin is touching the breast
- More of areola is visible above than below the baby's mouth.

Figure 3 shows the correct technique of breastfeeding.

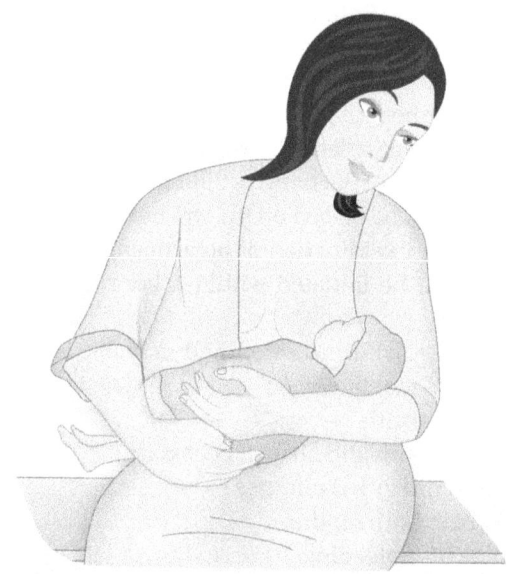

Fig. 3: Correct technique of breastfeeding.

How Frequently to Breastfeed?

A healthy newborn can be breastfed on demand. The interval between each feed is about 2–3 hours, i.e. 8–10 times in 24 hours, and importantly night feeds must not be omitted.

Assessing Adequacy of Breastfeeding

Breastfeeding is considered adequate if the baby:
- Passes urine 6–8 times in 24 hours
- Goes to sleep for 2–3 hours after feeds
- Gains weight at the rate of 10–15 g/kg/day.

Key Messages to Promote Exclusive Breastfeeding

- Put baby to breast as soon as possible after birth, preferably in the delivery room. Do not give any prelacteal feeds.

- Do not discard colostrum.
- Keep baby close to the mother.
- Breastfeed during day and at night, at least 8-10 times and on-demand.
- Allow baby to feed at and empty one breast completely before putting onto the other breast if needed. This allows the baby to get both foremilk and hindmilk, thus ensuring optimum nutrition.
- Do not feed ghutti, water, animal, or powdered milk before 6 months.
- Never use a bottle or pacifier.

PASSAGE OF MECONIUM

All babies must pass meconium within 24 hours, failure of which is an indication to rule out intestinal obstruction. The black tarry meconium is replaced after 2-3 days by greenish transition stools, which last for 1-2 days. Thereafter, most breastfed babies pass golden yellow stools 2-6 times/day. Top fed babies are relatively constipated.[3]

PASSAGE OF URINE

Most babies will pass urine on the first day, but all babies must void within 48 hours. Infants with delayed passage of urine must be investigated for obstructive uropathy and renal malformations. The normal frequency of urination is 6-12 times/day.[3]

NEONATAL JAUNDICE

Up to 25-50% term newborns will develop clinical jaundice.

Physiological Jaundice

- Appears after 24 hours
- Reaches a peak at 4-5 days, with light staining of trunk
- Gradually disappears by 10-14 days.

Pathological Jaundice

- Appearance of jaundice within 24 hours.
- Staining of palms and soles warrants immediate consultation to prevent acute bilirubin encephalopathy or kernicterus.
- Passage of clay-colored stools and/or yellow staining of diapers indicates conjugated hyperbilirubinemia and needs expert consultation.

PHYSIOLOGICAL PHENOMENON

Breast Enlargement

There is breast engorgement in both sexes on the third or fourth day that can last for days to weeks. It results from intrauterine maternal estrogen stimulation.[3] Massage or attempts to express milk can lead to cellulitis or abscess formation. Reassurance is all that is required.

Vaginal Bleeding

- High levels of placental estrogen stimulate growth of uterine endometrium. As this hormonal support wanes after birth, there may be light vaginal bleeding in up to one-fourth female infants.[3] The bleeding stops spontaneously in a few days and no treatment is required.
- Physiological responses like yawning, sneezing, and hiccups are normal.

IMMUNIZATION

Bacillus Calmette-Guérin (BCG) and first dose oral polio vaccines (OPV) and Hepatitis B are given at birth before discharge.

SUPPLEMENTS

- Vitamin K 1 mg intramuscular is given to all babies at birth to prevent hemorrhagic disease of the newborn.
- Vitamin D3 is given orally 400 IU/day till 1 year of age to all babies. There is no need to give iron or vitamin supplements to a normal newborn.

DISCHARGE

Before discharge, ensure that the baby is clinically stable and feeding well, has passed meconium, and is immunized. This typically occurs after 24 hours. The timing of discharge depends upon the health and stability of the mother and baby, the level of support she will receive at home and access to appropriate follow-up care.

FOLLOW-UP

In the first 6 weeks, all babies need at least four postnatal checkups, including the one after birth:[1]
- Day 1 (24 hours)
- Day 3 (48-72 hours)

- Between days 7 and 14
- 6 weeks.

During each visit, newborns should be assessed for key clinical signs of severe illness, adequacy of breastfeeding, and weight gain. Effort must be made to allay any fears and apprehensions in the mother.

DANGER SIGNS

The family should be advised to seek immediate healthcare if they identify any of the following signs in the baby:
- Poor feeding
- History of convulsions
- Fast breathing (rate of ≥60 per minute)
- Severe chest in-drawing
- No spontaneous movement
- Fever (temperature ≥37.5°C)
- Low body temperature (<35.5°C)
- Any jaundice in the first 24 hours of life or yellow palms and soles at any age.

REFERENCES

1. World Health Organization. Postnatal Care for Mothers and Newborns. Highlights from the World Health Organization 2013 Guidelines. Geneva: World Health Organization; 2013.
2. Ministry of Health and Family Welfare, Government of India. Module on Basic Newborn Care and Resuscitation. Navjaat Shishu Suraksha Karyakram.
3. Singh M. Care of the Newborn, 6th edition. New Delhi, India: CBS Publishers and Distributors Pvt. Ltd.

Chapter 52

Care of Preterm Newborns

Pancham Chauhan

INTRODUCTION

Preterm baby is defined as a baby born alive before 37 completed weeks of pregnancy.

There are subcategories of preterm birth based on gestational age:
- *Late preterm:* 34–36 weeks
- *Moderately preterm:* 32–34 weeks
- *Very preterm:* 28–32 weeks
- *Extreme preterm:* <28 weeks.

PRETERM BIRTHS RISING GLOBALLY[1]

- Every year estimated 15 million babies are born preterm—more than 1 in 10 babies around the world and this number is rising.
- Complications of preterm births are the leading cause of death for children under 5 years with estimated 1 million deaths in 2015 globally.

RISK FACTORS FOR PRETERM LABOR AND PREMATURITY

Maternal
- Maternal extremes of age (<18 years and >35 years)
- Multiple pregnancies
- *Infection:* Chorioamnionitis
- Pre-eclamptic toxemia and hypertension
- Incompetent cervix
- Malformations of uterus (bicornuate uterus or massive fibroids)
- *Antepartum hemorrhage:* Placenta previa or abruption
- *Amniotic fluid volume:* Polyhydramnios and oligohydramnios
- *Substance abuse:* Alcohol, cocaine, and cigarette smoking.

Fetal
- Fetal distress
- Congenital anomalies and trisomies.

Others
- Premature rupture of membrane
- Iatrogenic
- Trauma.

PREDICTION OF PRETERM DELIVERY

- Measurement of the length of cervix by ultrasound; cervical shortening is associated with preterm delivery.
- Presence of fetal fibronectin (biological glue) in vaginal/cervical secretions in mid-trimester is predictive of preterm labor.
- Duration and frequency of uterine contractions.

COMMON PROBLEMS IN THE PRETERM INFANTS

- *Pulmonary:* Immaturity
  - Respiratory distress syndrome (RDS)
  - Apnea

- Chronic lung disease (bronchopulmonary dysplasia)
- *Neurological:* Fragile capillary network in the subependymal area
  - Intraventricular hemorrhage (IVH)
  - Venous infarction
  - Hydrocephalus
  - Periventricular leukomalacia
- *Cardiac:*
  - Patent ductus arteriosus (PDA)
- *Hematological disorders:*
  - Anemia
  - Disseminated intravascular coagulation (DIC)
  - Bleeding from vitamin k deficiency
- *Thermal Instability:*
  - *Hypothermia:* More common
  - *Hyperthermia:* May be iatrogenic
- *Metabolic:*
  - Hypocalcemia
  - Hypoglycemia
  - Hyponatremia
  - Hypernatremia
  - Hyperkalemia
- *Gastrointestinal:*
  - Poor gut motility leads to feed intolerance
  - Necrotizing enterocolitis (NEC)
- Jaundice
- Renal Immaturity
- Infection
- *Surgical problems:*
  - Undescended testes, umbilical and inguinal hernias
- *Immature visual system:*
  - Retinopathy of prematurity
  - Myopia.

MANAGEMENT OF PRETERM LABOR

Prenatal Considerations

- Early identification and referral of women in preterm labor to a center equipped with good quality obstetrical and neonatal care facilities.
- Obstetrical management is a balanced decision between risks to mother and fetus of pregnancy continuation versus those of early delivery.
- Suppression of preterm labor with tocolytic agents such as atosiban (oxytocin receptor antagonist) or nifedipine (calcium channel blockers).
- These can delay preterm delivery by 2–7 days and gives time for corticosteroid therapy.
- Magnesium sulfate reduces the risk of cerebral palsy in preterm infants.

Antenatal Steroid Therapy

- The most cost-effective prenatal strategy.
- Reduce RDS (44%), IVH (46%), NEC, and neonatal death (37%).
- *Mechanism of action*: Glucocorticoids stimulate the fetal lung fibroblasts to produce a protein fibroblast-pneumocyte factor which in turn forms saturated phosphatidylcholine—lung maturity.

American College of Obstetricions and Gynecologists Recommendations

- A single course of corticosteroids is recommended for pregnant women between 24 0/7 weeks and 33 6/7 weeks of gestation who are at risk of preterm delivery within 7 days, including for those with ruptured membranes and multiple gestation.[2]
- Regularly scheduled repeat courses or serial courses (more than two) are not currently recommended.
- Betamethasone and dexamethasone are the most widely studied corticosteroids.
- Both cross the placenta and have identical biological activity and both lack mineralocorticoid activity.
- Betamethasone has a longer half-life. There is no difference in perinatal death or alterations in biophysical activity but there is decreased incidence of IVH with dexamethasone treatment.[3]
- *Betamethasone:* 12 mg given intramuscular two doses 24 hours apart.
- *Dexamethasone:* 6 mg given intramuscular four doses 12 hours apart.
- *Contraindications:*
  - Systemic infections
  - Tuberculosis
  - Chorioamnionitis.

Parental Education

- Senior experienced neonatologist along with obstetrician should discuss the survival rate, short- and long-term complications of preterm baby.
- When viability of preterm baby is questionable, parental desires or wishes should be determined.

MANAGEMENT OF PRETERM NEWBORNS (ALGORITHM 1)

Principle of gentle stabilization and minimal handling rather than aggressive resuscitation is beneficial in longer term.
- Stabilization at birth and golden hour management
- Transportation within the hospital or outside the hospital
- Supportive care in neonatal intensive care unit (NICU)
- Preparation for home discharge.

Stabilization at Birth and Golden Hour Management

- Experienced personnel should be present at delivery with prepared equipment.
- *Delivery room must be warm*: Temperature should be maintained at 28–30°C.
- Radiant warmer should be on 30 minutes before the delivery.
- Polyethylene bag can be used to wrap the baby immediately after delivery.
- Keep the head in a neutral position.
- Principles of preterm resuscitation and respiratory support after birth are fundamentally the same as for term newborns and should be as per neonatal resuscitation program (NRP) guidelines with following special considerations for preterm newborns:
  - Resuscitation usually starts with 21–30% oxygen and titrate oxygen concentration so as to achieve target oxygen saturation as per NRP.
  - During NICU care for all babies <32 weeks (suggested target of 88–92%).
  - Many preterm neonates require some degree of respiratory support after birth because of pulmonary immaturity and limited respiratory muscle strength. Room air or blow-by blended oxygen or continuous positive airway pressure (CPAP) or positive pressure ventilation is used depending upon respiratory efforts, distress, and oxygen saturation.
  - Low peak pressures (20–25 cm H_2O) and positive end-expiratory pressure (PEEP) (5–6 cm H_2O) must be maintained through the stabilization during CPAP or ventilator support.
  - Early surfactant therapy in preterm infants <26 weeks.
  - >28 weeks babies best managed with selective surfactant therapy and early elective nasal CPAP.

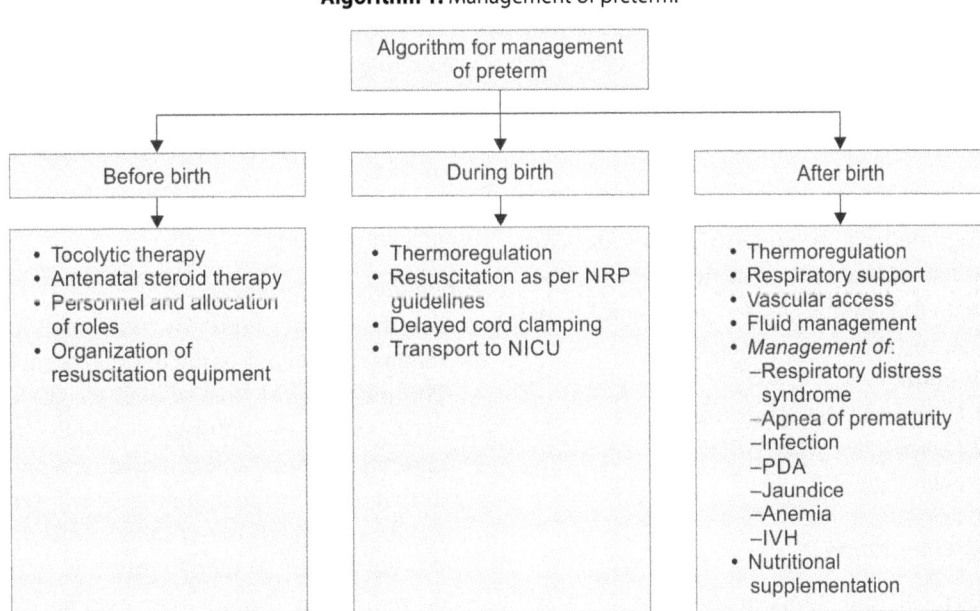

Algorithm 1: Management of preterm.

(IVH: intraventricular hemorrhage; NICU: neonatal intensive care unit; NRP: neonatal resuscitation program; PDA: patent ductus arteriosus)

Transport within the Hospital and between the Hospital

- Transport in a prewarmed incubator to the NICU.
- Transport incubator that provides warmth.

Supportive Care in Neonatal Intensive Care Unit

Nursing

- Nursing in a thermoneutral environment
- Maintaining asepsis
- Minimum possible sounds like low alarms, minimize conversation
- Shield baby eyes and use low lights
- Minimize pain and gentle handling
- Skin-to-skin contact wherever possible.

Monitoring

- Heart rate, respiratory rate, temperature, blood pressure (BP)
- Monitoring for apnea
- *Blood gas monitoring with targets as*: pH = 7.25–7.35, $PaCO_2$ = 40–50 mm Hg, and PaO_2 = 50–70 mm Hg.

Intravenous Fluids

- The goal is to maintain normoglycemia and normovolemia and to prevent fluid overload.
- *Start with 10% dextrose:* 60–100 mL/kg depending upon the gestation age. Later sodium and potassium are added on second or third day with close monitoring of their levels.

Feeding

- Initial feeding method in preterm babies depends upon gestational age rather than birth weight.
- Always evaluate the feeding skills expected for his/her gestational age and decide accordingly.
- *<28 weeks*: IV fluids
- *28–31 weeks*: Orogastric/nasogastric feeds
- *32–34 weeks*: Feeding by spoon/paladai
- *>34 weeks*: Breastfeeding.

Nutritional Supplementation

- *Calcium:* Start calcium supplementations (140–160 mg/kg/day) once the infant is on 100 mL/kg/day.
- *Phosphorus*: About 70–80 mg/kg/day

- *Vitamin D:* 400 IU/day
- *Iron:* 2 mg/kg/day at 4 weeks of life.

Management of Problems Encountered in Newborns

Respiratory distress syndrome:
- Antenatal steroids to decrease chances of RDS and use of postnatal surfactant.
- Continuous positive airway pressure or mechanical ventilation. Noninvasive ventilation (CPAP) is preferred over mechanical ventilation even in extreme premature.

Apnea of prematurity: It is related to immaturity of the central nervous system.
- Presents after 1–2 days but within first 7 days.
- Monitoring of preterm babies for bradycardia, cyanosis, and airway obstruction.
- Positioning of the neck in slightly extended position and gentle suctioning of oropharynx, if required.
- Apneic spells usually respond to tactile stimulation.
- Even after tactile stimulation if neonate continues to remain apneic, positive pressure ventilation should be initiated.
- Methylxanthine therapy is the mainstay of pharmacotherapy of apnea of prematurity.

Infection:
- Using standard methods for control of infection
- Hand washing
- High suspicion for sepsis so as to start early treatment.

Necrotizing enterocolitis:
- Antenatal steroids decrease the incidence of NEC.
- Probiotics have been showed to decrease the incidence of NEC.
- The risk of NEC decreases with breast milk compared to formula feeds.

Patent ductus arteriosus:
- Avoidance of fluid overload with careful fluid management is essential in preventing this condition.
- Pharmacological closure with the use of nonselective cyclo-oxygenase inhibitors which inhibits prostaglandin synthesis and causes ductal constriction.
- Both ibuprofen and indomethacin are equally effective. But ibuprofen has better safety profile.
- Persistence of hemodynamically significant ductus or reopening despite two courses defines medical treatment has been failed and need for surgical ligation of PDA.

Table 1: Phototherapy and exchange transfusion cut-off for preterm babies.[4]

Gestation in weeks	Phototherapy range (TSB mg/dL)	Exchange transfusion (TSB mg/dL)
<28 0/7	5–6	11–14
28 0/7–29 6/7	6–8	12–14
30 0/7–31 6/7	8–10	13–16
32 0/7–33 6/7	10–12	15–18
34 0/7–34 6/7	12–14	17–19

(TSB: total serum bilirubin)

Jaundice:
- Extremely common in preterm babies because of high red cell mass and poor liver conjugation.
- Increased risk of kernicterus because of poor blood-brain barrier.
- Phototherapy and exchange transfusion cut-off for preterm babies **(Table 1)**.

Anemia:
- Anemia of prematurity is an exaggerated response of premature infant during transition from relatively hypoxic state *in utero* to a relatively hyperoxic state.
- Prescribed iron supplementation
- Some preterm babies develop anemia as a result of frequent blood sampling which requires packed red blood cells (PRBCs) transfusion.

Intracranial Hemorrhage
- Intraventricular hemorrhage is the most common in premature babies.
- Arises from rupture of capillaries within the germinal matrix in the caudate nucleus.
- Maintenance of optimal blood pressure, oxygenation, acid-base status, and antenatal administration of antenatal steroids decreases the incidence of intracranial ventricular hemorrhage.

Preparation for Home Discharge

- Even after NICU care, preterm babies still need monitoring.
- Counseling of parents on feeding, nutritional supplementation, immunization, and introduction of complementary feeds.

REFERENCES

1. World Health Organization. Born Too Soon: The Global Action Report on Preterm Birth. Geneva: World Health Organization; 2012.
2. Periviable birth. Obstetric Care Consensus no. 4. Obstet Gynecol. 2016;127(6):e157-69.
3. Brownfoot FC, Gagliardi DI, Bain E, et al. Different corticosteroids and regimens for accelerating fetal lung maturation for women at risk of preterm birth. Cochrane Database Syst Rev. 2013;(8):CD006764.
4. Maisels MJ, Watchko JF, Bhutani VK, et at. An approach to management of hyperbilirubinemia in preterm infants less than 35 weeks of gestations. J Perinatol. 2012;32:660-4.

Chapter 53

Neonatal Resuscitation

Parveen Bhardwaj

INTRODUCTION

The goals of neonatal resuscitation are to prevent the morbidity and mortality associated with hypoxic-ischemic tissue (brain, heart, kidney) injury and to re-establish adequate spontaneous respiration and cardiac output. The fundamental principles include evaluation of the airway, establishing effective respiration, and adequate circulation. Rapid and appropriate resuscitative efforts improve the likelihood of preventing brain damage and achieving a successful outcome.

NEED OF RESUSCITATION

- Although the majority of babies undergo a smooth physiologic transition from intrauterine to extrauterine life and breathe effectively after delivery and hence do not require resuscitation.
- About 10% requires some active intervention to establish normal cardiorespiratory function.
- About 1% requires extensive resuscitative efforts for survival.
- High-risk situations should be anticipated from the history of the pregnancy, labor and delivery, and identification of signs of fetal distress.
- Decision regarding nonresuscitation of baby under special circumstances can be made by resuscitation team after detailed discussion with parents. Parents are generally considered the best surrogate decision-makers for their babies and should be involved in shared decision-making whenever possible.
- If there is agreement that intensive medical care will not improve the chances for the newborn's survival or will pose an unacceptable burden on the child, it is ethical to withhold resuscitation. Examples may include birth at a confirmed gestational age of less than 22 weeks' gestation and some severe congenital malformations and chromosomal anomalies.

PREPAREDNESS FOR RESUSCITATION (ALGORITHM 1)

- Every birth should be attended by at least one person who can perform the initial steps of newborn resuscitation and positive pressure ventilation (PPV) perfectly, and whose only responsibility is care of the newborn.
- When perinatal risk factors are identified, a resuscitation team should be present and a team leader identified. The leader should conduct a pre-resuscitation briefing, identify interventions that may be required, and assign roles and responsibilities to the team members.
- During resuscitation, the team should demonstrate effective communication and teamwork skills to help ensure quality and patient safety. Meconium-stained amniotic fluid (MSAF) is a risk factor for abnormal transition and team must ensure a member with advanced airway and resuscitation skills is in attendance.

Algorithm 1: Neonatal resuscitation algorithm—2015 update.

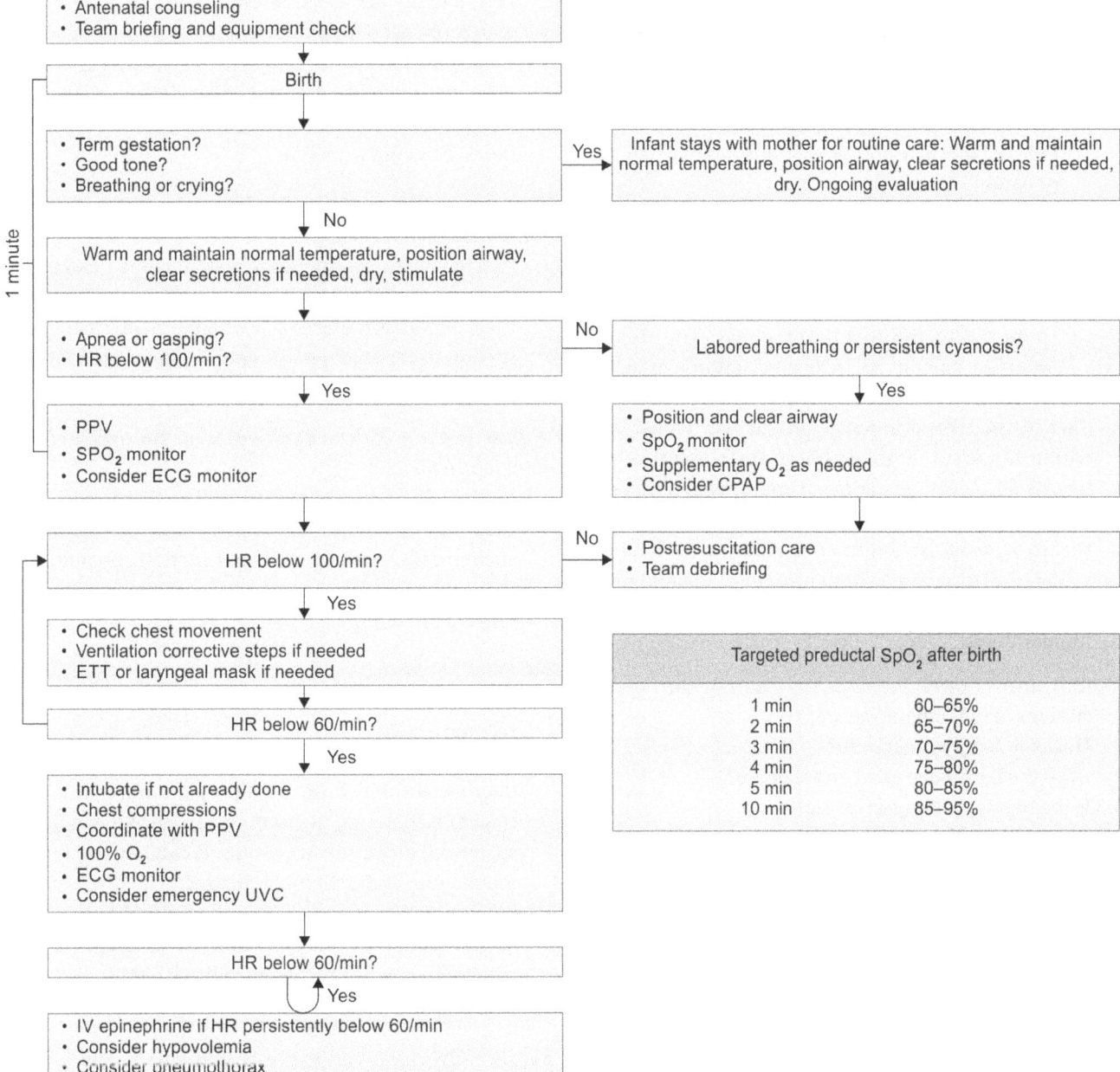

(CPAP: continuous positive airway pressure; ECG: electrocardiogram; ETT: endotracheal tube; HR: heart rate; IV: intravenous; PPV: positive pressure ventilation; SpO₂: saturation of peripheral Oxygen; UVC: umbilical venous catheter)

Thermal Management

- The room temperature should be increased to 23–25°C when the birth of a premature baby is expected.
- The baby's temperature should be maintained between 36.5°C and 37°C.
- A baby who is vigorous at birth should receive skin-to-skin care with the mother. Babies who are between 34 and 36 + 6 weeks' gestation, have good muscle tone, and are breathing or crying may have the initial steps completed while skin-to-skin with their mother.

- Use prewarmed caps for all babies. Ensure the head is dried before applying the hat.
- Use servo-controlled temperature probes as soon as possible on all babies positioned under radiant warmers for more than a few minutes.
- *For babies less than 32 week gestation*:
  - Put the baby in a food-grade transparent plastic bag or wrap.
  - Consider using the bag or wrap with or without a thermal mattress.
  - If using a thermal mattress, ensure it is placed under a prewarmed blanket so the baby is not in direct contact with the thermal mattress. The thermal mattress should be activated approximately 5 minutes before birth.
- *Therapeutic hypothermia* should be considered within the first 6 hours of life in the stabilized baby who is 35 weeks' gestation or more, who suffered a perinatal asphyxial event and develops moderate to severe hypoxic-ischemic encephalopathy. It is not initiated during resuscitation or initial stabilization and can be initiated only after consultation with a neonatologist.

At birth, answer *three questions* to determine the need for initial steps at the radiant warmer.
1. Does the baby appear term?
2. Does the baby have good muscle tone?
3. Is the baby breathing or crying?

Delay cord clamping for a minimum of 30 seconds while answering the above three questions and initiating the initial steps in the neonatal resuscitation program (NRP) algorithm.
- Current evidence suggests that cord clamping should be delayed for at least 30–60 seconds for most vigorous term and preterm newborns.
- Whenever possible, clear communication between providers must occur prior to the birth of the infant regarding cord clamping time.
- When there is a pulsatile cord, recommend delaying cord clamping for a minimum 30 seconds while initiating the initial steps in the NRP algorithm.
- Beneficial effects include less intraventricular hemorrhage (IVH), higher blood pressure (BP), blood volume, less need for transfusion after birth, and less necrotizing enterocolitis (NEC). No evidence of decreased mortality or decreased incidence of severe IVH. Slightly increased level of bilirubin is associated with more need for phototherapy.
- *Contraindications to delayed cord clamping include*: placental circulation is not intact (such as placental abruption, bleeding placenta previa, bleeding vasa previa), or cord avulsion.

If the answer to all three questions is yes then proceed to routine care which includes:
- Provide warmth—by skin-to-skin contact/Kangaroo mother care (KMC)/radiant warmer.
- Clear airway as required—wipe gently with clean cloth/suction using mucous sucker or suction apparatus.
- Dry and stimulate—if required.

If answer to any of these questions is no, proceed for initial steps which include:
- Provide warmth—shift under radiant warmer.
- Clear airway as required—wipe gently with clean cloth/suction using mucous sucker or suction apparatus.
- Dry and stimulate—by gently rubbing the back or flicking the soles.

Suction as needed:
- Routine suctioning of the mouth and nose is not recommended.
- Suction the oropharynx, mouth before nose (insertion depth measured from the tip of the nose to the ear tragus) if there are obvious secretions, known and or suspected airway obstruction secondary to secretions, meconium, and or before initiating PPV.
- Suctioning beyond the oropharynx should be avoided as stimulation beyond this area could trigger a vagal response causing or worsening bradycardia.

Care of babies born through meconium-stained liquor:
- No routine suctioning of the oropharynx while at the perineum.
- Tracheal suctioning for nonvigorous (poor tone, not breathing, or crying) babies born in the presence of meconium is not recommended.
- Meconium-stained amniotic fluid remains a risk factor for the need for resuscitation. A practitioner with intubation skill should be identified and immediately available as these babies may require intubation for tracheal suction or PPV later in the algorithm.

After clearing the airway (if necessary), dry and remove wet linen, reposition to open the airway, stimulate, and then *evaluate* respirations and heart rate (not color).
- Begin positive pressure ventilation if the baby is apneic or gasping, or the heart rate is less than 100 beats per minute (bpm).
- Consider continuous positive airway pressure (CPAP) for preterm babies if their breathing is labored and the heart rate is more than 100 bpm.

Approximately, 60 seconds (*"the Golden Minute"*) are allotted for completing initial steps, revaluating, and beginning ventilation if required.

Subsequently, evaluation and decision-making are based on respiration, heart rate, and oxygen saturation (per *pulse oximetry*):
- Auscultation and use of a cardiorespiratory monitor are the two recommended methods to assess the heart rate.
- Pulse oximeter can also be used to monitor the heart rate.
- *Indications for preductal pulse oximetry include*:
  - Preterm babies less than 34 weeks gestation.
  - Babies who appear cyanotic at 5 minutes or the perception of central cyanosis need to be confirmed.
  - Babies who require PPV.
  - While supplemental oxygen is being administered.
- The pulse oximeter should be set to the manufacturer's specified mode for neonatal resuscitation.
- The appropriately sized probe should be applied on the right hand or wrist first and then attached to the pulse oximeter in order to achieve the fastest readings.
- A compressed air source and oxygen blender must be available in the delivery room to enable titration of the oxygen dose.
- To avoid hyperoxemia, administration of supplemental oxygen should be titrated to achieve target oxygen saturation levels as shown in **Algoritham 1** for term and preterm babies.

Initiate resuscitation with 21% oxygen:
- For simplicity, the recommended initial oxygen concentration should be 21% for all babies.
- For babies less than 35 weeks' gestation, some facilities may choose to set the initial oxygen concentration between 21 and 30% as per their local guideline and/or team discussion.
- Oxygen concentration should be titrated based on pulse oximetry and target SpO_2.

Administer CPAP with 5 cm H_2O pressure to preterm babies with labored breathing or persistent central cyanosis and a heart rate greater than 100 bpm.
- The T-piece resuscitator is recommended as the device of choice to provide consistent CPAP during neonatal resuscitation. CPAP pressure should not exceed 8 cm H_2O.
- Persistent central cyanosis is defined as oxygen saturations less than the targeted level despite 40% or higher oxygen concentration.
- Mask or endotracheal PPV must be considered for all babies who have persistent central cyanosis despite 100% oxygen and or CPAP.
- Normally transitioning term babies can present with transient labored breathing, tachypnea, and/or grunting that do not require CPAP.
- Consider CPAP for babies demonstrating signs of moderate respiratory distress.

The most important intervention in NRP is *positive pressure ventilation*.
- *Devices used are*: Self-inflating bag, flow-inflating bag, and T-piece resuscitator
- Indications for PPV remain unchanged, that is heart rate less than 100 bpm or ineffective respirations despite initial steps.
- Initial peak inspiratory pressure (PIP) of 20 cm H_2O is recommended for term and preterm babies.
- Term babies who are apneic at birth may require an initial PIP of 30 cm H_2O for the first few breaths in order to inflate their lungs.
- Use positive end-expiratory pressure (PEEP) (5 cm H_2O) for all babies needing PPV.
- Ventilate at a rate of 40–60 breaths per minute.
- Consider attaching a CO_2 detector to the facemask when initiating PPV as it may provide a visual clue that the lungs are inflated.
- After 15 seconds of initial PPV, assess for chest movement, bilateral air entry, then rising heart rate. If an increase in heart rate does not occur, initiate ventilation corrective steps as **Table 1**.
- After 30 seconds of effective PPV if HR <100/ineffective respirations then continue PPV and reassess after every 30 seconds.

- After 30 seconds of effective PPV if HR <60, proceed to chest compressions.
- After 30 seconds of effective PPV if both HR >100 with good respiratory efforts, provide postresuscitation care.

Table 1: MRSOPPA

M	Mask adjustment (consider two-hand technique)
R	Reposition (head neutral or slightly extended). Once seal achieved, evaluate chest movement, air entry, then heart rate
S	Suction mouth (depth = nose tip to ear tragus)
O	Open mouth. Once seal achieved, evaluate chest movement, air entry, then heart rate
P	Pressure increase to 25–40/5 cmH$_2$O. Once seal achieved, evaluate chest movement, air entry, then heart rate
A	Airway alternative (ETT or LMA). Evaluate chest movement, air entry, CO$_2$ detector, then heart rate

The *endotracheal intubation* procedure ideally should be completed within 30 seconds.

- Intubation is strongly recommended when chest compressions begin, to help ensure effective ventilation. However, if intubation is not successful or not feasible, a laryngeal mask airway may be used.
- *Recommended endotracheal tube (ETT) sizes are*:
    - 2.5—if less than 1,000 g or 28 weeks' gestation
    - 3.0—if between 1,000 g and 2,000 g or 28–34 weeks' gestation
    - 3.5—if greater than 2,000 g or 34 weeks' gestation
    - 4.0—no longer recommended.
- The vocal cord guide on the ETT is an approximation for correct insertion depth.
- The use of 6 plus the baby's weight formula is a helpful formula for immediate assessment of insertion depth. This formula provides a good approximation for babies who weigh between 1,500 g and 2,500 g—it significantly overestimates the insertion depth for babies below and above this range.

Sudden Deterioration after Intubation

The mnemonic DOPE is useful in the event of a sudden deterioration following intubation. DOPE reflects possible causes:
- D—Displaced endotracheal tube
- O—Obstruction of the endotracheal tube
- P—Pneumothorax
- E—Equipment failure

Chest Compressions

- If the heart rate is still below 60 bpm despite 30 seconds of effective PPV, increase the oxygen concentration to 100%, and begin chest compressions.
- When the heart rate is below 60 bpm, the pulse oximeter may not function.
- The *two thumb technique* is preferred over two-finger method to administer chest compressions.
- Interruption of chest compressions to check the heart rate may result in a decrease of perfusion pressure in the coronary arteries. Therefore, continue chest compressions and coordinated ventilation for 45–60 seconds before stopping briefly to assess the heart rate, breath sounds, and oxygen saturation.
- The cardiorespiratory monitor is the preferred method for assessing the heart rate during chest compressions.

Medications

- The umbilical venous catheter (UVC) remains the preferred route for vascular access in the delivery room but the intraosseous (IO) needle is a reasonable alternative.
- Epinephrine is indicated when the heart rate remains below 60 bpm after 30 seconds of effective ventilation and another 60 seconds of coordinated chest compressions and effective ventilation with 100% oxygen.
- The preferred route for epinephrine is via a UVC or IO. The endotracheal route is associated with unreliable absorption and is unlikely to be effective.
- *The recommended dose of epinephrine (0.1 mg/mL concentration) is*:
    - *ETT route*: Dose is 0.1 mg/kg (1 mL/kg) of epinephrine 0.1 mg/mL (1:10,000). Maximum dose is 0.3 mg (3 mL). Draw up dose in a 3 mL syringe and label "for ETT." Administer rapidly. Do not follow with a flush.
- The first dose of epinephrine may be administered via ETT while the UVC is being inserted.
- *UVC/IV/IO route (these are the preferred routes)*: Dose is 0.01 mg/kg (0.1 mL/kg) of epinephrine 0.1 mg/mL (1:10,000). Draw up dose in a 1 mL syringe and label "for IV/UVC." Administer rapidly. Follow with a 3 mL 0.9% NaCl flush.

- The recommended flush volume of 0.5–1.0 mL from the tip of the line is required to ensure the medication enters into the circulation. Therefore, 3 mL of flush is recommended to account for line and valve dead space.
- A volume expander of 0.9% NaCl or unmatched type O Rh-negative packed red blood cells is indicated when the baby does not respond to resuscitation interventions and has signs of shock or history of acute blood loss.
- Volume expander can be administered IV or IO. The recommended dose is 10 mL/kg.
- Ringers lactate is no longer recommended as a volume expander.
- $NaHCO_3$ should not be administered to babies during resuscitation. There is no evidence to support this practice.
- Naloxone is no longer recommended for babies who have respiratory depression after maternal opiate exposure.

SUGGESTED READING

1. Accreditation Canada. Qmentum Program: Standards – Obstetric Services for Surveys Starting After January 01, 2017. February 01, 2016.
2. Canadian Paediatric Society. (2016). Medications for Neonatal Resuscitation Program – Canadian Adaptation. [online] Available from www.cps.ca/en/nrp-prn/provider-resources [Last accessed September, 2019].
3. Health Canada. Family-centered Maternal and Newborn Care: National Guidelines. Ottawa, Ontario: Health Canada; 2000.
4. Weiner G. Textbook of Neonatal Resuscitation, 7th edition. Evanston, IL: American Academy of Pediatrics; 2015.

Chapter 54

Neonatal Jaundice

Ram Krishan Kaushal

INTRODUCTION

Jaundice is the most common morbidity in neonates. Sixty percent full-term (FT) and 80% preterm (PT) newborns will have jaundice in the first week of life.[1] Mostly, it is *physiological jaundice*. About 6–10% of these babies will develop jaundice with total serum bilirubin (TSB) exceeding 15 mg/dL.

ETIOLOGY

Jaundice in a newborn could be due to elevation of unconjugated (indirect reacting) or conjugated (direct reacting) bilirubin in the serum **(Boxes 1 to 3)**. Unconjugated type of jaundice is more common.

PHYSIOLOGICAL JAUNDICE

Most common cause of neonatal jaundice in the first week of life is physiologic jaundice. Newborns are prone to develop physiologic jaundice due to following factors:
- *Increased bilirubin production:*
  - High-packed cell volume (PCV)
  - Shorter life span of red blood cells (RBCs)
  - Ineffective erythropoiesis
  - Increased enterohepatic circulation.
- *Transient limited hepatic metabolism:*
  - Poor uptake and glucuronidation of unconjugated bilirubin by hepatocytes
  - Poor excretory mechanism.

Box 1 Causes of unconjugated hyperbilirubinemia.

- *Physiological jaundice*
- *Hemolytic diseases:*
  - Blood group incompatibilities: Rh and ABO
  - Spherocytosis
  - Enzyme deficiency: G6PD, pyruvate kinase
  - Hemoglobinopathies: Severe α thalassemia
- *Extravasated blood:*
  - Cephalhematoma
  - Subaponeurotic bleed
  - Intracranial bleed
  - Severe bruises
- *Polycythemia:*
  - Small for date (SFD)/intrauterine growth retardation (IUGR)
  - Twin-to-twin transfusion (TTT)
  - Materno-fetal transfusion (MFT)
  - Delayed cord clamping
- *Increased enterohepatic circulation of biliburibin:*
  - Delayed passage of meconium
  - Small bowel obstruction
  - Pyloric stenosis
  - Poor/inadequate exclusive breast feeding
- *Poor binding or displacement of bilirubin from binding sites:*
  - Hypoalbuminemia
  - Sulfa group of drugs, moxalactum
  - Acidosis, starvation, hypoglycemia, hypothermia
- *Limited/deficient conjugation of bilirubin in the liver:*
  - *Transient*: Breast milk jaundice (BMJ)
  - *Endocrinal*: Hypothyroidism
  - *Genetic*: Crigler–Najjar syndrome, Gilbert's syndrome

Diagnosis of physiologic jaundice is made by its characteristics and exclusion of other known causes of jaundice **(Box 1)**.

| Box 2 | Causes of conjugated hyperbilirubinemia. |

- *Neonatal hepatitis:*
  - Infections: TORCHES group of infections—*Toxoplasma*, rubella, *Cytomegalovirus*, herpes, syphilis, sepsis, idiopathic hepatitis
- *Biliary atresia*
- *Choledochal cyst*
- *Caroli's disease*
- *Metabolic disorders:*
  - Galactosemia, hereditary fructose intolerance, α-1 antitrypsin deficiency
  - Tyrosinemia, glycogen storage type-IV
- *Inspissated bile plug*
- *Alagille syndrome*
- *Prolonged total parenteral nutrition (TPN)*
- *Chromosomal:* Trisomy 21

| Box 3 | Causes of prolonged/persistent jaundice beyond 2–3 weeks. |

- *Unconjugated type:*
  - Breast milk jaundice
  - Hypothyroidism
  - *Ongoing hemolysis*: Blood group incompatibilities, malaria
  - Crigler–Najjar syndrome, Gilbert's syndrome
- *Conjugated type:*
  - Neonatal hepatitis
  - Biliary atresia
  - Galactosemia

Characteristics of physiologic jaundice are:
- Appears after 24 hours of life
- Maximum intensity on 4th–5th day of life in FT and 7th day in PT
- Maximum TSB ≤12 mg/dL in FT and ≤15 mg/dL in PT
- *Self-limiting*: Disappears by day 10-14 in FT and 2–3 weeks of life in PT
- It is always unconjugated type
- Jaundice in neonates first appears on the face and with a further rise of TSB, it progresses in cephalocaudal direction. It is best detected by blanching the skin with digital pressure in revealing the underlying color of skin and subcutaneous tissue in a well-lighted room, preferably in daylight. TSB is usually ≥5 mg/dL when it is just detectable on the face. Based on extent of yellow staining, the body has been arbitrarily divided into five zones to predict the likely TSB **(Table 1)**.

However, visual estimation of TSB by the extent of skin staining is not always very reliable, particularly in babies with dark skin and those on phototherapy. Greatest risk of developing severe jaundice is around 72-96 hours of life because at this time the TSB is highest. So, follow-up review must be ensured in high-risk babies discharged

Table 1: Prediction of total serum bilirubin (TSB) by extent of yellow skin staining.

Zone	Area of body stained	TSB (mg/dL)
1	Face and neck	5–6
2	Chest up to umbilicus	6–9
3	Abdomen up to knees	9–12
4	Legs up to ankles	12–15
5	Palms and soles	≥15

Table 2: Time of follow-up of babies discharged early.

Age at discharge	Age of follow-up
Before 24 hours	72 hours
Between 24 and 48 hours	96 hours
Between 48 and 72 hours	120 hours

| Box 4 | High-risk factors for development of severe hyperbilirubinemia **(Fig. 1)**.[2] |

- Blood group incompatibility
- Known hemolytic disease such as G6PD deficiency
- Exclusive breast feeding with inadequate nursing (weight loss ≥10%)
- Extravasated blood like cephalhematoma, severe bruises
- Macrosomic infant
- Previous sibling received phototherapy
- Male gender
- Gestational age 35–36 weeks
- Predischarge TSB/transcutaneous bilirubin in high risk or high intermediate risk zone of hour specific serum distribution nomogram

(TSB: total serum bilirubin)

early for presence of jaundice and adequacy of feeding as per **Table 2**.

Some babies are at higher risk to develop jaundice **(Box 4)** and must have follow-up as per schedule in **Table 2**.

PATHOLOGICAL JAUNDICE

Based on the time of appearance, extent, and pattern of jaundice, presence of any of the following is indicative of it being pathological requiring further evaluation **(Box 5)**.

Bilirubin Encephalopathy (Kernicterus)

Clinical manifestations of indirect reacting bilirubin toxicity to basal ganglia and brainstem nuclei are referred to as kernicterus or bilirubin encephalopathy. To avoid any confusion, its manifestation in neonates is better

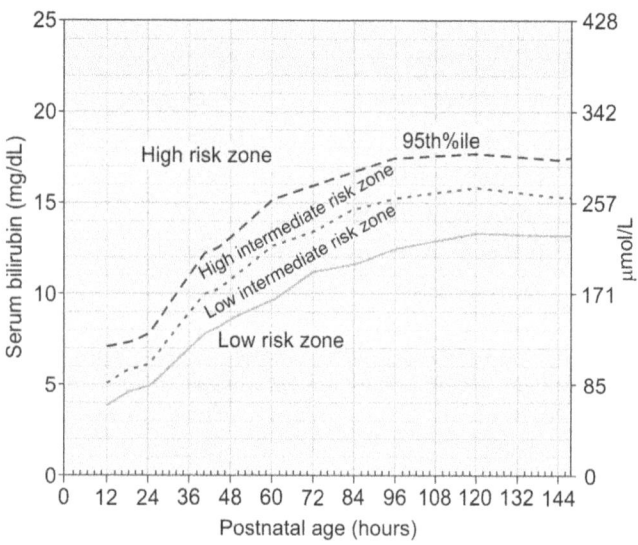

Fig. 1: Nomogram for designation of risk in well newborns ≥35 weeks gestation with birth weight ≥2,000 g based on the hour-specific TSB discharge.[2]

| Box 5 | Characteristics of pathological jaundice. |

- Jaundice appearing within 24 hours of life
- Jaundice persisting beyond 2–3 weeks of life
- Total serum bilirubin (TSB) ≥12 mg/dL in full-term (FT) and ≥10–14 mg/dL in preterm (PT)/low-birth weight (LBW)
- Rate of rise of TSB by ≥0.5 mg/dL/hr or 5 mg/dL/day
- Yellow urine positive for bilirubin
- Clay/white colored stool
- Conjugated serum bilirubin, ≥1 mg/dL if TSB ≤ 5 mg/dL or ≥20% of TSB if TSB ≥5 mg/dL
- Sick baby with presence of jaundice
- Jaundiced baby with signs of acute bilirubin encephalopathy (kernicterus)

called as acute bilirubin encephalopathy, whereas its chronic and permanent sequelae are called kernicterus. Acute bilirubin encephalopathy is characterized by lethargy, hypotonia followed by hypertonia (retrocollis and opisthotonus), poor sucking, irritability, moderate stupor, fever, and high pitched cry. It may get reversed by exchange blood transfusion. Advanced phase is irreversible and its manifestations include pronounced retrocollis/opisthotonus, shrill cry, no feeding, apnea, fever, deep stupor to coma and seizures.

ASSESSMENT OF NEONATE WITH JAUNDICE

Enquire the postnatal age in hours, gestational age at birth, birth weight, blood group of mother, type and adequacy of feeding, color of urine and stool, and history of significant jaundice in previous sibling. Examine the baby for extent of jaundice **(Table 1)**, any extravasated blood, stigmata of intrauterine infections, organomegaly, any signs of sepsis, or acute bilirubin encephalopathy **(Algorithms 1 to 5)**.

Clinical Assessment of a Neonate with Jaundice

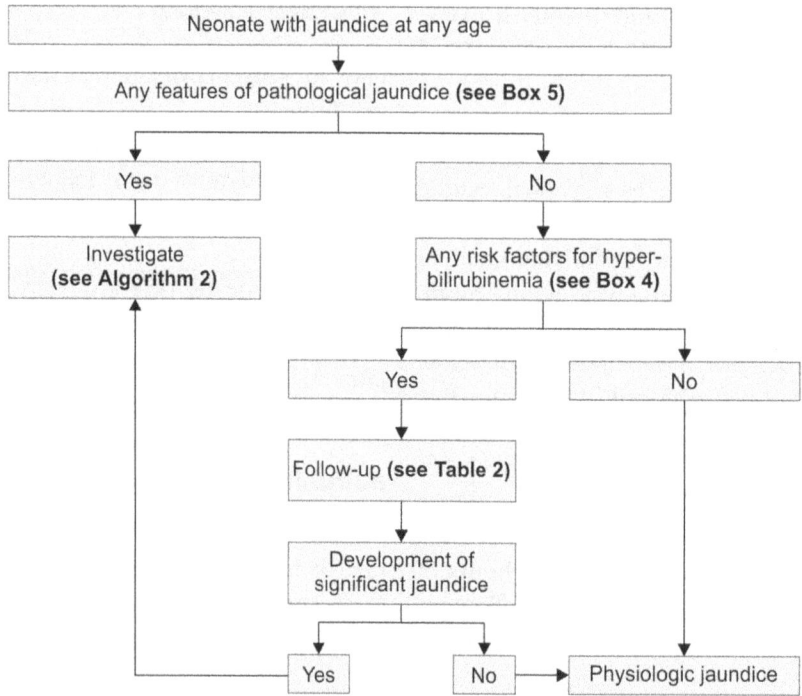

Algorithm 1: Clinical assessment of a neonate with jaundice.

Laboratory Evaluation of Neonatal Jaundice

Algorithm 2: Laboratory evaluation of neonatal jaundice.

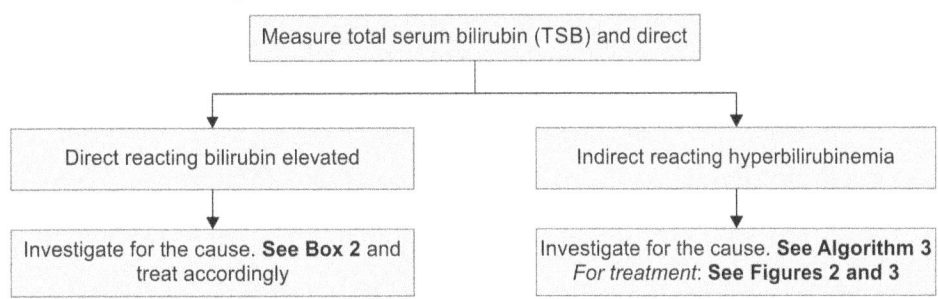

Laboratory Evaluation of Unconjugated Type of Jaundice

Algorithm 3: Laboratory evaluation of indirect reacting (unconjugated) hyperbilirubinemia.

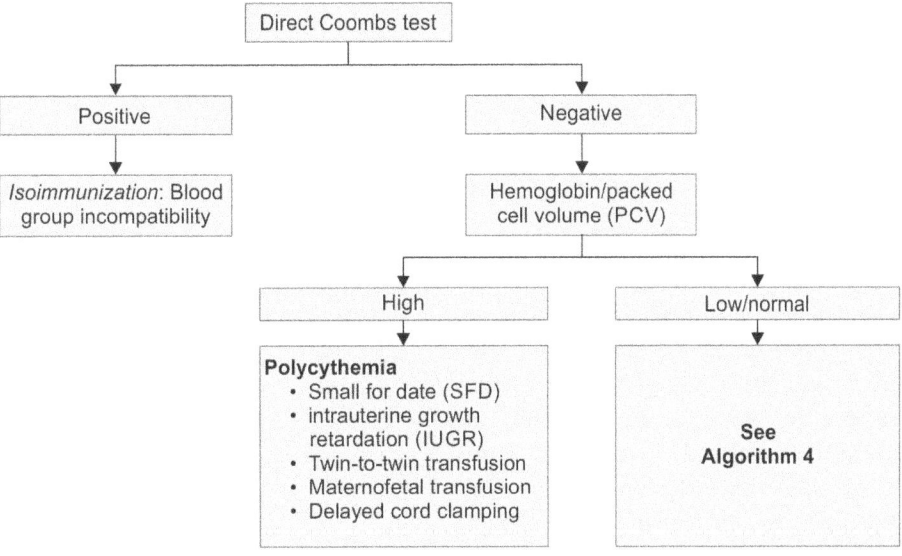

Laboratory Evaluation of Unconjugated Jaundice with Low or Normal Hemoglobin/PCV

Algorithm 4: Laboratory evaluation of unconjugated hyperbilirubinemia with low/normal Hb/PCV.

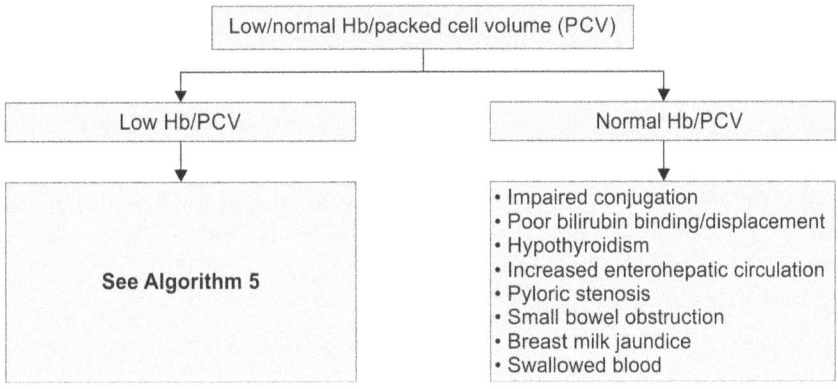

Laboratory Evaluation of Unconjugated Jaundice with Low Hemoglobin/PCV

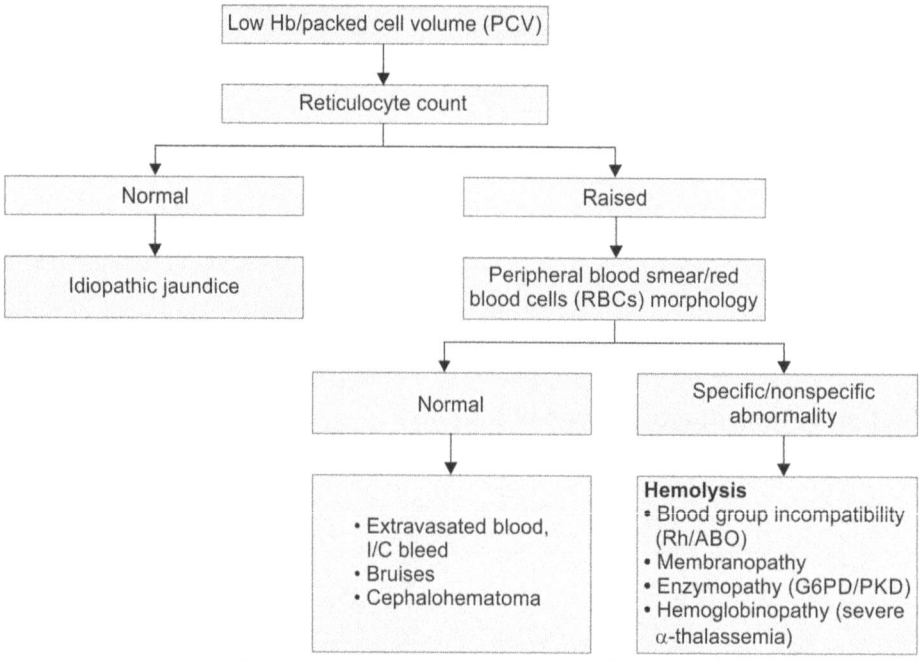

Algorithm 5: Laboratory evaluation of unconjugated hyperbilirubinemia in case of low Hb/PCV.

(I/C: intracranial; PKD: pyruvate kinase deficiency)

TREATMENT

The overall aim of prevention and treatment of indirect reacting hyperbilirubinemia is to prevent acute and chronic central nervous system (CNS) bilirubin toxicity. Safe and effective way to lower serum bilirubin is phototherapy and if the TSB is already in exchange zone or there are signs of acute bilirubin encephalopathy or phototherapy becomes ineffective, blood exchange transfusion (BET) is the only means of rapid lowering of TSB to safe level. None of the pharmacological agents investigated for treatment of hyperbilirubinemia have been found to be safe and effective. Intravenous ϒ-globulin has been used to reduce the need of exchange transfusion in isoimmune hemolytic disease in a dose of 0.5–1 g/kg over 2 hours if the TSB is rising despite intensive phototherapy or TSB is within 2–3 mg/dL of indication for BET. The general rule of thumb to guide the mode of treatment is to start phototherapy when TSB is 0.75% and do exchange transfusion when TSB is ≥1% of birth weight in grams. To be more precise, recommendations of American Academy of Pediatrics (AAP) for babies ≥35 weeks gestation are depicted in **Figures 2 and 3**.[3] Guidelines of treatment for low birth weight (LBW) babies are shown in **Table 3**.[4]

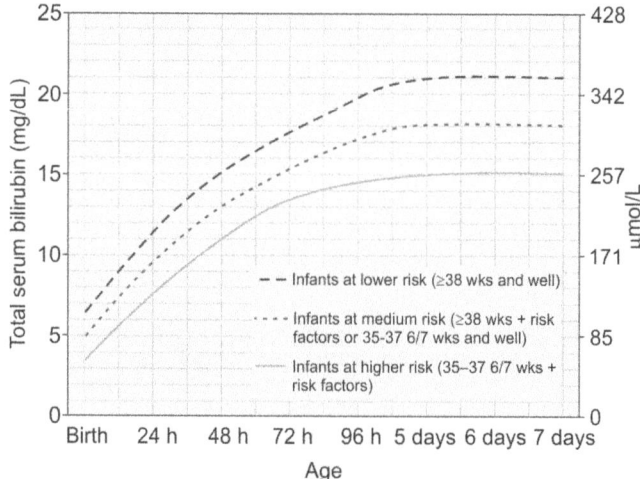

- Use TSB, do not subtract conjugated bilirubin.
- Risk factors—blood group incompatibilities, G6PD deficiency, birth asphyxia and suspected or proved septicemia.
- Adjust TSB levels for intervention around medium risk line in well infants of 35-37+ 6/7 weeks gestation.
- Conventional phototherapy may be given in hospital or at home with TSB 2–3 mg/dL below the actual TSB shown in well infants but home phototherapy is not recommended in infants with risk factors.

Fig. 2: Guidelines for phototherapy in newborns ≥35 weeks. Start phototherapy when total serum bilirubin (TSB) exceeds the line indicated for each category.[3]

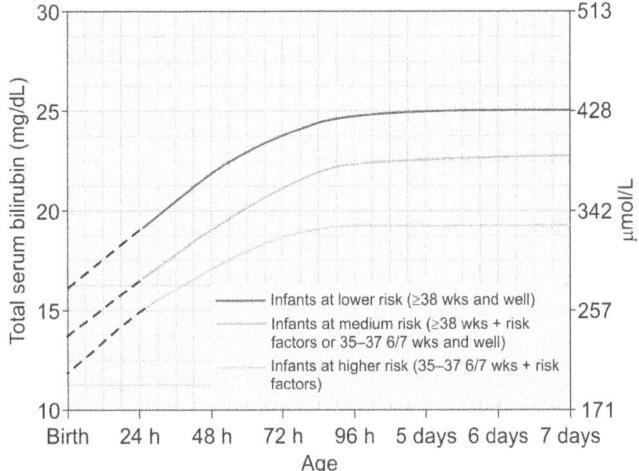

The dashed lines for the first 24 hours indicate uncertainty due to wide range of clinical circumstances and a range of responses to phototherapy.
- If TSB is ≥ 5 mg/dL (85 μmol/L) above these lines or there are clinical features of acute bilirubin encephalopathy immediate BET is recommended.
- Risk factors—blood group incompatibilities, G6PD deficiency, birth asphyxia, proved or suspected sepsis and acidosis.
- Measure serum albumin and calculate B/A ratio (see **Table 4**). B/A ratios can be used together with but not in lieu of the TSB level as an additional factor in determining the need for BET.
- Use TSB, do not subtract conjugated bilirubin.
- In a well baby with medium risk (35-37+ 6/7 week gestation), can individualize TSB level for ET on actual gestational age.
- At birth—hydrops fetalis, cord blood bilirubin ≥ 4.5 mg/dL, cord blood Hb ≤ 11 g/dL

Fig. 3: Guidelines for blood exchange transfusion in newborns ≥35 weeks gestation.[3]

Table 3: Guidelines for management of unconjugated hyperbilirubinemia in low-birth weight (LBW) babies.

Birth weight (g)	TSB (mg/dL)	
	Phototherapy	Exchange transfusion
≤1,500	5–8	13–16
1,500–1,999	8–12	16–18
2,000–2,499	11–14	18–20
(TSB: total serum bilirubin)		

Phototherapy

Intensive phototherapy with irradiance of at least 30 μw/cm²/nm in blue-green spectrum wavelength of approximately 430–490 nm delivered to as much of the baby's surface area as possible. Additional surface area exposure can be achieved by lining the sides of the bassinet with aluminum foil or a white cloth. The most effective light sources currently recommended for phototherapy are special blue fluorescent tubes (F20T12/BB or TL52/20w). These special blue tubes provide much greater irradiance than regular blue tubes (F20T12/B) in blue-green spectrum which penetrates the skin well and is absorbed maximally by the bilirubin. Devices with these tubes can be placed as close as within 10 cm of baby's skin without any risk of skin burn (cf. Halogen spot phototherapy which cannot be placed so close due to risk of burns). Maintain adequate hydration and good urine output to improve the efficacy of phototherapy in lowering TSB, because photoproducts of bilirubin are excreted in urine and bile. Unless there is dehydration requiring IV fluid, it is best to breastfeed more frequently.

Can Sunlight Exposure be Substituted for Phototherapy?

Sunlight does provide sufficient irradiance in 425–475 nm band but safety concerns exposing naked newborn to sun either inside or outside avoiding sunburn or hypothermia precludes it as a reliable and safe therapeutic tool of phototherapy.

When to Stop Phototherapy?

No definite standard can be fixed but generally when TSB falls below 13–14 mg/dL it can be stopped and follow-up check TSB after 24 hours should be done to see for any rebound rise of TSB.

Contraindications for Phototherapy

- Congenital porphyria
- Family history of porphyria.
 Concomitant use of drugs/agents that are photosensitizers.

Blood Exchange Transfusion

It is the most effective and rapid method to lower TSB level by physical removal of bilirubin, antibodies, sensitized RBCs and it also simultaneously corrects the anemia. Double volume exchange (80 × 2 × weight in kg = total blood in mL exchanged) replaces 87% of baby's blood volume and results in about 50% decline in pre-exchange TSB.

Indications for Blood Exchange Transfusion (Fig. 3)

- The dashed lines for the first 24 hours indicate uncertainty due to wide range of clinical circumstances and a range of responses to phototherapy.

Table 4: Total serum bilirubin (TSB) and serum albumin ratio (B/A) for consideration of blood exchange transfusion (BET).[3]

Risk category	B/A ratio at which BET should be considered	
	TSB (mg/dL)/ albumin (g/dL)	TSB (µmol/L)/ albumin (µmol/L)
Gestation ≥38 0/7 weeks	8.0	0.94
Gestation 35 0/7–36 6/7 and well	7.2	0.84
Or ≥38 0/7 week if higher risk or		
Isoimmune hemolytic disease		
Or G6PD deficiency		
Gestation 35 0/7–37 6/7 weeks if higher risk	6.8	0.80
Or isoimmune hemolytic disease or		
G6PD deficiency		

- Immediate ET is recommended if baby shows signs of acute bilirubin encephalopathy or if TSB is ≥5 mg/dL (85 µmol/L) above these lines.
- *Risk factors:* Isoimmune hemolytic disease, G6PD deficiency, asphyxia, significant lethargy, temperature instability, sepsis, and acidosis.
- Measure serum albumin and calculate B/A ratio **(Table 4)**. B/A ratios can be used together with but not in lieu of the TSB level as an additional factor in determining the need for BET.
- Use TSB, do not subtract directly reacting (conjugated) bilirubin.
- If the baby is well and medium risk (35–37 + 6/7 weeks gestation), can individualize TSB level for ET on actual gestational age.
- *At birth:* Hydrops fetalis, cord blood bilirubin ≥4.5 mg/dL, cord blood Hb ≤11 g/dL.

Choice of Blood for Exchange Transfusion

As fresh as possible, modified whole blood (red cells and plasma) cross-matched against the mother and compatible with the baby's blood. In Rh-incompatibility, Rh-negative cells, preferably O or AB of baby if the mother also has same type compatible with both baby and mother sera.

REFERENCES

1. Ambalavam N, Carlo WA. Jaundice and hyperbilirubinemia in the newborn. In: Kleigman RM, Stanton BF, St Geme III JW, Schor NF, Behrman RE (Eds). Nelson Textbook of Pediatrics, 20th edition (First South East Asian edition, Volume I). New Delhi: Elsevier; 2016. pp. 871-80.
2. Bhutani VK, Johnson L, Sivieri EM. Predictive ability of a predischarge hour-specific serum bilirubin for subsequent significant hyperbilirubinemia in healthy term and near-term newborns. Pediatrics. 1999;103:6-14.
3. American Academy of Pediatrics. Pediatric Clinical Practice Guidelines and Policies. A Compendium of Evidence-based Research for Pediatric Practice, 13th edition. New Delhi: Jaypee Brothers Medical Publishers (P) Ltd; 2013.
4. Gupta P. Textbook of Pediatrics, 1st edition. New Delhi: CBS Publishers and Distributors Pvt. Ltd; 2013.

Section 7

Miscellaneous

- **Teenage Pregnancy**
  Priti Samir Vyas

- **Blood and Blood Component Therapy**
  Dilpreet Kaur Pandher, Alok Sharma

- **Patient Communication**
  Girija Wagh, Aakanksha Kumar

- **Biomedical Waste Management Rules**
  Anuradha Sood, Smriti Chauhan, Subhash Chand Jaryal

- **How to Curb Maternal Mortality in India**
  Madhu Gupta, Kanica Kaushal

- **Needle-prick Injury**
  Madhuri Chandra

Chapter 55

Teenage Pregnancy

Priti Samir Vyas

INTRODUCTION

Adolescence, a unique developmental stage and teenage pregnancy (<20 years), deserves acknowledgment of its distinct inherent risks and an understanding of the relevant elements of care required for diagnosis, management of pregnancy during this time, for successful outcomes for mother, infant, and their surrounding social circle.

In our society, supposedly based on certain morals, teenage pregnancy is a kind of social taboo and in large parts of the world, society shuns it making it difficult for teenage mothers to survive in this world.

INCIDENCE: HIGH-RISK GROUP

(Number of pregnancies/1,000 females aged 15–19 years). In both developed and developing countries, teenage pregnancies are usually outside marriage and carry social stigma in many communities and cultures along with social issues, including lower educational levels, poverty, and other negative life outcomes in children of teenage mothers.

But, by contrast, in developing countries, teens are often also married and their pregnancies are often welcomed by family and society.

Worldwide:
- Highest is in the sub-Saharan African countries (143/1000)
- One of the lowest in South Korea (2.9/1000)
- Europe—ranges from 26.4/1000 in United Kingdom as per 2006 survey to 3.3/1000 in central parts of Italy.

Indian subcontinent:
- 62/1,000 teens.[1]
- Rural higher rate than urban.

In line with the incidence and needs of their population, guidelines have been given by bodies like NICE, SOGC, and AOCG.

High incidences are seen in:
- *Lower socioeconomic group.*
- *Social deprivation:* Teenagers from unskilled manual background are 10 times more likely than those from professional backgrounds.[2]
- *Low educational achievement.*
- *Having had teenage parents:* Children born to teenage parents are themselves at risk of teenage pregnancy due to:
  - Poor transition from school to work
  - Sexual abuse
  - Mental health problems
  - Early puberty
  - Culture; child marriages
  - Domestic violence and family strife.

CAUSES

UNICEF defines child marriage as a formal marriage or informal union before 18 years of age. UN Women' has proposed that child marriage be defined as a forced marriage because they believe children under age of 18 years are incapable of giving a legally valid consent.
- *Lack of education:* It has adverse impact on reproductive and sexual health awareness.

In age group of 15–19 years, only 7% of married women have higher secondary level of education, 17% have completed primary schooling, and 55% are illiterate (NFHS-2 data).

A study undertaken in urban slums of Mumbai to know impact of maternal biosocial determinants on birth weight found 52% of illiterate mothers gave birth to low birth weight (LBW) babies showing education plays a vital role in LBW prevention.

- *Poverty:* One of the leading cause—strong association with illiteracy, lack of awareness, lack of accessibility to contraceptive means, domestic violence, and social deprivation.
- *Child marriages:* UNICEF publications estimated India's child marriage rate at 47% (small sample surveys, 1998), UN reports at 30% (2005). Jharkhand has highest in India (14.1%)[3] while Kerala is the only state where rates have increased in recent years.[4]
- *Lack of supportive parents and family:* Resulting in psychological distress and thereby drug addictions, victims of sexual abuse/violence.
- *Peer pressure to have early sex and exposure to media:* Teen may be bullied for being coward and not having courage to take risks by peers.
- *Substance abuse:* Alcohol and inhibition-reducing drugs—cannabis, MDMA (ecstasy), etc.—encourage unintended sexual activity
- *Risk-taking behavior:* Increased independence, less adult supervision, experimentation with driving, substance abuse, and sexual activity, under the impression that they are not vulnerable.
- *Delay in seeking advice:* To abort or continue.
- *Inconsistent use of contraception.*
- *Exposure to sexual violence/abuse:* Multiple studies have indicated a strong link between early childhood sexual abuse and subsequent teenage pregnancy in industrialized countries. Up to 70% of women who gave birth in their teens were molested as young girls.[5]

CONSEQUENCES OF TEENAGE PREGNANCY (ALGORITHM 1)

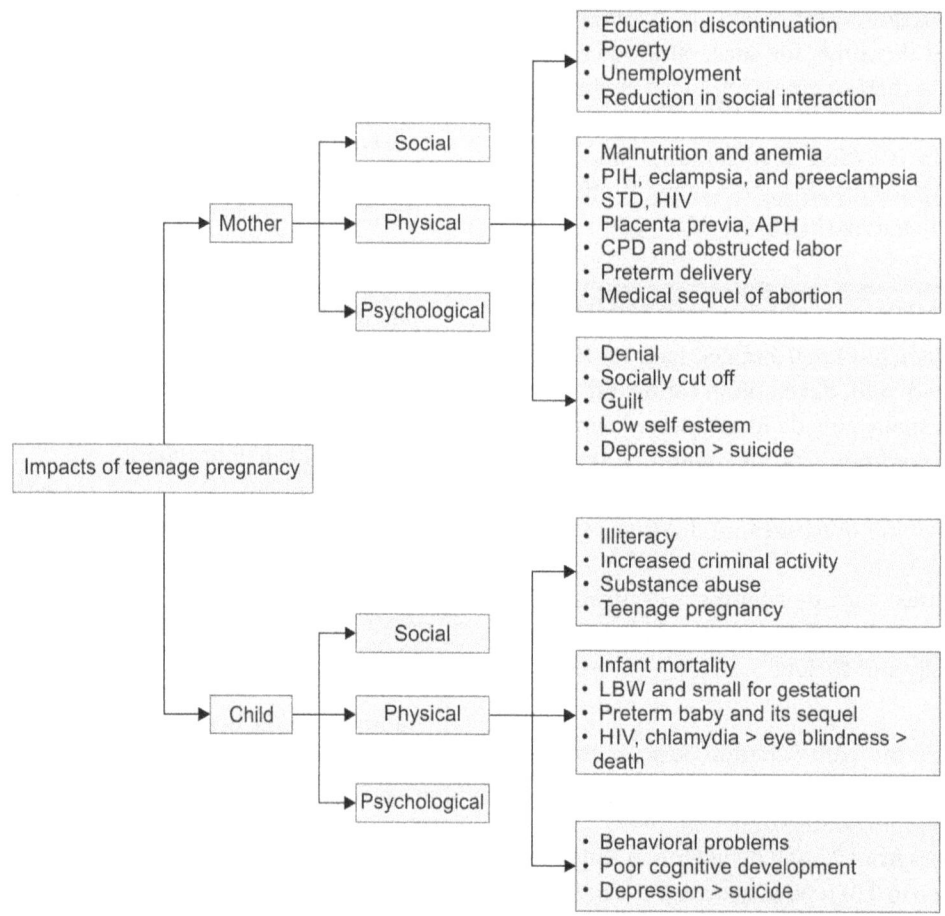

Algorithm 1: Impacts of teenage pregnancy.

(APH: antepartum hemorrhage; CPD: cephalopelvic disproportion; HIV: human immunodeficiency virus; LBW: low birth weight; PIH: pregnancy-induced hypertension; STDs: sexually transmitted diseases)

On Mother

Social

Domestic responsibilities, earning a livelihood at this age, lack of adequate nutrition, no rest, and increased demands of pregnancy result in medical and social complications:
- Discontinuation of education
- More likely to live in poverty
- Unemployment or having lower salaries due to lack of skills
- Limiting of social interaction
- Financial stress.

Physical

Risk for medical complications is greater under 15 years:
- *Anemia:* 56% teens are anemic in India.
- *Malnutrition:* Lower body mass index (BMI) leading to chronic energy deficiency.[6]
- *Pregnancy-induced hypertension (PIH):* Preeclampsia and eclampsia.[7]
- *Sexually transmitted diseases-human immunodeficiency virus (STDs-HIV):* Half of 20 million new cases. One in five sexually active teen girls resulting in infertility and even death. Pregnancy adds to the morbidities-mortalities of STDs.[8]

  Increased risk of catching any STD due to biological factors such as thin and immature and incompletely estrogenized cervix making it more susceptible to gonorrheal, chlamydial, and human papillomavirus (HPV) infections.
- More incidences of placenta previa and antepartum hemorrhage.
- *Premature delivery:* May be due to lower social class, poor economic condition, inadequate prenatal care, and a host of medical conditions such as preeclampsia, eclampsia, cardiovascular, and renal disorders may be responsible in part.
- *Obstructed labor:* The prepubertal pelvis is contracted from obstetric point of view. The younger patients experiencing shorter growth periods before conception exhibit greater proportion of contracted pelvis. Cephalopelvic disproportion (CPD) is the main indicator of lower segment cesarean section (LSCS) in teens.

  It is normally dealt by cesarean section in industrialized nations, in developing regions where medical services might be unavailable, it can lead to rupture uterus, obstetric fistula, infant mortality, or maternal death.[9]
- *Illegal abortions due to social stigma:* As compared to adults, adolescents are more likely to delay the abortion, resort to unskilled person to perform it, use dangerous methods, and present late when complications arise.

Psychological

In India, parents are rarely supportive of unmarried pregnant daughter and exert strong pressure for abortion or placing the child for adoption or forced marriage. The teenager goes through a varying phase of emotions. Her reaction to her condition is influenced by previous emotional health and the current circumstances; resulting in immediate and long-term sequel.

On Child

Physical, Social, and Psychological Implications

Infant mortality is high among this group maybe because of the combined effect of extreme prematurity, LBW, immature age of mother, and maternal complications. Inability to complete the education with the added burden of child-rearing and also lack of enough financial resources for the same results in the child suffering similar consequences.

MANAGEMENT OF TEENAGE PREGNANCY (ALGORITHM 2)

Managing a pregnancy for young adolescents is always a challenge from the point of view of obstetric, social as well as emotional issues. First, and foremost, they have to be counseled and all possible options have to be discussed with the girl and the parents, i.e. abortion, adoption, and parenting for the safety of both mother and child, keeping the laws of the land in mind.

During Pregnancy

There is higher rate of congenital anomalies, intrauterine growth restriction (IUGR), and complications such as PIH, preeclampsia, etc. so a strict watch and close monitoring, frequent visits in second and third trimester, and early referral to higher centers in complicated cases for less equipped healthcare centers is essential.

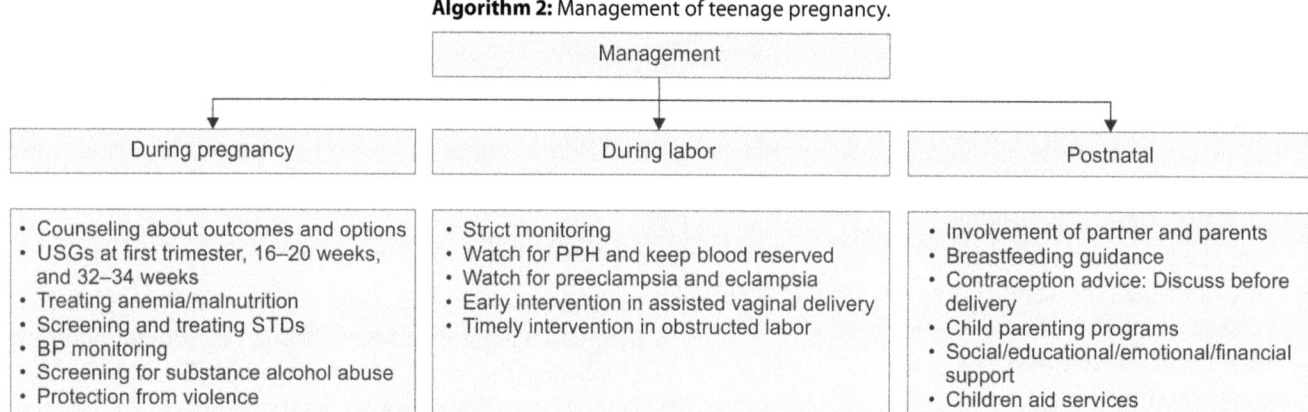

Algorithm 2: Management of teenage pregnancy.

(BP: blood pressure; PPH: postpartum hemorrhage; STDs: sexually transmitted diseases; USG: ultrasonography)

During Labor

There is increased risk of obstructed labor due to small and immature pelvis; timely intervention is to be done to prevent fatal outcomes.

Postnatal Management

Postpartum care programs to support adolescent parents, to improve mother's knowledge of parenting and give emotional, social, financial, and educational support especially, if secondary education to be continued, would help in the social upliftment.

PREVENTION OF TEENAGE PREGNANCY (ALGORITHM 3)

Unintended pregnancy is one which is unplanned, unwanted, and untimed. They have negative consequences not only on the mother and child but also the society, in general. Four out of five unintended pregnancies occur due to lack of access to modern effective contraception available. Hence, it is pertinent to educate the public and the society in general about health burdens and the consequences and also the available options to prevent the same.

A comprehensive approach through sex education, contraception education, and availability, and government plans and policies has to be followed.

Although abstinence is the most effective means of birth control, recent data suggest that abstinence-only programs are not as effective as those combined with contraceptive options. Knowledge, as well as, the accessibility to available methods of contraception, is most effective.

In the quest for the best contraceptive method, adolescents look for safety, convenience, privacy, and efficacy as the most important factors.

Barrier Method would help contraception and also protect against sexually transmitted infections, however in adolescents the use of condoms is not correct, continuous and consistent. The entire basket of options should be offered to them. It is important to *Communicate*—overcoming parent–child communication barrier.

POCSO ACT

The Protection of Children from Sexual Offences (POCSO). Act, 2012 is a comprehensive law to provide for the protection of children from the offenses of sexual assault, sexual harassment, and pornography, while safeguarding the interests of the child at every stage of the judicial process by incorporating child friendly mechanisms for reporting, recording of evidence, investigation, and speedy trial of offenses through designated special courts. It defines a child as any person below 18 years of age and defines different forms of sexual abuse including penetrative and nonpenetrative assault as well as sexual harassment and pornography.[10] If a girl less than 18 years of age comes for a medical abortion, the laws of POCSO need to be kept in mind; by the treating physician since it also becomes doctor's medico-legal responsibility to report to the concerned authorities before resorting to the abortion.

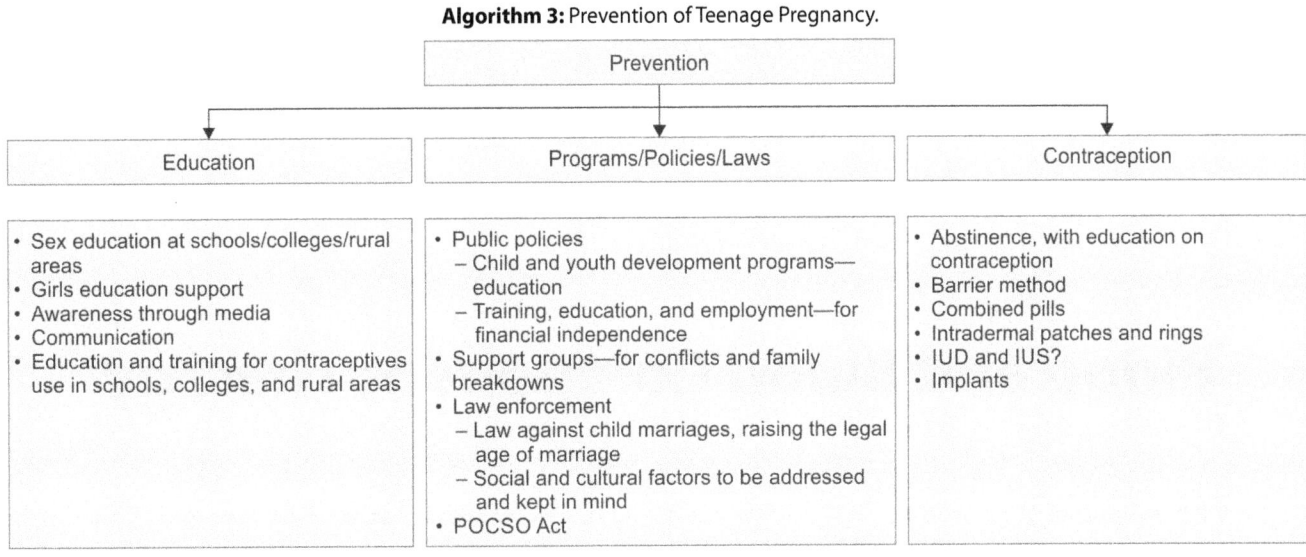

Algorithm 3: Prevention of Teenage Pregnancy.

(IUD: intrauterine device; IUS: intrauterine system)

CONCLUSION

Approximately, 80% of adolescent pregnancies are unintended and 50–60% of teens who are sexually active have had their first intercourse before the age of 18 years. There is an urgent need for education and increasing awareness among them as well as the society in general to improve not only their health but also benefit the society and the country at large.

REFERENCES

1. Dawan H. Teen pregnancies higher in India than even UK, US. The Economic Times (28 November 2008). Retrieved 2 May 2013.
2. Joshi SN. Effects of the maternal bio-social determinants on the birth weight in a slum area of greater Mumbai. Indian J Commun Med. 2002;3:106-9.
3. Sinha K. Nearly 50% fall in brides married below 18. The Times of India (February 10, 2012).
4. Gopakumar R. Child marriages high in Kerala. Deccan Herald (June 19, 2013).
5. Saewyc EM, Magee LL, Pettingell SE. Teenage pregnancy and associated risk behaviours among sexually abused adolescents. Perspect Sex Reprod Health. 2004;36(3): 98-105.
6. Kanani S. Nutrition health profile and intervention strategies for underprivileged adolescent girls in India: a selected review. Indian J Matern Child Health. 1990;1:129-33.
7. Singh N, Mishra C. Nutritional status of adolescent girls in a slum community of Varanasi. Indian J Public Health. 2001;45:128-34.
8. Centers for Disease Control and Prevention. Reported STDs in the United States. Atlanta, GA: National Center for HIV/AIDS, Viral hepatitis, STD & TB Prevention; 2014.
9. Konar H, Kushtagi P. The extremes of reproductive age: pregnancy in adolescence and advanced maternal age. Medical Disorders in Pregnancy: An Update. New Delhi: Jaypee Brothers Medical Publishers; 2006. p. 304.
10. The Protection Of Children From Sexual Offences Act, 2012 [No 32 OF 2012].

SUGGESTED READING

1. Gibbs RS. Danforth's Obstetrics and Gynecology.
2. Konar H, Kushtagi P. Medical Disorders in Pregnancy: An Update; 2006.
3. Krishna U. Pregnancy at Risk.
4. Ministry of Women and Child Development.
5. Model Guidelines under Section 39 of The Protection of Children from Sexual Offences Act, 2012.
6. Rayburn WF. Obstetrics And Gynecology Clinics of North America.
7. SOGC Clinical Practice Guideline—Adolescent Pregnancy Guidelines; 2015
8. Update on review of reviews on teenage pregnancy and parenthood December 2007 prepared by Trivedi D, Bunn F, Wentz R on behalf of the National Institute for Health and Clinical Excellence.

Chapter 56

Blood and Blood Component Therapy

Dilpreet Kaur Pandher, Alok Sharma

INTRODUCTION

Transfusion medicine guidelines for blood transfusion in pregnancy[1] suggest (level I evidence):

```
┌─────────────────────────────────────────────────────────────────────────────┐
│ Every obsteric unit should have their own guidelines for RBC transfusion    │
│ for the antenatal and postnatal cases not bleeding actively                 │
│ ABO-Rh typing and screening for antibodies to be done at first visit        │
│ and repeat at 28 weeks                                                      │
└─────────────────────────────────────────────────────────────────────────────┘
                                    ↓
┌─────────────────────────────────────────────────────────────────────────────┐
│ Reference to the higher center in case of:                                  │
│ Signs and symptoms of anemia                                                │
│ Severe anemia <7 g/dL                                                       │
│ Advanced gestation >34 weeks                                                │
└─────────────────────────────────────────────────────────────────────────────┘
                                    ↓
┌─────────────────────────────────────────────────────────────────────────────┐
│ Transfusion is recommended in nonbleeding patient with Hb <6 g/dL           │
│ after clinical assessment:                                                  │
│ Risk of bleeding, cardiorespiratory compromise, any symptoms                │
│ requiring immediate attention                                               │
└─────────────────────────────────────────────────────────────────────────────┘
                                    ↓
┌─────────────────────────────────────────────────────────────────────────────┐
│ No active bleeding, still transfusion seems necessary:                      │
│ Single unit RBC transfusion is done                                         │
│ Clinical reassessment and/or Hb decides further transfusion                 │
└─────────────────────────────────────────────────────────────────────────────┘
                                    ↓
┌─────────────────────────────────────────────────────────────────────────────┐
│ Fetal indication for maternal blood transfusion (ACOG, NICE 2008):[2-4]     │
│ Hb <6 g/dL:                                                                 │
│ Causes impaired fetal oxygenation, hence nonreassuring FHR and reduced      │
│ amniotic fluid volume and cerebral vasodilatation;                          │
│ blood transfusion should be given                                           │
└─────────────────────────────────────────────────────────────────────────────┘
```

(ACOG: American College of Obstetricians and Gynecologists; FHR: fetal heart rate; NICE: National Institute for Health and Care Excellence, England guidelines; RBC: red blood cell)

Red blood cells transfusion in nonbleeding patients:[1]
- One concentrate contains 240 mg iron.
- To treat deficiency and replenish stores, concomitant IV iron is recommended.
- Erythrocyte stimulating agent is advocated to maximize erythropoiesis.

In case of severe bleeding, blood transfusion is definitely proven to be beneficial whereas in nonbleeding anemic patients, role of blood transfusion is always doubtful. As per World Health Organization guidelines (2001a),[5] transfusion of blood and products should be undertaken only to treat a condition that would lead to significant morbidity or mortality and that cannot be prevented or managed effectively by other means. Women receiving blood transfusion should have full information regarding (WHO 2001B):[6]

- The indication of transfusion
- The alternatives available
- Informed consent for transfusion procedure must be obtained.

Risks of blood transfusion:[7]
- Infections like viral transmission
- Reactions
- Mismatch transfusion
- Transfusion-related acute lung injury (TRALI)
- Cardiac overload
- Allergic and febrile illness
- Hyperkalemia, hypocalcemia, iron overload, citrate toxicity
- Rare complications:
  - Emergent pathogen leading to infections
  - Immunomodulation, causing activation of cancer cells

MASSIVE HEMORRHAGE

Hemorrhage is said to be massive (ACOG 2016):[8]
- Anticipated need to replace 50% or more of blood volume within 2 hours
- Bleeding continues after the transfusion of 4 U of packed red blood cells within a short period of time (1–2 hours), or
- The systolic blood pressure is below 90 mm Hg and the heart rate is above 120 beats/min in the presence of uncontrolled bleeding.

Pathophysiological changes due to massive hemorrhage:[9]

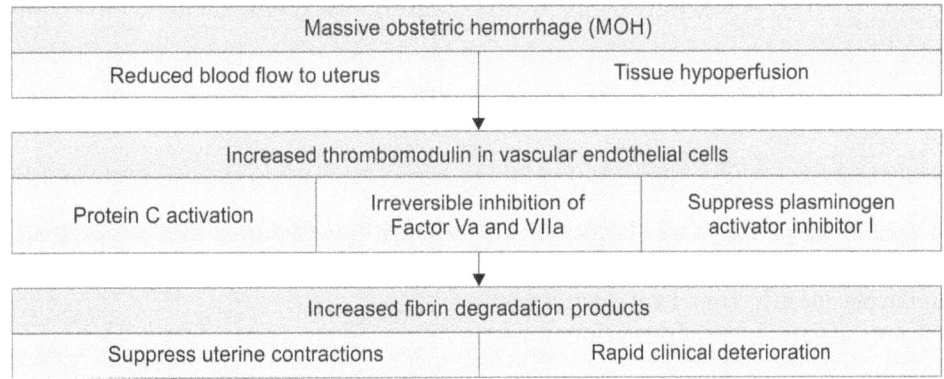

Management of Massive Obstetric Hemorrhage[10]

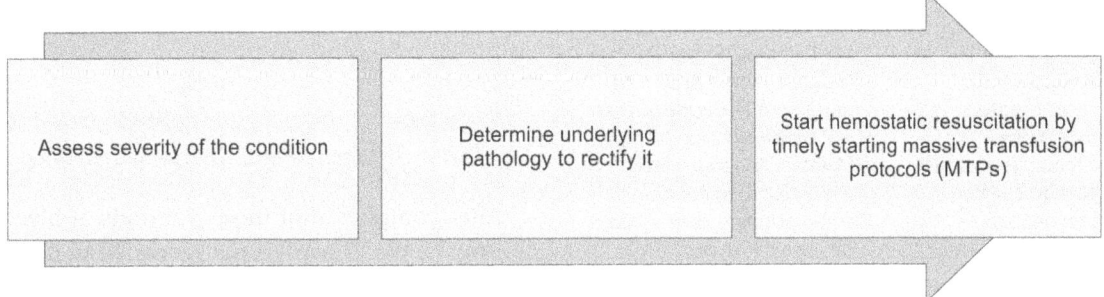

Massive transfusion protocols (MTPs) require multidisciplinary approach involving:[8]
- Obstetrician
- Anesthesiologist
- Hematologist
- Blood bank personnel: Provide blood and blood products at a predefined ratio.

Permissive Hypotension[11]

Systolic BP between 80 mm Hg and 100 mm Hg is found to be optimal to limit bleeding in postpartum hemorrhage by reducing blood flow due to low hydrostatic pressure and by preventing dislodgement of clots from the bleeding site. However, in cases prior to delivery, i.e. antenatal period, no data on this concept is available since blood flow to the fetus is also to be taken into consideration.

Earlier Concept of Resuscitation in Massive Obstetric Hemorrhage[8]

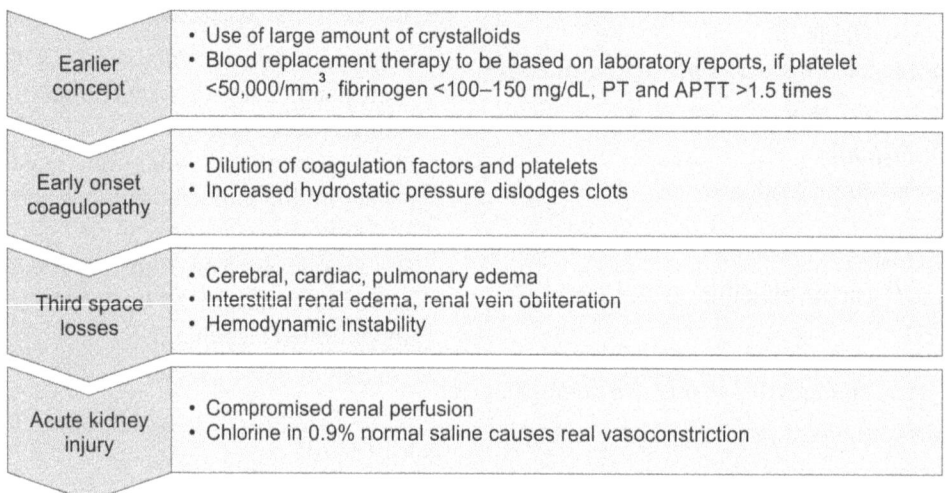

(APTT: activated partial thromboplastin time; PT: prothrombin time)

Crystalloids if required, Ringer lactate and PlasmaLyte or plasma-lyte (family of balanced crystalloid solutions that closely mimics human plasma in its content of electrolytes, osmolality and pH), are recommended by recent literature.

Recent Concept of "Hemostatic Resuscitation"

ACOG 2016[8]	RCOG 2015[12]
• Transfusion of RBC: FFP: Platelet in 1:1:1 ratio • Resolves coagulopathy, hypothermia, acidosis; the major contributors of maternal mortality • Targeted fibrinogen levels >150–200 mg/dL (value in normal pregnancy is 400–500 mg/dL)	• For every 6 units of red cells, administer FFP at a dose of 12–15 mL/kg body weight • Maintain PT and APTT ≤1.5 times normal; decide further FFP transfusion accordingly • Maintain fibrinogen level ≥150 mg/dL; transfuse cryoprecipitate as two 5 unit sets to achieve that

(APTT: activated partial thromboplastin time; FFP: fresh frozen plasma; PT: prothrombin time)

Massive blood transfusion protocols (ACOG 2016)[8]:

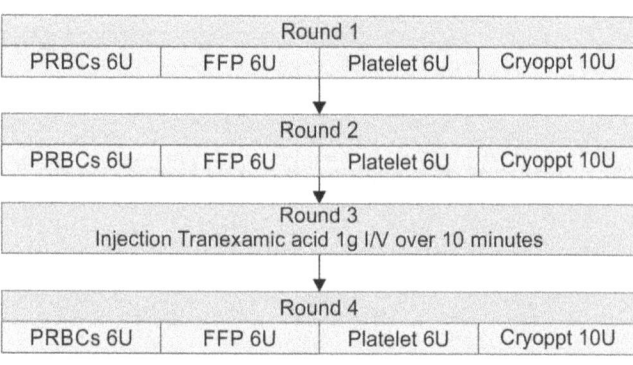

(FFP: fresh frozen plasma; PRBC: packed red blood cells)

After completion of these 4 rounds, if bleeding does not stop or blood bank is not informed to inactivate, the protocol restarts from round 1 as per American Journal of Obstetrics and Gynecology 2016.

BLOOD COMPONENTS

- *Platelet:*
  - One unit causes rise by 5,000–10,000/mm^3
  - Dose: 1 unit/10 kg body weight.
- *Fresh frozen plasma (FFP) (200–250 mL):* Made from plasma and stored at –35°C to preserve it. It contains all clotting factors and 2 g fibrinogen/1,000 mL.
  One unit increases fibrinogen level by 10 mg/dL.
  Fibrinogen is the first clotting factor to get depleted in massive obstetric hemorrhage (MOH). Under the effect of thromboplastin, it gets converted into the active form—fibrin.
  Usual time to release one RBC is 18 minutes, and for FFP (includes thawing) is 1 hour.
- *Cryoprecipitate:* Made from FFP to produce a concentrated source of clotting factors including factor VII, von Willebrand factor, and 2 g fibrinogen/100 mL. One unit increases fibrinogen level by 10 mg/dL. Adult dose is 10 U, for expected fibrinogen rise by 100 mg/dL. Side effect is that it needs thawing and risk of viral transmissions.
- *Fibrinogen concentrate:* Manufacturing process includes virus inactivation and removal of various antigens and antibodies. It can be stored at room temperature and contains 2 g fibrinogen/100 mL. Only drawback is that it is not yet widely available.
- *Tranexamic acid (TXA):* Found to be very effective particularly if used within 3 hours of hemorrhage. It is not associated with increased risk of thrombotic episodes. Viscoelastic tests to diagnose hyperfibrinolysis are not recommended before injection TXA.
  Combined use of TXA and cryoprecipitate improves outcome.
- *Recombinant activated factor VII (rFVIIa):*
  - Approved for use in hemophilia, inhibitory alloantibodies against factor VIII and IX.
  - Effective only after surgical hemostasis is achieved, not used as first line treatment.
  - Pre-requisites:
    - Platelets >50,000/mm^3
    - Fibrinogen >50–100 mg/dL
    - Temperature >32°C
    - pH >7.2
    - Normal ionized calcium levels.

Side effects: Increased risk of arterial thromboembolism, very high cost, and lack of survival benefit.

Contraindication: Amniotic fluid embolism; it increases mortality.

- *Prothrombin complex concentrates:* Human plasma derived concentrates of vitamin-K dependent clotting factors. Ideal use is emergency reversal of warfarin effect and can be used as a last resort in massive hemorrhage.

REFERENCES

1. Muñoz M, Peña-Rosas JP, Robinson S, et al. Patient blood management in obstetrics: management of anaemia and haematinic deficiencies in pregnancy and in the postpartum period: NATA consensus statement. Transfusion Medicine. 2017. pp. 22-39. doi: 10.1111/tme.12443.
2. Carles G, Tobal N, Raynal P, et al. Doppler assessment of the fetal cerebral hemodynamic response to moderate or severe maternal anemia. Am J Obstet Gynecol. 2003;188(3):794-9.
3. American College of Obstetricians and Gynecologists. ACOG Practice Bulletin no. 95: Anemia in pregnancy. Obstet Gynecol. 2008;112(1):201-7.
4. National Institute for Health and Care Excellence, London, UK. (2008). Antenatal care for uncomplicated pregnancies. NICE Guidelines [CG62]. [Online] Available from https://www.nice.org.uk/guidance/cg62 [Last accessed October, 2019].
5. WHO. The clinical use of blood in obstetrics, paediatrics, surgery and anaesthesia, trauma and burns. Geneva, Switzerland: World Health Organization; 2001(a).
6. WHO. Developing a National Policy and Guidelines on the Clinical use of Blood. Recommendations. Geneva, Switzerland: World Health Organization; 2001(b).
7. Goodnough LT, Shander A. Patient blood management. Anesthesiology. 2012;116(6):1367-76.
8. Pacheco LD, Saade GR, Costantine MM, et al. An update on the use of massive transfusion protocols in obstetrics. Am J Obstet Gynecol. 2016;214(3):340-4.
9. Brohi K, Cohen MJ, Davenport RA. Acute coagulopathy of trauma: mechanism, identification and effect. Curr Opin Crit Care. 2007;13(6):680-5.
10. J-MELS Advance Guidebook Editorial Committee. Maternal emergency lifesaving advance guidebook. 1st edition. Tokyo: Herusu Shuppan; 2017. pp. 135-6.
11. Ickx BE. Fluid and blood transfusion management in obstetrics. Eur J Anaesthesiol. 2010;27(12):1031-5.
12. RCOG. (2015). Green-top Guideline No. 47, Blood Transfusion in Obstetrics. [Online] Available from https://www.rcog.org.uk/en/guidelines-research-services/guidelines/gtg47/ [Last accessed October, 2019].

Chapter 57

Patient Communication

Girija Wagh, Aakanksha Kumar

INTRODUCTION

Communicating with patients is an important competency which the physician has to acquire along with the clinical skills. Patient communication is an essential component of obstetrical clinical practice and entails precision and clarity. In the current scenario, the changing social structure, access to digital media, and the litigation environment have made the obstetric practice more vulnerable to generalized dissatisfaction leading to many times adverse response and litigations in the community.

Unpredictability of certain outcomes especially in a high-risk situation need of privacy especially in the context of sexuality and relationship with a natural physiological phenomenon such as menstruation, pregnancy, and sexuality make it necessary that every obstetrician follows a structured plan while communicating with the patients. It is also imperative to maintain the dignity of the patient and her community while communication.

Effective communication with the patient is essential is for the following reasons:
- To gather correct information about the clinical situation
- To alleviate fear and anxiety
- To encourage cooperation from the patient for clinical examination and assessment
- To ensure compliance in order to deliver optimal care
- To educate and inform the patient about her communication and to encourage partnership in decision-making
- For documentation to avoid medicolegal litigation
- Financial issues.

Six Components of Communication

1. Gather information
2. Fearless participation
3. Cooperation
4. Compliance
5. Education and partnership
6. Documentation.

Special Situation Demands Special Attention

- Women seeking medical termination of pregnancy, sterilization operations, etc. need to be addressed with correct education, proper alternative, and a decision partnership between the clinician and the patient should be developed.
- Situations demanding swift compliance and readiness such as a need for urgent cesarean section, obstetric hysterectomy, intensive care unit (ICU) management, etc. require a sensitive and effective approach.
- Adverse outcomes and mishap communication requires special skills replete with empathy and should be based on correct knowledge about the condition.
- Patients such as unmarried women and teenagers or adolescent girls seeking termination of pregnancy require to be dealt with a nonjudgmental attitude.

ALGORITHMS

Primary clinical assessment of the patient is based on effective history of menstruation, obstetric events, and other confounding factors. Many patients are confused and scared and may not be able to correctly inform about their issues. A simple preclinical examination self-assessment card would help **(Box 1)**.

Box 1	Patient preassessment card or self-assessment card.

	• *To be filled by the patient or clinical assistant before actual consultation*
	• *Gross components:*
	  – Complaints, amenorrhea, menstruation, pain, any other complaints
	  – LMP
	  – Issues: Children, live miscarriage
	  – Birth control
	  – Medication
	  – Ailments/allergies
	  – Any other

(LMP: last menstrual period)	

Structured clinical assessment is essential as per the **Algorithm 1**.

Algorithm 1: Structured clinical assessment.

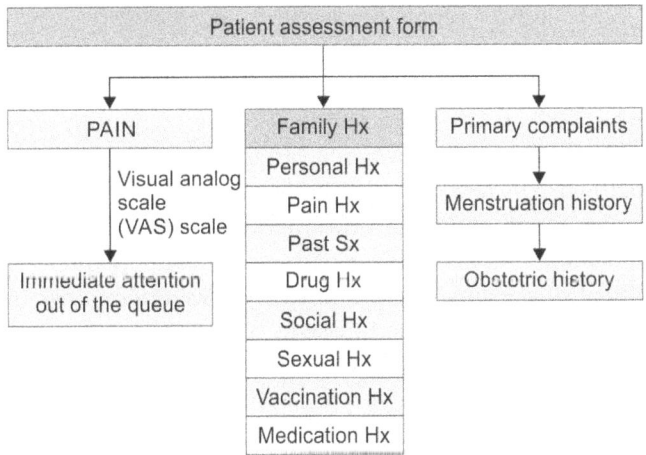

Empathic and nonjudgmental approach is essential. During the examination of the patient, the body language has to be of comfort and attention and not of anger and be perceived as harm by the patient. The gynecological examination has to be always performed in the presence of an attendant, a nurse, clinical assistant or the patient's relative. If not followed properly, may invite complaint and sometimes accusation from the patient.

Algorithm for Clinical Communication

- Inform the patient about the gynecological examination.
- After emptying the bladder, the appropriate position is guided by the clinician.
- Patient should be appropriately covered to ensure cooperation.
- Examination of the patient should be performed after due information to the patient and with the reason explained, e.g. palpation of the gravid uterus, examination of a bleeding (vaginal) patient, per rectal examination if necessary.

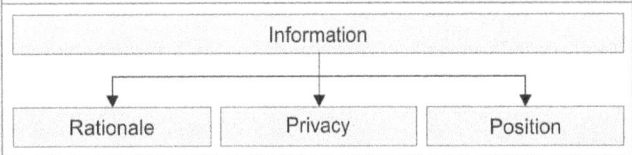

Investigations form an Important Component of Patient Communication

These consist of laboratory tests, imaging and some interventional tests, and some surgically performed tests such as endoscopy, etc.

Laboratory investigations are to be ordered with rationale and expected results discussed with the patient or the relatives. Timing of the tests is important, e.g. the double marker test [nuchal translucency (NT) + pregnancy associated plasma protein A (PAPP-A) and beta-human chorionic gonadotropin (β-hCG)] is time-specific and performed within 11 weeks to 12 + 6 weeks of pregnancy at the crown-rump length of 45–85 mm. The possible need for further evaluation has to be explained to the patient. Certain tests are mandatory such as blood group and are insisted upon with proper counseling. In tests such as HIV and HBsAg, screening has to be informed to the patient before and after the test as per the GOI guidelines. Investigations for the semen, even if one decided to do a postcoital test, are to be performed in the PCPNDT accredited center. The requisition for the same should be appropriately signed and labeled and dated. Some procedures are seemingly simple but necessary precautions, information to the patient, and documentation have to be done aptly. Insertion of intrauterine contraceptive device (IUCD) is a simple outpatient department (OPD) procedure but the possibility of syncope, pain exists, and patients need to be communicated regarding the possibilities of appropriate soft skills of communication.

Laboratory Test Requisitions Algorithm

Patient identification and contact details	*Timing*: Such as fasting/postmenstrual, etc.
The list of tests with rationale	Expected time of processing and results
Costs and preparation for the test	Postreporting counseling

Interventional Test Algorithm

Need and indication of the test	Expected discomfort	Documentation
Cost preparedness and consent	Anesthesia issues	Report handover
Associated complications	Anaphylaxis	Postprocedure counseling

Prescription is an important patient communication vehicle and has been recognized as an important medicolegal document and has to be written appropriately. This is what the patient carries, follows, and the pharmacist reads. It is thus a representation of your practice and style. It has to be completely clear and crisp.

Prescription Algorithm

Patients information and instructions	*Doctor information*
Name/age/address	Name
Diagnosis/weight	Qualification
Capital letters for medicines	Registration number
Dose/duration/route	Signature
Timings	Emergency contact number
Relation to food	Date of the prescription
Adverse effects, if any	
Follow-up visit	

Special situations demand special approach. In the case of obstetrics-gynecology practice especially, such situations are frequent, unpredictable, and emotionally challenging. Examples are a sexually active teenager, sexual abuse, fetal demise, critically ill mother, and on table mishaps. On one side, we deal with delivering good news regarding childbirth or a successfully performed surgery rendering the woman free of her illness but sometimes bad news are also a part of the practice and need to be communicated effectively.

Antenatal care is an important OB/GYN component and is a highly evolved time-based component of clinical practice involving communication with the patient.

Antenatal and Postnatal Counseling Algorithm

First trimester	Organogenesis	Excessive vomiting/hygiene
	Placentation	Bleeding spotting
	Medications/scans/review	What to expect next
Second trimester	Scans: TIFFA	Pain
	Nutrition counseling	Bleeding
	Vaccinations	What to expect next
Third trimester	Growth scans	EWS: Preeclampsia, preterm birth
	Vaccinations	Nutrition
	Birth plan discussion	Physical activity
At 37 weeks	Mode of delivery Painless labor Symptoms of labor	Need for intervention Information about process of delivery
Reporting to the facility	When	Contacts
Postdelivery	Lactation Neonatal care	Review visits

(TIFFA: targetter imaging for fetal anomalies; EWS: early warning signs)

Handling patients who are distressed and ill and the relatives is a challenge and necessitate communication skills. Also bad news comes in various types. Buckman has defined bad news as "Any information which adversely and seriously affects an individual's view of his/her future. In situations where there is either a feeling of no hope. A threat to persons, mental or physical well-being, risk of upsetting an established lifestyle." Bad news has medical as well as social, emotional, psychological, and legal aspects. Bad news can be typed as in the algorithm below.

True bad news	Unexpected malignancy, intrauterine death (IUD), tubal blocks, azoospermia, etc.
Imaginary bad news	To increase fear in the patient, e.g. squamous metaplasia is cancer, fetus is at risk, and cesarean section (CS) is mandatory
Malicious bad news	Conveyed to spoil the reputation of the other colleague

Bad news or expected adverse outcome is best dealt with the doctor himself. This communication should be based on true facts and the necessary after actions to be taken, e.g. IUD to be informed and the later management and consequence with baby disposal to be discussed.

Counseling Algorithm

Place: To sit and talk across the table
People: Relatives and your team members and patient if she can be around
Sometimes only the patient and her consort in case of personal issues
Discretion as to who to be involved in this session
Record: In a counseling diary or the paper record
Signatures: The counseling doctors and the relatives
Actions taken or decided

Postprocedure Counseling Algorithm

After every procedure, counseling of the patient is important.

Procedure schemata and indication
Intraoperative issues/need for interventions
Postoperative instructions and when to expect discharge
Symptoms for which emergency help be sought with contact numbers
Restrictions if any: For example, food, medicine combinations, sex, etc.

COMMUNICATION WITH ADOLESCENT PATIENTS

This has to be a little different from communication with the adult patient. Respect and dignity are prime most even in communication with a teenager. The communication has to ensure privacy, at the same time, the guardian needs to be taken into confidence in tricky situations such as sex and pregnancy. As a country, we are governed by the POCSO Act of 2012. The Protection of Children from Sexual Offenses Act of 2012 was formulated in order to effectively address sexual abuse and sexual exploitation of children. The act also provides for mandatory reporting of sexual offenses. This casts a legal duty upon a person who has knowledge that a child has been sexually abused to report the offense; if he/she fails to do so, he/she may be punished with 6 months' imprisonment and/or a fine. This is essential to note and comply with proper responsibility.

FINANCIAL COMMUNICATION

It is a good practice to document the financial counseling of the necessary treatments to ensure transparency and enhance faith in medical treatment. The doctor-patient relationship can be reinforced with trust and financial transparency. This can be done by the support staff but in any case, be documented to avoid mistrust. Documentation in the form of a written form signed with the estimated expense or CCTV camera recording can be done. The medical practice is currently a vulnerable entity as far as community displeasure is concerned and these are essential safety means that can be undertaken.

DOCTOR–PATIENT PARTNERSHIP FOR EFFECTIVE CARE

Effective patient communication can pave a road for fruitful outcomes and amelioration of adverse outcomes and resultant misgivings. Communication should encourage discussion and brainstorming and the consensus for therapy reached. With the current information technology, caution should be observed while communicating with the patient and the content has to be balanced effective and toward the betterment of the issue.

SUGGESTED READING

1. Brédart A, Bouleuc C, Dolbeault S. Doctor-patient communication and satisfaction with care in oncology. Curr Opin Oncol. 2005;17(14):351-4.
2. Brinkman WB, Geraghty SR, Lanphear BP, et al. Effect of multisource feedback on resident communication skills and professionalism: a randomized controlled trial. Arch Pediatr Adolesc. 2007;161(1):44-9.
3. Duffy FD, Gordon GH, Whelan G, et al. Assessing competence in communication and interpersonal skills: the Kalamazoo II report. Acad Med. 2004;79(6):495-507.
4. Hall JA, Roter DL, Rand CS. Communication of affect between patient and physician. J Health Soc Behav. 1981;22(1):18-30.
5. Van Zanten M, Boulet JR, McKinley DW, et al. Assessing the communication and interpersonal skills of graduates of international medical schools as part of the United States Medical Licensing Exam (USMLE) Step 2 Clinical Skills (CS) Exam. Acad Med. 2007;82(10 Suppl): S65-S68.

Chapter 58

Biomedical Waste Management Rules

Anuradha Sood, Smriti Chauhan, Subhash Chand Jaryal

DEFINITION

Biomedical waste (BMW) is any waste which is generated during diagnostic, treatment, or immunization of human beings or animals.

TYPES OF WASTE

- *Nonhazardous* or general waste (administrative, paper, kitchen, and housekeeping waste): 75–90%
- *Hazardous waste*: 10–25%

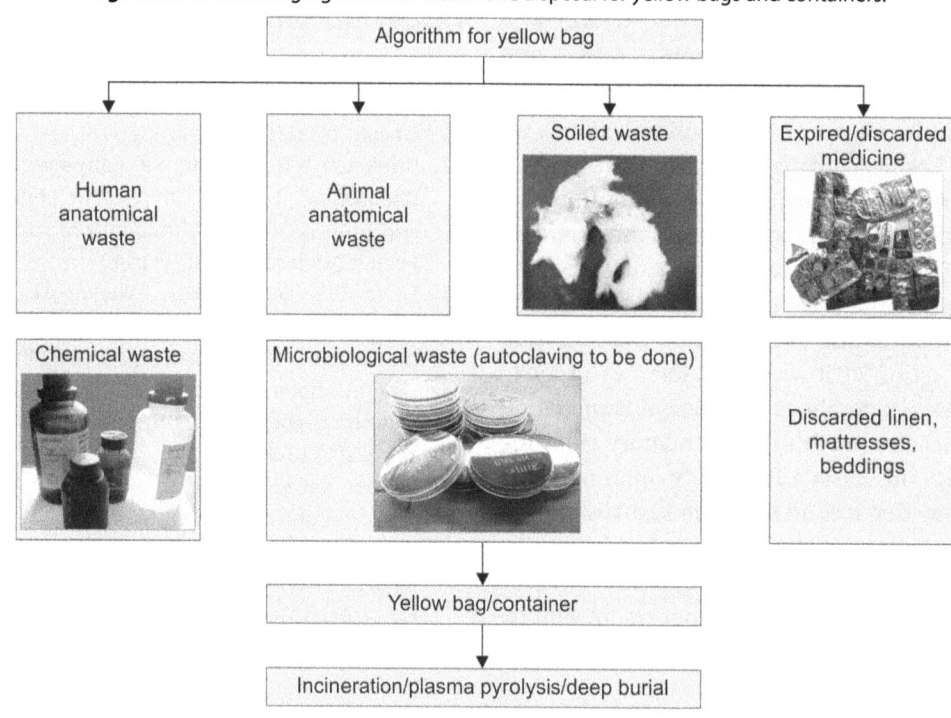

Algorithm 1: Waste segregation and treatment/disposal for yellow bags and containers.

- Infectious waste (waste contaminated with blood and body fluids, cultures and stocks of infectious agents, waste from infected patients in isolation wards): 10%
- Chemical/radioactive waste: 5%

Algorithm 2: Waste segregation and treatment/disposal for white containers.

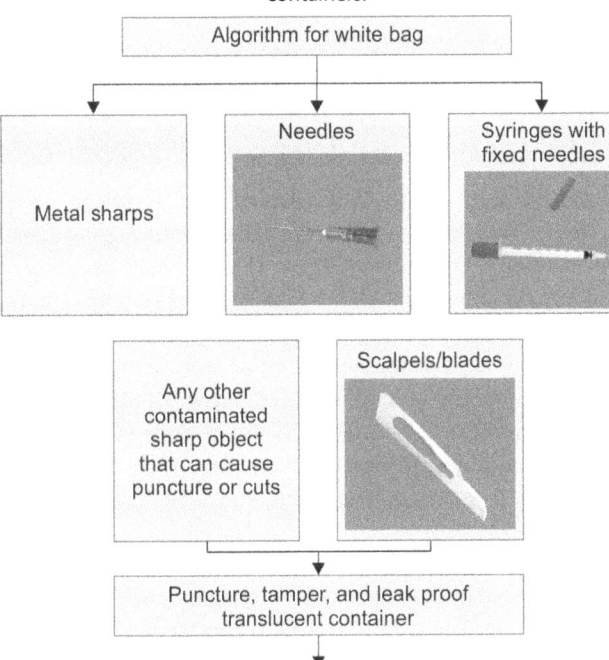

ACT—UNDER ENVIRONMENTAL PROTECTION ACT, 1986

- Biomedical Waste Rules, July 1998
- Amendments: 2003, 2011
- Newer rules: 2016, 2018.

RISKS ASSOCIATED WITH BIOMEDICAL WASTE

- Healthcare workers exposed to microbial infections
- Needle stick injury in healthcare workers and blood bank infections
- Cytotoxic, chemical, and radioactive waste—detrimental health effects
- Public health hazard.

SALIENT FEATURES OF BIOMEDICAL WASTE MANAGEMENT RULES, 2016

- Expanded to include vaccination, blood donation, and surgical camps.
- Categories of waste reduced from 10 to 4.
- Newer waste treatment facilities such as encapsulation, plasma pyrolysis, and inertization introduced.
- Cytotoxic drugs to be discarded in yellow bag with a cytotoxic sign.
- Metal sharps to be discarded in transparent puncture-proof box instead of blue/white bag.

Algorithm 3: Waste segregation and treatment/disposal for red bags/containers.

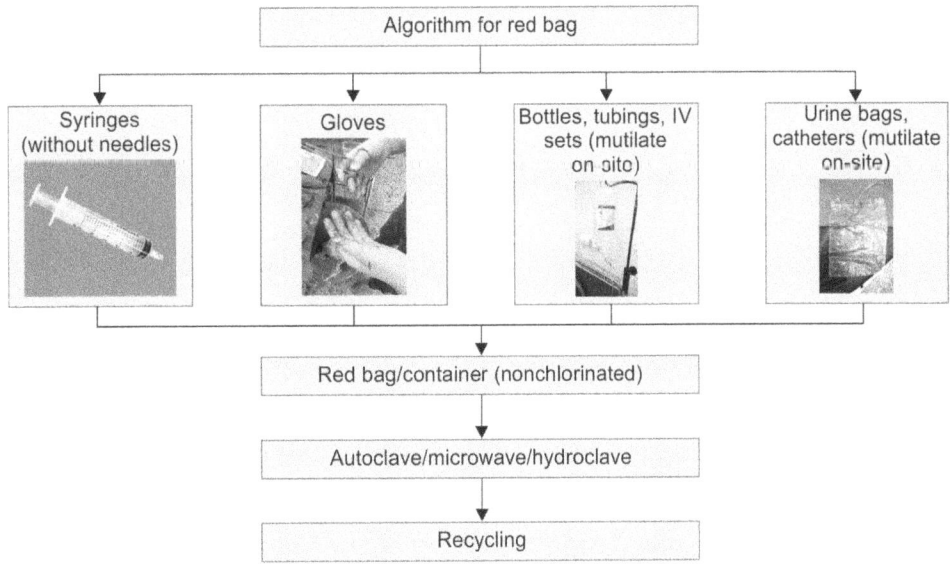

Algorithm 4: Waste segregation and treatment/disposal for blue containers.

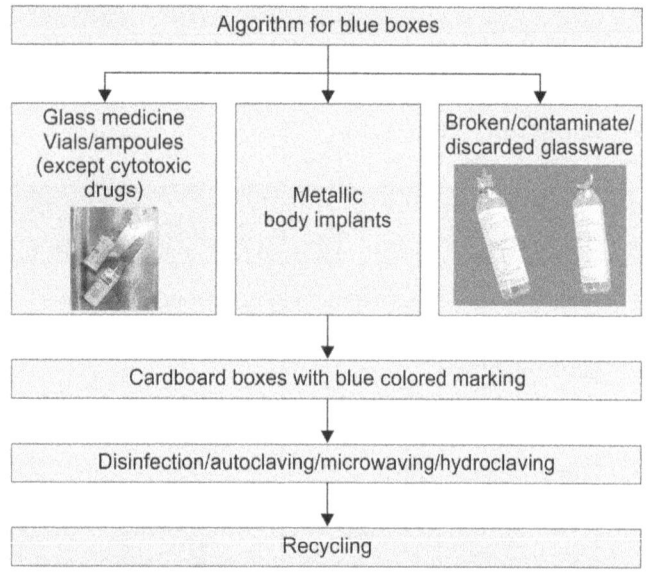

- Metallic implants to be discarded in transparent puncture-proof container.
- Pretreatment of laboratory waste, microbiological waste, etc. to be done at site as per National Aids Control Organization guidelines or as per WHO "Blue Book" 2014.
- To trace BMW by barcoding and GPS.

DO'S FOR BIOMEDICAL WASTE

- Fill only 3rd/4th bag/container
- Cytotoxic waste and all material used for cytotoxic drug administration is to be put in a nonchlorinated yellow container and labeled as cytotoxic.
- Liquid chemical waste to be collected separately and directed to effluent treatment plant.
- Separate trolleys for waste transportation to be used.

SUGGESTED READING

1. Bio-Medical Waste (Management and Handling 1998) Rules. New Delhi: Government of India Publications; 1998.
2. Chartier Y, Emmanuel J, Pieper U, et al. Safe Management of Wastes from Health Care Activities, 2nd edition. Geneva, Switzerland: WHO Blue Book, 2014.
3. Ministry of Environment, Forest and Climate Change (2018). The Bio-Medical Waste Management (Amendment) Rules (online). Available from http://www.indiaenvironmentportal.org.in/files/file/Bio%20medical%20waste%20management%20(amendement)183847.pdf. (Last accessed December, 2018).
4. Sastry AS, Deepashree R. Chapter 15: Waste Management in Healthcare facility. Essentials of Hospital Infection Control, 1st edition. New Delhi: Jaypee Brothers Medical Publishers; 2019. pp. 399-431.

Chapter 59

How to Curb Maternal Mortality in India

Madhu Gupta, Kanica Kaushal

INTRODUCTION

In this chapter, the authors have first described the definition, magnitude and causes of maternal mortality and then discussed the strategies to reduce maternal mortality especially in the context of India.

MATERNAL MORTALITY RATIO

Maternal mortality is the death of a woman while pregnant or within 42 days of termination of pregnancy, irrespective of the duration and site of the pregnancy, from any cause related to or aggravated by the pregnancy or its management but not from accidental or incidental causes. Maternal mortality ratio (MMR) is the number of maternal deaths during a given time period per 100,000 live births during the same time period.[1] The MMR is used as a measure of the quality of a healthcare system. Every day, approximately 830 women die from preventable causes related to pregnancy and childbirth around the world. Maternal mortality is higher in women living in rural areas and among poorer communities.[2] It was estimated that in 2015, roughly 303,000 women died during and following pregnancy and childbirth. Almost all of these deaths occurred in low-resource settings and most could have been prevented. As per sustainable development goals, the countries are now united to reduce the MMR to less than 70 per 100,000 live births by 2030.[3]

As far as India is concerned, the MMR is on a decline, and it reduced from 257 per 100,000 live births to 122 per 100,000 live births from 2004–2006 to 2015–2017 **(Table 1)**.[4,5] However, still, about five women die every hour in India from complications developed during childbirth. Also there are large geographical differences, with southern state having lower MMR (93 per 100,000 live births) as compared to other states. Assam has the highest MMR of 229 per 100,000 live births. MMR of empowered action group states together is 175 per 100,000 live births. The reason for these differences included differences in accessibility and availability of proper antenatal care including minimum of four antenatal check-ups, provision of iron-folic acid, tetanus toxoid injection, identification of high-risk pregnancies, timely referral of high-risk pregnancies, institutional delivery, proper intranatal, and postnatal care including management of complications.

CAUSES OF MATERNAL MORTALITY

Causes of maternal deaths are biological or medical and nonbiological or social causes. Globally, as per a systematic review, about 73% of all maternal deaths are due to direct obstetric causes and 27.5% are due to indirect causes.[6] Hemorrhage accounted for 27.1%, hypertensive disorders 14.0%, and sepsis 10.7% of maternal deaths. The rest of deaths were due to abortion (7.9%), embolism (3.2%), and all other direct causes of death (9.6%). In a nationally representative survey done in India, which is also known as Million Death Study, it was reported that one-quarter of maternal deaths were due to obstetric hemorrhage, with most deaths occurring in the intrapartum period,

Section 7
Miscellaneous

Table 1: Trend of maternal mortality ratio (MMR) (per Lakh five births) from 2004 to 2015-17.

Maternal Mortality Ratio: India, EAG* and Assam, Southern States and Other States (per 100,000 live births)	2004-06	2007-09	2010-12	2011-13	2014-16	2015-17
India total	254	212	178	167	130	122
Assam	480	390	328	300	237	229
Bihar/Jharkhand	312	261	219	208	165	165
Madhya Pradesh/Chhattisgarh	335	269	230	221	173	164.5
Odisha	303	258	235	222	180	168
Rajasthan	388	318	255	244	199	186
Uttar Pradesh/Uttarakhand	440	359	292	285	201	216
EAG and Assam subtotal*	375	308	257	246	188	175
Andhra Pradesh	154	134	110	92	74	74
Karnataka	213	178	144	133	108	97
Kerala	95	81	66	61	46	42
Tamil Nadu	111	97	90	79	66	63
South Subtotal	149	127	105	93	77	72
Gujarat	160	148	122	112	91	87
Haryana	186	153	146	127	101	98
Maharashtra	130	104	87	68	61	55
Punjab	192	172	155	141	122	122
West Bengal	141	145	117	113	101	94
Other states	206	160	136	126	97	96
Other subtotal	174	149	127	115	93	90

*EAG: Empowered action group

other one-quarter of maternal deaths were due to "other obstetric complications" including ill-defined cause of death in labor and the antenatal and postpartum period.[7] About 15% of maternal deaths were due to indirect causes. The remaining maternal deaths were pregnancy-related infection, abortion, hypertension, and anesthetic complications from obstetric surgery.

The social causes of maternal deaths are explained by the three-delay model, i.e. due to delay at three levels. Delay level one (delay-I), indicates the delay in taking the decision at home, that women are sick enough to be taken to the appropriate health facility due to ignorance, illiteracy, poverty, etc. Delay level two (delay-II) is at the level of arranging transport to take the women to the health facility once the decision has been taken to take her to the health facility, which could be either due to lack of availability of vehicle/ambulance or financial constraints to arrange a vehicle. Delay at level three (delay-III) is at the level of health facility in initiating the appropriate management to save the sick woman from dying. Dikid et al. reviewed the Maternal and Perinatal Death Inquiry and Response (MAPEDIR) process in selected districts of four states in India. They found that overall, 54% of the delays could be attributed to delay in deciding to seek care for an obstetric complication (delay-I), followed by 30% delay in coordinating transportation (delay-II), and 16% delay in obtaining care at the facility (delay-III). Major delay in seeking care was reported as the caregiver "did not think the deceased was sick enough to need healthcare" followed by "lack of finances to pay for care provider/facility." In most of the states, delay in coordinating transportation was either due to "inability to pay for transportation or nonavailability of transportation." The delay at facility level was due to "lack of blood or specialist doctor or equipment."[8] Kaur et al (2018), has also reported the contribution of social factors in leading to maternal

Table 2: Key interventions to reduce maternal deaths.

Direct causes of maternal death (percent reduction in mortality)	Cost-effective clinical interventions
Bleeding after delivery (24%)	• Active management of third stage of labor • Detect and treat anemia in pregnancy • *Skilled attendant at birth:* Prevent/treat bleeding with correct medicines, e.g. oxytocin, replace fluid loss by IV drip and transfusion if severe
Infection after childbirth (15%)	• *Skilled attendant at birth:* Clean practices • Antibiotic if infection arises
Unsafe abortion (13%)	*Skilled attendant:* Give antibiotics, empty uterus, replace fluids if needed, counsel and provide family planning/prevention. Access to safe abortion where not against the law
Obstructed labor	Use of partograph, cesarean section
High blood pressure, most dangerous when severe (eclampsia) (12%)	• Detect high blood pressure in pregnancy; refer to doctor at the hospital. Treat convulsions with appropriate anticonvulsive medicines ($MgSO_4$) • Refer unconscious woman for expert urgent assistance
Other direct obstetric causes (8%)	Refer ectopic pregnancy for operation

deaths and has used care pathways and delay models to explain their contribution.[9]

Hence, to prevent maternal mortality, both medical and nonmedical causes are to be addressed.

KEY INTERVENTIONS TO REDUCE MATERNAL MORTALITY

The key interventions to reduce maternal mortality are presented in **Table 2**.[10]

INITIATIVES TO REDUCE MATERNAL MORTALITY IN INDIA

In India, several steps have been taken in the last two decades to reduce MMR so as to achieve earlier the millennium development goal of reducing the MMR to below 100/100,000 live births till 2015, and now sustainable development goal till 2030 of reducing the MMR to below 70/100,000 live births. However, we still lag behind for achieving this goal till 2015. Under National Health Mission, Ministry of Health and Family Welfare, Government of India, there is Reproductive, Maternal, Newborn, Child and Adolescent Health (RMNCHA) program.[11] It has a five by five matrix (5 × 5), which indicates that there are five strategies which need to be implemented under each of its five components (reproductive, maternal, newborn, child, and adolescent health).

Under maternal health components, the strategies are:
1. Use of mother and child tracking system to ensure early registration of pregnancy and full antenatal care.
2. Detect high-risk pregnancies and line list including severely anemic mothers and ensure appropriate management.
3. Equip delivery points with highly trained human resource and ensure equitable access to emergency obstetric services through first referral units; and addition of Maternal and Child (MCH) wings as per need.
4. Review maternal, infant, and child deaths for corrective actions.
5. Identify villages with low-institutional delivery and distribute misoprostol to select women during pregnancy; incentivize auxiliary nurse midwives (ANMs) for domiciliary deliveries.

The Maternal Death Review (MDR) process initiated by Government of India in 2010, to improve the quality of obstetric care and reduce maternal mortality is revised as Maternal Death Surveillance and Response (MDSR) so that continuous cycle of identification, notification, review of maternal deaths and action taken to improve quality of care and prevent maternal deaths is followed.[12]

In 2017, health ministry launched an innovative scheme to provide free health check-ups to pregnant women at government health centers and hospitals by private doctors under *"The Pradhan Mantri Surakshit*

Matritva Abhiyan." Private sector was also invited to provide free antenatal services (ANC) on the ninth of every month on a voluntary basis to pregnant women, especially those living in underserved, semiurban, poor, and rural areas.

Other good initiatives under maternal health components include:

- *National guidelines for calcium supplementation during pregnancy and lactation:* Each pregnant women will receive 360 calcium tablets (500 mg twice daily) during antenatal period (after first trimester for 6 months), and 360 tablets during postnatal period (for 6 months) free of cost from the government supply to fulfill the calcium requirement of these ladies and also to prevent pregnancy-induced hypertension.
- *National guidelines for diagnosis and management of Gestational Diabetes Mellitus:* This stresses on the first testing during first antenatal contact as early as possible in pregnancy. The second testing is recommended to be done during 24–28 weeks of pregnancy if the first test is negative. All pregnant women who test positive for gestational diabetes mellitus (GDM) for the first time will be started on Medical Nutrition Therapy (MNT) for 2 weeks. After 2 weeks on MNT, a 2 hours PPPG (postmeal) will be done. Thus, GDM is managed initially with MNT and if it is not controlled with MNT, insulin therapy is added to the MNT.
- *National guidelines for screening of hypothyroidism during pregnancy:* The aim of these guidelines is to screen all pregnant women for hypothyroidism, facilitating early diagnosis and treatment thereby reducing maternal, fetal, and neonatal complications. Treatment has to get started with 25 µg of L-thyroxine/day if sensitive-thyroid-stimulating-hormone (sTSH) is more than 2.5 mIU/L in the first trimester and more than 3 mIU/L in second and third trimester and with 50 µg of L-thyroxine/day if sTSH is more than 10 mIU/L which has to be continued even postpartum.
- *LaQshay guidelines (Labor Room Quality Improvement Initiative):* These guidelines are meant to help the States' National Health Mission (NHM) Directors, Medical Education Departments, Heads of Department of Obstetrics and Gynecology in Medical Colleges, District Health Officials, Medical Superintendents, In-charge of Gynecology Departments, and teams engaged in the maternity care. Strategies are reorganizing/aligning labor room and maternity operation theater layout and workflow as per "Labor Room Standardization Guidelines" and "Maternal & Newborn Health Toolkit" issued by the Ministry of Health & Family Welfare, Government of India. Second is ensuring that at least all government medical college hospitals and high caseload district hospitals have dedicated obstetric High Dependency Units (HDUs) as per these guidelines, for managing complicated pregnancies that require life-saving critical care. Third, ensuring strict adherence to clinical protocols for management and stabilization of the complications before referral to higher centers.
- *National guidelines for deworming in pregnancy:* Albendazole is to be taken only once during the second trimester of pregnancy. The second dose is needed only in case the helminthic load is >40%. There is no specific contraindication/side effect except nausea, vomiting, rash, and abdominal pain, urticaria in some cases. It should not be used in the first trimester of pregnancy. Ideally, drug administration for deworming should be done under direct observation treatment (DOT).

Improving the maternal and child health and their survival are central to the achievement of national health goals under the National Health Mission, as well as to achieve sustainable development goals. However, improving maternal health also requires the involvement of other sectors than the health sector like education sector so as to improve the literacy level of the girls, road networks/connectivity in rural areas, the availability of electricity, sanitation facilities, and the use of new technology in health (m-health) like in Bangladesh, and employment so as to create and sustain an environment that supports the work of health systems and health partners, as is done in many other developing countries, which has better maternal health indicators than ours like Ethiopia, Egypt, Cambodia, China, and Vietnam.[13-17]

REFERENCES

1. Maternal mortality ratio. [online] Available from http://www.who.int/healthinfo/statistics/indmaternalmortality/en/ [Last accessed September, 2019].
2. Maternal mortality. [online] Available from http://www.who.int/mediacentre/factsheets/fs348/en/ [Last accessed September, 2019].
3. Alkema L, Chou D, Hogan D, et al. Global, regional, and national levels and trends in maternal mortality between

1990 and 2015, with scenario-based projections to 2030: a systematic analysis by the UN Maternal Mortality Estimation Inter-Agency Group. Lancet. 2016;387(10017):462-74.
4. Registrar General of India. Special Bulletin on Maternal Mortality in India. 2004-06. Sample Registration System. New Delhi; 2009.
5. Registrar General of India. Special Bulletin on Maternal Mortality in India. 2015-17. Sample Registration System. New Delhi. 2019. Available from http://www.censusindia.gov.in/vital_statistics/SRS_Bulletins/MMR_Bulletin-2015-17.pdf [Last accessed December, 2019].
6. Say L, Chou D, Gemmill A, et al. Global causes of maternal death: a WHO systematic analysis. Lancet Glob Health. 2014;2:e323-33.
7. Montgomery AL, Ram U, Kumar R, et al. Maternal mortality in India: causes and healthcare service use based on a nationally representative survey. PLoS One. 2014;9(1):e83331.
8. Dikid T, Gupta M, Kaur M, et al. Maternal and perinatal death inquiry and response project implementation review in India. J Obstet Gynecol India. 2013;63:101-7.
9. Kaur M, Gupta M, Pandara Purayil V, et al. Contribution of social factors to maternal deaths in urban India: Use of care pathway and delay models. PLoS ONE. 2018;13(10): e0203209. Available from https://doi.org/10.1371/journal.pone.0203209.
10. Campbell MRO, Graham WJ. Strategies for reducing maternal mortality: getting on what works. Lancet. 2006; 368(9543):1284-99.
11. A strategic approach to reproductive, maternal, newborn, child and adolescent health (RMNCH+A) in India. [online] Available from http://nhm.gov.in/images/pdf/RMNCH+A/RMNCH+A_Strategy.pdf [Last accessed September, 2019].
12. Guidelines for maternal death surveillance & response. [online] Available from http://nhm.gov.in/images/pdf/programmes/maternalhealth/guidelines/Guideline_for_MDSR.pdf [Last accessed September, 2019].
13. Ministry of Health. Ethiopia. Success factors for women and children's health. [online] Available from http://www.who.int/pmnch/knowledge/publications/ethiopia_country_report.pdf?ua=1 [Last accessed September, 2019].
14. Ministry of Health and Population. Success factors for women and children's health. Egypt. [online] Available from http://www.who.int/pmnch/knowledge/publications/egypt_country_report.pdf?ua=1 [Last accessed September, 2019].
15. Ministry of Health. Cambodia. Success factors for women and children's health. [online] Available from http://www.who.int/pmnch/knowledge/publications/cambodia_country_report.pdf?ua=1 [Last accessed September, 2019].
16. National Health and Planning Commission. China. Success factors for women and children's health. [online] Available from http://www.who.int/pmnch/knowledge/publications/china_country_report.pdf?ua=1 [Last accessed September, 2019].
17. Ministry of Health. Vietnam. Success factors for women and children's health. [online] Available from http://www.who.int/pmnch/knowledge/publications/vietnam_country_report.pdf?ua=1 [Last accessed September, 2019].

Chapter 60

Needle-prick Injury

Madhuri Chandra

INTRODUCTION

A needlestick injury or needle-prick (percutaneous) injury is the penetration of skin by a needle or other sharp object, which was in contact with blood, tissue, or other body fluid before the exposure. Needlestick injuries have the risk of transmitting infectious diseases like hepatitis B, hepatitis C, and human immunodeficiency virus (HIV). The capacity to transmit infection varies with the body fluid and **Table 1** lists the risk of HIV transmission of potentially infectious body fluids.

Occupational exposure refers to exposure to potential bloodborne viral infections (hepatitis B—HBV, hepatitis C—HCV, and human immunodeficiency virus—HIV) that occur during performance of job duties. Occupational needlestick injuries primarily affect the healthcare workers, of which obstetricians are at great risk, as they are liberally exposed to blood and other body fluids while conducting labor and delivery. Occupational exposures that may place a healthcare worker at risk of HIV infection, are percutaneous injury (needle prick or cut with a sharp instrument), contact with the mucous membranes of the eye or mouth, contact with nonintact skin, particularly when the exposed skin is chapped, abraded, or afflicted with dermatitis, or contact with intact skin when the duration of contact is prolonged with blood or other potentially infectious body fluids.

Needle-prick injuries with hollow needles can occur while drawing blood, giving intravenous (IV) or intramuscular drugs, needle recapping or improper disposal. Needle-prick injuries with solid needles occur during surgery while passing needles and suture material, tying knots, passing through tough fascia or deeper tissue. Improper technique, handling the needle with fingers, inexperienced surgeons, night time, high workload, and fatigue are other high-risk factors for needle prick and scalpel injuries.

Other professions at risk of needlestick injury are tattoo artists, the police, waste collectors, rag pickers, laborers, and agriculture workers. Accidental injury can occur in children while playing with syringes and needles.

Table 1: Potentially infectious body fluids.	
Exposure to body fluids considered "at risk"	Exposure to body fluids considered "not at risk"
• *Blood* • *Semen* • *Vaginal secretions* • Cerebrospinal fluid • Synovial, pleural, peritoneal, pericardial fluid • *Amniotic fluid* • Other body fluids contaminated with visible blood	• Tears • Nasal secretions • Sputum • Sweat • Urine and feces • Saliva • Unless these secretions contain visible blood

Blood on any sharp instrument whether fresh or dried can prove infectious. While HIV and hepatitis C virus remain viable for only a few hours after drying and exposure to sunlight and heat, hepatitis B is stable even when dried and is transmitted by fomites also. HIV can be transmitted by various routes **(Table 2)**—the most common being sexual intercourse, the risk of transmission is maximum after transfusion of contaminated or HIV-positive blood.

The risk of transmission of HIV after accidental exposure to body fluids from an HIV infected patient is generally low **(Table 2)**. Hepatitis B carries the greatest risk of transmission, with 10% exposed workers having seroconversion and 10% having symptoms of hepatitis B. Transmission rate of hepatitis C is about 1–10% and of HIV is 0.3% after needle-prick injury. Public awareness and hepatitis B vaccination have decreased the incidence of hepatitis B acquisition after accidental exposure.

MANAGEMENT OF NEEDLE-PRICK INJURY[1]

Management of Exposure Site: First Aid (Algorithm 1)

First aid involves the liberal washing of effected part, skin, or mucous membrane with running water. In case of needle prick, wash with soap and water, then remove gloves and rewash. It is advisable not to use spirit or any antiseptics as they are rubefacient.

Establish Eligibility for Postexposure Prophylaxis/Risk Evaluation

The risk of HIV transmission postexposure depends on the amount of HIV transmitted (amount of contaminated fluid and the viral load), the type of exposure, HIV status of source patient (terminal illness reflects high titer of HIV), and status of exposed individuals.

Types of Exposure (Algorithm 2)

- *Mild exposure (EC1):* To mucous membrane or nonintact skin with small volumes—a superficial wound (erosion of the epidermis) with a plain or low caliber needle, or contact with the eyes or mucous membranes, subcutaneous injections following small-bore needles.

Table 2: Risk of human immunodeficiency virus (HIV) transmission: different exposure routes.

Exposure route	Risk of HIV transmission
Blood transfusion	90–95%
Perinatal	20–40%
Sexual intercourse	0.1–10%
Injectable drugs	0.67%
Needlestick injury*	0.3%
Mucus membrane: eye, nasal splash	0.09%

*Risk of hepatitis B (HBV) 9–30% and hepatitis C (HCV) 1–10%.

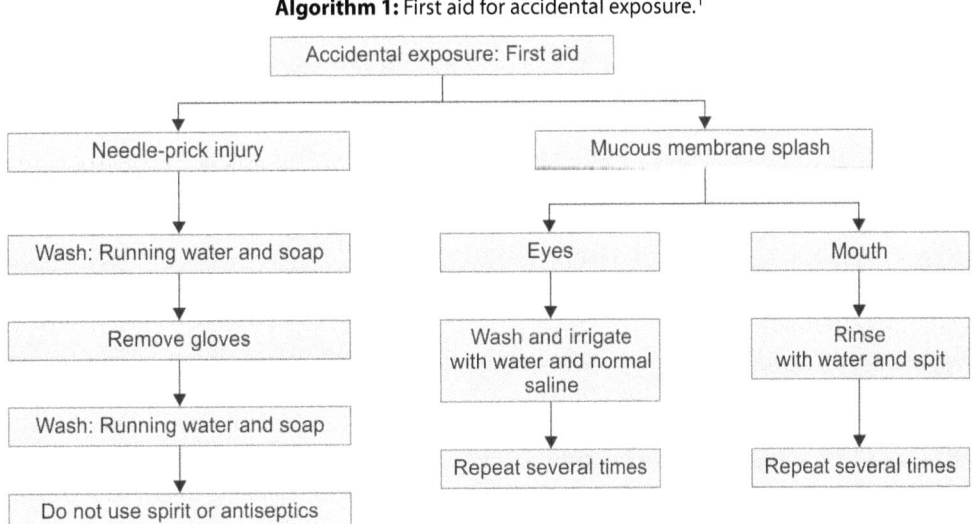

Algorithm 1: First aid for accidental exposure.[1]

Algorithm 2: Types of exposure.[1]

```
Source material blood, bloody fluid or other potentially infected
material or instrument contaminated with one of the substances
        │Yes                                    │No
        ▼                                       ▼
What type of exposure has occurred?      No PEP required
   │                │                │
   ▼                ▼                ▼
Mucous membrane   Intact skin      Percutaneous
or skin integrity only = No PEP    exposure
   │                                 │
   ▼                                 ▼
Volume                            Severity
   │                                 │
┌──┴──┐                           ┌──┴──┐
▼     ▼                           ▼     ▼
Few drops/short   Major splash/   Solid needle/   Hollow needle/
duration EC1      long duration   sup. scratch    deep injury EC3
                  EC2             EC2
```

(PEP: postexposure prophylaxis)

Algorithm 3: Source category.

```
            HIV status of exposure source
         │              │                │
         ▼              ▼                ▼
   HIV negative    HIV positive    HIV status/source unknown
         │         │        │              │
         ▼         ▼        ▼              ▼
   No PEP     Low titer   High titer    HIV SC unknown
   required   exposure    exposure
              Asymptomatic Advanced disease
              High CD4    Low CD4
                   │           │
                   ▼           ▼
              HIV SC1      HIV SC2
```

(HIV: human immunodeficiency virus; PEP: postexposure prophylaxis; SC: scenario)

- *Moderate exposure (EC2):* Mucous membrane/nonintact skin with large volumes *or* percutaneous superficial exposure with a solid needle, a cut or needlestick injury penetrating gloves.
- *Severe exposure (EC3):* Percutaneous with large volume—an accident with a high caliber hollow needle (>18G) visibly contaminated with blood, deep injuries, transmission of a significant volume of blood, an accident with material that has previously been used intravenously or intra-arterially.

The source of exposure must undergo voluntary testing for HIV antibody, HCV, and HBsAg. Unless the source is known to be HBV, HCV, and HIV-negative, postexposure prophylaxis (PEP) should be initiated, ideally within an hour of exposure. A positive rapid test for HIV requires confirmatory tests but initiation of PEP must not be delayed. If known to be HIV-positive, the WHO clinical stage, recent viral load, and antiretroviral therapy (ART) history must be ascertained.

Source Categories (Algorithm 3)

- *HIV negative:* Source is not HIV infected but considers HBV and HCV.
- *Low risk:* HIV positive and clinically asymptomatic.
- *High risk:* HIV positive and clinically symptomatic (see WHO clinical staging).
- *Unknown:* Status of the patient is unknown, and neither the patient nor his/her blood is available for testing (e.g. injury during medical waste management the source patient might be unknown). The risk assessment will be based only upon the exposure.

If source is hepatitis B positive, administer PEP for HBV. Administer hepatitis B vaccine and hepatitis B immunoglobulin as soon as possible after exposure, repeat hepatitis B vaccine at 1 and 6 months interval. If exposed person is vaccinated for hepatitis B, check anti-HBs levels, if over 10 mIU/mL, person adequate has immunity to HBV infection.

If source is HCV positive, monitor postexposure for seroconversion. There is no vaccine, immunoglobulin or antiviral recommended for HCV PEP.

Postexposure Prophylaxis Regime (Table 3)[2]

- *Wherever PEP is indicated and source is not on ART or unknown:*
  - Recommended regime is tenofovir 300 mg + lamivudine 300 mg + efavirenz 600 mg once daily for 28 days, as a single dose fixed drug combination (FDC).
  - The first dose of PEP regular should be administered as soon as possible, preferably within 2 hours of exposure, definitely within 72 hours and subsequently, dose should be given at bedtime with clear instruction to take it 2–3 hours after dinner and to avoid fatty food in dinner.
  - In case of intolerance to efavirenz, regime containing tenofovir + lamivudine + protease inhibitor (LPV/r) can be used after expert consultation.
- *In case of exposure where the source is on ART:*
  - Start TLE (Tenofovir 300 mg + Lamivudine 300 mg + Efavirenz 600 mg) first-line ART drugs immediately.

- *In case of sexual assault:*
  - PEP (TLE for 28 days) should be provided to exposed person as a part of overall package of postassault care.
- *Baseline laboratory investigations:*
  - Complete blood count (CBC)
  - Liver function tests (transaminases)
  - *Renal function test*: Urea, creatinine
  - HIV 1 and 2
  - HBV, HCV
  - Pregnancy test.

Follow-up

Clinical

- *For signs indicating an HIV seroconversion:* Acute fever, generalized lymphadenopathy, cutaneous eruption, pharyngitis, nonspecific flu symptoms, and ulcers of the mouth or genital area.
- An exposed person should be advised to avoid blood or tissue donations, breastfeeding, unprotected sexual relations, or pregnancy in order to prevent secondary transmission, especially during the first 6–12 weeks following exposure.
- Adherence and side effect counseling should be reinforced at every follow-up visit. Adverse effects are generally self-limited and include nausea, vomiting, and diarrhea.
- If exposed woman is pregnant, she must be counseled on the risks and benefits of PEP. The currently prescribed PEP drugs are category B and C drugs.

Table 3: Revised PEP recommendations (NACO December 2014).[2]

	Occupational exposure		
Exposure code	HIV-positive, source code	Postexposure prophylaxis (PEP) recommendations	Duration
1	1	Not required	28 days
1	2	Recommended	
2	1	Recommended	
2	2	Recommended	
3	1 or 2	Recommended	
2/3	Unknown	Consider, if human immunodeficiency virus (HIV) prevalence high in given population and risk categorization	

EC1: Intact skin or mucus membrane, low volume exposure
EC2: Intact skin or mucus membrane, high volume exposure or percutaneous exposure by solid needle
EC3: Percutaneous exposure by hollow needle or deep injury
HIV SC1: Low-titer exposure, asymptomatic, high CD4
HIV SC2: High-titer exposure, advanced disease, low CD4

Laboratory

- HIV antibody testing at 6, 12, and 24 weeks after exposure.
- Repeat CBC, renal function and liver function tests at 2 and 4 weeks after starting PEP.
- Repeat tests for hepatitis B and C at 12 and 24 weeks postexposure.

PREVENTION OF NEEDLE-PRICK INJURIES

- *Work practices:* Surgical techniques—using instruments to grasp needles and load scalpels, avoid hand-to-hand exchange of sharps.
- *Engineering controls:* Safety needles, needle removers, retractable needles, needle sheath, needleless IV kit.

Using Vacutainer to draw and collect blood samples. During surgery, use of blunt tip or taper tip suture needle.

Whether double gloves during surgery give extra protection or a false sense of security is uncertain.

REFERENCES

1. NACO. Antiretroviral Therapy Guidelines for HIV-Infected Adults and Adolescents including Post-Exposure Prophylaxis. New Delhi, India: NACO, Ministry of Health & Family Welfare Government of India; 2007.
2. NACO. Office memorandum, No. T-11020/52/2007 dated 2/Dec/14. Revised Guidelines for PEP for HIV. New Delhi, India: NACO, Ministry of Health & Family Welfare Government of India.

Index

Page numbers followed by *b* refer to box, *f* refer to figure, and *t* refer to table

A

Abdomen, computed tomography scan of 109
Abdominal examination 109, 111
Abdominal pain 107
    evaluation of 107, 109
    management of 108
Abortion 31, 99, 330
    illegal 315
    unsafe 331
Abruptio placenta 99, 117, 130
Abruption 133
    previous 117
Acid hematin 24
Acidosis
    maternal 188
    metabolic 182
Activated partial thromboplastin time 320
Adenomyosis 195
Adnexa, torsion of 107
Adnexal mass 107
Adolescent health program 331
Adult respiratory syndrome 198
Advanced trauma life support 56
    guidelines 57
Aedes aegypti 84
Aedes albopictus 84
Agonal breaths 257
Airway management 59
Alanine aminotransferase 39, 42
Alkaline 41, 42
    phosphatase, serum 125
Alkalosis 103
Allis forceps 266f, 267
Alpha-fetoprotein 125, 130
Alpha-thalassemia 29

American College of Obstetricians and Gynecologists 10, 11, 20, 53, 139, 144, 146, 152, 159, 318
    committee opinion 126
    criteria 124
        lung maturity 159
American Heart Association 20
Aminoglycosides 95
Amniotic fluid
    index 9-11, 13, 17, 35, 130
    meconium stained 192-194, 298
    spectrophotometric analysis of 72f
    volume 293
        measurement 135
Amniotomy 11, 175
Ampicillin 251
Analgesia
    central neuraxial 190
    epidural 20
        labor 190
    inhalational 189
    regional 190
Anemia 19, 23, 30, 94, 99, 297, 315
    aplastic 23
    causes of 25
    deficiency 23, 24
    effects of pregnancy on 28
    hemolytic 23, 71
    hemorrhagic 23
    late 74
    mild 24, 26
    moderate 24, 26
    physiological 32
    severe 24, 26, 31, 208
    types of 24
Anesthesia 49, 217, 232
    assistance 212
    general 32, 50, 217, 226, 240
    regional 240, 281

Angiotensin
    converting enzyme inhibitor 94
    receptor blockers 94
Anovulation 64
Antenatal
    care 13, 17, 66
    complications 49
    emergencies 101
    monitoring 9
    services 332
    steroid therapy 294
    surveillance 35
Antepartum
    management 20
    prophylaxis 54
    surveillance 6, 35
Antibiotics 95, 127
Anticoagulant, choice of 53
Anti-D immunoglobulin 73
Anti-D prophylaxis 116
Antiepileptic drugs 47-49
    and pregnancy, International registry of 48
    teratogenicity of 48
Antifibrinolytic agent 244
Antihypertensive 95
    agents 11*t*
Antiphospholipid antibody syndrome 3-5
    classification 3
    diagnostic criteria for 3, 4
    management 5
    pathophysiology 3
    secondary 3
Anxiety 158
Aorta, coarctation of 20
Aplastic crisis 31
Appendicitis 107
Arrhythmias 19

Arterial blood gas 59
Asherman syndrome 195
Aspartate aminotransferase 39, 42
Assisted reproductive technology 62, 163, 163b, 166
Asthma 77
Atherosclerosis 122, 135
Atonic postpartum hemorrhage 245
    management in 246
Atosiban 127
Atrial contraction 137
Atrial fibrillation 19
Atrial septal defect 19
Atropine 60
Auscultation, intermittent 182
Autoimmune diseases 133
Automated external defibrillator 258
Azathioprine 95
Azithromycin 132

B

Backache, low 124
Bacterial vaginosis 122
    screening 125
Bacteriuria, asymptomatic 25, 127
Bag and mask ventilation 258f
Balloon catheter 174
Barrier methods 21
Beta-human chorionic gonadotropin 113, 114, 164, 283, 323
    interpretation of 112t
    monitoring 112
    serum 110
Beta-thalassemia 29
    intermedia 30
    major 29
    minor 30
Bilirubin
    displacement of 304
    encephalopathy 305
    enterohepatic circulation of 304
    lower serum 308
    production 304
    total serum 305t, 308f, 310t
Biomedical waste 326-328
    management rules 326, 327
Biophysical profile 9-11, 13, 17, 136
    score 35
Birth
    asphyxia 135, 229
    canal 236
        injuries of 236
    weight, low 99, 163, 309t314
Bishop score, modifiers of 172

Bladder 212
    wall, posterior 196
Blake's cyst 88
Blastocyst culture 166
Bleeding 111, 117
    after delivery 331
    causes of 111
    diathesis 38
    in late pregnancy, management of 118
    management of 119, 120
Blood
    and blood component therapy 318
    components 321
    exchange transfusion 308, 309, 309f, 310t
        choice of 310
        indications for 309
    glucose 35
        monitoring 35
    lactate 187
    loss
        assessment of 57
        estimated 117
        excessive 206
        measurement of 58
        reduce 197
    oxygen 57
    pressure 7, 9-11, 13, 15, 17, 20, 66, 150, 166, 316
        control 11t
        diastolic 7
        high 300, 331
        monitoring 9, 10
        systolic 7, 57
    sugar monitoring 35
    transfusion 26, 28, 84, 318
        recommendations for 57
        risks of 57, 58, 319
    urea nitrogen 94
    volume of 73
Body
    fluids, infectious 334t
    mass index 33, 35t, 134
    temperature, assessment of 289t
    weight, expected 10
Bone marrow examination 25
Bounding peripheral pulse 18
Bradycardia 184
Brain 298
    damage 298
Brainstem 88
Breast enlargement 291
Breastfeeding 218, 290
    advantages of 290
    assessing adequacy of 290

    correct technique of 290f
    promote exclusive 290
    regular 74
Breathlessness 78
Breech 220
    clinical findings 220
    complications 222
    delivery 203
    etiology 220
    extraction 232
    fetus, management of term 221
    presentation 222, 223
    risk factors 220
    signs of 220
    symptoms of 220
    types of 221
Bupivacaine 190

C

Calcineurin inhibitors 95
Calcium channel blockers 126, 294
Campylobacter 279
Cancer cervix 284
Candidiasis 240
Carbetocin 244
Carbonyl iron 26
Carboprost 60
Cardiac arrest, signs of 257
Cardiac disease 18, 18b
    classification of 19t
    common 18
    signs in 18b
Cardiac failure 19, 208
    common risk period for 19b
    congestive 28, 56
Cardiac transplantation 20
Cardiomyopathy 18, 19, 21
    dilated 21
    hypertrophic 21
    peripartum 21
Cardiotocography 9-11, 132, 227
Cardiovascular disease 34, 122
Cardiovascular system 34
Care after operative vaginal birth 213
Cataracts 88
Catecholamines 188
Cavity, peritoneal 216
Ceftriaxone 95
Centers for Disease Control 86, 88
Central nervous system 34, 308
Central venous pressure 59, 272
Cephalopelvic disproportion 160, 180, 212, 314, 315
    severe 215

Cerclage
   indications of 148
   removal of 147, 148
   types of 148
Cerebellar atrophy 88
Cerebral
   artery
      middle 71, 74, 136, 137
      peak velocities 70
   atrophy 88
   calcification 88
   palsy 122
   venous sinus thrombosis 47
Cervical
   amputation 145
   cerclage 127
   changes 124
   competency 124
   conisation 145
   dysfunction 124
   incompetency 122, 124
   injuries 240
      causes of 241, 241*t*
      complications 241
      management 241
      prevention 241
   insufficiency 144-146
      pathophysiology of 145
   interleukin-6 125
   length 126
      measurement 126, 146*f*
   spine 222
   status 131
   tear 241
      exploration and repair 241*f*
      left lateral 241
Cervix 145, 212, 239*f*
   cauterization of 145
   length of 293
Cesarean delivery 66, 228
   previous 195
Cesarean section 28, 158, 163, 215, 268, 282, 284
   categories of 215
   classical 218
   extraperitoneal 218
   frequency of 195
   history of 211
   incidence, pregnancy after 159
   indications of 216
Chemoprophylaxis 132
Chest
   compressions 302
   X-ray 18
Chikungunya 84, 85
   prevalence of 84

Chlamydia trachomatis 129
Chlamydophila psittaci 279
Cholecystitis 107
Chorioamnionitis 107, 122, 158, 272
   clinical 122
   subclinical 122
Chorioangioma 133
Choriocarcinoma 284
Choroid plexus cysts 88
Chromosomal abnormalities 62, 133
Chronic obstructive pulmonary disease 77
Cisterna magna, enlarged 88
Clavulanic acid 283
Clindamycin 251, 281
Clostridioides difficile 281
Clostridium septicum 278
Coagulation disorder 154
Coagulopathy 246
Co-amoxiclav 281
Color Doppler 196
Combined spinal-epidural analgesia 190
Communication
   clinical 323
   financial 325
   six components of 322
Complete blood count 9-11, 13, 17, 110, 245, 283
Conception
   product of 108
   retained product of 108, 284
Condom catheter tamponade, steps of 250*f*
Congenital anomaly 66, 163
   history of 33
Congenital malformation 229
   rate 64
Conjunctival infection 85
Connective tissue 239
   disease 94
Continuous nonlocking technique 206
Continuous positive airway pressure 299
Contraception 21, 32, 51
Controlled cord traction 181
   steps of 181
Convulsions, neonatal 157
Coombs test, indirect 69-71, 74
Cord
   clamping, indications of early 181
   insertion, abnormal 133
   presentation 229
   prolapse 130, 229, 230
      diagnosis 230
      epidemiology 229
      management of 230, 231
      risk factors 229, 230

Cornual placenta 220
Corpus callosal 88
Cortisol 188
Coryza 78
Cough 78, 272
Coxiella burnetii 279
Crampy feeling 124
C-reactive protein 281, 283
Creutzfeldt-Jakob disease 59
Crown-rump length 113
Crystalloids 320
Cyanmethemoglobin 24
Cyanosis 18, 78
Cyclosporine A 95
Cystic fibrosis 77
Cystitis, acute 107
Cysts, periventricular 88
Cytomegalovirus 59, 135, 152

D

Daily fetal
   kick count 9-11, 13, 17
   movement count 136
Danger signs 292
Death, causes of 77
Deep venous thrombosis 52
Dehydration 103
   signs of 74
Delivery
   forceps 212
   method of 154
   mode of 9, 10, 132, 138
   premature 315
   room 295
      management 193
   timing of 9, 10, 73, 153
   vacuum 212
Dengue 83, 85
   prevalence of 84
Depot medroxyprogesterone acetate 21
Diabetes 33, 173
   complications of 34*t*
   family history of 33
   mellitus 66, 135
   pre-existing 67
   pregestational 133
Diamniotic twins 140
Diarrhea 78
Dinoprostone 175
   gel 175
   pessary 175
Direct fetal blood studies 72
Direct observation treatment 332
Disability-adjusted life years 23

Disseminated intravascular
    coagulation 9, 41
Dopamine 60, 61
Doppler studies 134
    role of 135
Down syndrome 62
    risk of 63
Drowsiness 78
Ductus venosus 136, 137
    abnormal Doppler flow velocity of
        137f, 243f
    normal Doppler flow velocity of 137f
Dyspnea 18
    paroxysmal nocturnal 18
Dysreflexia, autonomic 208

E

Early pregnancy 107, 108, 110
    bleeding 116
        assessment of 111
        diagnosis of 111
        issues 65
Echogenic mass 253f
Eclampsia 14, 122, 211, 270
Ectopic pregnancy 107, 114
Edema, pulmonary 7, 22
Eisenmenger syndrome 20
Electrocardiogram 18, 288, 299
Electrolyte imbalance 198
Electronic fetal monitoring 50, 182, 183
    indications for 182t
Elevated cervical fluid pH 125
Embolism, pulmonary 52
Encephalopathy, hepatic 41
Endocarditis 20
    infective 19, 20b
Endometrial cavity 253f
Endometritis 271, 278
Endomyometritis 158
Endotracheal tube 299, 302
Enterocolitis, necrotizing 135, 296, 300
Environmental Protection Act 327
Enzyme steroid sulfatase, absence of 157
Epilepsy 47-49
    diagnosis of 49
    sudden unexpected death in 48
    syndrome, classification of 47
Epinephrine 61, 302
    dose of 302
Episiotomy 203, 214
    advantages 203
    complications 206
    disadvantages 203
    incisions, types of 204f

indications 203
method of repair 205
order of repair 205
postoperative care 206
prerequisite 205
principles of repair 205
purpose of repair 205
repair of 205
scissors 204
steps of mediolateral 204
suture used 205
timing of repair 205
types of 203, 204t
Ergometrine 244
Erythrocyte 318
Erythropoietin 28
Estimated date of delivery 157
Estriol 125
Estrogen-containing pills 21
Ethnicity 33
Ethylenediaminetetraacetic acid 27
Exchange transfusion 28
Expected date of delivery 5
Exposure, types of 335, 336
External anal sphincter 236, 237
External cephalic version 122, 225, 227

F

Fainting 161
Fasciitis, necrotizing 206
Fasting plasma glucose 34
Fatigue 18
Fatty liver, acute 107
Febrile illness, acute 19
Feeding 290, 296
Feet, swelling of 38
Fern test 130
Ferric ammonium citrate 26
Ferric carboxymaltose 27
Ferrous ascorbate 26
Ferrous bisglycinate chelate 27
Ferrous fumarate 26
Ferrous gluconate 26
Ferrous succinate 26
Ferrous sulfate 26
Fetal
    acidemia 188
    activity 150
    anatomy, gross distortion of 153
    anomalies, targetter imaging for 324
    biometry 9
    blood sampling 72
    bradycardia 191
    cardiotocography, continuous 138

death 130, 152
echocardiography 20
fibronectin 124, 126, 130
growth 158
    restriction 13, 117, 135
heart
    absent 153
    gas shadow in 153
    rate 9, 11, 15, 113, 132, 158, 161,
        174, 179, 180, 182, 183, 193, 318
    restriction 17
    sound 10, 159, 230
hemolysis, severity of 72f
hemolytic disease 69, 69t
hypoxemia 193
hypoxia 182, 188, 228
infection 130, 131
    absence of 131
intestines 192
lung maturity 131
macrosomia 173
maturity, confirmation of 171
middle cerebral artery Doppler 137
monitoring 9, 10
morbidity 195
mortality 195
movements 149
    absent 149, 153
    maternal perception of 149
    number of 149
presentation 131
pulse oximetry 186
red blood cells 69
scalp blood
    lactate levels 187
    sampling 185
size, sonographic measurement
    of 135
surveillance during labor 182
transmittable infections 185
trauma 228
well-being 131
Fetus 71
    head of 133
    hydrocephalic 223
    presentation of 141
    preterm 120
Fever 78, 85
Fibrillation 18
Fibrinogen concentrate 321
Fibroids 163
    massive 293
    submucous 195
Flaviviridae family 83
Fluoroquinolones 95
Folic acid 26, 67, 159

Forceps 209, 212
   delivery 203
   operation, complications of 210
   right blade of 210*f*
Fothergill operation 145
Free erythrocyte protoporphyrin 25
Fresh frozen plasma 45, 59, 320, 321
Fundal height, symphysial 150
Fundus examination 10

G

Gastric delivery system 26
Gastrointestinal dysfunction 104
Gastrointestinal symptoms 78
Gastrointestinal tract 26, 34
Genetic
   counseling 22, 67
   predisposition 157
Genital tract 117, 129, 279
   trauma, lower 282
Gentamicin 251, 281
Gestation
   multifetal 122
   multiple 133, 139, 158, 221
   period of 87, 108, 134*f*, 135, 136
Gestational age 131, 132, 154
   miscalculated 122
   small for 93, 133, 134, 150, 163
Gestational diabetes mellitus 33, 34, 36, 163, 164, 277, 332
   diagnosis of 332
   incidence of 66
   major complication of 66
   management of 332
   pathophysiology of 33
   screening for 34
Glasgow coma scale 59
Glomerular filtration rate 92
Glucose, target values for 35*t*
Gonadotropin, human menopausal 105
Granulocyte colony stimulating factors 125
Graves' hyperthyroidism 100
Great vein of Galen 211
Growth restriction 172
   prevention of 135
Guillain-Barré syndrome 90

H

H1N1 79
   infection 76
      epidemiology of 76
   virus 76
      pathogenesis of 78*f*
      structure of 77*f*

H3N2 79
Haemophilus influenzae 280
Haultains method 267
Head
   circumference 133
   entrapment 223
Headache 78
Hearing impairment 122
Heart 298
   disease 211
      congenital 18, 20
   rate 57, 288, 299
   sound
      nonreassuring 215
      physiologic third 18
Hemangioma 133
Hematological disorders 294
Hematoma 191
   infralevator 240*t*
   supralevator 240*t*
   vulval 206
   vulvovaginal 240
Hematuria 25, 161
Hemodialysis, peritoneal 94
Hemoglobin 20, 24, 35
   low 307, 308
   mean corpuscular 25
   normal 307
Hemoglobinopathies 23, 29, 77
Hemolysis, elevated liver enzymes and low platelet count syndrome 38-41, 43, 107, 109
Hemolytic
   crisis 31
   diseases 304
   reactions 57
   uremic syndrome 41
Hemoptysis 18
Hemorrhage 85, 283, 319, 329
   alarming 236
   antepartum 28, 56, 117, 117*t*, 122, 163, 293, 314
   intracranial 297
   intraventricular 135, 295, 300
   late postpartum 282
   massive 319
   obstetric 329
   postpartum 21, 28, 41, 43, 45, 56, 99, 158, 159, 181, 210, 238, 244, 245, 263, 270, 282, 316
   primary postpartum 245
   secondary postpartum 251, 282-284
   severe 28
   subgaleal 212
   traumatic postpartum 246, 250
Heparin, unfractionated 5, 22, 53

Hepatic
   dysfunction 104
   failure, fulminant 40-42, 45
   metabolism, transient limited 304
   rupture 38
Hepatitis
   acute viral 38, 40, 42
   B 334, 337
      vaccine 337
   C 334
      virus 59
   E virus 44
   fulminant 45
Heterozygous β-thalassemia 29
High pulsatility index 137*f*
Home uterine activity monitoring 124
Hormone
   adrenocorticotropic 177
   corticotropin-releasing 125
Hpothalamic-pituitary-adrenal axis, dysregulation of 157
Human chorionic gonadotropin 94, 98, 103, 104
   test 159
Human immunodeficiency virus 59, 314, 315, 334, 336
   transmission of 335, 335*t*
Human leukocyte antigen 70
Human papillomavirus infections 315
Human placental lactogen 33
Huntington's method 267
Huntington's technique 267
Hydralazine 11
Hydrocephalus, internal 88
Hydronephrosis, acute 107
Hydrostatic pressure method 265
Hydroxychloroquine, antimalarial 95
Hyperbilirubinemia 135, 307, 308
   conjugated 305*b*, 309*t*
   severe 305*b*
   unconjugated 304*b*, 307, 308
Hyperechoic foci 253*f*
Hyperemesis 104, 116
   gravidarum 40, 100, 103, 104
   pathophysiology of 103
Hypertension 9, 15, 19, 66, 94, 122, 163, 330
   chronic 15, 66, 134
   gestational 12, 99
   portal 39
   pregnancy induced 66, 277, 314, 315
   pulmonary 20
      arterial 19
   risk of 135
   severe pregnancy-induced 122

Hypertensive disorders 7, 133, 163, 173, 329
Hypoglycemia, neonatal 135
Hypokalemia 103
Hypoproteinemia 25
Hypotension 21, 78, 161
   arterial 272
   permissive 320
Hypothalamic-pituitary-ovarian axis 94
Hypothermia 135, 289
   management of 289, 289t
   therapeutic 300
Hypothyroidism 98, 99, 332
   subclinical 99
Hypovolemia 21
Hypoxic-ischemic tissue 298

I

Idiopathic hypertrophic subaortic stenosis 20
Iliac artery, internal 239
Immunization 291
Immunoglobulin
   G 4
   M 4, 86, 88
Immunosuppressive agents 95
In vitro fertilization 105, 134, 163, 164, 171
Incision, extension of 206
Incubation period 77
Indian Council of Medical Research 24, 83
Indian Thyroid Society 98
Indomethacin 127
Induction, timing of 172
Infarction 133
Infection 28, 31, 58, 129, 206, 277, 296
   neonatal 130
   pregnancy related 330
   prevention of 290
     spread of 80, 81
Infectious diseases 133
Inferior vena cava 54
Infertility 64
   pregnancy after 163
Influenza 76, 81t
   categorization of 77
   infection, epidemiology of 76t
   management of 79
   strains 77
   virus 76
     symptoms of 78t
Infusion rate 35
Injury, obstetric 239

Insulin 35
   requirement during labor 35t
Intensive care unit 273
   management 322
Intensive phototherapy 309
Intermittent positive pressure ventilation 59
Internal anal sphincter 236, 237
Internal podalic version 227, 231
International normalized ratio 22, 39, 45
Intracytoplasmic sperm injection 163t, 164
Intraocular calcifications 88
Intrapartum fetal
   heart rate monitoring, methods of 185t
   surveillance 182, 186
Intrapartum management 20, 35, 49, 222
Intrapartum monitoring 127
Intrauterine contraceptive device 21, 32, 45, 109, 226, 317
   insertion of 323
   postpartum 161
Intrauterine death 157, 231
   diagnosis of 230
Intrauterine fetal
   death 152
   growth restriction 122
Intrauterine growth 11
   restriction 10, 11, 17, 34, 66, 133-135, 138, 315
     categorization of 133
     classification of 133t
Intrauterine pregnancy 113
   diagnosis of 113
Intrauterine system 317
Intravenous broad-spectrum antibiotic therapy 154
Intravenous fluids 296
Intubation, endotracheal 302
Iron 23, 26, 159
   deficiency anemia 25
   polymaltose complex 26
   prescription 27
   prophylaxis 26
   sorbitol citric acid complex 27
   sucrose 27
   therapy 26
Ischemia, myometrial 188

J

Japanese encephalitis virus 83
Jaundice 38, 39, 297, 304, 306
   causes of 38, 39
   clinical assessment of 306
   management of 44

   mild 41, 43
   neonatal 291, 304, 307
   pathological 291, 305, 306b
   persistent 305b
   physiologic 291, 304, 305
   prolonged 305b
   severe 42, 44, 45
   unconjugated 307, 308
     type of 307
Joint pains 85
Juvenile myoclonic epilepsy 48

K

Keilland forceps 210
Kernicterus 305
Ketosis 103
Kidney 298
   disease, chronic 93, 93b, 94, 134
   donors 95
   function test 13, 42, 92
   injury, acute 93

L

Labetalol 11
Labor 169, 177
   after cesarean, trial of 162
   analgesia 49, 188, 189t, 190
     history of 189
   and delivery 165
   and imminent preterm birth 127
   augmentation of 171, 177
   compound presentation in 226
   first stage of 140, 178, 188
   fourth stage of 181
   induction of 13, 17, 35, 158, 163, 171-174
   management of 140, 141, 161, 177
     first stage of 179
     second stage of 179, 180
     third stage of 142, 181
   mechanism of 177, 225
   obstetric 315
   pains 188
     physiology of 188
     reduce 188, 189f
   premature 34
   presence of 131
   room quality improvement initiative 332
   second stage of 20, 140, 188
   spontaneous onset of 171
   stages of 178
   third stage of 20, 161, 180, 252

Lactic dehydrogenase 41
   serum 38
Laparotomy 267
Laqshay guidelines 332
Last menstrual period 157
Late pregnancy 107, 108, 110
   issues 65
Left ventricular ejection fraction 19
Leiomyoma 221
Liley's graph 72f
Limb edema 85
Liquor, meconium-stained 193, 300
Listeria 152, 279
Liver
   dysfunction 41
   failure 44, 45
      fulminant 43
   function tests 9, 10, 11, 13, 17, 31, 43, 105, 109, 110, 245
Loop electrosurgical excision procedure 145
Low molecular weight heparin 5, 22, 53, 95
   higher dose 54
Lower segment cesarean section 9, 11, 13, 15, 17, 36, 159, 180, 226, 227, 259, 277
   pregnancy after 159
Lower uterine segment
   incision 216
   measurement of 160
Lumbar sympathetic block 191
Lung
   disease, chronic 122
   injury, transfusion-related 28, 57, 58
Lupus nephritis 94
Lymph node enlargement 85

M

MacAfee and Johnson regimen, elaboration of 118
Maceration 153
Macrosomia 158
Magnesium sulfate 126
Malnutrition 315
Mammary venous hum, internal 18
Marfan's syndrome 22, 62
Massive blood transfusion protocols 320
Massive obstetric hemorrhage 198, 320
   management of 319
Maternal age, advanced 33, 62, 117
Maternal collapse 256
   cause of 259

Maternal death 331
   causes of 330
   reduce 331t
Maternal fetal transmission 84
Maternal health components 331, 332
Maternal infection 130, 131
   absence of 131
Maternal mortality 329
   causes of 329
   ratio 329
   reduce 331
Maternal serum alpha-fetoprotein 125
McRoberts maneuver 234
Mean arterial pressure 59, 60
Mean corpuscular volume 25
Mean sac diameter 112, 113
Meconium 192
   aspiration syndrome 135, 157, 192, 194
      prevention of 193
   grades of 192
   nonparticulate 192
   passage of 291
Medical nutrition therapy 36
Megaloblastic crisis 31
Membranes
   artificial rupture of 15, 175, 230
   prelabor rupture of 129, 130, 163
   premature rupture of 10, 95, 174, 227
   preterm
      prelabor rupture of 129, 129b, 130, 131, 131b
      premature rupture of 45, 122, 130, 131, 146
Menopause 64
Metformin 165
Methotrexate regimen 114
Methyldopa 11
Methylergometrine 140, 244
Methylergonovine 60
Metronidazole 251, 281, 283
Micturition
   frequency of 272
   painful 272
Mimic cardiac diseases 18b
Miscarriage 107, 163
   general management of 115
   medical management of 115
Misoprostol 60, 161
Mitral regurgitation 19, 21
Mitral stenosis 19, 21
   management of 21b
   moderate 21
   severe 21, 21b
Mitral valve prolapse 19
Monochorionic diamniotic twins 140

Monochorionic twins 140
Monstress test 9
Morganella morganii 278
Multiparity 33, 117
Murmur
   diastolic 18
   functional systolic 18
   systolic 18
Muscle pains 85
Myalgia 78
Myocardial infarction 19, 56
Myoma, red degeneration of 107

N

Naked eye single tube red cell osmotic fragility test 29
National Centre for Disease Control 85
National Guidelines for Deworming in Pregnancy 332
National Institute for Health and Care Excellence 10, 11, 146, 318
Nausea 103, 105
   treatment of 105
   vomiting, management of 105
Needle-prick injury 334
   management of 335
   prevention of 338
Needlestick injury 334
Neonatal death 122, 130, 135, 228
Neonatal intensive care unit 160, 295
Neonatal Resuscitation Program 295, 300
Nephrolithiasis 107
Nerve injury 210
NESTROF test 29
New York Heart Association 19, 20
   classification 18t
Nifedipine 11, 127
Nitrazine test 129
Nitrofurantoin 95
Nonstress test 10, 11, 13, 17, 31, 35, 132, 136, 150, 158
Norepinephrine 61
Nuchal translucency 323
Nucleic acid test 88
Nutritional supplementation 296

O

Obesity 33, 157, 163, 165
   maternal 221
Obstetric care 47, 81
   part of 188
Obstetric emergency, acute 241
Obstetric management 5, 6, 193

Obstruction, intestinal 107
Oligohydramnios 172, 220
Operative delivery 34, 67
Operative vaginal delivery 209, 214
    classification of 209, 209t
    contraindications for 212
    indications for 208
Optical density 71, 74
Oral antihypertensive agents,
        common 11t
Oral contraceptive
    pills 161
    sterilization 161
Oral glucose tolerance test 34
Oral iron
    preparations 26t
    side effects of 27
    therapy 26
Oral pills 51
Organ
    dysfunction 270
    dysfunction, multiple 77
Orthopnea 18
Ototoxicity 95
Ovarian cyst
    hemorrhagic 107
    ruptured 107
Ovarian failure, premature 64
Ovarian hyperstimulation syndrome 107
Oxygen 272
    demand 188
Oxytocin 20, 60, 244
    infusion 176
    intraumbilical vein injection of 254
    receptor antagonist 294

P

Packed cell
    volumes 28
    blood cells 59, 320
Pain
    chest 78
    distressing 188
    low abdominal 124
    relief 188
    retro-orbital 85
    right lower quadrant 110
Painful crisis 31
Palpitation 18
Pancreatitis, acute 107
Paracervical block 191
Parenteral iron therapy 26, 27
Partial thromboplastin time 39
Parvovirus 152
Patent ductus arteriosus 19, 295, 296
Peak systolic velocity 71

Pedal edema 18
Pedunculated myoma, torsion of 107
Pelvic
    artery embolization 197
    examination 109
    floor repair 203
    inflammatory disease, risk for 277
    reconstructive surgery 203
    ultrasound 109
Periclitoral laceration 240
Perimenopause 64
Perimortem cesarean delivery 259
    section, role of 259
Perinatal
    morbidity 66, 157
    mortality 66, 157, 163
Perineal injuries 236, 238
    causes 238
    complications 238
    future pregnancies 239
    management 238
    prevention 238
Perineal laceration 158
Perineal membrane 239
Perineal tear
    causes of 238, 238t
    degrees of 237, 237t
    first-degree 237f
    fourth-degree 238f
    second-degree 237f
    third-degree 237f
Perineum 237f
    inelastic 203
    veins of 236
Peripartum period 277
Peripheral oxygen,
        saturation of 288, 299
Peritoneal dialysis 94
Periurethral laceration 240
Pessary removal 175
Pharyngitis 281
Phenylepinephrine 60, 61
Phototherapy 308f, 309
    contraindications for 309
Piperacillin 281
Placenta 246
    abnormal invasion of 196
    accreta 119, 195, 282
    accrete
        focal 195
        partial 195
        risk of 195t
        total 195
    anterior 221
    increta 195
    manual removal of 254, 254f, 282

    percreta 195
    previa 117, 119, 195, 220, 229
        classification of 118
        major 118
        minor 118
Placental abruption 107, 117, 120, 154
Placental adhesive disorders 195, 196
    classification of 195
    incidence of 195
    management of 196
    pathophysiology of 196
Placental insufficiency 3
Placental separation, mechanism of 252
Placental sulfatase deficiency 157
Plasma 310
    protein, pregnancy with 134, 164
Pneumonia 280
Polycystic ovarian syndrome 33, 163, 164
Polycythemia 304
Polydioxanone sutures 238
Polyhydramnios 34, 117, 172, 220, 221
    infections 122
Positive pressure ventilation 288, 298, 299
Posterior reversible leukoencephalopathy
        syndrome 47
Posterior wall rupture uterus 243f
Postexposure prophylaxis 336
    regime 337
Postpartum Care Programs 316
Pouch of Douglas 114
Povidone-iodine 204
Preassessment card 323b
Preconceptional counseling 15, 47, 48, 164
Preductal pulse oximetry,
        indications for 301
Preeclampsia 8, 15, 31, 34, 41, 43, 117, 270
    diagnostic criterion for 7t
    nonsevere 9t
    severe 10t, 38
Pregnancy 98, 104
    acute fatty liver of 38-43
    and postpartum 52
    complications in 49
    convulsions in 47
    drugs in 49
    effects of anemia on 28
    first seizure in 47
    intrahepatic cholestasis of 30, 38-41,
        43, 173
    loss 112
        recurrent 3
    medical termination of 30, 144
    molar 103, 116f
    multiple 19, 103, 163
    nutritional anemia in 24
    physiological changes of 92b

post-term 157
previous prolonged 157
prolonged 157
risk factors in 77
seizure in 48
termination of 74, 272
test, urine for 111
unintended 316
unwanted 125
Prematurity, apnea of 296
Prepregnancy 75
   counseling 22
Preterm birth 99, 122, 130, 146, 293
   previous 123
Preterm breech, management of 222
Preterm delivery 163
   prediction of 293
Preterm labor 107, 122, 146
   management of 294
Primary infertility, long period of 62
Primigravida 157
Progesterone 126, 127, 146, 147
   antagonists 126
   excess 103
   only pills 21
   serum 112
   types of 147
Proinflammatory cytokines, role of 123
Prominent neck veins 18
Prophylactic antibiotics 214
   use of 193
Prophylactic forceps 211
Prophylactic uterotonics, use of 244
Prostaglandin
   E1 60, 175
   E2 175
   synthetase inhibitors 127
Prosthetic valves 20, 21
Protection of Children from Sexual Offences Act 316
Proteins, serum 25
Proteinuria 7, 9, 9t, 15, 92
   test for 9
Prothrombin
   complex concentrates 321
   time 9, 39, 320
Proton pump inhibitor 105
Pudendal nerve block 191
Puerperium 67
Pulsatility index 134, 136
Pulse 150
   oximetry 301
   rate 15
Pyelonephritis 31, 107
Pyrexia, puerperal 277

Q

qSOFA score 270
QT syndrome 22

R

Radioactive iodine scanning 99
Rash, maculopapular 85
Rectal mucosa 206
Rectovaginal fistula 206
Rectus sheath hematoma 107
Red blood cell 24, 318
   transfusion 318
Reduced fetal movement 149
   causes of 150b
   intervention trial-2 151
Regurgitation, aortic 19
Renal biopsy 93b
Renal disease 77, 93b, 133
   absence of 7
   effect of pregnancy on 92
   end-stage 94
Renal disorders 92
Renal failure, acute 9, 198
Renal function test 9, 10, 11, 13, 15, 17, 31, 36, 245
Renal replacement therapy 94
   complications of 94b
   pregnancy with 94
Renal transplant, pregnancy in 95
Respiration, spontaneous 298
Respiratory disease, severe 78
Respiratory distress 99, 135, 192
   syndrome 296
Respiratory failure 77
Respiratory infection 19
Respiratory rate 57
Respiratory tract infection 127
Resuscitation 258, 298
   cardiopulmonary 257
   earlier concept of 320
   hemostatic 320
   neonatal 288, 298, 299
   preparedness for 298
Retained placenta 130, 246, 252
   complications of 254
   risk factors 253
   types of 253
Reticuloendothelial system 70
Retinopathy, proliferative 208
Reverse transcriptase-polymerase chain reaction 85-87
Rh hemolytic disease 72f
Rh isoimmunization 69, 72f
Rheumatic valvular disease 18
Ribonucleic acid 87
   virus 83
Ringer's lactate 15, 105
Ritodrine 126
Robert sign 153
Robson's classification 161
Royal College of Obstetricians and Gynecologists 53, 151, 152
Rugose vagina, limit of 265

S

Sac, gestational 108
Salbutamol 126
Saline, normal 15, 105
Salmonella 279
Salpingostomy 115
Salvage maneuvers 234
Sayeba's method 250f
See saw theory 126
Seizure
   co-recurrent 48
   eclamptic 50
   management of 50
   nonepileptic 50
   tonic-clonic 48
Self-assessment card 323b
Sepsis 270-273, 281, 290
   causes of 271
   development of 271
   management of 273
   maternal 193
   neonatal 193
   puerperal 67
   recognition of 271
   risk factors 271
   severe 270
   six bundle 272
Sequential organ failure assessment score 271t
Serum glutamic
   oxaloacetic transaminase 41, 42
   pyruvic transaminase 41, 42
Sexual abuse 314
Sexual assault 337
Sexual violence 314
Sexually transmitted diseases 314-316
Shock 56, 161
   anaphylactic 56
   cardiogenic 56
   causes of 262
   endotoxic 56, 60
   hemorrhagic 56, 57, 59, 61
   management of 61, 283
   neurogenic 56, 60
   refractory 77
   septic 56, 270, 273
   types of 56

Shoulder
   dystocia 203, 233, 234
      complications 234
      management of 233
      maternal complications 234
      neonatal complications 234
      signs of 233
   presentation, management of 226
Sickle cell
  anemia 31
  disorders 30
  hemoglobin 30
  syndromes 29
  trait 30
Sickle test 29
Sickling crisis 31
Silicon ventouse cup 266f
Single layer uterine closure 218
Single umbilical artery 133
Skin infection 280
Skull bones, overlapping of 153
Society of Maternal-Fetal Medicine 146
Society of Obstetricians and
      Gynecologists 53
Sodium feredetate 26, 27
Soft tissue infection 280
Sonogram-transvaginal ultrasound 160
Sore throat 78
Spalding sign 153
Spectrophotometry, indirect 71, 72
Sphincter 206
  injury 239
Spinal cord degeneration 88
Splenic rupture 107
Splenic sequestration crisis 31
Stenosis, aortic 20, 21
Steroid, antenatal 127
Stillbirth 31, 152, 228
   causes of 152
   diagnosis of 153
   history of 33
Stimulation, aympathetic 188
Streptococcus 129, 271
   pneumoniae 280
   pyogenes 278
Stress 122
  minimize 125
Substance abuse 133, 293, 314
Sulcus tear 210
Sulprostone 254
Suprapubic pressure 234
Surgery
  obstetric 330
  types of 114
Swiss-cheese appearance 196
Syphilis 152

T

Tachycardia 184, 271
  maternal 161
Tachypnea 78, 271
Tazobactam 281
Tears
  first-degree 238
  previous third-degree 239
  second-degree 238
  third- and fourth-degree 238
Teenage pregnancy 313
  causes 313
  consequences of 314
  impacts of 314
  management of 315, 316
  prevention of 316, 317
Teratogens 133
Terbutaline 126
Tetanus toxoid 159
Tetralogy of Fallot 19, 20
Thalami, agenesis of 88
Thalassemia 28, 29
  facies 30
Thermal
  instability 294
  management 299
Thoracic aorta, dissection of 19
Threatened preterm labor 126
  clinical features of 124
Thromboembolism 19
  risk factors for 165b
Thrombolysis indications 54
Thrombophilias 117
  testing for 54
Thromboprophylaxis 272
  role of 163
Thrombosis 3
  pathogenesis of 4
Thrombotic thrombocytopenic purpura 41
Thumb technique 302
Thyroglobulin antibody 99
Thyroid
  disorders 98
  dysfunction 98, 104
  function 98
    test ultrasonography 105
  peroxidase antibody 99
  screening, recommendations for 98
  stimulating hormone 98t, 104
    stimulation of 98
Thyrotoxicosis 19, 99
  diagnosis of 99, 100
  transient gestational 100
Thyroxine
  binding globulin 98
  serum total 98

Tocolytics 126
  role of 119
  use of 127
Total iron-binding capacity 25
Total leukocyte count 42
Traditional interrupted technique 206
Tranexamic acid 321
Transabdominal scan 112-114
Transcutaneous electrical nerve
      stimulation 49
Transferrin receptors 25
Transfusion
  immunomodulation 58
  reaction 28, 198
Transmission, dynamics of 84
Transurethral resection set 267f
Transvaginal cervical length
      assessment 146
Transvaginal scan 113, 114
Transverse lie 224, 224f, 226
  complications of 227
  diagnosis of 225
  fetal complications 227
  historical aspect 225
  incidence of 224
  management of 225, 226
  maternal complications 227
Trauma 117
  neonatal 213
Trisomy
  13, risk of 63
  18, risk of 63
Trophoblastic disease, gestational 116
Tubal blockage 277
Tubular necrosis, acute 93
Twin
  delivery of 139-142
  gestation 140
  pregnancy
    intrapartum monitoring of 140
    management of 222
    uncomplicated 173

U

Ulcer, duodenal 104
Ultrasonography 17, 35, 71, 108, 109, 130,
      151, 160, 227, 231, 284, 316
  grayscale 196
Ultrasound
  abdominal 109
  scan 112, 151
  transabdominal 160
  transvaginal 109
Umbilical artery 10, 11, 13, 17, 137f
  absent end-diastolic flow of 137f

Doppler 137
   abnormal 137
   normal Doppler flow velocity of 137f
Umbilical cord 288
   prolapse 229
Umbilical vein Doppler 137
Umbilical venous catheter 299, 302
Urinary retention, acute 107
Urinary tract 129
   infection 25, 31, 34, 104
      asymptomatic 122
      symptomatic 122
   injuries 197
Urine
   examination 25
   passage of 291
   pregnancy test 114
Uterine
   abnormality 220
   activity monitoring 124
   anomalies 163
      congenital 122
   artery
      blood flow, Doppler waveform of 134f
      Doppler 134
   closure, double-layer 218
   displacement, left 258f
   enlargement, excessive 116
   fibroids 107
   fundal height, measurement of 134
   hyperstimulation 174
   incisions 216, 218
   injuries 241
      causes 242
      complications 242
      diagnosis of 242, 242t
      future pregnancies 243
      management 243
      prevention 242
   inversion 260, 262
      classification of 260
      clinical features 263
      complications 268
      degrees of 260, 261
      diagnosis 261
      differential diagnosis 263
      etiology 261
      incidence 260
      management 263
      prevention 268
      timing of 261
      types of 260
   overdistension 123
   pathology 195
   prolapse, incomplete 262f
   rupture 107, 241
      causes of 242t
   scar 154
      dehiscence 243ff
      rupture 243ff
Uterotonic therapy 60
Uterus 239f
   bicornuate 195, 220, 293
   inversion 268
   malformations of 293
   manual replacement of 264, 264f
   retroverted gravid 107
   rupture 28
   septate 220
   subinvolution of 67

V

Vacuum
   application 209
   rotation, use of 214
Vagina 239, 239f
Vaginal birth after cesarean 159, 160
Vaginal bleeding 291
   abnormal 116, 161
Vaginal breech
   birth, management of 222
   deliveries 222
Vaginal delivery 198
   incidence 208
   instrumental 208
   spontaneous 20
   use of operative 208
Vaginal examination 111, 175, 225
Vaginal fluid 130
Vaginal fornix, posterior 265f
Vaginal injuries 239
   causes 240
   complications 240
   management 240
   prevention 240
Vaginal laceration 210, 240
Vaginal methods 267
Vaginal tears 240
Valvular lesions 18
Vasa previa 117
Vascular thrombosis 3
Vasopressin 61
Vasopressor therapy 272
Venous thromboembolism 52, 53
   treatment of acute 54
Venous thrombosis 53
Ventouse 211, 212
   delivery 203
Ventricular septal defect 19
Ventricular systolic flow 137
Ventricular tachycardia, pulseless 258
Vermian dysgenesis 88
Viral hepatitis 38
Virchow's triad 53
Virus infections 85t
Visceral peritoneum 216
Visual disturbances 7
Visual impairment 122
Visual inspection 131
Vital signs 38
Vitamin
   B_{12} 23
   D 94
   K 51
Vomiting 78, 103-105
   treatment of 105
von Willebrand disease 282

W

Warfarin, complications of 22
Waste
   segregation and treatment 326-328
   types of 326
Weight loss 103
West Nile virus 83
White blood cell 271
Wood's Corkscrew maneuver 234
Wound
   dehiscence 206
   repair and closure 218

X

X-linked recessive disorder 157

Y

Yellow fever 83

Z

Zavanelli maneuver 234
Zika virus 83, 85-87, 90
   diagnosis of 87
   disease 84, 85f
      clinical features of 84
      symptoms of 85f
   infection 86, 88, 90
      congenital 86, 87, 88b
      global spread of 84f
      prevention of 86, 89
      spread of 83f
   life cycle of 84f
   structure of 83f

EU GSPR Authorised Reprsentative
Logos Europe, 9 rue Nicolas Poussin
1700, La Rochelle, France
Phone: +33 (0) 6 67 93 73 78
E-mail: contact@logoseurope.eu

www.ingramcontent.com/pod-product-compliance
Ingram Content Group UK Ltd.
Pitfield, Milton Keynes, MK11 3LW, UK
UKHW050458150426
5217IPUK00025B/1746